Well-Controlled Diet Studies in Humans

A Practical Guide to Design and Management

Barbara H. Dennis, PhD, RD, Abby G. Ershow, ScD, RD,
Eva Obarzanek, PhD, MPH, RD, and Beverly A. Clevidence, PhD, Editors

THE AMERICAN DIETETIC ASSOCIATION

Cover image © 1997 PhotoDisc, Inc.

Acquisitions Editor: June Zaragoza, MPH, RD

Library of Congress Cataloging-in-Publication Data
Well-controlled diet studies in humans : a practical guide to
design and management / Barbara Dennis . . . [et al.]., eds.
   p.   cm.
  Includes bibliographical references and index.
  ISBN 0-88091-158-1
  1. Nutrition—Research—Methodology. 2.
Diet—Research—Methodology. 3. Human experimentation in
medicine—Methodology. I. Dennis, Barbara (Barbara H.)
  QP143.W44 1999
  613.2′072—dc21   98-48694
                     CIP

The views expressed in this publication are those of the authors and do not necessarily reflect policies and/or official
positions of The American Dietetic Association. Mention of product names in this publication does not constitute
endorsement by the authors or The American Dietetic Association. The American Dietetic Association disclaims
responsibility for the application of the information contained herein.

10 9 8 7 6 5 4 3 2 1

Contents

PART 5   ENHANCING THE OUTCOME OF DIETARY STUDIES

Foreword

Well-controlled diet studies in humans are challenging to plan and conduct because there are so many variables to control and so many details that demand attention. Such studies have been carried out in such diverse settings as hospital metabolic units and university and government research facilities. Many have provided the basis for our knowledge of nutrient requirements. The current scope of these studies has been expanded to include such disorders as hypertension, diabetes, dyslipidemia, obesity, cardiovascular disease, gallstones, kidney stones, osteoporosis, cirrhosis, and renal disease. Knowledge about how to carry out feeding studies has been imparted largely by word-of-mouth and on-site training. Until now there have been very few resources available to aid investigators.

The National Heart, Lung, and Blood Institute, with support and cooperation from The American Dietetic Association Foundation, organized a series of workshops in 1991 to address the practical issues of human feeding studies and to provide a unique opportunity to exchange specialized information that is seldom reported in journal articles. At the same time, nutritionists involved in clinical investigations carried out in the nationwide network of General Clinical Research Centers (GCRCs) were developing plans for updating the only manual currently available, *A Dietetic Manual for Metabolic Kitchen Units,* which was published in 1969 by the National Institutes of Health Clinical Center.

This happy coincidence led to a partnership of the NHLBI workshop organizing committee and GCRC nutritionists in collaboration with the Research Dietetic Practice Group of The American Dietetic Association to produce *Well-Controlled Diet Studies in Humans: A Practical Guide to Design and Management.* With its specific focus on controlled human feeding studies, this book complements the more general *Research: Successful Approaches,* published by the ADA in 1991.

Opportunities for conducting human nutrition research will continue to arise as we contemplate the role of nutrition in the prevention, management, and treatment of chronic and acute illnesses and in the optimization of human health through all life stages. *Well-Controlled Diet Studies in Humans: A Practical Guide to Design and Management* offers a most comprehensive and detailed discussion of the many topics that potential investigators must master, including study design, food chemistry, ethical protections, participant management, statistical methodology, food production and preparation, quality control, and physical and personnel resource allocation. The authors are experts in their subjects and offer the reader the best of their knowledge and experience.

Congratulations to the editors of this book, who have done an outstanding job of recognizing the need for this information and presenting it in a comprehensible and useful format. This publication makes a major advance toward the goal of conducting high-quality nutrition research.

Nancy D. Ernst, PhD, RD
Nutrition Coordinator, National Heart, Lung, and Blood Institute

Judith L. Vaitukaitis, MD
Director, National Center for Research Resources

Ronni Chernoff, PhD, RD, FADA
President, The American Dietetic Association, 1996–1997

Acknowledgments

The Editors would like to thank the many people whose help was instrumental in the development of this book:

Associate Editors Janis F. Swain, MS, RD, Ronni Chernoff, PhD, RD, FADA, and Phyllis E. Bowen, PhD, RD, whose suggestions shaped the contents and perspective;

Linda Lampe, Colleen M. Brown, Mary Maughlin, and Aluoch Ooro, who provided secretarial assistance;

Dennis Stanley, Thanh Du, and Tawanna Meadows, who lent their skill with computer graphics and literature searches;

Catherine Burke, whose fine editorial and organizational skills helped us to integrate the many parts of this very large and complex endeavor; and

June Zaragoza, MPH, RD, of The American Dietetic Association Publications Team, who was constant in her support and encouragement.

We also thank the National Heart, Lung, and Blood Institute, the General Clinical Research Centers Program of the National Center for Research Resources, and The American Dietetic Association for supporting the writing of this book, as well as the research programs and workshops that led to its inception.

Contributors

AUTHORS

*Member of Editorial Committee

Elaine J. Ayres, MS, RD
Office of the Director
National Institutes of Health Clinical Center
Bethesda, Maryland

Paul S. Bachorik, PhD
Departments of Pediatrics and Pathology
The Johns Hopkins University School of Medicine
Johns Hopkins Hospital
Baltimore, Maryland

David J. Baer, PhD
Diet and Human Performance Laboratory
Beltsville Human Nutrition Research Center
US Department of Agriculture
Beltsville, Maryland

Susan Learner Barr, MS, RD
Edelman PR Worldwide
New York, New York

Susan E. Blackwell
Collaborative Studies Coordinating Center
Department of Biostatistics
University of North Carolina
Chapel Hill, North Carolina

Phyllis E. Bowen, PhD, RD*
Department of Human Nutrition and Dietetics
University of Illinois at Chicago
Chicago, Illinois

Linda J. Brinkley, RD
General Clinical Research Center
The University of Texas Southwestern Medical Center
    at Dallas
Dallas, Texas

Marjorie Busby, MPH, RD
General Clinical Research Center
University of North Carolina—Chapel Hill Medical Center
Chapel Hill, North Carolina

I. Marilyn Buzzard, PhD, RD
Department of Preventive Medicine
    and Community Health
Medical College of Virginia
Virginia Commonwealth University
Richmond, Virginia

Catherine A. Chenard, MS, RD
General Clinical Research Center
University of Iowa
Iowa City, Iowa

Ronni Chernoff, PhD, RD, FADA*
Geriatric Research, Education, and Clinical Center
Central Arkansas Veterans Healthcare System
Little Rock, Arkansas

Beverly A. Clevidence, PhD*
Phytonutrients Laboratory
Beltsville Human Nutrition Research Center
US Department of Agriculture
Beltsville, Maryland

Elizabeth R. De Oliveira e Silva, MD
Laboratory of Biochemical Genetics and Metabolism
The Rockefeller University
New York, New York

Margo A. Denke, MD
Center for Human Nutrition
Department of Internal Medicine
The University of Texas Southwestern Medical Center
    at Dallas
Dallas, Texas

Barbara H. Dennis, PhD, RD*
Collaborative Studies Coordinating Center
Department of Biostatistics
University of North Carolina
Chapel Hill, North Carolina

Janice A. Derr, PhD
Statistical Consulting Center
Department of Statistics
Pennsylvania State University
University Park, Pennsylvania

Darrell L. Ellsworth, PhD
Division of Epidemiology and Clinical Applications
National Heart, Lung, and Blood Institute
Bethesda, Maryland

Patricia Engel, MS, RD
Metabolic Research Unit
Jean Mayer USDA Human Nutrition Research Center
    on Aging at Tufts University
Boston, Massachusetts

Nancy D. Ernst, PhD, RD
Division of Epidemiology and Clinical Applications
National Heart, Lung, and Blood Institute
Bethesda, Maryland

Abby G. Ershow, ScD, RD*
Division of Heart and Vascular Diseases
National Heart, Lung, and Blood Institute
Bethesda, Maryland

Alice K. H. Fong, EdD, RD
Western Human Nutrition Research Center
US Department of Agriculture
Presidio of San Francisco, California

Darlene Fontana, MS, RD
Fred Hutchinson Cancer Research Center
Seattle, Washington

Susan E. Gebhardt, MS
Nutrient Data Laboratory
Beltsville Human Nutrition Research Center
US Department of Agriculture
Riverdale, Maryland

Carla R. Heiser, MS, RD
StatScript Pharmacy
Chicago, Illinois

David J. Jenkins, MD, PhD, DSc
Department of Nutritional Sciences
Faculty of Medicine
University of Toronto
Toronto, Ontario, Canada

Wahida Karmally, MS, RD
Irving Center for Clinical Research
College of Physicians and Surgeons
Columbia University
New York, New York

Mary Ann Tilley Kidd, MS, RD
Nutrition Department
Flagler Hospital
St Augustine, Florida

Penny M. Kris-Etherton, PhD, RD
Nutrition Department
The Pennsylvania State University
University Park, Pennsylvania

Alice H. Lichtenstein, DSc
Lipid Metabolism Laboratory
Jean Mayer USDA Human Nutrition Research Center
    on Aging at Tufts University
Boston, Massachusetts

Beena Loharikar, MS, RD
Naperville, Illinois

Colleen Matthys, RD
Clinical Research Center
University of Washington
Seattle, Washington

Ruth McPherson, MD, PhD
Department of Medicine
Division of Cardiology and Endocrinology
University of Ottawa Heart Institute
Ottawa, Ontario, Canada

Vikkie A. Mustad, PhD
Ross Products Division
Abbott Laboratories
Columbus, Ohio

Janet A. Novotny, PhD
Diet and Human Performance Laboratory
Beltsville Human Nutrition Research Center
US Department of Agriculture
Beltsville, Maryland

Eva Obarzanek, PhD, MPH, RD*
Division of Epidemiology and Clinical Applications
National Heart, Lung, and Blood Institute
Bethesda, Maryland

Mary Joan Oexmann, MS, RD
Department of Pharmacology
Medical University of South Carolina
Charleston, South Carolina

Katherine M. Phillips, PhD
Department of Biochemistry
Virginia Polytechnic Institute and State University
Blacksburg, Virginia

Henry J. Pownall, PhD
Department of Medicine
Baylor College of Medicine
Houston, Texas

T. Elaine Prewitt, DrPH, RD
Department of Preventive Medicine and Epidemiology
Loyola University School of Medicine
Maywood, Illinois

Keren Price, MS, RD
Minneapolis, Minnesota

Helen Rasmussen, MS, RD, FADA
Metabolic Research Unit
Jean Mayer USDA Human Nutrition Research Center
    on Aging at Tufts University
Boston, Massachusetts

Patti Riggs, RD
Nutrition Department
National Institutes of Health Clinical Center
Bethesda, Maryland

Arline D. Salbe, PhD, RD
Clinical Diabetes and Nutrition Section
Phoenix Epidemiology and Clinical Research Branch
National Institute of Diabetes
    and Digestive and Kidney Diseases
Phoenix, Arizona

Michelle Sandow-Pajewski, MS, RD
General Clinical Research Center
University of Virginia
Charlottesville, Virginia

Cynthia Seidman, MS, RD
General Clinical Research Center
Rockefeller University Hospital
New York, New York

Madeleine Sigman-Grant, PhD, RD
University of Nevada Cooperative Extension Service
Las Vegas, Nevada

Jane E. Stegner, MS, RD
Winston Salem, North Carolina

Kent K. Stewart, PhD
Department of Chemistry
The University of Texas
Austin, Texas

Sachiko T. St Jeor, PhD, RD
Nutrition Education and Research Program
University of Nevada School of Medicine
Reno, Nevada

Phyllis J. Stumbo, PhD, RD
General Clinical Research Center
University of Iowa
Iowa City, Iowa

Janis F. Swain, MS, RD*
General Clinical Research Center
Brigham and Women's Hospital
Boston, Massachusetts

Karen Todd, MS, RD
General Clinical Research Center
University of California at San Francisco
San Francisco, California

Rita Tsay, MS, RD
General Clinical Research Center
Massachusetts Institute of Technology
Cambridge, Massachusetts

Judith L. Vaitukaitis, MD
Office of the Director
National Center for Research Resources
Bethesda, Maryland

Marlene M. Windhauser, PhD, RD, FADA
Pennington Biomedical Research Center
Louisiana State University
Baton Rouge, Louisiana

REVIEWERS

Wanda Chenoweth, PhD, RD
Department of Food Science
  and Human Nutrition
Michigan State University
East Lansing, Michigan

Ann M. Coulston, MS, RD, FADA
General Clinical Research Center
Stanford University Medical Center
Stanford, California

Patricia J. Elmer, PhD, RD
Kaiser Permanente Center for Health Research
Portland, Oregon

Barbara Howard, PhD, RD
Medlantic Research Institute
Washington Hospital Center
Washington, DC

D. Yvonne Jones, PhD, RD
Pine Brook, New Jersey

Penny M. Kris-Etherton, PhD, RD
Nutrition Department
Pennsylvania State University
University Park, Pennsylvania

Michael Lefevre, PhD
Pennington Biomedical Research Center
Baton Rouge, Louisiana

Martha McMurry, MS, RD
General Clinical Research Center
Oregon Health Sciences University
Portland, Oregon

Cheryl Rock, PhD, RD, FADA
Program in Human Nutrition
University of California, San Diego
San Diego, California

Carol Stollar, MEd, RD
General Clinical Research Center
Beth Israel Deaconess Medical Center
Boston, Massachusetts

Introduction

BARBARA H. DENNIS, PHD, RD

> WANTED
> Experienced investigator to conduct research in nutrition and disease utilizing rigorously controlled human feeding studies. Successful candidate will have training and experience in clinical dietetics, medical nutrition, food chemistry, biostatistics, computer programming, word processing, psychology, clinical chemistry, and public relations. Must be highly skilled and creative chef with knowledge of food technology, food safety, and food composition. This position requires excellent organizational skills and stamina. Requires approximately 280 hours per week. No time off during feeding periods. Excellent fringe benefits.

If this advertisement appeared in the classified section of a newspaper or journal, it is unlikely that any applicants would qualify. The job description illustrates the complexity of skills and talents that go into the design and management of successful human feeding studies. It is, in fact, the job description for a team so well integrated that it functions as a single entity.

Although controlled diet studies have many similarities to controlled clinical trials, there are several characteristics that set them apart. These characteristics fall into two categories: (1) the participants are mobile human beings who are accustomed to considerable autonomy in their daily lives, and they are required to surrender a major portion of that autonomy—control over food choice—to follow a rigid protocol; and (2) the "treatment" is a complex chemical matrix called food, which is also endowed with social meaning.

A controlled diet study places more severe constraints on a person's lifestyle than almost any other type of protocol. It removes a great deal of personal freedom surrounding the choice of one's food and the social dimensions associated with it. Other requirements, such as collection of urine and fecal samples, are burdensome and not aesthetically accommodated in most social interactions. Human relationships also may become strained during the study because the participant cannot partake of any food offered in the context of entertainment and socialization.

Food in these studies becomes the medium for delivering the nutrient treatment. The food must be defined (that is, assayed), and variability in its composition must be minimized among participants and over time. Assay methods need to be accurate and appropriate for the particular food matrix. Sources of variability, not all of which can be controlled, include season, growing and storage conditions, formulation, and handling. To minimize this variability, detailed specifications for the food must be developed. If possible, the food for an entire study should be formulated at one time. This can be done for synthetic diets and liquid formulas, but is not practical when diets are made up of ordinary foods prepared in familiar ways.

Food is perishable. Enzymatic activity or bacterial growth can change its composition, its acceptability, and ultimately its safety. Thus, food cannot be produced with the same batch-to-batch precision as pharmaceuticals. In addition, the handling of food in a feeding study requires special procedures. Cooking and portioning must be carried out with a higher degree of precision than occurs in most foodservice operations, although newer methods employed in large-scale commercial food production to control portion size and quality provide a level of precision that may be acceptable in some studies. Staff need additional training to follow procedures exactly and report any deviations from protocol, and must be supervised more closely than in conventional foodservice.

Masking the participant to the treatment assignment is difficult in feeding studies. The staff members who prepare and serve the food need to know the assignment, but they must not reveal the diet assignment to participants or other study staff, nor should they manage participants on one regimen differently from those on another. This may be difficult if the treatment diet is less well accepted than the "placebo" (control) diet.

Food has social and emotional meaning; "treatment" is not a meaning most people would apply to the food they eat. Thus, in the context of feeding studies, variety, taste, texture, temperature, appearance, and meal pattern become important. Food connotes family life and hospitality. The social setting of the dining room becomes important, as do interactions with staff and dining partners. Holidays and other major social occasions must be accommodated by thoughtful scheduling of feeding periods or by providing special foods. All of these considerations contribute to the uniqueness of human feeding studies and require particular attention.

The contents of this book provide a level of detail that is not generally available in the peer-reviewed literature but is essential for planning and managing studies. Wherever possible, the authors have used experience-based data to support their recommendations. They also provide guidance concerning recruitment, compliance, diet validation, documentation, quality assurance, and efficient use of resources. This information can help nutrition researchers not only to meet their scientific objectives but also to obtain adequate financial support. The most scientifically sound and well-thought-out study cannot be initiated unless it is funded. Human feeding studies are expensive precisely because of the level of detail required to control the diet and manage the participants. If the budget required to meet the scientific objectives is not adequately justified, the study may not be funded at all or the budget may be reduced to a degree that compromises the study's integrity.

This book focuses primarily on those factors that distinguish well-controlled feeding studies from other types of nutrition research. The chapters are designed to lead the reader from the general issues (Part 1) through the particular—the human factors (Part 2), food factors (Part 3), kitchen factors (Part 4), and laboratory factors (Part 5). The final chapter looks at the multicenter trial, a new model for controlled diet studies.

PART 1

STUDY DESIGN

CHAPTER 1

THE SCIENTIFIC RATIONALE OF HUMAN FEEDING STUDIES

MARGO A. DENKE, MD; AND EVA OBARZANEK, PHD, MPH, RD

Half of all the chronic illness in America is estimated to be a direct consequence of the national diet (1, 2). This is a remarkable figure, given that the most common chronic illnesses and debilitating conditions—cancer, coronary heart disease, arthritis, gallstones, obesity, osteoporosis, diabetes, hypertension, and liver disease—have widely differing causes and treatments. Although our understanding of the relevant biological processes is incomplete at present, diet probably acts through multiple mechanisms to enhance or diminish the propensity for disease in susceptible individuals. This chapter reviews the various types of research designs involved in postulating and testing relationships between diet and disease, or between diet and metabolic effects. The chapter also describes the specialized but essential role of human feeding studies in providing evidence for these relationships.

RESEARCH METHODOLOGY FOR TESTING DIET-DISEASE RELATIONSHIPS

Concluding that some aspect of diet causes a disease requires a diverse body of information collected by epidemiologists, laboratory scientists, and clinical researchers. These individuals use the specialized methods of their scientific disciplines to assess a variety of outcomes, including measures of early pathology, occurrence of subclinical and clinical disease, and, for some diseases, death. Nondisease (intermediate) outcomes are also assessed; these are sometimes referred to as *risk factors* if they have been associated with

likelihood of disease or are good predictors of disease (3–6). The following are some lines of scientific evidence used to generate and test a diet-disease hypothesis:

- Between-country data demonstrating relationships between food balance sheets or food disappearance data and national rates of disease.
- Studies of migrants demonstrating that the disease rates of migrants gradually shift toward the rates typical of the adopted country.
- Studies of identical twins demonstrating greater concordance of disease in twins reared together than in twins reared apart.
- Case-control studies suggesting that diet-related risk factors and characteristics of diet differ between cases with disease and controls without disease.
- Prospective cohort studies demonstrating that individuals with differing dietary intakes have different levels of a risk factor or different rates of disease.
- Animal studies describing dietary effects on the development of disease and the mechanisms involved.
- Human feeding studies examining the effects of intake of specific dietary constituents on risk factors or other intermediate outcomes.
- Large, randomized controlled trials demonstrating that altering dietary intake alters risk factors, disease incidence, or mortality.

Each research method has its strengths and limitations for assessing the relationship between diet and disease. In particular, the various lines of research differ in their ability to demonstrate strong associations between diet and disease risk. Doing so requires the investigators to establish the following: proper temporal sequence (ie, the postulated cause precedes the effect); independence of effect through control of confounding and other sources of experimental error; consistency of results; and biological plausibility. In addition, the various types of studies differ in the generalizability of their findings (7–10). All of the lines of research described in this section can contribute information to the totality of evidence that allows for conclusions about causality.

EPIDEMIOLOGIC STUDIES

Observational Investigations

Observational epidemiologic studies can be classified as ecologic (observations are made on groups of people); cross-sectional (information on individuals is obtained in a defined population at 1 point in time); case-control (individuals are selected on the basis of their disease status); or prospective (individuals from a defined population are selected, exposure such as diet is determined, and the individuals are observed over time).

Observational studies comparing disease rates between genetically similar migrant and nonmigrant populations, or comparing twins reared together or apart, can evaluate the relative importance of genetic and environmental factors (11–13). Epidemiologic studies can also be experimental in character, in which case they are called *randomized controlled clinical trials* or *intervention trials.*

Types of Observational Studies

Ecologic studies compare disease rates in populations and are useful in generating hypotheses. For example, ecologic studies have found that countries characterized by different dietary intakes also experience different rates of disease; those nations whose populations have diets high in saturated fat and cholesterol and low in polyunsaturated fat have correspondingly high rates of coronary heart disease (14–16). *Cross-sectional epidemiologic observations,* in which information is obtained on individuals at one point in time, also can identify associations between diet and disease or risk factors. For example, cross-sectional studies have shown that blood pressure is related directly to dietary salt intake and inversely to dietary potassium intake (17, 18). In *case-control studies,* the nutrient intakes of individuals who have disease are compared with those who do not have disease. For example, blood levels of homocysteine, which are strongly related to folate intake, are higher in patients with coronary heart disease (cases) than in healthy individuals (controls), supporting the hypothesis that hyperhomocysteinemia is a risk factor for coronary heart disease (19, 20).

Prospective cohort studies gather information on a population sample (cohort) at baseline (the beginning of the study period) and then make sequential observations for an extended period of time, usually years (the follow-up period). For example, research on a cohort of men living in Framingham, Massachusetts, has found that a diet high in fruits and vegetables is associated with a reduced risk of stroke after 20 years of follow-up (21).

Strengths and Limitations of Observational Studies

Because epidemiologic investigations typically study large numbers of individuals and because the study sample often is chosen to be representative of the underlying population, the results usually are widely applicable and generalizable. Prospective cohort studies also can provide strong evidence of causality in the relationship between diet and disease risk because dietary intake is measured at the start of the study, prior to any disease onset, and disease rates are measured prospectively (4, 6, 7, 14). This allows the temporal sequence of cause and effect to be established.

Observational studies have several limitations, however. One problem is that, in cross-sectional and some case-control studies, the temporal sequence is unknown; that is, it cannot be determined whether the postulated causal factor (such as dietary exposure) preceded the disease, or whether diet was altered in response to the diagnosis or initial symptoms. Associations identified solely from these study designs cannot be used to draw conclusions about causality, but they are useful for generating hypotheses. They also provide some evidence that can contribute to causal inference (ie, drawing conclusions concerning cause and effect). Another limitation of observational studies is the inability to characterize or otherwise control the many relevant genetic, behavioral, and environmental factors that could influence the interpretation of the results. Differences among populations or individuals in these factors, which may be unmeasured or unknown, could account for observed differences in disease rates.

It therefore is desirable, in both cross-sectional and prospective observational studies, to measure as many diet- and disease-related characteristics and factors as possible in order to adjust for them in the data analysis and avoid drawing wrong conclusions.

EXPERIMENTAL STUDIES

Randomized Controlled Trials

Randomized controlled trials, which also are called *clinical trials,* are studies in humans that provide strong evidence of causality. In these studies, individuals are assigned in random order to one or more experimental treatments or to a control condition or treatment, and disease or risk factor outcomes are measured prospectively. (Also see Chapter 2, "Statistical Aspects of Controlled Diet Studies.")

Dietary Counseling Trials

The most common method of delivering a dietary intervention in a randomized controlled setting is by counseling participants to follow the diet. Adherence to the diet is assessed in order to confirm that dietary exposure or treatment differs between the intervention and control groups. Intervention trials using dietary counseling have the potential for long treatment periods and large sample sizes. An example is the Trials of Hypertension Prevention (TOHP) study, which tested the effects of sodium reduction and weight loss, singly and in combination, on blood pressure and risk of hypertension over a 3- to 4-year period in 2,382 men and women (22). Another example is the Dietary Intervention Study in Children (DISC) study, a nutrition counseling trial that followed 663 children for as long as 7 years and examined the effects of a reduced-fat diet on blood cholesterol concentration (23).

Human Feeding Studies

Another method of delivering a dietary intervention using a randomized controlled design is the feeding study, wherein participants consume prepared foods of specified composition. Two main approaches are used for assignment of participants to treatment: (1) random assignment to a control diet or a test diet (note: there may be several such diets) (parallel-arm design); and (2) assignment to a random sequence of test and control diets (crossover design). In addition to diet, many other aspects of the participants' lives, such as physical activity and medications, are also tightly regulated during the study. Specific dietary effects on pathologic processes or on risk factors, rather than on development of disease, are the primary outcomes. For example, in a study of the effects of salt and potassium intake on blood pressure, 20 men received, in random order for 2 weeks at a time, each of 4 diets: a control (typical) diet low in potassium and high in salt, and 3 test diets—high-potassium/high-salt, low-potassium/low-salt, and high-potassium/low-salt (24). Primarily for feasibility, a feeding study often has small numbers of participants and a short duration, typically ranging from days to months, but occasionally as long as one year. (Also see A Study Design to Test the Hypothesis later in this chapter.)

Strengths and Limitations of Randomized Controlled Trials

The randomized controlled trial design has the cardinal feature of ensuring that the exposure (such as diet) precedes the disease-related outcome, thus providing strong evidence of causation. In addition, all other factors, either known or unknown, that may influence the outcome are equally likely to be found in the intervention or treatment group(s) as well as in the control group(s). Therefore, any differences in disease rates or risk factors observed between the study groups can be attributed to the diet and not to other factors (25), pro-vided other sources of bias are also minimized during the study. Results that are generalizable to a target population generally require trials that have large sample size and long duration, such as dietary counseling trials; achieving large sample size in the context of feeding studies usually requires multicenter designs or the enrollment of successive cohorts (see the discussion of study design later in this chapter and in Chapter 25, "The Multicenter Approach to Human Feeding Studies").

Other Types of Human Feeding Studies

Many feeding studies are conducted as clinical investigations that do not require a randomized controlled design. Either the control group is lacking or the test diets are not assigned to the participants in random order. The sample sizes of clinical studies are generally small, their duration is limited, and the outcomes usually relate to some biological parameter or risk factor rather than disease risk. The population sample for clinical studies tends not to be broadly representative of the general population, and the lack of randomization limits the ability to draw definitive cause-and-effect conclusions (26). Instead, the value of these studies lies in their ability to provide detailed information about specific dietary components and about physiologic processes and mechanisms. For example, one clinical study gave 10 women sequentially increasing doses of vitamin B-6 during 4 test diet periods of 12 days each; although the design was not randomized, the study provided useful information regarding the relationship between vitamin B-6 status and the dietary vitamin B-6:protein ratio (27).

Animal Studies

Animal research conducted by laboratory scientists contributes other types of information, especially for elucidating the mechanisms whereby diet may exert biological effects, such as: high sodium intake → hypertension → arterial wall stress → arterial wall injury → atherosclerotic plaque. The advantage of such studies is that, in a relatively short period of time (several weeks to several years, depending on the animal model), a diet → mechanism → disease relationship can be tested, wherein outcomes consist of pathologic changes confirmed by necropsy examination (28). Just as with the human studies described earlier, the ability to draw definitive conclusions is limited if the animals are not randomly assigned to the experimental conditions.

DIETARY ASSESSMENT METHODOLOGY

Apart from experimental design, an important feature of the various types of research methods is the procedure for ascertaining dietary intake (29, 30). Ecological studies typically use food balance data for this purpose (31, 32). The intake estimates are calculated from food supply statistics, such as foods grown or processed in the country, foods imported and exported, and changes in food stocks. The amounts of food used for other purposes, such as livestock feed, are then subtracted. To calculate per capita consumption, the mean available quantities are divided by the population size (31, 32). It can be difficult to estimate average per capita intake of populations because data on food supply and population size may be incomplete.

For observational and intervention studies, the unit of observation is not a population but rather an individual. Thus, the available information on diet is based primarily on the individual's recall of foods consumed. Several methodological approaches for the collection of dietary intake data are available; the intake estimates that they yield have varying degrees of precision, reliability, and accuracy (32–37). The intake of some nutrients (such as energy, fat, or protein) may be relatively easy to estimate. Estimating the intake of other nutrients (such as certain vitamins or minerals) may be more difficult, especially if the nutrient is found in a large number of foods or in greatly varying concentration. The methods also depend on the availability of high-quality food composition databases (38). Nutrient intake in feeding studies can be measured with relatively high accuracy because the food provided to the participants has been purchased by the study staff and has been prepared, weighed, and measured in a research kitchen. Furthermore, the nutrient composition of the menus is often verified by chemical analysis.

LINES OF SCIENTIFIC EVIDENCE: THE EXAMPLE OF DIET AND CORONARY HEART DISEASE

Studies of the relationship between diet and coronary heart disease provide a good example of the process of examining the totality of the evidence based on various types of research to provide evidence of causality. Virtually the full scope of research methods has been used. Early ecologic investigations of dietary intake in different countries yielded observations that average dietary fat intake is correlated with coronary heart disease rates (14). Studies of Japanese migrants who moved to Hawaii or San Francisco and adopted the dietary habits of their surroundings showed that those individuals experience coronary heart disease rates typical of their adopted, rather than of their native, environments (39). Case-control studies provided suggestive evidence, and longitudinal cohort studies provided strong evidence, that risk factors such as high blood cholesterol, high blood pressure, and smoking are associated with, precede, and increase the probability of developing the disease (40, 41). Cross-sectional and longitudinal epidemiologic studies further showed that intakes of saturated fat, cholesterol, and sodium

are associated with various risk factors, notably serum cholesterol levels and blood pressure, as well as disease (42–46). Human feeding studies indicated that specific dietary saturated fatty acids, as well as the cholesterol content of the diet, play a major role in determining serum cholesterol levels (47, 48). Animal and human pathology studies provided information about mechanisms of disease development by demonstrating clear influences of diet on blood cholesterol levels and blood pressure, and subsequent anatomical changes in disease progression when these factors are modified (49, 50). Lastly, intervention trials of individuals with hypercholesterolemia demonstrated that lowering serum cholesterol levels with either diet or drug therapy can lower disease rates (51–54).

KEY ASPECTS OF CONDUCTING A HUMAN FEEDING STUDY

Four broad conceptual and practical issues must be considered before researchers embark on a human feeding study: a testable, well-founded hypothesis; a study design that can test the hypothesis; appropriately selected outcome measures; and a feasible study protocol.

A Testable, Well-founded Hypothesis

Hypotheses amenable to testing with feeding studies are those for which one or more dietary constituents, given in a known amount, are expected to alter one or more outcome variables. The variables usually are risk factors or surrogate measures for disease. It must be both necessary and possible to test the efficacy of the dietary variable under conditions of high adherence to the diet. In addition, the effects of diet must be expected to occur in a relatively short time frame—days, weeks, or months—and must be unlikely to cause harm to long-term health.

The tight dietary control and adherence conditions of a feeding study yield a high probability that the participants will receive the intended experimental treatment (ie, diet). These conditions lead to high precision in determining the effects of specific dietary constituents.

A Study Design to Test the Hypothesis

Feeding studies are hypothesis-testing studies. (Note: As mentioned earlier, the strongest evidence for a cause-and-effect relationship is provided by a randomized design.) Because feeding studies provide conditions of high adherence, they can quantify precisely the independent effects of a small number of dietary constituents on one or more outcome variables. The specific study design and the characteristics of the experimental diets are purposefully chosen to allow a specific hypothesis to be tested. Following are examples of design elements that must be defined by the study's hypothesis:

Participants

Disease status
  Healthy volunteers
  Individuals with established risk factors
  Individuals with disease
Special populations
  Demographic subgroups
  Older adults
  Children
  Pregnant women

Diet

Type of diet: liquid formula or conventional food
Dose of test nutrient needed to achieve desired effect
Sources of test nutrient and how they are integrated into diet
Macronutrient content of diet
Distribution of energy sources
Micronutrient content of diet
Other nutrient requirements
Dietary and nondietary factors balanced across feeding periods or diet groups to avoid confounding

Time Factors and Statistical Issues

Length of study needed to achieve steady state in endpoint measurements
Need for washout periods
Anticipated effect size
Variability and reliability of endpoint measurements
Sample size calculations to estimate number of participants and measurements
Number of participants feasible to study at one time
Concurrent or successive cohort enrollment

Defined test and control diets are fed to individuals over a specified period of time and all known factors that might alter measured outcomes are balanced across the treatment groups. For example, the foods comprising the diet must be selected in a way that controls for constituents that may alter nutrient absorption (such as the dietary content of vitamin D and oxalate in calcium studies). Extraneous sources of nutrients also must be controlled because they may accidentally influence the results of the study (such as water and toothpaste in calcium studies, or sunlight exposure in a calcium study with controlled vitamin D intake).

The hypothesis of a diet study can be generally phrased as follows: In subjects Q, compared to subjects R, or compared to a control condition, what are the effects of a change in nutrient X on outcome Y, while the confounding variables P, S, and T, known to influence X and Y, are controlled? The hypothesis should have biologic plausibility and should generate data that would fit the time sequence of a causal relationship. The experimental design should be simple, able to produce definitive information, and amenable to standard statistical approaches. Study designs enrolling a relatively small number of participants need to provide sufficient statistical power to detect effects of defined magnitude. (See Chapter 2, "Statistical Aspects of Controlled Diet Studies.")

The type of diet administered should be the one that best fits the hypothesis. For example, liquid formula diets can be effectively used to test a hypothesis requiring a direct comparison of proteins or fats but may be inappropriate when a study compares natural dietary fibers. The dose of the nutrient may deliberately be set to be higher than is commonly consumed in order to detect small biological effects. Conversely, a smaller difference in dose could be used to evaluate effects of typical intakes.

The statistical power for testing the hypothesis can be enhanced by appropriate criteria for participant selection. For example, if the anticipated effect of the test diet is relatively small, it may be desirable to use participants who exhibit a more marked response to dietary modification. Study participants also can be specifically selected to help demonstrate particular biological effects or applications of research. Participants fitting specific entry criteria (such as high-normal blood pressure) may be preferred if the experimental diets (with varying sodium levels, for example) offer information on how to alter disease risk. Participants with established disease (such as osteoporosis) may be chosen when the goal of the intervention is to obtain specific information about how to modify existing disease (such as prevention of subsequent fractures).

The duration of the diet periods should be chosen so that there is sufficient time to achieve first a nutritional steady state for each diet and then a change in outcome measurements. Studies of lipoprotein metabolism might require a feeding period of 2 to 5 weeks to achieve steady state. Other studies may be shorter (such as 5-day periods for sodium balance) or longer (such as a year to evaluate dietary effects on bone mineral density).

Feeding studies tend to enroll small numbers of participants because usually only 5 to 25 individuals can be brought into the facility at one time (although there are a small number of facilities with higher capacity). If larger sample sizes are needed to achieve adequate statistical power, successive cohorts can be studied using the same protocol. Another approach is to use a concurrent multicenter protocol of the type developed for large clinical trials. (Also see Chapter 25, "The Multicenter Approach to Human Feeding Studies.")

Appropriately Selected Outcome Variables

In feeding studies the diet itself is the primary independent design variable: the diet is "well-controlled." The effects of the diet are measured as dependent outcome variables, which may include biochemical assays of blood or tissue samples, physical characteristics of the study participants, objective or subjective assessments of behavior, or clinical symptoms of disease confirmed by physical examination or tissue pathology. Although certain rapidly progressing diseases or metabolically labile conditions may allow researchers to make short-term assessments of diet effects on observable clinical outcomes, chronic diseases generally are symptomatic only after decades-long pathologic processes have taken place (50). This time lag obviously makes it difficult to study dietary effects on chronic diseases in a prospective manner during the lifespan of the investigator. Sometimes this problem can be circumvented with methods that detect occult or early disease (such as exercise tolerance testing or coronary angiography for coronary heart disease; or colonoscopy or barium enema to evaluate the presence of colonic polyps, precursors of colon cancer). Alternatively, study participants can be selected who are at high risk for developing disease within a few years. The typical time course of a feeding study, however, is usually too brief to produce measurable changes in preclinical disease status. Yet another approach (discussed earlier in Research Methodology for Testing Diet-Disease Relationships) is to identify intermediate outcomes or risk factors for the biological process of interest. Risk factors also can suggest plausible mechanisms by which disease processes become manifest.

Outcome parameters are useful in the conduct of a human feeding study only if the available measurement techniques are reliable and precise. In addition, the study design should address how often the outcome variable must be measured after achieving the steady state to reduce imprecision from both analytic and biologic variation. For example, bone densitometry measurements are relatively constant within individuals or with repeated observations. Plasma cholesterol levels, however, have 3% to 5% analytic variation and 9% to 19% within-individual biologic variation and require multiple measurements to estimate true effects (55). The need for multiple measurements can extend the length of the study and greatly increase the cost of the project.

A Feasible Study Protocol

The distinguishing features of a feeding study are the high degree of precision in executing the diet and the ability to monitor adherence. In a dietary counseling study, the participant is instructed about how to select a diet to achieve study goals, but it can at best only be estimated how well those goals are achieved. In a feeding study, however, all of the food given to the participant is of known composition, the participant is observed while consuming the food, and energy intake is adjusted if needed to maintain the patient's weight. Thus, dietary counseling studies only approximate the desired diet due to varying levels of adherence, whereas feeding studies literally define the diet. These elements of control establish feeding studies as providing the best estimate in quantifying the relationship between a specific dietary constituent and a specific outcome.

It must be practical to execute the experimental diet design. An adequate nutrient database must be available to determine sources of the test nutrients, and methods must be available to confirm dietary composition. Essential information about the nutrients includes their natural variability in specific foods (such as the vitamin C content of tomatoes)

and whether their biologic effects can be altered through processes such as storage (such as the antioxidant content of vegetable oils) or food preparation (such as the fatty acid profile in oils used for frying). It is also necessary to calculate the nutrient dose needed to produce an outcome effect (such as the amount of fiber from psyllium vs other natural sources) and whether this designated dose can be reasonably consumed by participants with typical energy requirements for their age, sex, and state of health. Nutrient-nutrient interactions (such as vitamin C enhancement of nonheme iron absorption) must be considered, so that they can be controlled for when study designers construct the test diets. The diets must be visually attractive, pleasing in taste, and reasonably varied, yet within the production capabilities of the kitchen. The composition of the diet must meet study goals, yet also be nutritionally adequate in other respects.

CONCLUSION

A strong association between diet and disease or measured intermediate outcome is determined through multiple lines of investigation, including epidemiologic studies, animal studies, dietary counseling intervention studies, and human feeding studies. Each line of investigation has its strengths and weaknesses. Epidemiologic studies poorly quantify diet but carefully quantify manifest disease, whereas feeding studies precisely quantify diet but can only approximate disease through risk factors or surrogate endpoints for disease. Because there are many problems inherent in estimating the nutrient intake of individuals consuming self-selected diets, animal and clinical studies are used to identify more precisely which dietary factors, in which quantities, might be implicated in altering disease processes or disease risk. Large randomized controlled trials, such as dietary counseling trials, usually provide the best generalizable test of whether altering diet can alter risk factors and subsequently risk of disease.

Because their great precision demands great effort, human feeding studies are undertaken only when the weight of the scientific evidence is sufficiently strong to justify hypothesis-testing research concerning the biological effects or mechanisms of dietary constituents, individually and in combination, on given outcomes. Feeding studies thus will always be essential in clarifying how diet influences risk factors and disease processes, even though many other types of research will also be needed to define cause-and-effect relationships between diet and disease, and to determine the populations to which the results may be generalized. Feeding studies with well-controlled diets provide a scientific viewpoint that is like looking at the world through a keyhole: the perspective may be narrow but the picture is clear.

REFERENCES

1. *The Surgeon General's Report on Nutrition and Health.* Washington, DC: US Dept of Health and Human Services, Public Health Service; 1988. DHHS (PHS) publication 88–50210.

2. Committee on Diet and Health, Food and Nutrition Board, Commission on Life Sciences, National Research Council. *Diet and Health: Implications for Reducing Chronic Disease Risk.* Washington, DC: National Academy Press; 1989.

3. Keys A. Dietary epidemiology. *Am J Clin Nutr.* 1967;20:1151–1157.

4. Stamler J. *Lectures in Preventive Cardiology.* New York, NY: Grune & Statton, Inc; 1967.

5. Steinberg D. The cholesterol controversy is over. Why did it take so long? *Circulation.* 1989;80:1070–1078.

6. Sherry B. Epidemiologic analytic research. In: Monsen ER, ed. *Research: Successful Approaches.* Chicago, Ill: American Dietetic Association; 1992:133–150.

7. Rothman KJ. Causal inference in epidemiology. In: *Modern Epidemiology.* Boston, Mass: Little, Brown and Co; 1986:7–12.

8. DeAngelis C. *An Introduction to Clinical Research.* Oxford, UK: Oxford University Press; 1990.

9. Gehlbach SH. *Interpreting the Medical Literature.* Lexington, Mass: DC Heath & Co; 1982.

10. Fleiss JL. *The Design and Analysis of Clinical Experiments.* New York, NY: John Wiley & Sons, Inc; 1986.

11. Yano K, MacLean CJ, Reed DM, et al. A comparison of the 12-year mortality and predictive factors of coronary heart disease among Japanese men in Japan and Hawaii. *Am J Epidemiol.* 1988;127:476–487.

12. Stunkard AJ, Foch TT, Hrubec Z. A twin study of human obesity. *JAMA.* 1986;256:51–54.

13. Stunkard AJ, Harris JR, Pedersen NL, McClearn GE. The body-mass index of twins who have been reared apart. *N Engl J Med.* 1990;322:1483–1487.

14. Stamler J. Population studies. In: Levy R, Rifkind B, Dennis B, Ernst N, eds. *Nutrition, Lipids and Coronary Heart Disease—A Global View.* New York, NY: Raven Press; 1979:25–88.

15. Liu K, Stamler J, Trevisan M, et al. Dietary lipids, sugar, fiber and mortality from coronary heart disease: bivariate analysis of international data. *Arteriosclerosis.* 1982;2:221–227.

16. Keys A. *Coronary Heart Disease in Seven Countries.* New York, NY: American Heart Association, Inc; 1970. AHA Monograph No. 29.

17. Intersalt Cooperative Research Group. Intersalt: an international study of electrolyte excretion and blood pressure. Results for 24 hour urinary sodium and potassium excretion. *BMJ.* 1988;297:319–328.

18. Khaw K-T, Barrett-Connor E. Dietary potassium and blood pressure in a population. *Am J Clin Nutr.* 1984;39:963–968.

19. Mason JB, Miller JW. The effects of vitamins B_{12}, B_6, and folate on blood homocysteine levels. *Ann NY Acad Sci.* 1992;669:197–204.

20. Verhoef P, Stampfer MJ, Buring JE, et al. Homocysteine metabolism and risk of myocardial infarction: relation with vitamins B_6, B_{12}, and folate. *Am J Epidemiol.* 1996;143:846–859.

21. Gillman MW, Cupples LA, Gagnon D, et al. Protective effect of fruits and vegetables on development of stroke in men. *JAMA.* 1995;273:1113–1117.

22. Trials of Hypertension Prevention Collaborative Research Group. Effects of weight loss and sodium reduction intervention on blood pressure and hypertension incidence in overweight people with high-normal blood pressure. The Trials of Hypertension Prevention, Phase II. *Arch Intern Med.* 1997;157:657–667.

23. The Writing Group for the DISC Collaborative Research Group. Efficacy and safety of lowering dietary intake of fat and cholesterol in children with elevated low-density lipoprotein cholesterol. The Dietary Intervention Study in Children (DISC). *JAMA.* 1995;273:1429–1435.

24. Skrabal F, Aubock J, Hortnagl H. Low sodium/high potassium diet for prevention of hypertension: probable mechanisms of action. *Lancet.* 1981;2:895–900.

25. Bulpitt CJ. *Randomized Controlled Trials.* The Hague, The Netherlands: Martinus Nijhoff; 1983.

26. Silverman WA. *Human Experimentation: A Guided Step into the Unknown.* Oxford, UK: Oxford University Press; 1985.

27. Hansen CM, Leklem JE, Miller LT. Changes in vitamin B-6 status indicators of women fed a constant protein diet with varying levels of vitamin B-6. *Am J Clin Nutr.* 1997;66:1379–1387.

28. Clarkson TB, Shively CA, Weingand KW. Animal models of diet-induced atherosclerosis. Comparative animal nutrition. In: Beynen AC, West CES, eds. *Use of Animal Models for Research in Human Nutrition.* Vol 6. Basel, Switzerland: Karger, AG; 1988:56–82.

29. Pennington JAT. Associations between diet and health: The use of food consumption measurements, nutrient databases, and dietary guidelines. *J Am Diet Assoc.* 1988;88:1221–1224.

30. Hankin JH. Dietary intake methodology. In: Monsen ER, ed. *Research: Successful Approaches.* Chicago, Ill: American Dietetic Association; 1992:173–194.

31. *Food Balance Sheets: 1979–81 Average.* Rome, Italy: Food and Agriculture Organization of the United Nations; 1984.

32. Peterkin BB. Nationwide food consumption survey, 1977–1978. In: *Nutrition in the 1980's: Constraints on Our Knowledge.* New York, NY: Alan R Liss; 1981: 59–69.

33. Sempos CT, Briefel RB, Flegal KM, et al. Factors involved in selecting a dietary survey methodology for national nutrition surveys. *Austr J Nutr Diet.* 1992; 49(3):96–105.

34. Karkeck JM. Improving the use of dietary survey methodology. *J Am Diet Assoc.* 1987;87:869–873.

35. Basiotis PP, Welsh SO, Cronin FJ, et al. Number of days of food intake records required to estimate individual and group nutrient intakes with defined confidence. *J Nutr.* 1987;117:1638–1641.

36. Briefel RR, Flegal KM, Winn DM, et al. Assessing the nation's diet: limitations of the food frequency questionnaire. *J Am Diet Assoc.* 1992;92:959–962.

37. Willett W. *Nutritional Epidemiology.* New York, NY: Oxford University Press; 1990.

38. Pennington JAT. Development and use of food composition data and databases. In: Monsen ER, ed. *Research: Successful Approaches.* Chicago, Ill: American Dietetic Association; 1992:195–203.

39. Kagan A, Harris BR, Winkelstein W Jr, et al. Epidemiologic studies of coronary heart disease and stroke in Japanese men living in Japan, Hawaii, and California: demographic, physical, dietary and biochemical characteristics. *J Chron Dis.* 1974;27:345–364.

40. Rosenberg L. Case-control studies of risk factors for myocardial infarction among women. In: Eaker ED, Packard B, Wenger NK, et al, eds. *Coronary Heart Disease in Women.* New York, NY: Haymarket Doyma; 1987:70–77.

41. Stokes III J, Kannel WB, Wolf PA, et al. The relative importance of selected risk factors for various manifestations of cardiovascular disease among men and women from 35 to 64 years old: 30 years of follow-up in the Framingham study. *Circulation.* 1987;75:V65-V73.

42. Posner BM, Cobb JL, Belanger AJ, et al. Dietary lipid predictors of coronary heart disease in men: the Framingham study. *Arch Intern Med.* 1991;151:1181–1187.

43. Kushi LH, Lew RA, Stare FJ, et al. Diet and 20-year mortality from coronary heart disease: the Ireland-Boston Diet-Heart study. *N Engl J Med.* 1985;312:811–818.

44. Elliott P. Observational studies of salt and blood pressure. *Hypertension.* 1991;17(suppl 1):I3–I8.

45. Keys A. *Seven Countries: A Multivariate Analysis of Death and Coronary Heart Disease.* Cambridge, Mass: Harvard University Press; 1980.

46. Shekelle RB, Shyrock AM, Paul O, et al. Diet, serum cholesterol, and death from coronary heart disease: the Western Electric study. *N Engl J Med.* 1981;304:65–70.

47. Keys A, Anderson JT, Grande F. Prediction of serum-cholesterol responses of man to changes in fats in the diet. *Lancet.* 1957;ii:955–966.

48. Hegsted DM, McGandy RB, Myers ML, et al. Quantitative effects of dietary fat on serum cholesterol in man. *Am J Clin Nutr.* 1965;17:281–295.

49. Pathobiological Determinants of Atherosclerosis in Youth (PDAY) Research Group. Relationship of atherosclerosis in young men to serum lipoprotein cholesterol concentrations and smoking. *JAMA.* 1990;264:3018–3024.

50. McGill HC. Persistent problems in the pathogenesis of atherosclerosis. *Arteriosclerosis.* 1984;4:443–451.

51. Hjermann I, Velve Byre K, Holme I, Leren P. Effect of diet and smoking intervention on the incidence of coronary heart disease. Report from the Oslo Study Group of a randomised trial in healthy men. *Lancet.* 1981; 2:1303–1310.

52. Ornish D, Brown SE, Scherwitz LW, et al. Can lifestyle changes reverse coronary heart disease? *Lancet.* 1990;336:129–133.

53. Watts GF, Lewis B, Brunt JNH, et al. Effects on coronary artery disease of lipid-lowering diet, or diet plus cholestyramine, in the St. Thomas Atherosclerosis Regression Study (STARS). *Lancet.* 1992;339:563–569.

54. Lipid Research Clinics Program. The Lipid Research Clinics Coronary Primary Prevention Trial results. I. Reduction in incidence of coronary heart disease. *JAMA.* 1984;251:351–364.

55. *Recommendations for Improving Cholesterol Measurement, National Cholesterol Education Program.* Washington, DC: US Dept of Health and Human Services, Public Health Service; 1990. DHHS (PHS) publication 90–2964.

CHAPTER 2

STATISTICAL ASPECTS OF CONTROLLED DIET STUDIES

JANICE A. DERR, PhD

The proper planning of a research study and its data management and analysis involve many decisions. What type of experimental design should be used? How many participants should be studied and for how long? How should test diets be assigned to participants? How should the data be analyzed when a participant drops out or fails to comply with a protocol? A statistician can help investigators in the planning of the study by addressing these questions. This chapter provides information about the advantages and disadvantages of different experimental designs and discusses issues related to sample size and power, study implementation, and data analysis.

PLANNING THE STUDY

A good experimental study is organized around a set of research questions originating from the scientific objectives of the project. The purpose of the initial project-planning sessions should be to identify and prioritize the research questions that the study will be designed to answer. A statistician should be involved even at this early stage. By participating in the project-planning sessions, the statistician gains a better understanding of the scientific issues motivating the study.

Several issues that have an impact on study design and data analysis can be clarified at the project-planning stage. These include the major objectives of the study, the variables and comparisons of primary interest, secondary or exploratory variables and comparisons, policy on the exclusion of data, and the population to which generalizations about the study are to be extended. Clarifying these issues during the planning phase will provide a good basis for making statistical decisions throughout the remainder of the study.

Experimental Designs

Once the research questions are clarified, it is time to consider possible experimental designs that could be used to achieve the study objectives. The statistician should be able to present the relative advantages and disadvantages of several options and discuss them with the investigators. To do so requires a good understanding of the research setting and any practical limitations it may have. A statistician gains this understanding through regular contact with the scientist and exposure to the study setting—the laboratories, the kitchens, and the areas where participants and dietitians will be interacting.

Crossover and Parallel-arm Designs

An example of the way in which a statistician might discuss different options for the experimental design of a study is given by the comparison between a crossover design and a parallel-arm design. In a *crossover design,* each participant receives all test diets in a randomized order. In a *parallel-arm design,* each participant is assigned at random to only one test diet; different groups of participants receive different test diets. Table 2-1 illustrates these two designs. The advantages and disadvantages associated with each design are summarized in Table 2-2 and discussed here.

The main advantage of a crossover design is that the sample size required to detect a given experimental effect is smaller than with a parallel-arm design. The reduced sample size is feasible because each participant receives each test diet; the statistical comparison among test diets is made using the within-participant error. In a parallel-arm design, the comparison between test diets is made using the between-

TABLE 2-1

Crossover and Parallel-arm Designs

Crossover design: Each subject receives all test diets in randomized order. This example shows three diets and three periods.

Subjects	Period 1	Period 2	Period 3
Subject 1	Diet A	Diet B	Diet C
Subject 2	Diet B	Diet C	Diet A
Subject 3	Diet C	Diet A	Diet B
Subject 4	Diet A	Diet C	Diet B
Subject 5	Diet C	Diet B	Diet A
Subject 6	Diet B	Diet A	Diet C
⋮	⋮	⋮	⋮
Subject n	Diet C	Diet A	Diet B
Subject Totals	**Period 1**	**Period 2**	**Period 3**
Diet A	n/3	n/3	n/3
Diet B	n/3	n/3	n/3
Diet C	n/3	n/3	n/3

Parallel-arm design: Each subject receives only one test diet. Only one time period is required.

Diet A	Diet B	Diet C
Subject 1	Subject 2	Subject 3
Subject 4	Subject 5	Subject 6
Subject m-2	Subject m-1	Subject m

TABLE 2-2

Crossover and Parallel-arm Designs: Advantages (A) and Disadvantages (D)

Study Feature		Crossover Design		Parallel-arm Design
Sample size	A	Smaller	D	Larger
Duration of study	D	Longer	A	Shorter
Use of facilities and resources	A	More evenly distributed across time	D	Effort concentrated in a shorter time period
Expectation of subjects	D	Requires greater commitment	A	Requires less commitment
Design considerations	A	Balanced randomization	A	Balanced randomization
	D	Not suitable when carryover effects are expected	A	No adverse consequences of carryover
	D	Low % dropouts required	A	Moderate % dropouts acceptable
	D	Susceptible to confounding from Period X Test Diet interactions	A	Free of confounding from Period X Test Diet interactions
Data analysis	D	More complex	A	Less complex

participant error, which is generally larger than the within-participant error. Table 2-3 shows an example of sample size calculations for a diet study having either a parallel-arm or a crossover design. This will be discussed in more detail later in Selection of Design.

Counterbalancing the crossover design's advantage of reduced sample size are several considerations that add to its complexity. Because each participant must be given all of the test diets, the participants in a crossover design must be enrolled for a much longer period of time than in a parallel-arm design. In addition, the crossover design relies on *balance* to partition the effects of time period (see Table 2-1) from the effects of test diet. When a participant drops out before the study is finished, that balance is threatened. Therefore, well-worked-out strategies for participant retention should be incorporated in the protocol of a crossover design.

If the crossover design is to retain its increased efficiency relative to the parallel-arm design, the response to a diet given in one test period should not affect the response to diets given in subsequent test periods (referred to as a *carryover effect*). Data from prior or pilot studies can identify the length of time required for the measures of interest to stabilize under test diet conditions. One strategy often

TABLE 2-3

Example of Sample Size Requirement for a Parallel-arm Design Compared to a Crossover Design

Minimum Detectable Difference Total Cholesterol (mg/dL)[1,2]	Two-group parallel-arm design Total number of subjects	Two-period crossover design Total number of subjects
6.5[3]	156[3]	51[4]
8.0	102	34
10.0	71	22
16.0	27	9

[1]For 80% power with one-tailed $\alpha = 0.05$:
the variance calculation for the parallel-arm designs uses: $\sigma^2_{among} + \sigma^2_{within} = 89.3 + 173.7 = 263.0$; the variance calculations for the crossover designs uses: $\sigma^2_{within} = 173.7$.
[2]These estimates were derived from data reported in Kris-Etherton et al (12).
[3]For number of subject per group, divide total in column by 2. Each group is assigned one test diet.
[4]Each subject experiences both test diets in random order.

employed to minimize the carryover effect is to include interim periods, known as *washout periods* (Figure 2-1), between test periods. The purpose of the washout period is to allow each participant's measurements to return to a baseline level before the participant begins the next test diet. Measurements taken at baseline can be used to assess carryover effects. Jones and Kenward (1) offer a more technical treatment of crossover designs and carryover effects.

Washout periods can be designed in one of two ways. This period can serve as a "break" from the experimental regimen during which time the participant's diet is not under experimental control. Alternatively, the participants may all be fed a standard diet such as one following the Dietary Guidelines for Americans (2), or the National Cholesterol Education Program (NCEP) guidelines (3). Another strategy for minimizing carryover effects does not make use of a washout period. Rather, the test diets follow each other in sequence without a break, and the test diet periods are long enough so that the endpoint measurements are not influenced by the previous diet. This strategy would be employed when there is no interest in the values of variables at the beginning of each test diet period.

Prior to the first test period, feeding studies can also incorporate a *run-in period* (Figure 2-1) during which the participants experience the protocol of the study. A run-in period helps investigators achieve several objectives important to the successful conduct of the study: (1) familiarizing participants with the feeding protocol used during the study; (2) allowing participants who discover they cannot tolerate the protocol to drop out prior to randomization; and (3) allowing participants to achieve a baseline value of the measurements of interest while on a common diet. The specific diets fed to the participants during the run-in period and the washout period, and the possibility that participants' diets are not under experimental control during these periods, are important issues that should be discussed among scientists and the project statistician.

In comparison with a crossover design, the parallel-arm design offers a relatively straightforward means of comparing the response to a set of test diets. However, there are two important issues that must be addressed with the parallel-arm design. First, the random assignment of participants to test diets must be done with care in order to ensure that the groups have a similar profile with respect to key variables prior to the test period. This is discussed in more detail later in Randomization. Second, because of the larger sample size requirement of the parallel-arm design relative to the crossover design, some parallel-arm designs will require more participants than can be processed at once at any one research facility. It thus may be necessary to conduct the parallel-arm design in *blocks,* or replicates of the design. The composition of the blocks must be carefully considered. Each block should contain a complete replicate of the design (that is, all of the test diets under consideration in all of the

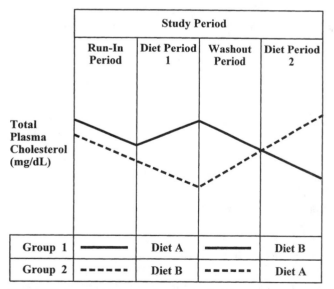

FIGURE 2-1. Schematic of a two-period crossover design. Two groups of subjects are treated with hypothetical diets A and B. Total plasma cholesterol is measured at the beginning and/or end of each study period.

different orders) and the randomization of participants to test diets should be balanced within each block. Blocks of the design can be conducted by different facilities, as is done in a multicenter study, or by the same facility over a period of time.

Designs to Avoid

Every statistician's nightmare is the *confounded* design. This is a design in which it is not possible to distinguish between a response to treatments, such as a set of test diets, and some other factor in the design. An example of a confounded design is a crossover design in which all participants receive Diet A during test period one, Diet B during test period two, and Diet C during test period three. In this design, the effect of test period is indistinguishable from the effect of diet. A second example of a confounded design is a parallel-arm design in which females receive Diet A and males receive Diet B. In this second example, it is not possible to distinguish between a diet effect and a gender effect. Confounded designs produce uninterpretable results, and there is no miracle of data analysis that can remedy the problem. It therefore is in everyone's best interest to discuss potential confounding factors with the statistician on the research team and to make sure that the critical factors are identified and accounted for in the design.

Control Groups

In feeding studies, the definition of a control is problematic. What is a *control diet?* Is it the participant's free-living diet? Is it the NCEP Step One diet? (3) The only way a statistician can help to answer this question is to enter the discussion about the objectives of a proposed feeding study. Do the scientists want to examine the response of a test diet as a *difference* from a baseline value? If so, then perhaps a standard reference diet can be used to establish a baseline. Are the scientists interested only in comparing a set of test diets, using as measurements only the values at the end of each test diet period? If so, then perhaps there is no need for a reference diet.

However, the strategy of not using a reference diet should be adopted with care. Seasonal effects, if there are any, become critically important for crossover designs as well as for parallel-arm designs conducted in blocks over periods of time. For example, effects of increasing sunlight exposure from winter to summer must be addressed in studies that examine calcium and vitamin D metabolism. Designs can become unbalanced because of dropouts or slightly uneven numbers in the original demographic categories. Including a reference diet in these designs can permit a seasonal adjustment in the comparison among test diets.

Including a control group in the design is important when participants are recruited from population extremes. For example, consider a study in which participants in the 95th to 99th percentile for total cholesterol are recruited. In this hypothetical study, there is a test diet that is thought to lower total cholesterol. Plasma total cholesterol will be mea-

sured at baseline and after participants consume the test diet for a specific time period. To provide a valid estimate of the cholesterol-lowering effect of the test diet, a proportion (usually half) of the eligible participants should be assigned at random to a control diet. This is because participants whose first blood sample puts them in an extreme percentile group will tend to have a second measurement closer to the population mean even with *no* intervention at all. This effect is known as the *regression to the mean*. Without a control group, the regression to the mean effect can be misinterpreted to be a treatment effect.

The true effect of the test diet is the *net* difference between change in total cholesterol for the group given the test diet and the change in total cholesterol for the control group. (See Figure 2-2 for an illustration of this net difference.) Davis (4) discusses the regression to the mean effect in lipid studies and gives suggestions for ways in which this effect can be reduced, such as using the mean of several baseline blood samples to classify participants prior to a dietary intervention.

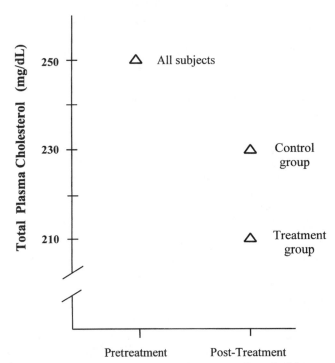

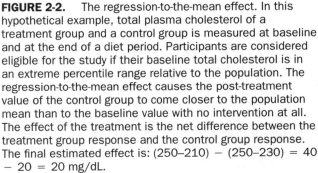

FIGURE 2-2. The regression-to-the-mean effect. In this hypothetical example, total plasma cholesterol of a treatment group and a control group is measured at baseline and at the end of a diet period. Participants are considered eligible for the study if their baseline total cholesterol is in an extreme percentile range relative to the population. The regression-to-the-mean effect causes the post-treatment value of the control group to come closer to the population mean than to the baseline value with no intervention at all. The effect of the treatment is the net difference between the treatment group response and the control group response. The final estimated effect is: $(250–210) - (250–230) = 40 - 20 = 20$ mg/dL.

Sample Size and Power

How many participants should be used in the research study? This is a crucial issue that will be closely examined by the institutional review board and the agency providing the funds for the research study. The institutional review board must consider two mandates that influence the choice of sample size: (1) the benefits of the research study must justify the potential risk to the participants, and (2) human participants should not be exposed to an excessive amount of risk. On one hand, a study with an inadequate number of participants exposes these participants to an unjustifiable amount of risk, because the study will fail to meet its objectives. On the other hand, a study with more participants than are needed to address the research questions exposes some participants to an unnecessary amount of risk. Therefore, considerations of human safety require the investigators to justify that they are including an adequate number of participants, but no more, to meet their research objectives.

From the perspective of the funding agency, the cost of processing each participant through a feeding trial also suggests that the number of participants should be the minimum that is adequate to address the research objectives. With these pressures in mind, the estimation of sample size should be carried out with great care and with the highest quality of information available.

The best number of participants for a feeding study is influenced by several factors: (1) the study design; (2) the size of the experimental effect that the investigators wish to detect; (3) the desired level of statistical power and significance; (4) the amount of variation within and among participants; and (5) the number of dropouts and the level of compliance for participants in the study. The statistician on the research team should compute and illustrate the statistical properties of the range of sample sizes and circumstances under consideration.

The statistician can also use previous data from similar studies in order to determine sample size requirements for different candidate designs. If no such data are available from either the research team or the published literature, it may be necessary to conduct a pilot study.

Selection of Design

The decision about sample size is inseparable from the decision about design. For example, a crossover design will generally require fewer participants but greater time commitment per participant than will a parallel-arm design. (See the earlier discussion in Experimental Designs.) Table 2-3 shows sample sizes that were computed during the planning stages of a feeding study. These estimates were calculated so that the investigators could make an informed decision between using a two-period crossover design and a parallel-arm design. Using estimates of within- and among-participant error from a previous study of a similar participant population, the calculations showed that a total of 102 participants would be required for a parallel-arm design (51 participants in each of two groups) in order to detect a min-

imum difference of 8.0 mg/dL total cholesterol between the two test diets at 80% power and 5% significance. The same statistical characteristics could be achieved in a crossover design with 34 participants, with each participant receiving both test diets in randomized order.

Size of Experimental Effect

Sample size requirements also depend on the size of the effect that the investigators want to detect with high probability. This effect size, often called the *minimum detectable difference,* is the smallest difference between means (eg, the mean response on each test diet) that the investigators would consider important. The criteria of "importance" must be determined from the clinical or research perspective. For example, consider the study discussed in Selection of Design, in which 8.0 mg/dL total cholesterol was determined to be the smallest difference between test diets that was important from a clinical perspective. A parallel-arm design with 156 participants would be able to detect a difference of 6.5 mg/dL total cholesterol with high probability. This difference, although statistically significant with 156 participants, might not be considered clinically important in the context of this hypothetical study.

The objective in computing sample size is to provide a match between an effect size that is meaningful to the investigators and the effect size that can be detected in the data analysis as statistically significant. It is not possible to estimate sample size without a criterion for effect size; the p-values generated from a study without any criteria for sample size are meaningless.

Statistical Power and Significance

Power refers to the probability of detecting a significant effect if one exists. Having high power, such as 80% or 90%, to detect a significant effect means that a correct conclusion is likely to be made about whether a dietary variable causes a change in an outcome variable such as blood pressure or blood lipids. The statistical properties of power and significance are components in the calculation of sample size. These properties determine the probability that the study results are truly representative of the entire reference population. Hypothesis testing is the basis of power and significance, but a detailed description is beyond the scope of this chapter. A very clear explication of these concepts can be found in Zar (5), Meinert (6) and Friedman, Furberg, and DeMets (7).

Variation

A reliable estimate of sample size depends on good estimates of variation for the response variables of interest. Data from previous studies or from a pilot study can be used to estimate variation. The participant population from previous studies should be as similar as possible to the participant population in the proposed study.

It also is critically important to choose which estimate of variance is the correct one for each sample size estimation.

For example, the variation *among* participants is used in a parallel-arm design, and the variation *within* participants is used for a crossover design. If the value of an outcome variable will be estimated from an average of several samples (for example, the mean total cholesterol from blood samples taken on three consecutive days), then the sample size formula should incorporate the variance of this mean.

Resources

Computational formulas for sample sizes vary according to the design and the type of variables to be measured. Reliable formulas and tables for sample size calculations can be found in Kraemer and Thiemann (8) and Cohen (9). Computer software can be purchased to automate the computations. One product is PASS® (10), which computes sample size and power for a broad range of experimental designs and types of response variables. Users of computer software are strongly cautioned to compare the computer output with hand-calculated and tabled values in order to make sure that the program is being used and interpreted correctly.

Dropout Rate and Compliance

When participants drop out of a study or do not completely follow the protocol for a test diet, the statistical power of the design is reduced. Investigators should estimate dropout rate and compliance from previous similar studies and inflate the sample size estimates accordingly. The question of whether and how to use data from dropouts or noncompliant participants will be discussed in Analyzing the Data.

IMPLEMENTING THE STUDY: STATISTICAL ISSUES

Randomization

One of the statistician's tasks is ensuring that a valid randomization procedure is used to assign participants to test diets in a way that protects against selection bias. A randomization can also provide balance in the design so that the main effects of interest will not be confounded with other factors. For example, in a parallel-arm design, the randomization scheme should provide balance across gender, race, and age group for each test diet. In a crossover design, the test diet sequences should be balanced across time period and carryover effects from one diet to the next.

For example, Table 2-4 shows a set of test diet sequences that were used in a feeding study having a four-period crossover design. In this example, the statistician discussed the study with the investigator and learned that dropouts were most likely to occur within the first week of the first test period (these were participants who discovered they could not tolerate the protocol). Therefore, the statistician devised the randomization in two steps: First, participants were assigned to test diets for Period 1. The scientist then reported which participants had dropped out by the end of Period 1. Once the dropouts were eliminated from Period 1, the sequence of test diets for Periods 2, 3, and 4 were then computed for the remaining participants. This strategy achieved the best balance of diets in each period and of pairs of diets across the whole design.

A great variety of randomization schemes can be devised to meet the requirements of a feeding study. Meinert (6) and Friedman, Furberg, and DeMets (7) provide detailed descriptions of methods for assigning participants at random to groups.

Data Management

The development of a data management system should begin during the early project-planning stages. Data management encompasses the entire process from information gathering to data analysis: (1) the design and testing of all forms used to gather data; (2) the development of systems for labeling samples, identifying participants, and masking (ie, "blinding") certain processes; (3) data entry and error checking; (4) online storage plus offline archiving and retrieval of files; (5) the production of summary statistics at interim stages of the project; and (6) the development of data files to be used for analysis. A good data management system is essential to producing high-quality information that can be readily analyzed, and to ensure the security, safety, and confidentiality of the data.

The first responsibility of the data management team is to develop and test the forms that will be used in data collection. In feeding studies this generally involves forms that track variables stemming from many activities, such as participant characteristics and participant responses during recruitment and throughout the study, laboratory assays of biologic samples, and nutrient analysis of the diets. The data management team needs to work with the investigators and the project staff to develop a system that accommodates not just data management but also clinic, laboratory, and kitchen procedures. The timing of each measurement and the nature of each variable should be planned in advance. Adequate identification and labeling systems need to be developed to facilitate the collection of data. The data management team should develop a system for tracking laboratory samples and data as well as a coding system for information that must be kept masked. All forms must be tested (and revised) before the study begins. Meinert (6) provides a comprehensive reference to good practices in data management.

Another task of the data management team is to create a central database with a high level of security, protection, and quality control. For the data to be useful not just during the life of the project but also for a wide range of future research investigations, the issues of quality control, storage, security, access, and reporting are of paramount importance. Appropriate system security features need to be implemented to ensure that access to data, forms, and reports is restricted to authorized personnel and investigators. Frequent backups of data protect the database from possible data loss or corruption caused by electronic or power irregularities.

TABLE 2-4

Randomization Scheme for a Four-Period Crossover Design[1]

Subject ID	Period 1	Period 2	Period 3	Period 4
1	D	B	C	A
2	C	A	D	B
3	C	A	B	D
4	D	C	B	A
5	A	B	C	D
6	A	C	D	B
7	D	A	B	C
8	C	B	D	A
9	A	D	B	C
10	B	A	C	D
11	D	C	A	B
12	C	D	A	B
13	C	B	A	D
14	B	—[1]	—	—
15	A	—[1]	—	—
16	B	D	C	A
17	B	D	A	C
18	A	—[1]	—	—

Totals	Period 1	Period 2	Period 3	Period 4
A	3[2]	4	4	4
B	3[2]	4	4	4
C	5	3	4	3
D	4	4	3	4

Individual ordered diet pairs

—A	AB	AC	AD	—B	BA	BC	BD	—C	CA	CB	CD	—D	DA	DB	DC
4	5	3	3	4	3	4	4	5	5	3	4	4	4	4	3

[1]Diet treatment groups are indicated by letters A–D.
[2]For Period 1 there were originally 5 subjects in Diet Group A and 4 subjects in Diet Group B. Several subjects dropped out before Period 2.

Data quality control should include review and error checking at a number of stages of data entry and management. All forms should be reviewed for unusual events or missing information before data are entered. Programs for identifying out-of-range values can be executed once the data are entered. It is necessary to develop a system for querying missing information and out-of-range data that keeps the project staff in communication with the data management team. At regular intervals, the data management team should produce summary reports with descriptive information from the database. The data management team is also responsible for producing files in the appropriate format for data analysis.

ANALYZING THE DATA

Exclusion of Data

In any clinical study, the investigators must decide which data from which participants should be included in the analysis. For example, there may be reason to believe that not everybody complied fully with the protocol. Some responses may appear atypical. Some participants may have dropped out before the study was finished. A well-planned feeding study will include a discussion of these issues and a statement of policy in advance of the trial.

It is likely that the statistician on the research team will bring to this discussion the *intent-to-treat paradigm*. This paradigm, well established in the clinical trials literature, directs the investigators to analyze data from all participants that were randomized into the study. Excluding participants according to compliance, errors in delivering the test diet, or other criteria can lead to an unknown amount of bias in the results. However, the intent-to-treat paradigm relates most directly to clinical trials in which noncompliance and inaccurate delivery of the treatment are considered valid aspects of the treatment regimen as it may be applied to the population at large. Friedman, Furberg, and DeMets (7) provide a discussion of the intent-to-treat paradigm from the clinical perspective.

There is room for discussion about the way in which unusual observations or departures from treatment will be handled in feeding studies. This discussion should be held in advance of any data analysis and should result in a carefully documented policy on criteria for excluding participants or data from analysis. This policy should be fully described in the publications resulting from the study. Regardless of the approach taken, the policy should be sufficiently well-considered and valid to withstand the scrutiny of peer review.

The Analytical Approach

Before any analysis, the statistician inspects the data through various graphical, descriptive, and diagnostic routines to ensure that the assumptions of the proposed analytical approach are satisfied. For linear models such as analysis of variance and linear regression, these assumptions include normality of errors and constant error variance. For crossover designs the structure of the covariance matrix should also be evaluated. Data *outliers,* or extreme values that do not appear to belong to the distribution of the majority of the data, will be evaluated. Some response measures may require a transformation, such as a logarithmic transformation for skewed data, before they are analyzed.

It is the responsibility of the statistician to select the most powerful statistical analysis compatible with the nature of the data. This is because the use of human participants requires that exposure to risk be balanced with maximal benefit from the acquired data. Several aspects of feeding studies suggest that the best statistical analysis is likely to be complex:

1. Many experimental designs have more than one test diet. A simple two-sample procedure such as a t-test comparison of one test diet to a control diet will generally be less powerful than an analysis of variance, which includes data from all of the test diets with follow-up comparisons of pairs of test diets.
2. A study design may involve a number of factors such as population subgroups, replicates, or centers that should be represented in the analysis.
3. Covariates such as baseline values may need to be incorporated in the analysis.
4. Crossover studies require the investigation of carryover effects and "test diet by time period" interactions that are not of direct interest but affect the analytical approach and results.
5. It may be necessary to provide a seasonal adjustment for designs that include blocks of time.
6. The occurrence of dropouts in the study generates incomplete data, which adds to the complexity of the analysis.

There are a wide variety of statistical approaches that can incorporate complex information, and more refinements in methodology are always appearing in the literature. It is a good idea to identify the probable analytical model at the project planning stages and to nominate alternatives to use if key assumptions are not met.

Multiple Tests of Significance

Most feeding studies involve a multiplicity of response measurements and comparisons of interest. For example, several plasma lipid measurements such as total cholesterol, LDL cholesterol, and HDL cholesterol may be included in the study. There may be several test diets in the study and an interest in comparing all possible pairs of test diets. It is important to determine in advance of the data analysis how this multiplicity will be managed because each statistical test carries with it an error rate given by the α level of the test. The error rates of each test within the same study are additive, which means that if the error rates for statistical tests are uncontrolled, there is a high chance that one or more false conclusions will result from the data analysis of the entire study.

A well-planned study provides not only an investigation of the major research questions of interest but also an exploratory analysis of other factors that could lead to the next research study. A good way to manage multiplicity in tests of significance is to make a well-defined distinction between these two phases. At the project planning stage, the study team should define the measurements and comparisons of interest comprising the primary aims of the study. Other measurements and comparisons should then be designated as "secondary" or exploratory. One approach to multiplicity is for each primary measurement (such as total cholesterol, LDL cholesterol, and HDL cholesterol) to be analyzed without mutual adjustment for multiplicity. Within each primary measurement, a multiple comparison procedure with good statistical properties should be used to adjust the significance level of comparisons of primary importance, such as comparisons in the level of total cholesterol between pairs of test diets. The best multiple comparison procedure will depend on the design and the structure of the comparisons. Neter, Wasserman, and Kutner (11) describe several frequently used procedures for making multiple comparisons.

The exploratory analysis of secondary measurements and comparisons can be treated in a number of ways. One option is to make a single Bonferroni adjustment to the p-values of all of the secondary tests. Another option is to report the unadjusted p-values of secondary tests in the literature without using the language of statistical inference. This means that secondary tests would be treated in a section on "exploratory data analysis" and discussed without using the terms *significantly different* or *not significantly different.*

There are many statistical approaches to multiplicity, and this topic is a matter of active debate in the statistical literature. As a guiding principle, the reader of the study's results should be able to determine how many statistical tests were conducted and what adjustments were made to account for multiplicity. Reporting only the unadjusted p-values of the few "significant" tests obtained from a vast search of the database and hundreds or thousands of tests—known as *data-dredging*—not only misleads the reader but also is likely to lead to the embarrassment of researchers who produce unreplicable results.

When a careful approach to multiplicity is used, the manuscript can indicate future analysis plans suggested by exploratory approaches. The same cautious approach will allow the investigators to report their primary results with confidence.

CONCLUSION

The proper planning of a research study requires statistical insight into study design, implementation, and data analysis. Consultation with a statistician during the planning phase is essential for proper planning. The hypotheses must be specified a priori and are the keystone to the experiment and subsequent data analysis. The choice of experimental design is based on a number of factors, including the number of participants needed to show a prespecified effect size with a specified degree of confidence to detect that effect size and some assessment of likelihood of adherence and dropout. Inclusion of a control group is highly desirable and in many cases essential. Implementation of a well-designed study includes developing randomization procedures, study forms that have been pretested, methods for masking data collectors from knowing the treatment assignment of the participants they are measuring, plans for quality control of data collection and transmission, and methods for data management. The statistical analysis should be appropriate for the study design and should in advance address statistical issues such as adjusting significance levels for multiple comparisons, analytic approaches for dealing with dropouts, and conditions for excluding data.

Careful attention paid to the statistical aspects of design, implementation, and analysis in designing a human feeding study will result in a well-designed study with results that are readily interpretable.

REFERENCES

1. Jones B, Kenward MG. *Design and Analysis of Cross-Over Trials.* London, UK: Chapman and Hall; 1989.

2. US Dept of Agriculture and US Dept of Health and Human Services. *Dietary Guidelines for Americans.* 4th ed. Washington, DC: US Government Printing Office; 1995. Home and Garden Bulletin No 232.

3. *The Second Report of the Expert Panel on Detection, Evaluation, and Treatment of High Blood Cholesterol in Adults.* Washington, DC: National Cholesterol Education Program; 1993. NIH publication 93–3095.

4. Davis CE. The effect of regression to the mean in epidemiologic and clinical studies. *Am J Epidemiol.* 1976; 104:493–498.

5. Zar JH. *Biostatistical Analysis.* 2nd ed. Englewood Cliffs, NJ: Prentice-Hall, Inc; 1984.

6. Meinert CL. *Clinical Trials: Design, Conduct, and Analysis.* New York, NY: Oxford University Press; 1986.

7. Friedman LM, Furberg CD, DeMets DL. *Fundamentals of Clinical Trials.* 2nd ed. Littleton, Mass: PSG Publishing Co, Inc; 1985.

8. Kraemer HC, Thiemann S. *How Many Participants?* Newbury Park, Calif: SAGE Publications; 1987.

9. Cohen J. *Statistical Power Analysis for the Behavioral Sciences.* New York, NY: Academic Press; 1977.

10. *PASS: Power Analysis and Sample Size.* Kaysville, Utah: NCSS Statisticcal Software; 1991.

11. Neter J, Wasserman W, Kutner MH. *Applied Linear Statistical Models.* 2nd ed. Homewood, Ill: Richard D Irwin, Inc; 1985.

12. Kris-Etherton PM, Derr JA, Mitchell DC, et al. The role of fatty acid saturation on plasma lipids, lipoproteins, and apolipoproteins. I. Effects of whole food diets high in cocoa butter, olive oil, soybean oil, dairy butter, and milk chocolate on the plasma lipids of young men. *Metabolism.* 1993;42:121–129.

CHAPTER 3

COMPUTER APPLICATIONS IN CONTROLLED DIET STUDIES

PHYLLIS J. STUMBO, PHD, RD; KEREN PRICE, MS, RD;
CATHERINE A. CHENARD, MS, RD; I. MARILYN BUZZARD, PHD, RD;
AND ALICE K. H. FONG, EDD, RD

Computers were first applied in dietetics to nutrient calculations (1–6), a tedious task that readily lent itself to the new technology. Foodservice management and communication applications developed gradually as computer hardware became more accessible. This chapter will focus primarily on computer applications for nutrient calculations in research. Applications for foodservice management are discussed next, followed by a brief discussion of communication applications.

COMPUTER APPLICATIONS FOR CALCULATING RESEARCH DIETS

Research diet studies may include a feeding component, an *ad libitum (ad lib)* component, or both. During the *feeding component* stage, the dietitian develops a research diet that meets specific nutrient goals and then provides these foods

and beverages to participants. The foods and recipes that are included in research diets are typically those that can be carefully controlled and have a known nutrient content. The number of foods used is relatively small, as is the size of the corresponding food composition database. During the *ad lib component* stage, participants select and prepare their own foods and beverages; sometimes their choices must meet specific criteria. Because participants can choose from the wide variety of foods available in the marketplace and may prepare any of numerous recipes at home, a large food composition database may be needed.

Feeding Components of Research Diet Studies

The primary nutrient-calculation task during feeding components is determining the correct proportions of foods to produce diets that meet specific nutrient goals. Research diet construction is an iterative process. Software is used to repeatedly calculate the nutrient content of a menu as types and amounts of foods are adjusted and readjusted to achieve specific nutrient goals.

It is critical for foods in the database to be clearly and completely described so that foods served on the research ward can be matched to foods in the nutrient database. Values should be available for the nutrients studied, as well as for overall nutrient indicators, such as iron, calcium, and vitamin A, to evaluate the nutritional adequacy of the research diet. Nutrient values should be available for every nutrient and food in the database, if possible, and any missing values should be identified on calculation reports. Because research diets typically contain unique foods and recipes and can involve rarely studied nutrients, the user should be able to add additional foods and nutrients to the database.

The purpose of the study will determine the degree of precision required for the nutrient content of the research diets. (See Chapter 11, "Designing Research Diets.") In studies using estimated, weighed, controlled nutrient, or constant diets (7), the calculated nutrient content of the diet may suffice. For example, in studies of gastric motility, total meal volume and macronutrient content are precisely controlled, but micronutrient content is not. In studies of drug absorption, wide fluctuations in diet composition must be avoided, but it may not be necessary to verify nutrient composition with chemical analysis of the diet. Chemical verification of calculated diets may be especially important, however, when the different experimental diets must be statistically distinguishable from each other. (See Chapter 22, "Validating Diet Composition by Chemical Analysis.")

In metabolic balance studies as well as in many other types of controlled diet studies, the actual nutrient content of the diet is determined by chemical analysis so that intake can be compared with excretion. Food composition tables are used in this type of study primarily for planning the research diets.

Food tables are also used in research diet studies to help ensure that other dietary variables do not affect the metabolic data collected. For example, when researchers conduct studies of zinc nutrition, the fiber content of the diet should not vary markedly from one diet period to another because mineral absorption could be affected. Alternatively, when investigators study nitrogen balance, if energy is extremely high during one time period and inadvertently lower in another, this difference may influence protein metabolism. Therefore, estimates of intake calculated from food composition tables play an important role in controlling for any nutrients that will not be chemically analyzed.

Ad Lib Components of Research Diet Studies

In ad lib components of research diet studies, nutrient intakes are assessed using food records, 24-hour recalls, and food frequencies. These ad lib diets may be an unexpectedly important component of the protocol, because nutrient intake prior to the study may influence nutrient metabolism during the experimental period. For sodium or potassium, a 5- or 6-day period with a constant diet will bring the participant into a state of equilibrium, ensuring that experimental conditions will have the desired effects on subsequent days.

When extended periods of time are needed, however, as for calcium (8), it is not feasible to employ an equilibrium period to acclimate participants to a new level of intake. One way to simplify the study of calcium balance is to determine the participant's habitual calcium intake through standard dietary recall methods and provide this level throughout the balance period (9–11).

SOFTWARE REQUIREMENTS FOR CALCULATING RESEARCH DIETS

Understanding software features helps users determine whether existing software can satisfy their research requirements or whether they must develop their own. Specific requirements will depend on the research protocol and whether there is a feeding component, an ad lib component, or both. If both components are present, two different programs may be necessary.

Nutrient-calculation programs may be categorized as having data entry features, database features, and reporting features. Weaknesses in any one of these three categories can seriously limit a software package's usefulness. For example, the most accurate and complete database will be of little value if data entry is time consuming and error prone. On the other hand, the most user-friendly software will be of little value if its database is poorly maintained or incomplete. Finally, user-friendly software with a sound database will only be of value if the dietitian can generate the reports needed.

Data Entry Features

Entering Food Descriptions

Most of the early nutrient-calculation software packages required the user to enter food descriptions by numeric code. This meant locating the food in a code book, determining the appropriate code, and entering the code into the computer. This process is tedious and error prone, especially if participants eat a wide variety of foods or the database is large. Most nutrient-calculation software packages now allow food descriptions to be entered by typing the first few letters of the food name. Some packages offer the option of entering food descriptions either by food name or numeric code. It still may be efficient to enter food descriptions by code when the study protocol involves feeding participants a cycle of menus in which the same foods are served repeatedly.

In feeding studies, it is critical that database food descriptors be sufficiently detailed so that foods selected from the nutrient database will match what is served in the research ward or dining room. Abbreviations and descriptors should be used consistently throughout the database to facilitate locating the appropriate database entry.

Entering Food Amounts

Because database nutrient values usually are expressed per 100 g food, almost all nutrient-calculation programs allow entering amounts by weight (eg, ounces, pounds, and grams). If the research protocol involves only a feeding component, this may be sufficient. An ad lib diet component requires software that allows a wider variety of units because participants eating ad lib diets are often unable to describe amounts of food in terms of gram weights. Unit options may include:

- Volume (eg, cups, fluid ounces, tablespoons, and pints).
- Volume with multiple forms (eg, 1 cup sliced vs 1 cup mashed).
- Volume or weight before cooking (this is especially helpful when calculating the nutrient content of a recipe because many include raw ingredients that are ultimately cooked).
- Weight with refuse (eg, when the weight of a piece of meat includes the weight of the bone).
- Standard piece (eg, a "fun size" candy bar, a "medium" banana, or a "Nasco©" model-size muffin model).
- Shape (eg, a 2″ × 3″ × 1″ brownie).
- Nonstandard units (eg, bite, sip, handful).
- Not specified or not further specified (ie, no details about amount).

If more of these unit options are offered, fewer manual conversions are needed and there are fewer chances of error. The advantage of the "not specified" category is that missing information is handled in a standardized way.

Entering Demographic Information

A research protocol may require demographic or other information to characterize participants. Some nutrient-calculation software will prompt for entries about age, sex, height, weight, activity level, anthropometric or laboratory measurements, and medication use. Other packages may allow the user to add customized fields for the specific information needed. If the data in these fields and subsequent calculations can be saved in ASCII field-delimited format, the values can be exported to statistical or spreadsheet software. ASCII (American Standard Code for Information Interchange) is a standard code that represents letters, numbers, and keyboard characters and enables information from 1 computer or software package to be interpreted by information from another computer or software package. These data can then be used for other calculations (eg, energy requirements), for grouping records (eg, mean nutrient intakes of males and females), or for merging with other datasets.

Edit Checks for Data Entry

Software developers can incorporate automated edit checks at most points of data entry. These checks help to minimize data entry errors. For example, automated food description edit checks will indicate whether entered letters or code numbers fail to match any of the food descriptions in the database. A user-friendly software package will then suggest alternatives. An automated food quantity edit check will prompt the user to verify or change unusually large values. Some systems may also provide for "double-keyed" data entry, wherein two users enter the same dataset. Any differences between the two are tagged for further verification. This feature is useful for large datasets to prevent errors in entering within-range values (ie, incorrect values that are not unusually large or small).

Database Features

Sources of Data for Databases

Most database developers use one of three United States Department of Agriculture (USDA) data sets as their primary source of data (Table 3–1): The Nutrient Database for Standard Reference (Release 12) (SR-12)(12), the Nutritive Value of Foods (Home and Garden Bulletin 72) (13, 14), or the Survey Nutrient Database (15). The Standard Reference Database is extensive, containing up to 81 nutrient fields for more than 5,000 foods, but there are many missing values. (Earlier versions of the Standard Reference Database were released to the public in print form as Agricultural Handbook No. 8 [16].) Home and Garden Bulletin 72 is available in printed and electronic form (13, 14); all versions include 20 nutrient fields and 960 foods, and have relatively few missing values. The Survey Nutrient Database is the main database used to calculate the nutrient content of dietary intake records collected in the Continuing Survey of Food Intakes by Individuals and the Nationwide Food Consumption Survey, and the National Health and Nutrition Examination Survey III (NHANES III) (17). This database includes 30 nutrient fields and 6,010 foods, and has no missing values.

Other sources of nutrient data may include provisional USDA information (eg, the Provisional Table on the Vitamin K Content of Foods) (18), information released by food manufacturers, foreign food composition tables, and research published in scientific journals.

Data obtained from food manufacturers present special challenges. The amount of information provided by a manufacturer may range from an extensive list of nutrient values, ingredient lists, densities, and preparation instructions to the minimal number of nutrient values required on the product label (19). In addition, the nutrient values may be based on chemical analysis or nutrient calculations of formulations, or they may be the rounded values printed on the product label. As a result, it may be hard to compare nutrient values reported for different brand name products.

Because database developers may obtain their information from many places, the source of each value in a da-

TABLE 3-1

Datasets Maintained by the USDA

Print Version	Machine-Readable Version	Number of Nutrients	Approximate Number of Foods	Missing Values (Yes/No)
Composition of Foods: Raw, Processed, Prepared (Agriculture Handbook 8)	*Nutrient Database for Standard Reference* (SR-12)	81	5,975	Yes
Nutritive Value of Foods (Home and Garden Bulletin 72)	*Dataset 72–1* (Release 3.2)	20	960	Yes
Survey Nutrient Database	*Survey Nutrient Database*	30	6,010	No

tabase should be documented. Some software provide this information to the user on screen (Nutritionist V®) but most maintain it in other formats. A few programs have only one source of data. For example, the Food Intake Analysis System® (FIAS) uses only USDA survey data. When many sources are maintained the source may be catalogued by category. If this is the case, source categories should be specific enough to include the different types of data provided by food manufacturers or the different scientific journals and USDA publications from which nutrient data might be obtained (20). It is important that the people responsible for maintaining the database be experts in food composition and use standardized criteria to evaluate sources of data.

Foods Included in Databases

Food records for ad lib components are evaluated by summarizing the nutrient content of all foods consumed by the participant. Because the participant is free to choose among some 50,000 products in the consumer market as well as hundreds of recipes or variations of recipes, developing a representative database can be daunting.

In general, the more foods the database contains, the better. A database that contains many foods will require fewer substitutions and "judgment calls" during data entry. Several techniques have been used to create nutrient databases to evaluate varied intakes. For example, USDA uses a database of approximately 6,000 foods to assess the intake of the entire US population (ie, the *Survey Database* [15]), but many of the 6,000 foods are listed in both salted and unsalted form (increasing the database to about 9,000 entries) and many are also listed several times to reflect about nine different fats that might be used. The grand total is over 30,000 entries. Most programs combine USDA food values with manufacturers' data for commercial foods. The University of Minnesota Nutrition Data System (NDS) database probably has the most extensive database providing nutrient information by brand name. Many other programs also can provide the user with the tools needed to estimate nutrient intake during ad lib periods, particularly when a limited number of nutrients are required.

In addition to listing foods by generic food type and by brand name, databases may also include a "not specified"

category for some foods. For example, databases often contain descriptions for different forms of the same food, eg, french fries cooked from fresh potatoes, frozen french fries (baked), frozen french fries (fried), and fast-food french fries. It is helpful if the database also includes an "unknown" choice (eg, "unknown type" of french fries) to use when the participant cannot provide sufficient detail about a food. Food descriptions should be mutually exclusive, so that the user does not have to make judgment calls and data collection is standardized.

When an "unknown" choice is selected for a food, the calculated nutrient content typically defaults to either the worst case (eg, the food description with the highest fat content) or to the most common practice (eg, 2% fat milk vs whole or skim milk). The software developer should use consistent criteria in assigning default choices. It is important for the user of the program to be aware of the principles underlying the developer's choice of default options.

Public or commercial databases can be used to calculate the composition of diets developed for feeding studies, but dietitians often choose to develop a center-specific database for their particular research unit. These unique databases are seldom shared because they represent foods favored by the local staff and participants and contain recipes whose preparation has been standardized in that particular kitchen. The data generally consist of USDA values for basic foods, calculated values for recipes developed in the research kitchen, and (occasionally) chemically analyzed values for foods prepared at the center.

The preferences of the people included in a research study and the nutrients of interest will determine the types of foods needed in the database. When studies include specific ethnic groups (eg, Mexican Americans or Native Americans), the database should include the foods indigenous to those cultures. To support studies of infants and young children, the database must include infant formula and baby foods. When fat is the nutrient of interest, the software should allow changes in preparation method. If sodium is an important study variable, the database should include both salted and unsalted foods.

Regardless of the study population or nutrient of interest, databases that include foods by brand name have two important advantages. First, in the ad lib diet component of a study, participants may tend to report many of the foods they eat by brand name, and it may be difficult to match brand name foods to a generic database entry. Brand-specific data are also helpful when commercial products are purchased for feeding studies. Second, there may be significant differences in the nutrient content of different brands of the same food. For example, the saturated fat content of various brands of margarine may vary from 0.15 to 1.5 grams per teaspoon. The growing availability of lower-fat and lower-sodium products makes the inclusion of foods by brand name in a database increasingly important. For example, in 1989 there were more than 5,600 reduced-fat products for sale in retail grocery stores (21).

Including brand names in the database also has two disadvantages. First, it becomes necessary to update the database frequently, perhaps as often as every 6 months, to keep pace with new products on the market. Second, no matter how complete the database may be, brand name data will not be available for every product.

Because it is unlikely that any database will contain all foods needed, nutrient-calculation programs should allow additional foods to be added to the database. This is particularly necessary for the feeding component of research studies because the research diet may contain special foods (such as low-protein noodles) or ingredients (such as lyophilized egg-yolk powder) and specially modified recipes not found in commercial databases. If unique foods or recipes are added to the database, software must have a facility for retaining additions when users upgrade to a new version of the software or else the data will be lost.

Recipe Calculations

Both the feeding and ad lib components of research studies may require recipe calculations. Some nutrient-calculation programs (eg, FIAS) allow the user to apply specific nutrient retention factors to raw ingredients to calculate the vitamin and mineral content after cooking (22). Other software packages (eg, NDS) include nutrients for the cooked forms of ingredients, so use of retention factors is not necessary. A third method is to use nutrient values for the raw ingredients and a retention factor for the whole dish (23). For the ad lib component, database builders must consider ways to specify amounts eaten when researchers calculate recipes without accurate yield determinations (eg, expressing amount eaten as a fraction of the whole recipe).

Nutrients Included in the Database

It may seem obvious that the database must include the nutrients addressed in the research hypotheses, but this is sometimes less than straightforward. For example, literature describing a software package may list "fiber" as one of the nutrients included in the database, but upon further inspection, the values actually represent crude fiber instead of dietary fiber. This is sometimes the case, because most database developers take the majority of their data from the older USDA Agricultural Handbook No. 8 series, which included crude fiber but not dietary fiber (16). USDA's 1988 "Provisional Table on the Dietary Fiber Content of Selected Foods" (24) and 1989 supplement to Handbook No. 8 listed dietary fiber values for only 300 to 350 foods. Current forms of the database (12) have more complete data.

Even if a database does include the nutrients addressed in the research hypothesis, it is essential to verify that the database is complete for all those nutrients. Many common databases include an extensive set of nutrients but provide little actual data in some nutrient fields. For example, the brochure for a software package may indicate that the database includes values for total saturated fatty acids. However, these values may be missing for a large percentage of the foods because values for some nutrients are not readily available. For example, the software developer may request information from a manufacturer about the nutrient content of frozen entrees. The manufacturer may not provide data for total saturated fatty acid content, however, because the chemical analysis can be costly. Therefore, the database developer might include the products in the database but leave the fields for total saturated fatty acids blank. Problems of this kind can cause a gross underestimation of total saturated fatty acid intake. This characteristic is sometimes referred to as *database sparseness* (its converse is *database completeness*), and it is a critical feature when databases are evaluated for use in a study.

Software developers sometimes replace missing values with estimated values. These are imputed from the nutrient content of similar foods, the nutrient content of different forms of the same food, other nutrients in the same food, published recipes, food formulas, or product ingredient lists (20). In the case of brand name products, the use of ingredient lists may provide the most accurate results. For example, to impute the total fatty acid content of a frozen entree, the software developer can use existing entries in the database to develop a "recipe" based on the ingredient list and nutrient values provided by the manufacturer. The software developer then adjusts the amount of each ingredient in the recipe until the calculated nutrient totals match those reported by the manufacturer as closely as possible (19). Imputing requires the knowledge of highly trained and experienced nutrition scientists. Adding one or more nutrient fields to a database is a job that requires formal training in food science and nutrition, as well as criteria for evaluating different sources of data (25).

In research the need for data often precedes its availability. For example, researchers wishing to study the effect of boron or choline intake on health parameters are hampered by the lack of data on the choline or boron content of foods. Investigators working in the forefront of these areas must develop their own databases and are best off choosing software that can be customized to incorporate additional data. This feature is also useful for conducting feeding studies when nutrient data are available for foods that have been chemically analyzed. As mentioned earlier, it is important to retain added nutrient fields when an updated version of software is installed.

It is important for the user to compile a complete dataset for the added nutrient field, particularly for ad lib components of research diet studies. For studies having only a feeding component, the dataset should be complete for at least the foods being fed (see the previous discussion of missing nutrient values). In either case, the nutrient-calculation program should highlight missing values when they arise.

Updating and Database Integrity

It is critical that software developers update their databases frequently to reflect the most recent analytic data available from the USDA and other sources. Up-to-date information on new and reformulated grocery items must be obtained directly through regular correspondence with the manufacturers; data on products served in fast-food franchises are obtained in a similar fashion. Standard database recipes may also require updating to reflect changes in typical preparation techniques or in the nutrient values of ingredients.

All updates and additions to a database should be cross-checked by a second person trained in database maintenance. Prior to the release of an updated database, there are a series of additional quality control procedures to use in order to minimize data entry errors. These include

1. Computerized edit checks that flag values falling outside of specified ranges for each food category in the database.
2. Validation queries, where calculated algorithms are compared with expected values for each database entry (eg, comparing the sum of soluble and insoluble fiber to the values for total fiber).
3. Comparison of repeated calculations of a set of test records to verify that differences between database versions are caused by intended modifications and not data entry errors (25).

Time-Related Databases

Dietary intake data from long-term studies are sometimes calculated or recalculated months or even years after the original data were collected. Because the composition of food products may change over time, consideration is usually given to using a database appropriate for the time when the feeding period occurred. Investigators may decide to "freeze" the database, meaning they do not adopt updated versions of the databases throughout the study, so study results are not altered by database changes. However, if time-related maintenance procedures are used by a database developer, each version of the database can be used to calculate nutrients for dietary data collected in the past as well as the present (26). This is particularly relevant for labor-intensive inpatient studies, which may accrue their participants during a period of several years.

With time-related databases, nutrients for each food can have more than one value, each for a specific time period, to account for changes in the formulations of products over time. Depending on the date of the food record, the software selects appropriate nutrient values. No foods are deleted from the database, so food records may be recalculated even though they contain food products no longer manufactured. The manager of a time-related database must assign new values to all foods in the database (both historical and current entries) when improved data become available. This was the case when cholesterol data were updated because of better analytical technology, or when previously unavailable values, such as for the selenium content of foods, are published for the first time.

Reporting Features

Calculations Needed for Research Diet Studies

Common to almost all nutrient-calculation software packages is a report of total daily nutrient intake. The number of nutrients for which intake can be calculated usually reflects the number of nutrients in the software's database. Many packages also report the nutrient content of each food eaten, with subtotals for each meal, as well as totals for the day. Some software packages calculate diabetic exchanges. Others compare intake to a standard, such as the Recommended Dietary Allowances (27) or the daily values developed by the Food and Drug Administration for use in food labels (28), and may allow users to enter customized standards to reflect specific research objectives. Some software translates frequency information into average daily nutrient intake.

The feeding intervention component of research studies requires special calculation features unique to the menu development process. Some nutrient-calculation software packages are able to sort a menu or the entire database by a specific nutrient. This feature is useful when investigators select food items rich or poor in certain nutrients to construct a research diet. Because the menu is repeatedly adjusted and recalculated, a screen displaying the diet's composition, user-established target values, and the absolute difference or percent difference between the two values shows how well the diet matches the nutrient prescription. Other helpful features include computing nutrient intake per kilogram body weight and average nutrient intake for multiple days. Because some research studies use the same menu for all participants but serve different amounts depending on energy needs, an important feature is *scaling,* ie, the ability to adjust all food weights on a menu by a factor to produce menus with different energy levels. The ability to calculate basal energy expenditure and total energy need is essential during the menu development phase of a study. (See Chapter 17, "Energy Needs and Weight Maintenance in Controlled Diet Studies.")

Features that support copying menus and editing food quantities simplify the process of calculating participants' actual intakes for the duration of feeding studies in which the same menus are served repeatedly. When investigators

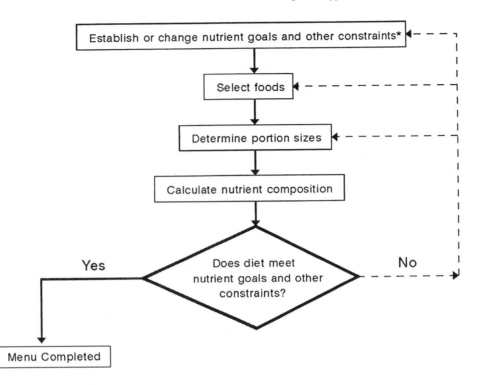

*Constraints include palatability, cost, minimum and maximum portion sizes, and production logistics.

FIGURE 3-1. Research diet development process.

work with research diets that have different nutrient goals, a time-saving printing feature records the user's request for the entire array of specific nutrients; future printing requests then can "call up" this list and do not require the individual nutrients to be specified.

Reporting Capabilities and Output Files

Most software packages can display reports on the computer monitor or on paper and sometimes as files in ASCII format. It is helpful for investigators to view reports on the computer monitor when determining the nutrient content of a single food, developing a menu that meets certain criteria, and at other times when a printed report is not needed. Reports saved as ASCII files can be edited or merged with other files to incorporate nutrient values into written materials without retyping the information. ASCII files can also be merged with other software for statistical analysis.

Developing In-house Nutrient-Calculation Software

Nutrition studies may require features not included in commercial software packages. When existing programs do not meet the nutrient-calculation or reporting requirements of a research study, users may develop customized databases and programs. Nutrient-calculation programs have been developed using database managers, Statistical Analysis System (SAS®), Fortran®, and other computer languages. These

custom applications are generally not distributed outside the unit where they were developed. Diet Planner is one such custom program, however, that has been shared among the units of the General Clinical Research Center (GCRC) program.

Developing customized programs requires a computer programmer or other staff member with programming skills. Database management software may be one of the easiest ways to develop a custom program if the software is user-friendly enough for novice developers. In practice, however, developing and managing a database and computer program require tremendous effort. The benefit of having a custom-designed program should outweigh, by a substantial margin, the additional time and personnel required to develop and maintain the database and program. See Chapter 11, "Designing Research Diets," for further discussion of developing customized menu analysis programs.

COMPUTER-ASSISTED MENU PLANNING

During research diet development, dietitians use nutrient-calculation software to repeatedly calculate the nutrient content of the diet as they adjust foods and amounts to achieve nutrient goals. Nutrient calculation, however, is just one step in the development process. As outlined in Figure 3–1, the process begins with determining nutrient goals and other constraints and ends with a menu that satisfies them. Dietitians can benefit from software that automatically adjusts the menu to match the goals; for example, algorithmic and mathematical methods such as linear programming can automate food and portion size selection (29, 30). Software with these more sophisticated capabilities is sometimes called a *computer-assisted menu planning (CAMP) program.*

CAMP programs that assist with both food and portion selection can produce palatable, nutritionally adequate, and least-cost regular and modified menus for institutional food service (31), as well as menus and grocery shopping lists for patients with diabetes (32) and other dietary needs. Early CAMP programs developed for institutional foodservices during the 1960s and 1970s were inconvenient because it was difficult and time consuming to quantify all variables influencing menu satisfaction (33). In addition, factors influencing foodservice implementation could not be considered (34).

Current CAMP programs require users to select a menu before the computer determines the portions required to achieve nutrient goals. Examples include programs calculating the quantity of special formulas required to provide the phenylalanine and protein needs of patients with phenylketonuria (35), the weights of foods required to meet nutrient goals of research diets (4, 5), and the proportion of ingredients in mixed dishes that match manufacturer's nutrition label information (36, 37).

Research Diets as Mathematical Problems

Although CAMP programs are not widely used, they have the potential to reduce the time required to develop research diets. CAMP programs typically use complex mathematical techniques, such as matrix arithmetic and linear or integer programming, to develop menus meeting specific criteria. Some spreadsheet programs, such as Quattro Pro® and Microsoft Excel®, have matrix, linear, and/or integer programming tools that could be used to perform these calculations.

Complex calculations typically performed by CAMP programs are shown in Figure 3–2. Consider developing a formula diet containing lard, safflower oil, and olive oil and providing 19.5 g saturated, 23.0 g monounsaturated, and 7.5 g polyunsaturated fatty acids. Determining the correct fat proportions by trial and error can be time consuming and frustrating. Mathematical techniques, on the other hand, produce an answer more quickly. To compute the answer manually, a set of equations is first developed. Each equation relates the three ingredients' nutrient composition to the target goal or prescription. Coefficients in the equations are simply the nutrient values per gram of fat (eg, lard contains 39.2 g saturated fat per 100 g and the coefficient is 0.392). (Because other formula ingredients—sugar, cornstarch, vanilla, casein, and water—are fat-free, they are not included here.) To find the solution, the equations are solved for three unknowns—amounts of lard, safflower oil, and olive oil— that satisfy all three equations. By varying the equations and adding new ones, this process can be used to determine the amount of other formula ingredients required to match other nutrient goals, such as protein, carbohydrate, and minerals.

CAMP Programs in Research

Linear programming has been used in research settings to calculate formula diets (38) and rat chows (39). CAMP programs are more readily used for developing formula diets than for mixed-food diets because of the greater range of ingredients and proportions that will produce a palatable formula. CAMP applications have been used successfully for mixed-food diets (4), however, to calculate the amounts of foods required to satisfy as many as 23 nutrient goals and maximize or minimize food cost or nutrient level without violating predetermined maximum and minimum portion sizes.

Prescription[1]				Sat, g	Mono, g	Poly, g
				19.5	23.0	7.5
Data	Fat Source			Amount of Fatty Acids Per Gram of Fat		
		Fat, g		Sat, g	Mono, g	Poly, g
	Lard	x		.392	.451	.112
	Safflower Oil	y		.091	.121	.745
	Olive Oil	z		.135	.737	.084
Equations	Prescription	= Lard	+ Safflower Oil	+ Olive Oil		
	19.5 g Sat	= .392x +	.091y	+ .135z		
	23.0 g Mono	= .451x +	.121y	+ .737z		
	7.5 g Poly	= .112x +	.745y	+ .084z		
Solution[2]		x = 48.83 g lard				
		y = 2.63 g safflower oil				
		z = 0.90 g olive oil				

[1] Sat(urated), Mono(unsaturated), and Poly(unsaturated) fatty acids.
[2] Satisfies all three equations.

FIGURE 3-2. Sample CAMP problem, solving 3 equations for 3 unknowns (the amounts of lard, safflower oil, and olive oil required to match a fatty acid prescription).

The CAMP program Interactive Diet Construction (IDC) calculates the composition of foods entered into a menu and determines portion sizes needed to achieve the nutrient goal(s) specified (5). The dietitian determines the menu, declares the portion size of each food as "fixed" or "variable," and sets the desired level of key nutrient(s). The program then determines the weight of variable foods required to match the nutrient prescriptions. Foods on the menu can be all fixed, all variable, or any combination of fixed and variable where the number of nutrient goals meets or exceeds the number of variable foods. If the computer solution yields an unreasonably large or small portion or calculates a negative portion, the dietitian must add or delete foods or change amounts until the answer is acceptable. This software calculates food amounts to match nutrient goals but not to maximize or minimize a nutrient level.

Because the IDC program was developed for in-house use at one particular research center, it lacks some features commonly found in commercially developed software, such as a sophisticated search procedure, comprehensive user's manual, database documentation, data entry windows, and display and printing options. IDC could nevertheless be a timesaver when investigators are developing formulas or traditional food menus to achieve complex diet prescriptions.

CHOOSING A NUTRIENT-CALCULATION SYSTEM FOR FEEDING STUDIES

In summary, the most important features of software for research diet design are: (1) a validated database and (2) a calculation module that facilitates iterative calculations as diets are adjusted and readjusted to achieve the research prescription. So far we have discussed the advantages of developing in-house programs and have given two examples of this type of software: Diet Planner and IDC. In most situations, however, it will be more efficient to purchase programs. Two commercially available programs designed for research (FIAS and NDS) have been described. Other programs frequently used for research diet design include CBORD Diet Analyzer, Nutritionist V, and Food Processor.

The MENu database is a new program developed at the Pennington Biomedical Research Center to facilitate the design of diets for metabolic feeding studies. This system, which uses the ETNV (Extended Table of Nutrient Values) database developed by Margaret Moore in the late 1950s, features easy transition between data entry and nutrient totals to support the many revisions required as research diets are adjusted to match study goals.

Another new software package is the ProNutra Analysis System for Metabolic Studies. This system readily lends itself to essentially every type of setting in which controlled diet studies are conducted, although it originally was designed to meet the particular needs of the General Clinical Research Center nutrition program. ProNutra provides diet design and nutrient-calculation functions, as well as kitchen management tools and modules for setting up clinic and kitchen schedules, performing anthropometric calculations, and tracking body weight.

CITING NUTRIENT DATABASES AND SOFTWARE

Whether the nutrient-calculation program is commercial or custom designed, it is important to document the database and software in published reports. To help researchers be consistent, Monsen (40) and Murphy (41) recommend including the following information when reporting nutrient data:

- Software name.
- Software developer or vendor's name and address.
- Copyright year, year updated.
- Version number, if applicable.
- Nutrient data source (eg, USDA, manufacturer), if appropriate—especially if the nutrient database is not commercially available. (If the list is extensive, indicate it is available upon request.)
- Database additions or modifications made by user and all sources of data.
- How missing data (eg, nutrient values and foods) were handled by user and their impact on dietary totals, if applicable.

Providing this information in published reports will help investigators evaluate the validity of new research.

OTHER COMPUTER APPLICATIONS IN FEEDING STUDIES

In addition to calculating the nutrient composition of research diets and ad lib dietary intakes, computers can also expedite management and educational tasks associated with nutrition studies. These tasks include: producing kitchen food production sheets and food labels, monitoring inventory and food budgets, tracking numbers of meals served, producing written materials for participants, and generating graphs and slides for presentations. This section briefly outlines personal computer software that research dietitians may find useful, discusses computerizing foodservice tasks, and describes computer communications (eg, electronic mail).

General Software Applications

Many general-purpose programs can streamline research activities and improve the appearance of printed materials.

Word Processors

Word processing programs used with laser printers offer investigators valuable resources for preparing patient education materials, training and management documents, and research reports. Such software also can simplify mass mailings for recruitment activities. These programs can be used for instant revision, reformatting, and error correction, and they allow typefaces and type sizes to be mixed within a text. Some packages have special options to enhance writing, such as a thesaurus; they also check for spelling mistakes and literacy level (ie, readability). Some software will also print labels (42). Common word processing programs include WordPerfect®, Microsoft Word®, and Lotus Word Pro® (43).

Desktop Publishing

Desktop publishing programs combine word processing and graphic design features. They enable the user to change typefaces and layout, incorporate diagrams and graphs into the text, and shade sections of text for emphasis. These are complex programs that require considerable training, but they can make educational materials, newsletters, and handouts attractive and effective. Popular desktop publishing software includes Adobe PageMaker® and Microsoft Publisher® (43).

Spreadsheets

Spreadsheets are electronic tables that support entering, deleting, and modifying data. Mathematical formulas are entered and stored so that calculations may be performed instantly when data are entered or modified. Spreadsheets are commonly used for budgets and cost comparisons. They also may be used for manipulating nutrient or other dietary data. As shown in Table 3–2, spreadsheets can be used for "what if" calculations (42), such as "what happens to energy requirements if age is increased or decreased by 10 years?"

Spreadsheets are especially useful for repetitive calculations. For example, some research studies serve the same menu to all participants but scale the food amounts proportionately for each participant to provide the required energy level. For this purpose, spreadsheet programs can automatically calculate larger or smaller weights for each food. Spreadsheets have also been used to store data on the number of meals served and produced daily, monthly, and year-to-date reports (44).

Spreadsheets generally do not have word processing features, but some word processors can "import" spreadsheet data. Spreadsheets have multiple reporting options and may also have graphics capabilities that enhance printed materials. Popular spreadsheet programs include Lotus 123®, Microsoft Excel®, and Corel Quattro Pro® (43).

Database Management Systems

In general, database management systems (DBMSs) are like electronic filing cabinets for storing information. Data are entered in rows (records) and columns (fields) similar to a spreadsheet. Groups of records with the same type of information are called *tables* or *data files*. Information can be entered, deleted, and modified quickly. Databases can be searched and a subset of files with specific characteristics retrieved without physically manipulating or moving records. For instance, all protein studies with more than 40 meals served in January can be selected from a file containing data about many studies. Reporting options enable the user to determine how the data are printed, such as in columns, free-form reports, or labels (45). Popular programs include Microsoft Access®, Corel Paradox®, and dBase® (43).

DBMSs in cost and features offered. Some products require the user to write computer programs to use the software and others do not. "Flatfile" databases store all related data in a single file, whereas other DBMSs allow multiple tables that are linked through one or more common fields. Multitable databases are flexible, easily updated, and more easily perform complex data tasks (46), but an easily learned flatfile or nonprogrammable database package may be all that is needed for most foodservice uses (47).

Statistical Analysis

It may be necessary to summarize the dietary information that has been collected during a study. Spreadsheet and DBMS programs can perform some statistical calculations and facilitate printing data summaries. More sophisticated analyses can be performed on a personal computer with pro-

TABLE 3-2

Using a Spreadsheet to Calculate the Energy Requirement for a Male at Different Ages

Column	1	2	3	4	5	6	7
Name	Height (cm)	Weight (kg)	Age (yr)	Gender	BEE*	Activity Factor	Energy Requirements (Kcal/day)
Doe, John	178	80	36	Male	1,815	1.5	2,723
When age is:							
Increased	178	80	46	Male	1,747	1.5	2,621
Decreased	178	80	26	Male	1,883	1.5	2,825

*BEE = Basal Energy Expenditure:
If male, then BEE = $66 + (13.8 \times \text{weight}) + (5 \times \text{height}) - (6.8 \times \text{age})$.
If female, then BEE = $655 + (9.6 \times \text{weight}) + (1.8 \times \text{height}) - (4.7 \times \text{age})$.
Energy requirement (kcal/day) = BEE $\times$ Activity Factor.

grams such as SPSS/PC+®, SAS®, BMDP/PC®, and Systat® (48). Applications designed for clinical research, such as Prophet 5.0 (which runs on current Windows® and UNIX® [Sun OS, Solaris, SGI IRIX, and Digital UNIX]), offer convenient data management tools and are user-friendly. Consulting with a statistician during the design phase of a study as well as during data analysis can help in the choice of appropriate software. (See Chapter 2, "Statistical Aspects of Controlled Diet Studies.")

If nutrient data will be statistically analyzed, the nutrient-calculation program should export the data in a row and column format suitable for statistical, spreadsheet, or DBMS programs.

Graphics for Presentation of Data

Graphs provide a "picture" of data and help the reader understand large amounts of information (49, 50). At the same time, the researcher should not be tempted to generate a fancier picture than is needed to portray the data accurately and efficiently. (Helpful discussions of this topic are found in two books by Tufte [51, 52].) Graphs can be generated either by programs specifically designed for this purpose or by spreadsheet and DBMS programs. Programs for use with Microsoft Windows include Microsoft PowerPoint for Windows®, Corel Presentations®, Harvard Graphics®, and Lotus Freelance Graphics.

Graphics software packages vary in features but most, including those mentioned, can produce simple word, bar, and line graphs. (Pie charts are not recommended because they are visually complex and do not foster good quantitative comparisons [49].) Programs such as SigmaPlot® generate bar and line graphs with error bars for presenting scientific data. For three-dimensional, contour, and trajectory technical graphs, or graphs with large amounts of data, specialized programs are available (50). Graphs also facilitate management and training activities in the context of feeding studies. Production staff can benefit from graphic presentation of inventory and food census data; students can learn much from graphic displays of food composition and metabolic balance data.

Other Software

Other specialty programs are available for checking grammar, producing calendars for research participants or kitchen staff (53), making departmental or project organizational charts (54), and scheduling employees (55, 56).

COMPUTER-ASSISTED FOODSERVICE MANAGEMENT

The computer can assist with many foodservice tasks in the research diet kitchen, such as budgeting, conducting food inventories, and generating kitchen food production sheets and food labels. The following should be considered before automating foodservice tasks because not all such tasks will benefit from computer assistance (57):

- What problems decrease the effectiveness of the foodservice (eg, frequently running out of food supplies)? Would computerizing the task increase effectiveness?
- What routine, repetitive tasks do not require human judgment (eg, writing labels)? These are ideally suited to computerization.
- What data or information are needed quickly (eg, food production information) to avoid delays in implementing the diet? Would effectiveness increase if this information were available sooner?
- What data are needed for decision making (eg, projected food costs for a new study)? Would effectiveness increase if data were available when needed?
- Are the required data and procedures readily available for input (eg, is there a standardized version of every recipe)?
- Is the benefit of computerization greater than the time and cost of development (ie, should custom software be developed to meet on-site needs or can those needs be adjusted to fit existing software)?

Foodservice tasks form a complex interrelated system with the menu at its core (58). The simplified diagram in Figure 3–3 shows how the research diet directs many foodservice tasks. The ideal software package would integrate all nutrient-calculation and foodservice functions by using one or more linked databases or passing shared data among programs. Once research diet foods and amounts are entered, nutrient composition can be calculated and food production sheets or menus can be generated without manually reentering or transferring the diet data into another program or data file.

The most efficient way to computerize foodservice tasks is to purchase existing software. Users may need to be creative, however; it may be necessary to modify the commercial package. Some institutional market software integrates foodservice and nutrient-calculation features. These programs support typical activities such as cycle menus, inventory and purchasing management, bid analysis, menu costing, forecasting, recipe database, scaled recipes and production sheets, diet order tracking, menus for participants, and employee scheduling (59).

Bar code technology has the potential for widespread application in research kitchen management. Bar code technology may be used in foodservices for ordering, receiving, keeping inventory, and tracking supplies. A bar code is a series of black bars and white spaces of varying widths that correspond to letters, numbers, and symbols and can be read by a machine (scanner) that shines light across the bars. Because black absorbs light and white reflects light, the patterns of light can be decoded and translated into information the computer understands. For example, the universal product code (UPC) found on nearly all grocery items is used at the supermarket to calculate grocery bills and subtract food from

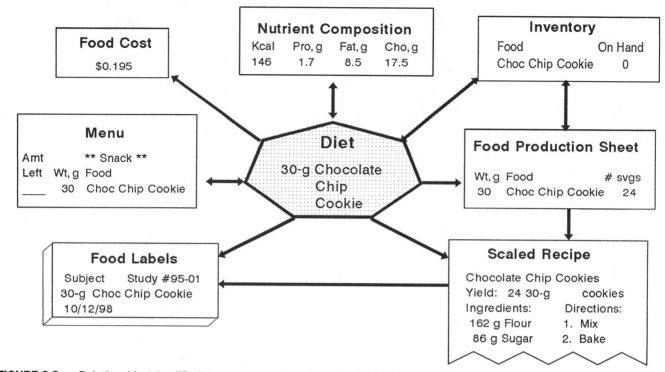

FIGURE 3-3.   Relationship (simplified) among research diet, nutrient calculation, and foodservice tasks. (Abbreviations: Amt, amount; CHO, carbohydrate; Choc, chocolate; kcal, kilocalories; Pro, protein; svgs, servings; wt, weight)

the store's inventory (60). Bar codes are quick and accurate because they eliminate manual data entry and its associated errors. Bar code labels can be purchased or made on site with printers having a bar code option (60). For more information about this technology, contact Director, Research Kitchen, USDA Human Nutrition Research Center, Houston, Tex; Computype Inc, Millersville, Md; and Intermec Technologies Corp, Everett, Wash.

Although research and institutional foodservices have much in common, research units seldom use commercial foodservice software. Some units have customized programs; others use nutrient-calculation software, word processors, desktop publishers, spreadsheets, and DBMSs alone or in combination. Because some programs—but not all—enable the export and import of data, software packages should be carefully evaluated before purchase (42). Because developing specialized applications requires considerable time and expertise, potential users should discuss the software with researchers who have achieved satisfactory results. Examples of customized applications are given in the following examples.

Example 1. Food Production Sheets for Cooks

After a research menu is planned, all food must be prepared and exact portions weighed and stored for service. Detailed production sheets may be printed to guide kitchen workers.

Generating the lists of foods to weigh and recipes to make is a repetitive task used for all diet studies. It has been cost effective for some research units to develop customized programs.

A sample computergenerated food production sheet is shown in Exhibit 3–1. The software uses a previously entered research diet data file and a database that classifies foods as "weighed fresh daily," "weighed in bulk" before the study begins, or "prepared from recipes." The production sheet in Exhibit 3–1 lists the foods weighed prior to the study and those with special recipes. Foods weighed fresh daily, such as brewed coffee, are listed separately (not shown). The foods are listed in a format that documents the food preparer (who initials each item under "Init"), the kitchen storage location (location is recorded under "Store" when food is placed in storage), and the number of servings remaining after the study is over (recorded under "Post-Study Inventory"). A word processor is used to add special directions, such as "Weigh egg whites and yolks together." The program also automatically generates a file for printing self-adhesive food labels.

If developing a custom program is not feasible, spreadsheets or DBMSs can be used to generate food production sheets. Alternatively, the output from nutrient-calculation software can be imported to a word processor and modified. The production sheet shown in Exhibit 3–2 lists the total weight of foods required for one study day. To facilitate fluid intake estimates, the weights of "fluid" and "solid" foods are listed in separate columns.

EXHIBIT 3-1

Food Production Sheet from Custom-Designed Program (University of Iowa GCRC)

Dr. Casey's Diet Study #99–99
    Constant Diet
    Foods to Weigh for: Ima Sample   Needed by (Date): _____

Done[1]	Init[2]	Weight (g)/Food	Servings[3]	Store[4]	Post-study[5] Inventory
Foods to Weigh					
☐	———	65.0 Egg whites (weigh with yolks)	12	———	———
☐	———	7.0 Egg yolks, fresh (weigh with whites)	12	———	———
☐	———	3.0 Butter	12	———	———
☐	———	5.0 Butter	24	———	———
☐	———	10.0 Butter	12	———	———
☐	———	4.0 Butter	12	———	———
☐	———	0.5 Salt	12	———	———
☐	———	0.2 Salt	12	———	———
☐	———	25.0 Cracked-wheat bread	12	———	———
☐	———	25.0 40% Bran Flakes, Kellogg's	12	———	———
☐	———	40.0 Hamburger bun	12	———	
☐	———	95.0 Turkey brst #1260 Plantation brand	12	———	———
☐	———	25.0 Milk chocolate candy (Hershey's)	12	———	———
☐	———	20.0 Potato chip w/soy oil (hydrogenated)	12	———	———
Recipes					
☐	———	45.0 Grd beef, cooked, lean (20% fat)	12	———	———
☐	———	45.0 Brownie	12	———	———
☐	———	110.0 Mashed potatoes w/milk	12	———	———
☐	———	100.0 Sage stuffing	12	———	———
☐	———	10.0 Tea beverage	12	———	———

CMDSIP:SAMPLE.KIT[6]   DATA FILE:SAMPLE.DAT[7]
10-JAN-98

---

[1]Done = Checked off after food is weighed and stored.
[2]Init = Initialed by staff member completing task.
[3]Servings = Number of servings required.
[4]Store = Kitchen location to store food.
[5]Post-study inventory = Number of servings remaining at end of study; used to verify that appropriate number of servings were consumed (excess is prepared for unexpected needs).
[6]CMDSIP: SAMPLE.KIT = Text filename.
[7]DATA FILE: SAMPLE.DAT = Data file containing code is used for nutrient calculations and to generate food production sheet and food labels.

Example 2. Food Labels

Printed food labels are much appreciated by kitchen staff. The labels eliminate the problem of illegible handwriting and smeared ink and save considerable amounts of time. Food labels may include items such as the participant's name or identification number, investigator's name, food description, portion size, date prepared, and intended meal. Label files can be printed directly onto adhesive labels. The labels must have an adhesive backing that sticks to storage containers or vials for extended time periods and withstands extremes of heat, cold, dryness, or moisture. Labels that ad-

here in the kitchen refrigerator may fall off in –20°C freezers. If the study design requires *blinding*, the labels must not include any information that would indicate which experimental diet the participant is receiving.

Example 3. Recipes

Nutrient-calculation software seldom supports the printing of scaled recipes, but this is a common feature of institutional foodservice software. Recipe databases in institutional software include recipe name, recipe number, ingredient

EXHIBIT 3-2

Low-Protein Diet-Production Sheet
(Generated by Downloading Input from Nutrient-Calculation Program into Word Processor)

Food	Fluid	Solid
Orange juice 240 g	240	
Coffee—brewed 400 g (200 + 200)	400	
White sugar 35 g		35
Sugar-frosted flakes 25 g		25
Low-protein corn bread 70 g		70
Peaches 135 g		135
Cream—half & half 100 g + distilled H_2O 100 g	200	
Butter 45 g (15–15–15)		45
Jelly 45 g (15–30)		45
Diet Coke 355 g	355	
Diet mandarin orange slice 355 g	355	
Potato chips 28 g		28
Bagel 85 g		85
Low-protein rigatoni 80 g (dry weight)		80
Low-protein spaghetti sauce 120 g		120
Low-protein DP[1] bread 64 g		64
Iceberg lettuce 100 g		100
Tomato 75 g		75
Olive oil 30 g		30
Red wine vinegar 15 g	15	
Low-protein cinnamon cookies 40 g		40
Low-protein butterscotch cookies 40 g		40

BREAKFAST	LUNCH	DINNER
Orange juice 240 g	Bagel 85 g	LP rigatoni 80 g dry
Coffee 400 g	Butter 15 g	LP spaghetti sauce 120 g
White sugar 35 g	Jelly 30 g	Iceberg lettuce 100 g
Sugar-frosted flakes 25 g	Potato chips 28 g	Tomato 75 g
LP[2] corn bread 70 g	Diet Coke 355 g	Olive oil 30 g
Peaches 135 g	LP cinnamon cookies 40 g	Red wine vinegar 15 g
Half & half 100 g +		LP DP bread 64 g
distilled H_2O 100 g		Butter 15 g
Butter 15 g		Diet mandarin orange slice 355 g
Jelly 15 g		LP butterscotch cookies 40 g

New York Hospital-Cornell Medical Center GCRC.
[1]DP = dp brand.
[2]LP = low-protein.

names and code numbers, ingredient quantity, recipe directions, yield, and other information (61). Research units without this computer support sometimes use spreadsheet or DBMS programs to store recipe data and print scaled recipes. Exhibit 3–3 shows a recipe printed from a spreadsheet program. Research recipe directions can also be manually prepared and revised using a word processor.

Example 4. Research Menus, Diet Setup, Foodservice, and Compliance Monitoring

Kitchen staff need a menu to guide research diet setup and service, but typing menus can be tedious. This task is even more difficult if the protocol calls for blinding (masking), because one must be on guard against inadvertently breaking the treatment code in menus, instructions, or messages for staff or participants. Some units have developed programs that automatically generate kitchen menus from their nutrient-calculation software. Exhibit 3–4 is a computer-generated menu from one such customized program. The program uses a data file from a previously entered research diet to produce a menu to document diet setup, monitor participant compliance, and make a duplicate diet preparation for laboratory analysis. Food storage locations, meal times, and directions for kitchen staff are added with a word processor.

Other research units copy the nutrient-calculation program output into a word processing file and modify it to produce a menu for kitchen use. Exhibit 3–5 shows a sample menu that was generated with this method. Foods for the day are listed at the top; to facilitate fluid intake estimates, the weights of "fluid" foods are listed in a separate column.

EXHIBIT 3-3

Scaled Recipe Generated from Spreadsheet Program

RK[1]—APPLE OR CHERRY CRISP	Nutrient Data:		Diabetic Exchanges:
	Kcal	220	Fruit 1
	PRO (g)	2	Bread 2
	CHO (g)	37	Fat 2
	Fat (g)	8	
	Na (mg)	96	
	K (mg)	119	RECIPE 4967

Portion size 120 g or ½ c (1-g scoop)

Ingredients:	Amt for 1[2]	Amt for 3	Amt for 5	Amt for 7	Amt for 10	Amt for 12	Amt for 15
Granulated sugar	20 g	¼ C	½ C	⅔ C	¾ C	1 C	1¼ C
Margarine	10 g	2 Tbsp	3½ Tbsp	¼ C	⅓ C	½ C	⅔ C
Flour	10 g	¼ C	½ C	⅔ C	¾ C	1 C	1¼ C
Apple slices, canned, OR Sweet cherries, canned	80 g	1½ C	2½ C	3½ C	5 C	6 C	7 C

Preparation Instructions:

1. Mix sugar, margarine, and flour until crumbly.
2. Spray small casserole dishes with PAM®.
3. Weigh 80 g fruit into each casserole.
4. Top with 40 g crumb mixture.
5. Bake at 375° until topping is brown (approximately 15 minutes).
6. Serve immediately or freeze.
7. To freeze: Cover with aluminum foil, label with name and date; freeze until needed.
   To reheat: Place in oven at 350° for 5–7 minutes or microwave for 1½ minutes.

Modifications

Research diets:	Prepare as listed.
Regular diets:	Prepare as listed.
Diabetic diets:	NOT ALLOWED.
Low-sodium diets:	USE SALT-FREE MARGARINE
(sodium content 1.3 mg per serving).	

[1]RK = Research kitchen.
[2]"Amount for 1" is used for weighed diets; multiple-serving recipes are for general use (University of North Carolina at Chapel Hill GCRC).

The box at the bottom lists foods per meal with a "Taken" column for recording actual food intake.

Menus may also be printed from a spreadsheet or DBMS program using a reporting option. Exhibit 3–6 is a spreadsheet that shows menus for two participants and includes columns for recording the weight of refused (uneaten) food.

Example 5. Inventory

A food inventory system may be helpful, especially when researchers deal with large volumes of food or with long-term studies for which it is impractical to purchase all the food for the entire study at one time. Some centers use custom programs to monitor their perpetual inventories. When a case of food is received, the quantity is entered onto the computer and a label, such as shown in Figure 3–4, is affixed to each case. As the case is opened, the label is removed and the food subtracted from the computerized inventory. Reorder points are established for each food, and reports showing items to reorder are printed once a week. A *reorder point* is the minimum number of cases in an inventory list before food is reordered. For example, if the reorder point = 2 (cases), additional food is reordered when all but

2 cases are removed from inventory. A sample reorder point report is shown in Exhibit 3–7. A similar system could also be developed using a DBMS program.

Example 6. Budget and Food Costs

Research dietitians may be required to forecast, monitor, and document food costs and other expenses. Budget and food cost data can be stored and manipulated using spreadsheet, DBMS, or statistical packages. Exhibit 3–8 shows a sample spreadsheet for calculating food costs. The total cost was calculated by dividing the total items received by the items per purchasing unit (PU) and multiplying by cost per PU.

COMPUTER NETWORKS AND COMPUTER-MEDIATED COMMUNICATION

The computers that operate nutrient-calculation and food-service software are sometimes connected to other computers (nodes) and peripheral computer equipment (eg, printers) as part of a computer network. Networks allow resource sharing (eg, storage media, databases, programs, printers)

EXHIBIT 3-4

Research Menu Corresponding to Food Production Sheet from Exhibit 3-1
Generated from Custom-Designed Program (University of Iowa GCRC)

Name: Ima Sample
Dr. Casey #99–99
Constant Diet
CMDSIP: Sample.Men[a]

Date: _____
Period: 1   2
Day: 1   2   3   4   5

_____ g/2761.7g = _____

Diet wt + 250[b]/Calc wt + 250 H_2O[c]   = .98 – 1.02[d]

Blended Wt[e]: _____ g Init[f]

Code No[g]	(X) CRC Done[h]	(X) ATE All[i]	(X) Left Some[j]	Reason Left Code #[k]	AMT Left g[l]	(g)	BREAKFAST @?[m]
1032	☐	☐	☐	——	——	120	Orange juice?
				——	——		Scrambled eggs:
710	☐	☐	☐	——	——	65	Egg whites, fresh
720	☐	☐	☐	——	——	7	Egg yolks, fresh
280	☐	☐	☐	——	——	3	Butter?
1290	☐	☐	☐	——	——	0.5	Salt?
210	☐	☐	☐	——	——	25	Cracked-wheat bread?
280	☐	☐	☐	——	——	5	Butter?
399	☐	☐	☐	——	——	25	40% Bran Flakes, Kellogg's?
944	☐	☐	☐	——	——	180	2% Milk
500	☐	☐	☐	——	——	180	Brewed coffee

Code No	(X) CRC Done	(X) ATE All	(X) Left Some	Reason Left Code #	AMT Left g	(g)	LUNCH @?
274	☐	☐	☐	——	——	40	Hamburger bun?
280	☐	☐	☐	——	——	5	Butter?
391	☐	☐	☐	——	——	11	Catsup, reg
960	☐	☐	☐	——	——	4	Yellow mustard
1020	☐	☐	☐	——	——	10	Onion, raw
1130	☐	☐	☐	——	——	10	Dill pickle?
840	☐	☐	☐	——	——	45	Hamburger, lean (20% fat), panfry, well?
1290	☐	☐	☐	——	——	0.2	Salt?
370	☐	☐	☐	——	——	40	Carrot, raw
400	☐	☐	☐	——	——	40	Celery, raw
269	☐	☐	☐	——	——	45	Brownie?
480	☐	☐	☐	——	——	300	Coca Cola

(continued)

and computer-mediated communication. A metanetwork of many interconnected computer networks may eventually be as common as telephone networks are today (62).

There are several ways to communicate with others via computer. One way is through a local area network (LAN). Computers in a LAN are connected in a closed circuit network by a set of cables; the network is maintained by a system manager. This configuration usually occurs among personal computers in the same building and is useful for communicating within and among departments. A LAN enables everyone to transfer information and to have access to the same programs and equipment, such as printers (63).

Another way to communicate via computer is using larger networks. Such networks support communication across a wider area. The Internet is the world's largest group of interconnected networks. The Internet is accessed through a university connection or an Internet service provider (ISP)

such as CompuServe® or America Online®. The Internet facilitates transfer of data files and machine-readable documents, an important consideration in research endeavors. Two other useful Internet features are electronic mail and the World Wide Web (WWW or Web).

E-mail is probably the most commonly used Internet feature. Researchers may find e-mail useful (62, 64, 65) for many reasons. Some of these are improvements to traditional surface mail. For example, e-mail allows simultaneous mass mailing, eliminates stamps, eliminates paper copies unless needed, and is usually faster and less expensive than surface mail. E-mail also circumvents certain difficulties with telephone communications, such as time zone differences, work interruptions, and missing phone calls and return calls. Security in e-mail is usually low; encryption is necessary for confidential messages or messages including otherwise restricted information about study participants (62, 66).

EXHIBIT 3-4 (cont.)

Code No	(X) CRC Done	(X) ATE All	(X) Left Some	Reason Left Code #	AMT Left g	(g)	DINNER @?
1526	☐	☐	☐	——	——	95	Turkey breast w/o skin?
1203	☐	☐	☐	——	——	110	Mashed potatoes?
280	☐	☐	☐	——	——	10	Butter?
804	☐	☐	☐	——	——	45	Canned chicken gravy?
1475	☐	☐	☐	——	——	100	Sage stuffing?
125	☐	☐	☐	——	——	75	Green bean, CANNED W/SALT, drained?
280	☐	☐	☐	——	——	4	Butter?
	☐	☐	☐	——	——		Tossed salad:
910	☐	☐	☐	——	——	40	Lettuce, crisphead
1520	☐	☐	☐	——	——	40	Tomato, raw
1350	☐	☐	☐	——	——	17	French dressing?
1056	☐	☐	☐	——	——	110	Peach, juice pack, drain?
1510	☐	☐	☐	——	——	200	Tea beverage

Code No	(X) CRC Done	(X) ATE All	(X) Left Some	Reason Left Code #	AMT Left g	(g)	HS SNACK @?
342				——	——	25	Hershey's Milk Chocolate?
35				——	——	100	Apple w/o core
1204				——	——	20	Potato chips?
19				——	——	360	Diet 7-UP

[a]SAMPLE.MEN = Text filename.

[b]Diet wt + 250 = Actual weight of foods plus 250 g distilled water used to rinse containers. Notes b-f refer to duplicate diet prepared for laboratory analysis.

[c]Calc wt + 250 H_2O = Sum of all food weights on menu plus 250 g water for rinsing containers. Total weight is generated from nutrient data file and menu program and adjusted manually if needed (eg, to account for moisture loss during cooking eggs).

[d].98–1.02 = Ratio of actual duplicate weight to calculated weight; duplicate diets not within this range are discarded.

[e]Blended wt = Weight of duplicate diet after blending.

[f]Init = Initialed by staff completing task.

[g]Code no = Code identifying food in nutrient database.

[h]CRC done = Checked when food has been retrieved from storage or weighed fresh for this study day.

[i]Ate all = Checked if subject ate each specific food.

[j]Left some = Checked if subject did not finish food.

[k]Reason left code no = Reason subject did not finish food; codes are listed on menu back and include items such as "too much food," "didn't like food," and "forgot."

[l]Amt left g = Weight of uneaten food in grams.

[m]? = Foods weighed in bulk before the study are identified with question mark. Using a word processor, the ? is replaced with the food storage location. The ? after the meal name is replaced with the meal time.

The WWW is an information retrieval system. It is a multimedia portion of the Internet supporting pictures and sound and using page layout concepts. Web documents and menus contain hyperlinks that "link" to other documents on the Web. A tool called a *browser* enables the user to connect to a specific site by specifying its location (eg, http://www.nih.gov for the National Institutes of Health). Exam-

Date Arrived	Food	Date Pulled
8/10/98	Apples	☐

Lot #	Box #	Staff Initials
3587-46	1–5	☐

FIGURE 3-4.   Sample label attached to food cases and used to monitor food inventory at the Grand Forks Human Nutrition Research Center.

ples of browsers include Netscape Communicator, Mosaic, Lynx, Microsoft Internet Explorer, Hot Java, and Opera. Researchers can find valuable research and grant information at the various private and public Web sites.

Many useful resources providing information related to nutrient-calculation software are summarized in Table 3–3. Whenever possible, software should be tested before purchase. Some vendors demonstrate their software at meetings such as the National Nutrient Data Bank Conference and The American Dietetic Association Annual Meeting or offer demonstration disks to potential buyers. A few universities have nutrient-calculation programs for review. The National Agricultural Library in Beltsville, Md, maintains a listing of nutrient analysis, foodservice, and health and nutrition education software that is updated regularly. This list can be viewed at the Web site: http://www.nal.usda.gov/fnic/software/software.html. USDA nutrient data are also

EXHIBIT 3-5

Research Menu Generated by Downloading Output from Nutrient Calculation Program into Word Processor (Cornell University Medical College GCRC)

Balance Diet: Daily Menu   Dates: _____

Patient Name: _____

Food/Amount	Solid	Fluid
Coffee, Inst Max[1] 4 g + 800 g dist[2] H_2O	4 g	800 g
Half & half 50 g + 50 g dist H_2O		100 g
White sugar 20 g	20 g	
Uns[3] bread white 40 g + 40 g + 40 g	120 g	
FTWT[4] red raspberry preserves 20 g	20 g	
Ardmore juice, apple 120 g		120 g
Ardmore juice, pineapple 120 g		120 g
Uns butter 40 g	40 g	
FTWT Familia[5] original 45 g	45 g	
FTWT UNS tunafish 120 g	120 g	
FTWT Soyamaise 20 g	20 g	
Lettuce 50 g + 50 g	100 g	
Tomato 50 g + 50 g	100 g	
Corn oil 10 g + 10 g	20 g	
Vinegar 10 g + 10 g		20 g
Coca Cola Classic 355 g + 355 g		710 g
Balance chicken 120 g	120 g	
FTWT apricot preserves 15 g	15 g	
White rice (cooked) 175 g	175 g	
FTWT green beans 150 g	150 g	
FTWT corn chips 30 g	30 g	

MENU

Breakfast	Taken	Lunch	Taken	Dinner	Taken
40 g uns bread, toasted + 20 g FTWT red rasp preserves	____	SANDWICH: 40 g uns bread + 120 g FTWT uns tuna + 20 g FTWT soyamaise	____	120 g bal chicken + 15 g apricot pres + 20 g uns butter	____
4 g coffee + 800 g dist H_2O + 20 g white sugar	____	SALAD: 50 g lettuce + 50 g tomato + 10 g corn oil + 10 g vinegar	____	SALAD: 50 g lettuce + 50 g tomato + 10 g corn oil + 10 g vinegar	____
45 g FTWT Familia original	____	355 g Coca Cola Classic	____	40 g uns bread + 20 g uns butter	____
120 g Ardmore pineapple juice	____			355 g Coca Cola Classic	____
120 g Ardmore apple juice	____			175 g white rice (cooked)	____
50 g half & half + 50 g dist H_2O	____			150 g FTWT green beans	____
				30 g FTWT corn chips	____

[1] Inst Max = Instant Maxwell House coffee.
[2] Dist = Distilled.
[3] Uns = Unsalted.
[4] FTWT = Featherweight brand.
[5] Familia = Familia grain and fruit cereal.

EXHIBIT 3-6

Research Menu for Two Subjects Generated from Spreadsheet (University of North Carolina at Chapel Hill GCRC)

PROJECT 753 DIET RECORD SHEET   DATE:

Patient: _____   Patient: _____

Food and Beverages	Intake (g or PKT)	Refusal (g or PKT)	Intake (g or PKT)	Refusal (g or PKT)
BREAKFAST: (Mo[1]) IN UNIT				
RK[2] orange juice	240	——	240	——
Corn flakes	20	——	30	——
Whole-wheat toast	40	——	56	——
Redi-Pat margarine	15	——	12	——
Jelly	15	——	25	——
Sugar (weigh into medicine cup)	15	——	10	——
Decaf coffee	200	——	200	——
Whole milk	240	——	240	——
LUNCH: PACK AT & GIVE AT BREAKFAST				
RK grape juice	240	——	240	——
RK turkey breast	45	——	47	——
Whole-wheat bread	50	——	50	——
Kraft Mayonnaise	22	——	25	——
RK pineapple	150	——	150	——
Sugar (add to pineapple)	8	——	8	——
Salt	1 PKT	——	1 PKT	——
Pepper	1 PKT	——	1 PKT	——
DINNER: IN UNIT				
RK apple juice	240	——	240	——
RK ham	50	——	60	——
RK sweet potatoes	100	——	100	——
RK green beans	75	——	75	——
Redi-Pat margarine (add to vegetable)	10	——	10	——
CRU[3] yeast rolls	0	0	27	——
Redi-Pat margarine (for dinner roll)	0	0	5	——
RK peaches	150	——	150	——
Sugar (add to peaches)	16	——	16	——
Decaf iced tea	200	——	200	——
Salt	1 PKT	——	1 PKT	——
Pepper	1 PKT	——	1 PKT	——
NOURISHMENT: GIVE AT DINNER				
Graham crackers	28	——	28	——
RK grapefruit juice	240	——	240	——
Sugar (add to juice)	0	0	15	——

[1]Mo. = Monday.
[2]RK = Research kitchen.
[3]CRU = Clinical research unit.

available through the National Agricultural Library's Web site at http://www.nal.usda.gov/fnic/foodcomp/ (Table 3–3).

CONCLUSION

Computers are an invaluable aid to the dietitian in supporting controlled diet research. Nutrient-calculation systems are the most developed software application for this purpose. Linear programming or other mathematical procedures promise further assistance in the design of defined diets for metabolic research. Developing cost-effective computer support for research diet foodservice requires nutrition managers to carefully define their needs if they wish to use programming designed for a broader audience. The most successful future applications will be flexible enough to accommodate a variety of foodservice needs and methods of operation.

EXHIBIT 3-7

Inventory Reorder Point Report Generated from Custom-Designed Program (USDA Grand Forks Human Nutrition Research Center)

DIETARY INVENTORY SYSTEM REORDER POINT REPORT
03/05/93 09:50:45
LOCATION = Metabolic Kitchen / food item
PAGE : 1

Potato, canned		BRAND = Butter Kernal	VENDOR = Hugos	
LOT: SPN1N63	UNIT/CASE = 24	UNIT WT. = 16 oz	REORDER PONT = 2	QTY ON HAND = 2

Butter, salted		BRAND = Bridgemans	VENDOR = Bridgemans	
LOT: MARCH0993D	UNIT/CASE = 36	UNIT WT. = 1 lb	REORDER POINT = 1	QTY ON HAND = 1

Cinnamon, ground		BRAND = Schilling	VENDOR = Hugos	
LOT: 7462B	UNIT/CASE = 6	UNIT WT. = 1 oz	REORDER POINT = 2	QTY ON HAND = 2

Cornflakes		BRAND = Kellogg's	VENDOR = Hugos	
LOT: OCT301993	UNIT/CASE = 24	UNIT WT. = 12 oz	REORDER POINT = 1	QTY ON HAND = 1

Drink mix, wild strawberry		BRAND = Wyler's	VENDOR = Hugos	
LOT: 1F28FA12	UNIT/CASE = 144	UNIT WT. = .18 oz	REORDER POINT = 1	QTY ON HAND = 0.5

Ice cream, vanilla		BRAND = Bridgemans	VENDOR = Bridgemans	
LOT: TG2344M	UNIT/CASE = 4	UNIT WT. = ½ gal	REORDER POINT = 2	QTY ON HAND = 1

Mayonnaise, real		BRAND = Kraft	VENDOR = Hugos	
LOT: to order	UNIT/CASE = 12	UNIT WT. = 32 oz	REORDER POINT = 1	QTY ON HAND = 0

Oil, vegetable		BRAND = Crisco, soybean	VENDOR = Hugos	
LOT: 12283AA2	UNIT/CASE = 12	UNIT WT. = 32 oz	REORDER POINT = 1	QTY ON HAND = 1

Parmesan cheese, grated		BRAND = Kraft	VENDOR = Hugos	
LOT: to order	UNIT/CASE = 12	UNIT WT. = 8 oz	REORDER POINT = 1	QTY ON HAND = 0

Peas, frozen		BRAND = Birdseye	VENDOR = Hugos	
LOT: to order	UNIT/CASE = 12	UNIT WT. = 16 oz	REORDER POINT = 2	QTY ON HAND = 0

[1]Qty = Quantity.

PRODUCTS CITED

Food and Nutrition Software

Auto Nutritionist IV, CAMP Program: One commercial program with this function is Auto Nutritionist IV®, First DataBank. The Hearst Corp, 1111 Bayhill Dr, San Bruno, CA 94066–3035. (800) 633–3453; http://www.firstdatabank.com.

Diet Analyzer: The CBORD Group, Inc, 61 Brown Road, Ithaca, NY 14858. (607) 257–2410.

Food Intake and Analysis System (FIAS): University of Texas Houston Health Science Center, Human Nutrition Center, PO Box 20186, Houston, TX 77225. (713) 500–9343.

Food Processor: ESHA Research, 4263 Commercial St, SE, Suite 200, Salem, OR 97302–3938. (503) 585–6242 or (800) 659–3742, e-mail: esh@esha.com.

Interactive Diet Construction (IDC) (CAMP Program): General Clinical Research Center, Medical College of South Carolina, Charleston, SC 29425. (803) 792–3357.

Moore's Extended Nutrient (MENu) Database: Database Manager, Pennington Biomedical Research Center, 6400 Perkins Rd, Baton Rouge, LA 70808–4124. (504) 763–2500, e-mail: Champacm@mhs.pbrc.edu.

Nutrition Data System (NDS): Nutrition Coordinating Center, University of Minnesota, 1300 South Second St, Lower Level, Minneapolis, MN 55414. (612) 627–9429.

Nutritionist V: First DataBank. The Hearst Corp, 1111 Bayhill Dr, San Bruno, CA 94066–3035. (800) 633–3453; http://www.firstdatabank.com.

ProNutra: ProNutra Nutrient Analysis System for Metabolic Studies. Princeton, NJ: Princeton Multimedia Technologies, 145 Witherspoon Street, Princeton, NJ 08540. System development was supported by a Small Business Innovation Research Grant (R44-RR11678) from the National Center for Research Resources, Bethesda, Md.

EXHIBIT 3-8

Food Cost Spreadsheet (University of North Carolina at Chapel Hill GCRC)

CRU[1] DIETARY EXPENSE 7/98

Category	Description	Purchase Unit	Cost/PU[2]	Units/PU	7/7/ 98	7/14/ 98	7/22/ 98	7/28/ 98	7/31/ 98	Total Cost
CANNED	SOUP-TOMATO-IND[3]	24/7.3OZCN[4]/CS[5]	$ 7.87	24	15		8			$7.54
CANNED	SOUP-VEGETABLE-IND	24/7.3 OZ CN/CS	$ 7.59	24						$0.00
COND[6]	SEASON-MRS.DASH-IND	300 PKG[7]/CS	$13.02	1						$0.00
COND	SALT SUBSTITUTE-IND	2/1000/CS	$18.00	2						$0.00
COND	SUGAR SUB-IND	2/1250 BX[8]/CS	$11.34	2						$0.00
CANNED	TUNA-DIET	24/6.5 OZ CN/CS	$29.79	24						$0.00
CANNED	APPLESAUCE-UNSWT[9]	24/16 OZ CN/CS	$10.16	24						$0.00
CANNED	FRUIT COCKTAIL-UNSWT	24/16 OZ CN/CS	$20.19	24						$0.00
CANNED	PEACH HALVES-UNSWT	24/16 OZ CN/CS	$18.89	24						$0.00
CANNED	PEACHES SLICED-UNSWT	24/16 OZ CN/CS	$18.89	24						$0.00
CANNED	PEAR HALVES-UNSWT	24/16 OZ CN/CS	$16.89	24						$0.00
CANNED	PINEAPPLE-SLI[10] UNSWT	24/20 OZ CN/CS	$17.50	24						$0.00
STAPLES	GELATIN-CHERRY SF[11]	12/3.4 OZ PKG/ CS	$33.75	12			1			$2.81
STAPLES	GELATIN-LIME-SF	12/3.4 OZ PKG/ CS	$31.97	12						$0.00
CANNED	JUICE-TOMATO-SF	24/18 OZ CN/CS	$11.71	24						$0.00
STAPLES	PICKLES-CHIPS-SF	12/16 OZ JR[12]/ CS	$18.60	12						$0.00
CANNED	SOUP-CHIX[13] NOODLES-SF 24	24/7.3 OZ CN/CS	$ 8.73	24	3		4			$2.55
CANNED	SOUP-TOMATO-SF	24/7.3 OZ CN/CS	$ 7.70	24	4					$1.28
CANNED	SOUP-VEGETABLE-SF	24/7.3 OZ CN/CS	$ 7.97	24		3		4		$2.32
STAPLES	BROTH-BEEF-SF	6/50 PKG BX/CS	$29.19	6						$0.00
STAPLES	BROTH-CHICKEN-SF	6/50 PKG BX/CS	$29.20	6						$0.00
STAPLES	GRAVY/BRN[14] SCE[15] MIX-SF	24/3 OZ BX/CS	$51.57	24						$0.00
STAPLES	GRAVY/CHIX MIX-SF	24/4 OZ BX/CS	$54.08	24						$0.00

[1]CRU = Clinical research unit; [2]PU = Purchasing unit; [3]IND = Individual; [4]CN = Can; [5]CS = Case; [6]COND = Condiment; [7]PKG = Package; [8]BX = Box; [9]UNSWT = Unsweetened; [10]SLI = Sliced; [11]SF = Salt free; [12]JR = Junior; [13]CHIX = Chicken; [14]BRN = Brown; [15]SCE = Sauce.

General Applications Software

Version 1: Full-length URLS and publishers

Access (98): Microsoft (http://www.microsoft.com/access/)

America Online: America Online, Inc (http://www.aol.com)

BMDP/PC: SPSS (http://www.spss.com/support/Documents/BM-122995-03.html)

CompuServe: CompuServe Interactive Services, Inc (http://www.compuserve.com)

Digital UNIX: Digital Equipment Corporation (http://www.unix.digital.com/)

Excel: Microsoft (http://www.microsoft.com/office/excel/)

Freelance Graphics: Lotus (http://www.lotus.com/home.nsf/welcome/freelance)

GroupWise: Novell, Inc (http://www.novell.com)

Harvard Graphics (98): SPC Software Publishing (http://www.harvardgraphics.com)

Hot Java (1.1.4): Sun Microsystems, Inc (http://www.java.sun.com/products/hotjava/)

Internet Explorer (4.0): Microsoft (http://www.microsoft.com/ie/ie40/)

IRIX (6.5): Silicon Graphics, Inc (http://www.sgi.com/software/irix6.5/)

TABLE 3-3

Sources of Additional Information

Resource	Description	Contact
Journals		
Foodservice Information Systems Report (previously *Byting In*)	Computer newsletter for food and nutrition professionals	Center Publications Cyntergy Corporation 656 Quince Orchard Road Gaithersburg, MD 20878-1409 (301) 926-3726
Food and Nutrition News	Includes reviews of several commercially available nutrition-related software packages in alternate issues	National Cattlemen's Beef Association 444 N Michigan Ave Chicago, IL 60611 (312) 467-5520
Journal of The American Dietetic Association	Includes reviews of several commercially available nutrition-related software packages in alternate issues	The American Dietetic Association 216 W Jackson Blvd Suite 800 Chicago, IL 60606-6995 (312) 899-0040
Nutrition Today	Includes reviews of several commercially available nutrition-related software packages in alternate issues	Williams & Wilkens, Publishers 351 West Camden St Baltimore, MD 21201-2436 (800) 638-6423 Editor: (814) 237-1078
Catalogs		
Microcomputer Software Collection	List of approximately 180 software packages and a brief description of each	Food and Nutrition Information Center National Agricultural Library 10301 Baltimore Blvd Beltsville, MD 20705-2351 (301) 504-5719 http://www.nal.usda.gov/fnic/software /software.html
National Nutrient Databank Directory	Annotated listing of nutrient-calculation software	Department of Nutrition and Dietetics 238 Alison Hall University of Delaware Newark, DE 19716 (302) 831-8729
US Department of Agriculture Nutrient Database	Food composition tables	Food and Nutrition Information Center National Agricultural Library 10301 Baltimore Blvd Beltsville, MD 20705-2351 (301) 504-5719 http://www.nal.usda.gov/fnic/foodcomp
Meetings		
International Conference on Dietary Assessment Methods	Biannual meeting to address the diverse needs of nutrient database users and developers	Department of Preventive Medicine and Community Health Medical College of Virginia PO Box 980212 Richmond, VA 23298-0212 (804) 828-3258
National Nutrient Databank Conference	Annual meeting to address the diverse needs of nutrient database users and developers	Research Leader Nutrient Data Laboratory USDA Agricultural Research Service Beltsville, MD 20705 (301) 734-8491

Lotus 1-2-3: Lotus (http://www.lotus.com/)
Lynx: University of Kansas (http://www.cc.ukans.edu/lynx help/Lynx users guide.html)
Mosaic for Windows (3.0): NCSA (http://www.ncsa.uiuc.edu/SDG/Software/WinMosaic/HomePage.html)
MSWord X.X: Microsoft Corportation (http://www.microsoft.com/office/word/)
Netscape Communicator: Netscape Communications (http://www.netscape.com)
Opera (3.21): Opera Software (http://www.operasoftware.com)
PageMaker (6.5): Adobe (http://www.adobe.com/prodindex/pagemaker/main.html)
Paradox (8.0): Corel Corporation (http://www.corel.com/products/wordperfect/paradox8/index.htm)
PowerPoint (97) for Windows: Microsoft (http://www.microsoft.com/office/powerpoint/)
Presentations (7.0): Corel Corporation (http://www.corel.com/products/wordperfect/cp7/index.htm)
Prophet (5.0): GTE Internetworking (http://www-prophet.bbn.com/prophet-home.htm)
Publisher (98): Microsoft (http://www.microsoft.com/products/business.htm)
Quattro Pro (6.0): Corel Corporation (http://www.corel.com/products/wordperfect/cops/index.htm)
SAS: SAS Institute Inc (http://www.sas.com)
SigmaPlot: SPSS (http://www.spss.com/software/science/sigmaplot)
Solaris (2.6): Sun Microsystems, Inc (http://www.sun.com/solaris/)
SPSS: Statistical Product & Service Products, Inc (http://www.spss.com)
Sun OS: Sun Microsystems, Inc (see Solaris above)
Systat (8.0): SPSS (http://www.spss.com/software/science/systat/systat8.htm)
Visual dBase (7): Inprise (http://www.inprise.com/VdBASE/)
Windows 98: Microsoft Corporation (http://www.microsoft.com/windows98/)
Wordperfect (8.0): Corel Corporation (http://www.corel.com/products/wordperfect/wp8dragon/index.htm)
Word Pro: Lotus Development Corporation (http://www.lotus.com/)
World Wide Web Consortium (http://www.w3.org)

Version 2: Short URLS and publishers

Access (98): Microsoft (http://www.microsoft.com)
America Online: America Online, Inc (http://www.aol.com)
BMDP/PC: SPSS (http://www.spss.com)
CompuServe: CompuServe Interactive Services, Inc (http://www.compuserve.com)
Digital UNIX: Digital Equipment Corporation (http://www.unix.digital.com)

Excel: Microsoft (http://www.microsoft.com)
Freelance Graphics: Lotus (http://www.lotus.com)
GroupWise: Novell, Inc (http://www.novell.com)
Harvard Graphics (98): SPC Software Publishing (http://www.harvardgraphics.com)
Hot Java (1.1.4): Sun Microsystems, Inc (http://www.java.sun.com)
Internet Explorer (4.0): Microsoft (http://www.microsoft.com)
IRIX (6.5): Silicon Graphics, Inc (http://www.sgi.com)
Lotus 1-2-3: Lotus (http://www.lotus.com)
Lynx: University of Kansas (http://www.cc.ukans.edu)
Mosaic for Windows (3.0): NCSA (http://www.ncsa.uiuc.edu)
MSWord X.X: Microsoft Corportation (http://www.microsoft.com)
Netscape Communicator: Netscape Communications (http://www.netscape.com)
Opera (3.21): Opera Software (http://www.operasoftware.com)
PageMaker (6.5): Adobe (http://www.adobe.com)
Paradox (8.0): Corel Corporation (http://www.corel.com)
PowerPoint (97) for Windows: Microsoft (http://www.microsoft.com)
Presentations (7.0): Corel Corporation (http://www.corel.com)
Prophet (5.0): GTE Internetworking (http://www-prophet.bbn.com)
Publisher (98): Microsoft (http://www.microsoft.com)
Quattro Pro (6.0): Corel Corporation (http://www.corel.com)
SAS: SAS Institute, Inc (http://www.sas.com)
SigmaPlot: SPSS (http://www.spss.com)
Solaris (2.6): Sun Microsystems, Inc (http://www.sun.com)
SPSS: Statistical Product & Service Products, Inc (http://www.spss.com)
Sun OS: Sun Microsystems, Inc (http://www.sun.com)
Systat (8.0): SPSS (http://www.spss.com)
Visual dBase (7): Inprise (http://www.inprise.com)
Windows 98: Microsoft Corporation (http://www.microsoft.com)
Wordperfect (8.0): Corel Corporation (http://www.corel.com)
Word Pro: Lotus Development Corporation (http://www.lotus.com)
World Wide Web Consortium (http://www.w3.org)

Other Products

Bar Code Technology

Computype, Inc: 1120C Benfield Boulevard, PO Box 987, Millersville, MD 21109-0987. (800) 437-5712; http://www.computypeinc.com.
Intermec Technologies Corporation: 6001 36th Avenue West, PO Box 4280, Everett, WA 98203-9280. (800) 347-2636; http://www.intermec.com.

Food Models

Nasco, Inc: 901 Janesville Ave, Fort Atkinson, WI 53538 (414) 563–2446 and Nasco West, 4825 Stoddard Rd, Modesto, CA 95356. (209) 545–1600.

REFERENCES

1. Hjortland MC, Duddleson WG, Porter C, French AB. Using the computer to calculate nutrients in metabolic diets. *J Am Diet Assoc.* 1966;49:316–318.

2. St Jeor STD, Millar R, Tyler FH. The digital computer in research dietetics. *J Am Diet Assoc.* 1970;56:404–408.

3. Mo A, Peckos PS, Glatky CB. Computers in a dietary study. *J Am Diet Assoc.* 1971;59:111–115.

4. Wheeler ML, Wheeler LA. Nutrient menu planning for clinical research centers. *J Am Diet Assoc.* 1975;67:346–350.

5. Oexmann MJ. Automated diet construction for clinical research. *J Am Diet Assoc.* 1983;82:72–75.

6. Dare D, Al-Bander SY. A computerized diet analysis system for the research nutritionist. *J Am Diet Assoc.* 1987;87:629–632.

7. St Jeor ST, Bryan GT. Clinical research diets: definition of terms. *J Am Diet Assoc.* 1973;62:47–51.

8. Lentner C, Lauffenburger T, Guncaga J, et al. The metabolic balance technique: a critical reappraisal. *Metabolism.* 1975;24:461–470.

9. St Jeor ST, Guthrie HA, Jones HB. Variability in nutrient intake in a 28-day period. *J Am Diet Assoc.* 1983;83: 155–162.

10. Basiotis PP, Welsh SO, Cronin FJ, et al. Number of days of food intake records required to estimate individual and group nutrient intakes with defined confidence. *J Nutr.* 1987;117:1638–1641.

11. Cummings SR, Block G, McHenry K, et al. Evaluation of two food frequency methods of measuring dietary calcium intake. *Am J Epidemiol.* 1987;126:796–802.

12. US Department of Agriculture. *Nutrient Data Base for Standard Reference.* Release 12 (SR-12). Agricultural Research Service, Beltsville, Md; 1998.

13. US Department of Agriculture. *Nutritive Value of Foods.* Home and Garden Bulletin No. 72. Available in print version from National Technical Information Service, Springfield, Va. Agricultural Research Service, Beltsville, Md; 1991.

14. US Department of Agriculture. *Home and Garden Bulletin No. 72–1, Nutritive Value of Foods* (Release 3.2). Data Tape or Disk, National Technical Information Service, Springfield, Va; 1990.

15. US Department of Agriculture. *Nutrient Data Base for Individual Food Intake Surveys.* Data Tape, Release 4. National Technical Information Service, Springfield, Va; 1990.

16. Consumer and Food Economic Institute. *Composition of Foods—Raw, Processed, Prepared.* Washington, DC: US Government Printing Office; 1976–91. Agriculture Handbook 8. (Revisions: 8-1 through 8-21).

17. Life Sciences Research Office, Federation of American Societies for Experimental Biology. *Third Report on Nutrition Monitoring in the United States.* Prepared for the US Department of Agriculture and the US Department of Health and Human Services. DHHS (PHS) Publication 89-1255. Washington, DC: US Government Printing Office; 1995.

18. US Department of Agriculture. *Provisional Table on the Vitamin K Content of Selected Foods.* Washington, DC: USDA Agricultural Research Service; 1994.

19. Schakel SF, Warren RA, Buzzard IM. Imputing nutrient values from manufacturers' data. *Proceedings of the Fourteenth National Nutrient Databank Conference, June 1989, University of Iowa.* Ithaca, NY: The CBORD Group, Inc; 1990.

20. Schakel SF, Sievert YA, Buzzard IM. Sources of data for developing and maintaining a nutrient database. *J Am Diet Assoc.* 1988;88:1268-1271.

21. Sievert YA, Schakel SF, and Buzzard IM. Maintenance of a nutrient database for clinical trials. *Control Clin Trials.* 1989;10:416–425.

22. US Department of Agriculture. *Table of Nutrient Retention Factors,* Release 3. Springfield, Va: National Technical Information Service; 1992.

23. Marsh A. Problems associated with recipe analysis. In: Tobelmann R, ed. *Proceedings of the Eighth National Nutrient Databank Conference.* Minneapolis, Minn: Nutrition Coding Center, University of Minnesota; 1983.

24. US Department of Agriculture. *Provisional Table on the Dietary Fiber Content of Selected Foods.* Washington, DC: USDA Human Nutrition Information Service; 1988.

25. Perloff BP, LaComb R. Nutrient data banks—their role in nutrition today: nutrient data base considerations. *Cereal Foods World.* 1990;35:653–659.

26. Buzzard IM. Maintaining time-related databases for dietary data collection and nutrient calculation. In: Murphy SP, ed. *Proceedings of the 16th National Nutrient Databank Conference.* Ithaca, NY: CBORD; 1991.

27. Food and Nutrition Board, National Research Council. *Recommended Dietary Allowances.* 10th ed. Washington, DC: National Academy of Sciences Press; 1989.

28. Nutrition Labeling and Education Act of 1990. Pub L No 101–535. 21 CFR (1993). Washington, DC.

29. Balintfy JL. Menu planning by computer. *Commun ACM.* 1994;7:255–259.

30. Gue RL. Mathematical basis for computer-planned nonselective menus. *Hospitals.* 1969;43:102–104.

31. Gelpi MJ, Balintfy JL, Dennis LC, et al. Integrated nutrition and food cost control by computer. *J Am Diet Assoc.* 1972;61:637–646.

32. Wheeler ML, Wheeler LA. Computer-planned menus for patients with diabetes mellitus. *Diabetes Care.* 1980;3:663–667.

33. Connell B. Applications: food and labor productions services in health care services. In: Kaud FA, ed. *Effective Computer Management in Food and Nutrition Services.* Rockville, Md: Aspen Publications, Inc; 1989.

34. Hoover L. Personal communication with Phyllis Stumbo, January 1993.

35. Anderson K, Kennedy B, Acosta PB. Computer-implemented nutrition support of phenylketonuria. *J Am Diet Assoc.* 1985;85:1623–1625.

36. Marcoe KK, Haytowitz DB. Estimating nutrient values of mixed dishes from label information. *Food Technology.* 1993;47:69–75.

37. Westrich BJ. *Development and Evaluation of Mathematical Optimization Software for Estimation of Nutrient Values in Food Products.* Minneapolis, Minn: University of Minnesota; 1993. Dissertation.

38. Fong AKH. Food composition data banks: important considerations in designing metabolic research diets. *Proceedings of the 17th National Nutrient Databank Conference.* Washington, DC: International Life Sciences Institute; 1992.

39. Wilcke HL, Hopkins DT, Reutzel LF, et al. Evaluation of linear programming techniques in formulating human diets with rat-feeding tests. *J Nutr.* 1973;103:179–188.

40. Monsen ER. Publishing and citing papers concerning nutrient data. In: Murphy SP, ed. *Proceedings of the 16th National Nutrient Databank Conference.* Ithaca, NY: CBORD; 1991.

41. Murphy SP. Recommendations for describing nutrient databases used in published research. *Proceedings of the 18th National Nutrient Databank Conference.* Ithaca, NY: CBORD; 1993.

42. Owen B. *Personal Computers for the Computer Illiterate.* New York, NY: Harper Perennial; 1991.

43. Asbeck C. Software update for dietetics professionals. Presented at American Dietetic Association Annual Meeting; October 22, 1992.

44. Coulston AM, Schaaf PM, Mukensnable G. Use of a single system to predict research dietary effort for protocols and to track daily meal census and dietary activities. Poster presented at General Clinical Research Center meeting, December 9, 1992, in Reston, Virginia.

45. Smith J. Databases for nonprogrammers. *PC/Computing.* 1992;5:223–252.

46. Kalman D. 15 relational databases: easy access, programming power. *PC Magazine.* 1991;10:101–108.

47. Alford Powers M. Database software for food and nutrition services. *Byting In.* 1991;2(1):1,10–12.

48. Raskin R. Statistical software for the PC: testing for significance. *PC Magazine.* 1989;8:103–116.

49. Miller R. To inform and convince: ten presentation graphics programs. *PC Magazine.* 1992;11:113–125.

50. Simon B. Stanford Graphics: technical presentations arrive in the 20th century. *PC Magazine.* 1992;11:122–123.

51. Tufte E. *The Visual Display of Quantitative Information.* Cheshire, Conn: Graphics Press; 1983.

52. Tufte E. *Envisioning Information.* Cheshire, Conn: Graphics Press; 1990.

53. Review. Calendar Creator Plus ver. 4.0. *Byting In.* 1992;3(5):13–14.

54. Barr C. Five programs for making organizational charts. *PC Magazine.* 1991;10:339–368.

55. Special report: employee scheduling. *Byting In.* 1992; 3(2):1,45.

56. Comparing scheduling software. *Byting In.* 1992; 3(2):610.

57. Ostenso GL. Concepts of food systems management. In: Moore AN, Tuthill BH, eds. *Computer-Assisted Food Management Systems.* Columbia, Mo: Technical Education Services; 1971.

58. Leinen SK. A menu-focused computer system for health care. In: Kaud FA, ed. *Effective Computer Management in Food and Nutrition Services.* Rockville, Md: Aspen Publications, Inc; 1989.

59. Food/nutrition software shapes up for '93. *Byting In.* 1992;3 (6): 2–24.

60. Kaud FA. Bar coding technology. In: Kaud FA, ed. *Effective Computer Management in Food and Nutrition Services.* Rockville, Md: Aspen Publications, Inc; 1989.

61. Baltzer LE, Sawyer CA, Gregoire M. Food service database management. In: Kaud FA, ed. *Effective Computer Management in Food and Nutrition Services.* Rockville, Md: Aspen Publications, Inc; 1989.

62. Quarterman JS. *The Matrix. Computer Networks and Conferencing Systems Worldwide.* Bedford, Mass: Digital Press; 1990.

63. Schrock JR, Schrock JM. Local area network systems. In: Kaud FA, ed. *Effective Computer Management in Food and Nutrition Services.* Rockville, Md: Aspen Publications, Inc; 1989.

64. Krol E. *The Whole Internet User's Guide & Catalog.* Sebastopol, Calif: O'Reilly & Associates, Inc; 1992.

65. Userlink. *Byting In.* 1992;3(2):2–3.

66. Scura L, Klensin JC. Using electronic mail (e-mail) for database communications. In: Murphy SP, ed. *Proceedings of the 16th National Nutrient Databank Conference.* Ithaca, NY: CBORD; 1991.

Chapter 4

Genetic Effects in Human Dietary Studies

Elizabeth R. De Oliveira E Silva, MD; Ruth McPherson, MD, PhD; and Darrell L. Ellsworth, PhD

Interactions Between Genes and Nutrition

Metabolic responses to dietary change are complex and vary considerably among individuals. Genetic factors are known to account for a portion of the normal population variation in parameters ranging from fasting serum cholesterol concentration to basal metabolic rate. Genetic variables thus are likely to contribute to individual responses to dietary change and must be considered during in-depth analyses of the biochemical effects of specific nutritional interventions. Studies on the genetic basis of variable dietary response in humans are complicated, however, by the inability to adequately control for a number of confounding environmental factors. For example, the background (prestudy) diet is often difficult to quantify but may have important effects on the response to a specific dietary intervention. Also, although diet can be rigorously controlled if resources permit, other environmental variables that affect the dietary response are more difficult to quantify and regulate.

The biochemical nature of the interactions between dietary response and genetic factors is not well understood, although nutrients have been shown to exhibit specific effects on various levels of gene expression including transcription and messenger RNA (mRNA) processing and stability (1). More research is needed on the effects of individual nutrients on the expression of specific genes and on modulation of gene expression by other genes in order to understand the metabolic basis of individual differences in nutritional responses.

Major gene disorders such as familial hypercholesterolemia have been well characterized despite the fact that they account for only a small percentage of the total population variability in dietary response. Polygenic diversity is also of primary importance in nutrition studies, because multiple genes likely account for a significant portion of the total genetic variance contributing to response *phenotypes*. For example, individual susceptibility to the hyperlipidemic effects of dietary cholesterol and saturated fatty acids, excess alcohol intake, and obesity is believed to have a considerable genetic component. Despite their potential importance, progress in the identification and characterization of the many genes contributing to variability in dietary response has been limited.

Genes Influencing Obesity and Body Fat Distribution

Factors influencing obesity and body fat distribution may be important considerations in dietary studies because of the increasing prevalence of obesity in developed countries (2) and associations between weight gain and increased susceptibility to cardiovascular disease (3). The distribution of body fat appears to be an important determinant of the morbidity that is associated with obesity, and abdominal visceral fat in particular is believed to play a critical role in the metabolic complications that are commonly observed in obese patients (4–6).

Genetic (7) and environmental (8) factors are both important determinants of interindividual variability in abdominal visceral fat levels and total body fat content. Intervention studies using identical twins first suggested the influence of genetic factors on body fat storage and mobilization (9), and subsequent research has identified numerous candidate genes that may influence the level and distribution of body fat. A summary of all genes and anonymous genetic markers potentially related to obesity syndromes and obesity-related phenotypes is presented within the human obesity gene map (10). To date approximately 133 candidate loci have been identified from various lines of evidence, including association and linkage studies as well as cross-breeding experiments and animal models of obesity. Identifying susceptibility genes associated with candidate loci and evaluating the relative contributions of known candidate genes to obesity in different human populations will likely be an important focus of future research (11).

STUDY DESIGNS IN GENETIC RESEARCH

Ascertainment of Study Subjects

The purpose and goals of a genetic study examining various phenotypes associated with diet will determine the selection strategy for subjects as well as the type of data that will be collected. Unrelated individuals in matched case-control designs can provide useful genetic information and can be used in association studies to detect relationships between specific measures of a particular phenotype and polymorphisms in candidate genes. However, it is often important to observe the transmission of the phenotype of interest from parents to their children and to identify regions of the genome that are shared by siblings or family members who exhibit similar response phenotypes.

Family studies are often crucial to defining the contributions of genetic factors to complex phenotypes (such as dietary response). Such studies may evaluate as few as two affected siblings or as many as several hundred individuals spanning multiple generations. The goals and specific aims of the research, however, are what dictate the type and number of families that would be optimal. Different family structures have advantages and limitations (see Table 4–1) that must be considered before investigators commit to the expensive and time-consuming tasks of recruitment and screening (12). The method of ascertainment to be used in an investigation must be specified a priori and will be dependent on the research questions being investigated (Table 4–2). Commonly used family groups include monozygotic (MZ) and dizygotic (DZ) twins, sibling pairs, nuclear families (parents and their children), multiplex (multiple-

generation) families, and extended pedigrees containing more distant relatives. (Also see Chapter 9, "Children as Participants in Feeding Studies.")

Initial Genetic Analyses

Before researchers conduct DNA-based studies with the ultimate goal of localizing and characterizing genes that influence dietary response, it is prudent to determine as much as possible about the genetic basis of the trait of interest. An obvious first step is to define the relative contributions of genetic and environmental factors to the phenotype(s) under study. *Heritability analyses* estimate the proportion of the total phenotypic variance that is caused by genetic variation, as opposed to environmental variation and measurement error. Twin studies, which compare MZ and DZ twins, are used for estimating the proportion of a complex phenotype that is attributable to genetic factors (13, 14). The basic premise is that MZ twins, which result from the division of a single fertilized ovum, share 100% of their genes and are thus genetically identical, whereas DZ twins are expected to share only about 50% of their genes and hence are no more genetically similar than siblings of the same parents born after separate pregnancies. Greater concordance (ie, similarity with respect to the phenotype) between MZ twin pairs relative to DZ twin pairs is believed to reflect a genetic contribution to the trait (15, 16). This is a particularly important issue for complex phenotypes, which may be significantly influenced by the environment. It may be an oversimplification to assume that the greater similarity between MZ twins relative to DZ twins is solely attributable to genetic factors.

Environmental influences may differ between MZ and DZ twins even though twin pairs are generally assumed to share a common environment. Even the concordance of the prenatal environment may not be the same for MZ and DZ twins. MZ twins are formed from a division of a single fertilized ovum. If the division occurs at an early stage—between the zygote and the formation of the embryonic disc— the two embryos will have separate sets of fetal membranes, resulting in dichorionic-diamniotic twins. More commonly, the division occurs after the blastocyst has been formed, resulting in monochorionic-diamniotic twins. Rarely, if the division occurs much later, it results in monochorionic-monoamniotic twins. All dizygotic twins, however, are dichorionic-diamniotic, because they result from the separate fertilization of two ova by two spermatozoa, and each embryo develops within its own set of fetal membranes. Because the placenta develops from the chorionic structures, those MZ twins who share a single placenta will experience a greater similarity of maternal/paternal effects than DZ and MZ twins who develop with separate placentas.

Further studies on the genetics of nutrition and dietary response may be able to delineate models of inheritance to determine the number of genes (and their relative magni-

TABLE 4-1

Population Sampling Strategies for Genetic Research in Dietary Studies

Study Group	Attributes and Applications
Twins	Monozygotic (MZ) and dizygotic (DZ) twins are useful for estimating the proportion of a complex phenotype that is attributable to genetic factors (in heritability and concordance analyses), because they share different proportions of their genes (MZ 100%, DZ 50%) but are assumed to experience similar environmental exposures. Discordant twin pairs provide information regarding environmental influences on complex traits. Environmental influences, however, may differ between MZ and DZ twins and may complicate comparisons.
Nuclear families	Children and their parents are perhaps the easiest family structure to obtain and tend to be most representative of a particular phenotype in the general population. Nuclear families have traditionally been used to localize genes responsible for single-gene (Mendelian) diseases but may not be appropriate for complex phenotypes. This is because it may be labor intensive to identify complete nuclear families in which to observe hereditary transmission for traits with late age of onset, and it may be difficult to detect major genes if multiple genes contribute significantly to the phenotype.
Extended pedigrees	Such pedigrees are often ascertained through a single proband and then extended to more distant relatives. A single large pedigree may provide evidence for linkage, thereby reducing the potential problem of genetic heterogeneity (genetic differences) among families. Transmission of the phenotype of interest and inheritance of genetic markers may be traced across several generations, providing important information for segregation, linkage, and mapping studies. Extended pedigrees may not be representative of most families because the gene(s) contributing to a particular phenotype in a single pedigree may be relatively rare in the general population. Genetic heterogeneity may complicate phenotypic expression if additional genes influencing the phenotype are introduced by spouses into the extended family.
Siblings	Affected sibling-pair methods have recently become popular for localizing disease susceptibility genes because these methods are amenable to nonparametric (model-free) methodologies; they use allele-sharing methods that are conceptually and computationally simple. Discordant siblings provide significant power to detect linkage, which reduces the number of individuals needed in the analyses. Despite their popularity, sib-pair methods have several disadvantages, including reliance on identity-by-state (IBS) estimates of allele sharing rather than identity-by-descent (IBD), and potentially large sample sizes because many sibling pairs may be required to detect genes having relatively modest effects on complex phenotypes.
Inbred or isolated populations	Inbred or genetically isolated populations may facilitate the identification of genes influencing a complex trait due to reduced genetic heterogeneity—only a small number of genes influencing the trait may be present in that population. Conversely, genes affecting the trait may not be identifiable because many of the susceptibility genes that affect the general population may not be present in the isolate.
Unrelated individuals	Unrelated individuals may be used in association studies that compare the frequency of alleles between affected individuals (cases) and healthy individuals of similar age and gender (controls). Subjects are typically recruited based on the phenotype of interest which may be present or absent (in the case of disease). However, recruitment may also sample individuals from the extremes of the population distribution for a given trait. Unrelated individuals do not provide information on the transmission of genes or phenotypes from parents to children and thus are not suitable for linkage analyses.

TABLE 4-2

Study Designs for Genetic Research in Dietary Studies[1]

Objective	Potential Study Groups
Estimate the proportion of a complex phenotype that is attributable to genetic factors.	Monozygotic (MZ)/dizygotic (DZ) twins Siblings raised separately

Explain inheritance patterns and the number of genes contributing to a particular trait.	Nuclear families ascertained through
	    (1) an affected parent
	    (2) two or more affected siblings
	Extended pedigrees

Localize genes influencing a complex phenotype.	Affected sibling pairs Nuclear and extended families Inbred or genetically isolated populations
Examine relationships between DNA variants and phenotypes of interest.	Unrelated individuals (cases vs controls) Trios (a subject and his or her parents)

[1]Adapted from DS Postma and DA Meyers, in SB Liggett and DA Meyers, eds, *The Genetics of Asthma* (New York: Marcel Dekker, Inc; 1996), p 447, by permission of Marcel Dekker, Inc.

tude) influencing a particular trait. *Segregation analyses* attempt to explain the inheritance patterns of a given trait in families (pedigrees) by "fitting" various models to the observed patterns of inheritance and expression (17). Models range from simplistic, in which a single gene is sufficient to account for the observed familial correlations, to highly complex, in which many genes interact in controlling inheritance and phenotypic expression.

Localizing and Identifying Genes

Two basic approaches may be implemented to identify genes influencing individual metabolic responses to diet. The study of *candidate genes* is restricted to examining known genes of presumed metabolic relevance (18). Genes become candidates for involvement in complex traits when detailed biological and physiological information about the phenotype suggests that the action or product of the gene may be involved in early developmental pathways (presymptomatic), in the biochemical and cellular processes of progression, or in clinical manifestations (19). Complex phenotypes that may be pertinent to dietary studies include metabolic processes (such as thrombogenesis, the regulation of plasma low-density lipoprotein [LDL] kinetics, or calcium absorption), and may extend to common chronic diseases such as atherosclerosis and heart disease. The candidate gene approach is often limited because many important genes involved in regulating dietary response are unknown or have not been well characterized, and because investigators often have differing opinions regarding which genes should be considered viable candidates for influencing a particular phenotype. (See Figure 4–1 for an example of gene structure.)

An alternate approach for localizing genes associated with complex phenotypes such as metabolic response to diet involves a *genome-wide scan* in families or affected sibling pairs using genetic markers at regularly spaced intervals throughout the genome (eg, 20, 21). Linkage statistics can help to define initial candidate regions that must be further characterized by fine-mapping and physical mapping techniques to locate the gene(s) of interest.

Linkage analyses are commonly used to identify genes contributing to a particular phenotype or disease; the strength of the evidence for linkage is compared to the strength of the evidence for no linkage (22). Linkage is caused by the close proximity of two genes (or markers) along a chromosome and is inferred to exist when cosegregation is detected more often than would be expected by chance between a genetic marker and a gene affecting the phenotype of interest.

Traditional linkage approaches for localizing genes contributing to single-gene disorders may not be appropriate for the study of complex phenotypes such as dietary response, which is likely influenced by many genes. This is because *alleles* (alternate forms of a gene that differ in their DNA sequence) associated with individual differences in response may be common in the general population and any one gene may contribute only modestly to the response phenotype. Affected sib-pair methods have become popular for localizing genes that confer increased susceptibility to complex diseases. Such methods have increased in popularity because they are amenable to nonparametric (model-free) statistical methodologies and use techniques that are relatively simple from both conceptual and computational standpoints (23–25). For these reasons, nonparametric methods may generally be appropriate for nutrition studies, which often examine complex phenotypes.

A

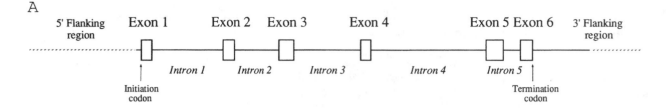

B

```
                                    Met Gly Leu Thr Val Ser Ala Leu Phe Ser Arg Ile Phe Gly Lys Lys Gln Met Arg
ccgcgtcggtgcccgcgcccctccccgggccccgcc ATG GGC CTC ACC GTG TCC GCG CTC TTT TCG CGG ATC TTC GGG AAG AAG CAG ATG CGG
Ile Leu Met Val>
ATT CTC ATG G gtgaggcagatcgagcgcgcggcccggaccggggcgccggccccggcgcagcccttccgccccgcgtccctccagccccgctcacctgggtctctggc
cccgagtcacccacctcataacgccccgggcctctgctctcgggcgggtcccggtctgcatcgccgaccccgggggcctgacaccggagctgcgggcctgggtggggtgaag
ctccctccgccccagcccggctggtaagaagggaggattccgccctttggagacgacttttaaaacgagcgcggcctacctcccgtgcccttgcctccagtcctctcccgctc
cgcgccctctttggagttggctcacgcaccgactgccctccaggcctcaaaggtagataacgacgcgcacctggaggcgtccccgctctccgccccagtcaccatcagctg
                                                                                          Gly Leu Asp Ala Ala Gly Lys Thr
ttgtggcctctccctttccctggtctctaggggggctccctcgctcccatctccatccctgtgcccctttccgttgcag TT GGC TTG GAT GCG GCT GGC AAG ACC
Thr Ile Leu Tyr Lys Leu Lys Leu Gly Glu Ile Val Thr Thr Ile Pro Thr Ile Gly>
ACA ATC CTG TAC AAA CTG AAG TTG GGG GAG ATT GTC ACC ACC ATC CCA ACC ATA G gtgagcccgggggacgaagcagggagcgggagcgccgcgg
ncgggccctcgcggggtctgctcccagttctgccacttttctggagctgacccgtgacaccagntacagctatttgagaagtggcttcaggggtatctctacgtggataccggagg
cagggtggatgtgacctagccccgccctgttgaccgccagttctggggttctgttcccctgggccttgatcattgccttctggtttttgtgtccctgctgaaatctaagtagtt
                                                                     Phe Asn Val Glu Thr Val Glu Tyr Lys Asn Ile Cys
ttagtgagttcctttctttcaggagttttctcatccttttttttttttccaattatctgcag GC TTC AAT GTA GAA ACA GTG GAA TAT AAG AAC ATC TGT
Phe Thr Val Trp Asp Val Gly Gly Gln Asp Lys Ile Arg Pro Leu Trp Arg His Tyr Phe Gln Asn Thr Gln>
TTC ACA GTC TGG GAC GTG GGA GGC CAG GAC AAG ATT CGG CCT CTG TGG CGG CAC TAC TTC CAG AAC ACT CAG gtggagtgttgggaggg
gactttctaacccacgggaaaaggtgttaggggcgggagaacagaattgttggcctaggctgggcccccaggcaaggaaaaaacccttcccacttctacccccttctgtttg
gctatcccctactcactcttcagaactcaccttagtcttccccagcttggacttctcttttagaagcaggattctgggacaggctgcctgatttagccctcataacatgtctt
tatttccttgcacatctttggataaactacttcctctttgcagtggggtctctctagtttgtgccatgactcctgtagagcttctatagagttctgtaaacttctgtagagttta
ctagatgagaaggattgacacaattacaaatgggaagaaaacagaaagggccacactacggtatgtcccaggcagaagtgattgcttctccttctcctttcctttcctgccca
     Gly Leu Ile Phe Val Val Asp Ser Asn Asp Arg Glu Arg Val Gln Glu Ser Ala Asp Glu Leu Gln Lys Met>
g GGC CTC ATC TTT GTG GTG GAC AGT AAT GAC CGG GAG CGG GTC CAA GAA TCT GCT GAT GAA CTC CAG AAG ATG gtgagtacccagagc
cctgggaactgagccctcagcttggggacagagtgatctctgcagtggtatagaagtcagggagccccaacaggcattgaagacctggaatataagttttttctttgtggaca
gacacattgtgtatctcaccctgtttggatgggagtgacttttttcacttttctgtgcattgtcttgtcttttttttttttttgaaatgggagttttgctgttgttgcccagg
ctggagttgcaatggtgcaatctcggctcactgcaacctccgtctcccgggttcaagcaattctccggcctcagcctcccaagtagctgggattacaggcgcccgctgccatg
cccagttaattttgtatttttagtanagacgggggtttcaccatgttggccaggctggtcttgaacccccaacctcaggtgatccacccgtcttggtctcccaaagtgctggg
attacaggagtgagccactgcgcccggccgcattctcntgtccttttacatctgagtctgagaagttgtgggagagatgggacttatatgtgcaaagagaaacattttacattc
ctgcctttttccatttggaaatgttgtcatttgtgcctaggcaagtactcaaattaggaaaaggtctttcttttctggacttatgggctcaggtcacctcaagctcatttacaac
tatgtcttgtcttcaacggcagactgcacaatactttttttttccaatcaagatgctaggaggtagaaagggagttccccaacacgatagaggagacgcagcctgggtcccac
                   Leu Gln Glu Asp Glu Leu Arg Asp Ala Val Leu Leu Val Phe Ala Asn Lys Gln Asp Met Pro Asn Ala
cttctcttctcctctcag CTG CAG GAG GAC GAG CTG CGG GAT GCA GTG CTG CTG GTA TTT GCC AAC AAG CAG GAC ATG CCC AAC GCC
Met Pro Val Ser Glu Glu Leu Thr Asp Lys Leu Gly Leu Gln His Leu Arg Ser Arg Thr>
ATG CCC GTG AGC GAG CTG ACT GAC AAG CTG GGG CTA CAG CAC TTA CGC AGC CGC ACG gtagggtcctgcccacctggtgctgaatcctgcctc
                                                                     Trp Tyr Val Gln Ala Thr
ttgagggaagctgcaggctgggacagagatataaaggcattcctttgttcctggttgctgacctcttcttttccttttccccacag TGG TAT GTC CAG GCC ACC
Cys Ala Thr Gln Gly Thr Gly Leu Tyr Asp Gly Leu Asp Trp Leu Ser His Glu Leu Ser Lys Arg ***
TGT GCC ACC CAA GGC ACA GGT CTG TAC GAT GGT CTG GAC TGG CTG TCC CAC GAG CTG TCA AAG CGC taa ccagccaggggcaggcccctg
atgcccggaagctcctgcgtgcatccccggggtgaccagactcccggactcctcaggcagtgcccttctctcccacttttcctcccccatagccacaggcctctgctcctgct
cctgcctgcatgttctctctgttgttggagcctggagccttgctctctgggcacagaggggtccactctcctgcctgctgggacctatggaaggggcttcctggccaaggccc
cctcttccagaggaggagcagggatctgggtttcctttttttttttctgtttgggtgtactctaggggccaggttgggaggggggaagggcttcgggtggtgctataat
gtggcactggatcttgagtaataaatttgctgtggtttg
```

FIGURE 4-1. (A) Schematic drawing representing the overall structure of a typical gene. The gene depicted is the human ADP-ribosylation factor 5 (ARF5) gene with exon and intron sizes drawn approximately to scale. Nucleotide sequence has been determined for the main portion of the gene (solid line) but is unavailable for part of the flanking regions (dashed line). The 5' flanking region contains the promoter—the region of the DNA to which an RNA polymerase binds to initiate transcription (production of messenger RNA). Exons contain the information that is translated into the amino acid sequence of the gene product (protein), whereas introns (intervening sequences) are removed from the messenger RNA and thus do not encode amino acid sequence. The 3' flanking region contains the polyadenylation signal that functions in processing the messenger RNA transcript once it has been synthesized. (B) Nucleotide sequence of the human ARF5 gene with exons depicted in uppercase letters and introns/flanking regions in lowercase letters. The predicted amino acid sequence (abbreviated) is listed above the corresponding DNA sequence, the termination codon is indicated by asterisks, and the polyadenylation signal (aataaa) is underlined. Reprinted with permission of Academic Press from McGuire et al (94).

Identification and Analysis of DNA Sequence Variation

Once potential candidate genes have been identified, through either a compilation of genes of known function or a genome scan, genetic polymorphisms (variations in the DNA sequence) within these genes may be examined. In the event that the candidate genes have not been well characterized, an exhaustive search must be conducted for DNA variation within the candidate gene region. A variety of scanning techniques is available for the initial detection of unknown mutations (26).

Characterized genetic polymorphisms may be genotyped in a particular study population in one of several ways. *Restriction fragment length polymorphisms (RFLPs)* are genetic variants that occur within a restriction site, a short DNA sequence recognized by restriction enzymes that cut the DNA only at that specific sequence (Figure 4–2). Many copies of the region can be generated by *polymerase chain reaction (PCR)* amplification, followed by restriction enzyme digestion and resolution of the resulting fragments on acrylamide or agarose gels (eg, 27, 28). Polymorphisms that do not occur within restriction sites can be assayed with allele-specific oligonucleotides and the *oligonucleotide*

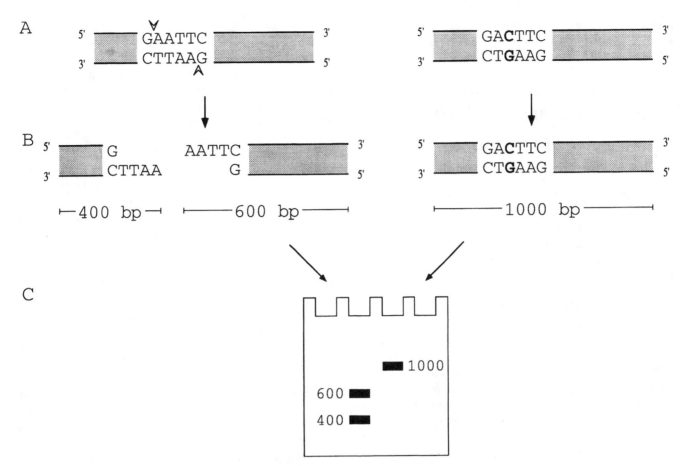

FIGURE 4-2. Representation of a restriction fragment length polymorphism (RFLP). To characterize an RFLP genetic marker, many copies of the DNA region containing the RFLP can be generated using the polymerase chain reaction. (A) A short DNA sequence (5'-GAATTC-3') that is recognized by the restriction enzyme *Eco* RI (isolated from the bacterium *Escherichia coli*) is located within the amplified fragment of DNA on the left. The restriction enzyme will cut both strands of the DNA within this sequence between the bases indicated by open arrowheads. A single base substitution (in bold) has altered the restriction site (5'-GACTTC-3') such that *Eco* RI will not cut the DNA fragment on the right. (B) The fragment on the left has been cut into two smaller fragments. One fragment is 400 base pairs in length whereas the other fragment is 600 base pairs long. The fragment on the right has not been cut and remains 1,000 base pairs long. (C) The fragments resulting from the restriction digestion can be separated and visualized on an agarose or polyacrylamide gel. The DNA is applied to the gel in the wells at the top and migrates toward the bottom of the gel when an electric current is applied. Fragments are separated by size and when visualized produce a characteristic banding pattern.

ligation assay (OLA) (29). Emerging techniques such as genetic bit analysis (GBA) (30) and DNA chip technologies (31, 32), which use miniaturized arrays of custom DNA fragments (DNA chips), are automated, high-throughput methodologies that have the capacity to rapidly generate *genotype* and DNA sequence information.

Genetic polymorphisms can then be analyzed by statistical methods in populations or families with respect to particular outcomes (such as lipoprotein response to diet). For example, association studies compare the frequency of alleles between unrelated individuals who exhibit the phenotype of interest (cases) relative to those who do not (controls). An allele is considered to be associated with a given phenotype if that allele occurs at a significantly higher frequency in the case group relative to the controls (17).

Many genetic polymorphisms identified in population surveys do not alter gene function or expression either be-

cause they do not result in an amino acid substitution in the corresponding protein (silent or synonymous substitutions) or because they occur in noncoding regions of the gene such as introns. However, such markers may be statistically associated with a particular phenotype because they are in *linkage disequilibrium* with true functional mutations. Alleles exhibiting linkage disequilibrium often occur at loci that are physically close to one another (tightly linked) and tend to be inherited together because they are located on the same chromosome.

Transmission disequilibrium tests (TDT) may help avoid some of the potential problems that may be encountered in simple association studies as a result of linkage disequilibrium. Most TDT statistics examine the transmission of alleles from heterozygous parents to those children exhibiting the phenotype of interest. The transmission of an allele associated with the phenotype will be greater than that expected under random (Mendelian) segregation if the marker is located close to the phenotype-associated gene (33, 34).

Dietary and Genetic Influences on Plasma Lipids and Lipoproteins

Metabolic and Genetic Basis of Dietary Cholesterol Responsiveness

Variability among individuals in response to diet-induced hypercholesterolemia has been observed in numerous animal species and has been attributed to a variety of genes that regulate lipid and lipoprotein metabolism. Insights from animal models first suggested the influence of genetic factors in cholesterol responsiveness to diet (35) and have subsequently identified biochemical mechanisms and novel candidate genes that may alter dietary sensitivity (36, 37).

Cholesterol absorption efficiency and alterations in bile acid synthetic capacity appear to be significant correlates of the hypercholesterolemic effect of dietary fat and cholesterol in animals. For example, an inbred substrain of New Zealand white rabbits (CRT/mlo) can markedly upregulate or increase bile acid synthesis in response to a cholesterol challenge. By increasing expression of cholesterol 7 α-hydroxylase, the putative rate-limiting enzyme in bile acid synthesis, CRT/mlo rabbits are able to dispose of excess dietary cholesterol and thus resist hypercholesterolemia and atherosclerosis (38).

Similarly, elevated expression of sterol 27-hydroxylase, another important enzyme regulating bile acid synthesis, appears to mitigate diet-induced hypercholesterolemia in baboons (*Papio* spp.) subjected to a high-cholesterol, high-fat diet (39). African green monkeys (*Cercopithecus aethiops*) may downregulate intestinal cholesterol absorption by reducing bile acid production in response to increased dietary cholesterol. Regulation of cholesterol 7 α-hydroxylase activity and abundance may attenuate bile acid secretion; this may be an important adaptive strategy for reducing cholesterol absorption in nonhuman primate species (40).

Early metabolic studies in humans recognized variability in dietary response among individuals and attempted to quantify intrinsic cholesterol responsiveness to diet (41, 42). Marked heterogeneity of response to dietary cholesterol and fatty acid intake has been consistently observed in virtually all dietary studies despite rigorous dietary control (43–47). For example, increases in LDL-cholesterol (LDL-C) varied from 0% to 62% in young men consuming 80 or 320 mg cholesterol per 1,000 kcal in an otherwise constant diet (47). Similarly, Mistry et al (43) demonstrated that consumption of 1,500 mg cholesterol per day for 2 weeks increased plasma total cholesterol concentrations by 4 to 75 mg/dL in 32 subjects, but in 5 subjects the diet produced no change or a slight decrease in cholesterol. Most studies indicate that approximately 10% of individuals are hyperresponders (ie, show significant changes), whereas a similar proportion exhibit little or no change in plasma cholesterol in response to specific alterations in dietary fat and cholesterol.

Although dietary responsiveness appears to be inversely correlated with habitual cholesterol consumption (a greater response is typically associated with lower baseline cholesterol levels) (48), investigations of individual response to dietary cholesterol suggest that multiple metabolic variables may play a role. These variables may include: failure to downregulate endogenous cholesterol synthesis in response to dietary cholesterol (43, 45, 49); linear increases in cholesterol absorption with increasing dietary cholesterol intake (50); and, in individuals most sensitive to the hypercholesterolemic effects of dietary fat (51), low fractional catabolic (degradation) rates of LDL apoB, suggesting a marked downregulation of hepatic LDL receptors.

The numerous genes involved in the complex pathways of lipoprotein metabolism are likely to contribute to variation in dietary responsiveness (52). Individual responses to changes in dietary fatty acid and cholesterol intake may be driven by genetic factors regulating cholesterol absorption and excretion, chylomicron remnant clearance, and downregulation of the LDL receptor and HMG-CoA reductase. In addition, metabolic responses to dietary change, including alterations in apolipoprotein A-I (apoA-I) and apoB synthesis and the activity of hepatic lipase and lipoprotein lipase, are subject to genetic variation. Increasing knowledge of the human genome and advances in molecular biology are anticipated to uncover novel genes and genetic mechanisms that influence complex phenotypes (53) and provide the framework for testing the involvement of putative candidate genes in dietary response.

Candidate Genes Regulating Plasma Lipid Response to Diet

Numerous studies have reported associations between common genetic variation at the apolipoprotein E (apoE) gene and variation in plasma lipid levels, atherosclerotic involvement, and cardiovascular disease (54–56). ApoE is a key component of plasma lipid metabolism and plays a central role in the catabolism of triglyceride-rich lipoprotein remnants (57). The variant forms of apoE have been shown to effect differences in total serum cholesterol levels because of differential binding affinities for lipoprotein receptors in the liver and differences in the metabolism of lipoproteins.

The average effect of the ε4 allele is to raise total plasma cholesterol levels, possibly through efficient uptake and conversion of lipoprotein particle remnants to LDL (58, 59). Substantial data indicate an association between the ε4 allele and elevated levels of LDL-C and total cholesterol that are strongly related to atherosclerotic potential (60, 61). Conversely, the ε2 allele is often associated with lower plasma cholesterol levels and may thus have a protective effect against the development of coronary disease (62, 63).

Clinical and population studies on the effects of the apoE gene on sensitivity to dietary fat and cholesterol report that the ε4 allele is associated with marked increases in LDL-C in response to dietary cholesterol (64–66). Although Kesaniemi et al (67) reported an increase in cholesterol absorption in subjects with an apoE ε4 allele, inconsistent results have been reported from a number of additional studies, such as Lefevre et al (68), suggesting that multiple genes are involved in determining dietary sensitivity and that the relative physiological effects of these genes may differ among populations (69, 70).

Additional genes that may affect dietary fat and cholesterol absorption and/or influence lipoprotein metabolism include apolipoprotein A-IV (apoA-IV), apolipoprotein B (apoB), and lipoprotein lipase. A glutamine → histidine substitution (Gln360His) near the C-terminus of the apoA-IV protein distinguishes apoA-IV-1 and apoA-IV-2 alleles that are present in white populations at frequencies of approximately 90% and 8%, respectively (71). The glutamine (in the apoA-IV-1 form) → histidine (in apoA-IV-2) amino acid substitution adds a positive charge to the apoA-IV protein but does not appear to alter its primary or secondary structure. The average effect of the A-IV-2 allele is to raise high-density cholesterol (HDL) and to lower triglyceride levels (72). A recent dietary-modification study (73) suggested that the A-IV-2 allele may attenuate short-term hypercholesterolemic responses to high levels of dietary cholesterol.

Genetic variation within the apoB gene is associated with alterations in plasma lipid and triglyceride levels and is also linked to obesity, high cholesterol levels, and an increased risk of coronary artery disease (74, 75). Specific mutations in apoB may alter the binding affinity of low-density lipoproteins for the low-density lipoprotein receptor and thus significantly affect rates of LDL catabolism and clearance (76, 77). Individuals homozygous for the absence of an *Xba* I restriction site in the apoB gene appear to exhibit the greatest sensitivity to dietary saturated fat and cholesterol (69). However, the precise mechanism for the relationship between the *Xba* I polymorphism and dietary sensitivity remains unclear because the site does not appear to alter the receptor binding region of apoB.

Susceptibility to hypertriglyceridemia in response to obesity and alcohol intake also appears to be influenced by genetic factors. For example, a mutation in the lipoprotein lipase gene that causes asparagine to be replaced by serine at position 291 may predispose individuals to elevated plasma triglyceride levels in conjunction with certain physiological characteristics such as increased body mass index (BMI) (78).

High-Density Lipoprotein Turnover Studies

Environmental and hormonal influences account for a significant fraction of the variance for HDL-cholesterol (HDL-C) in the general population; however, family studies provide evidence that genetic factors are also important. Twin studies have shown a much higher correlation between HDL-C levels in MZ twins (0.68–0.74) relative to DZ twin pairs (0.34–0.46) (79–81).

A series of lipoprotein turnover studies in the laboratory of one of the authors (De Oliveira) has been examining the genetic and environmental influences of HDL-C response to diet by studying HDL turnover (a measure of HDL metabolism) under metabolic ward conditions in MZ and DZ twins. Intrapair correlations can be more accurately estimated in an inpatient setting because environmental variables can be minimized and repeat sampling can be conducted. The HDL turnover studies evaluate healthy individuals with various HDL levels to determine the relative contributions of synthesis and catabolism of HDL proteins in determining plasma HDL levels. During the 4-week trials, subjects consume a carefully controlled (metabolic) diet, receive a protein tracer injection, and donate blood and urine samples on an approximately daily basis during the final 2 weeks of the diet period. Information about the logistical aspects of conducting dietary studies with twins is provided in Tables 4–3 and 4–4.

Differences in the intrapair correlations for a given parameter such as the rate of HDL metabolism between MZ and DZ twins can be used to estimate heritability. Heritability estimates use MZ and DZ twins to determine the relative contribution of genetic factors to a particular phenotype under the assumption that the environments for both identical and fraternal twins are similar. However, this assumption may not be valid because identical twins are often subjected to more similar microenvironments (diet, activity, education) than fraternal twins and may even have a greater similarity of dietary habits. In fact, food and nutrient intake may be influenced by the genetic background of the individual. Dairy products, for example, are eaten less often by persons with lactase deficiency. Genetic mechanisms also may affect food selection apart from the components of total energy intake that are related to body weight and energy requirement; the distribution of dietary energy among macronutrient sources (ie, protein, fat, and carbohydrate) has been reported as more similar in MZ twins than in DZ twins (82). (Also see reference 81.)

Furthermore, twin studies have traditionally been conducted with free-living individuals not subject to dietary control or repeat sampling. Violation of the identical environments assumption and lack of dietary control may affect the intrapair correlations and may bias (inflate) estimates of genetic heritability. Despite the possibility that MZ twins may share a more similar environment than DZ twins, twin studies are highly suggestive of genetic influences on HDL-C levels.

Heritability Estimates, Sample Sizes, and Power Calculations

Heritability estimates have been used extensively to examine the genetic components of a broad range of phenotypes, and a variety of complex traits and disease syndromes have been

TABLE 4-3

Challenges of Conducting Controlled Diet Studies with Twins

Issues and Implications	Relevant Information and Potential Solutions
Twins are relatively rare in populations: It can be difficult to recruit adequate numbers to achieve sufficient statistical power within a satisfactory time frame. Recruiting activities may require extra time, money, and labor.	Twins comprise about 1% of live births. The rate of twinning varies according to ethnic group and geographical region, a factor that can affect recruitment strategies.
	Demographically diverse study populations should be recruited for twin studies, as for other research projects, unless justified on scientific grounds.
	Recruitment techniques for twin studies include: advertisements in local and national newspapers, magazines, and radio stations; signs posted at colleges and hospitals; informal "word-of-mouth" referrals from enrolled participants; recruitment materials included in mailings from twins organizations; and materials distributed at information booths at national twins meetings.
	Accrual of twin pairs can be slow, with consequences for budget, personnel, data collection, and interpretation and publication of results. Slow accrual indicates that recruitment efforts, and possibly the scientific goals of the protocol, should be evaluated.
	Recruitment materials can highlight (in realistic terms) the unique opportunities and benefits of participation, such as: confirming zygosity status, learning about personal health and medical situations, experiencing once more a common living situation with their twin (perhaps after years of being geographically separated).
	Twins may be surprisingly receptive to participation in research protocols because they often have long experience of other people's curiosity and may even have a sense of being a part of a "natural experiment."
Study outcomes usually require complete data for both twins: If one twin leaves the study, the partial data for both twins would not be usable in most cases. Screening procedures thus must ensure that both twins are eligible and likely to complete the study. Management techniques to enhance compliance and retention are critical to prevent loss of data.	Recruitment for twin studies is rendered more difficult than for other types of controlled diet studies by the requirements that both members of the pair must fit the eligibility criteria and be able and willing to participate.
	The obstacles to enrollment of twins are similar to those faced by other individuals. These include family commitments, financial problems, work schedules, reluctance to undergo study procedures, and unwillingness to eat the study food.
	Logistical support with arrangements may help potential participants to overcome difficulties in enrollment. This support structure may include providing transportation subsidies, allowing spouses and relatives to visit periodically and to stay nearby, providing long-distance telephone services, and covering other expenses associated with participating.
	Financial incentives may be helpful if allowed by the research institution.
	Family social obligations (such as weddings and graduations) or emergencies (such as sickness or death) are likely to affect both members of a twin pair. Allowing a one-day absence with prepacked study meals can help to address such situations.

Continued

shown to have significant heritable components. These estimates are expressed as h^2, which is derived from the fraction of trait variance caused by heritable factors. Values range from 0 (no genetic contribution) to 1 (complete genetic control). Assuming a trait is 100% genetic ($h^2 = 1$), the correlation between DZ twins would be 50% of the correlation between MZ twins. However, if a trait were not influenced by genetic factors ($h^2 = 0$), correlations between MZ and DZ twins would be identical. To estimate statistical power in the HDL-C study mentioned earlier, the heritability

TABLE 4-3

Issues and Implications	Relevant Information and Potential Solutions
	Particular care must be exercised in the initial selection of participants. A thorough medical and social history often will help researchers in identifying which twins can be considered for enrollment, and whether problems are likely to develop. The twin pair must be considered as the unit of recruitment, and both individuals must be good candidates for compliance and retention. It is prudent to require a series of "run-in" activities that will evaluate the cooperation of both members; these may include attending clinic visits, participating in interviews, filling out questionnaires, and eating several sample study meals.
	The potential subjects should be provided with a detailed explanation of all study protocols. The importance of good compliance should be discussed in detail.
Identification errors are likely to occur: Monozygotic twins are expected to be visually identical, but dizygotic twins also can look very much alike. Twins also often have similar-sounding names with identical first and last initials. Misidentification errors thus can occur during the distribution of food and medication and during the collection and labeling of biological samples such as blood or urine.	Conduct rigorous training for staff regarding the rationale of the protocol and the procedures involved. This should include advance consideration of procedures and activities susceptible to error.
	Hold a joint briefing for subjects and staff before the study begins, including question and answer sessions. This enhances the psychological "investment" of the subjects in the outcome of the study.
	Expand the role of subjects to include an appropriate degree of responsibility for their own protocols. This can include checking labels and procedure times and telling the staff about misidentifications.
	Build safeguards into the protocol, study materials, and procedures, including: double-checking labels and verifying names before distributing food and medications and conducting procedures; using full first and last names, rather than initials, for labeling food items, sample tubes, etc; establishing unique identifiers for collected samples; color-coding dietary treatments, food and medicine labels, and other items.
	Labeling or identification errors made with one twin probably will be repeated with the other twin (for example, in providing food items or timing blood draws).
Each twin has individual rights as a research subject: Decisions to participate or withdraw must be made independently by each twin.	Investigators must guard against coercive pressures either from the co-twin or from members of the research team.
	Respect for the individual integrity of each member of the twin pair must be maintained; staff should avoid referring to participants as "the twins" or "the set."

The information presented in this table draws on the experience of one of the authors (De Oliveira) at the General Clinical Research Center, Rockefeller University, New York, NY, in conducting controlled feeding studies in twins.

of HDL-C was hypothesized to be 0.5–1.0. Given this assumption, a sensitivity analysis ensured that the study possessed adequate power to detect differences between MZ and DZ twin intrapair correlations at a significance level of $P < 0.05$.

Fisher's Z transformation may be used to evaluate the null hypothesis (H_0: $r_{MZ} = r_{DZ}$) that the intrapair correlation coefficients for MZ (r_{MZ}) and DZ (r_{DZ}) twins are identical (83). The distribution of this quantity is approximately normal with a mean of $\frac{1}{2}\log_e[(1 + r)/(1-r)]$ and a variance of $1/(n-3)$. H_0 represents a simple test that compares two

normally distributed statistics with known variances $1/(n_{MZ}-3)$ and $1/(n_{DZ}-3)$ using the following formula:

$$Z = \frac{\frac{1}{2}\log_e \left(\frac{1 + r_{MZ}}{1 - r_{MZ}} \right) - \frac{1}{2}\log_e \left(\frac{1 + r_{DZ}}{1 - r_{DZ}} \right)}{\sqrt{\frac{1}{n_{MZ}-3} + \frac{1}{n_{DZ}-3}}}$$

The experimental design used equal numbers of MZ and DZ twins. Assuming $r_{MZ} > r_{DZ}$, the Z for the one sided al-

TABLE 4-4

Registries and National Organizations for the Identification and Recruitment of Twins

Organization Name and Address	Telephone/Fax/E-mail Address/Internet Address
International Twins Association (ITA) 6898 Channel Road Minneapolis, MN 55432	Telephone: (612) 571-3022
The Twins Foundation PO Box 6043 Providence, RI 02940-6043	Telephone: (401) 729-1000 Fax: (401) 751-4642 E-mail: twins@twinsfoundation.com Internet: http://www.twinsfoundation.com
National Organization of Mothers of Twins Clubs (NOMOTC) PO Box 23188 Albuquerque, NM 87192-1188	Telephone: (505) 275-0955 or (800) 243-2276 Internet: http://www.nomotc.org
Parents of Multiple Births Association of Canada (POMBA) 240 Graff Ave, Box 22005 Stratford, Ontario, Canada N5A 7V6	Telephone: (519) 272-2203 Fax: (519) 272-1926 E-mail: office@pomba.org Internet: http://www.pomba.org
Twins Days Festival Committee, Inc PO Box 29 Twinsburg, OH 44087	Telephone: (330) 425-3652 Fax: (330) 426-7280

Note: Many twin registries and other similar organizations require that information provided for research purposes be kept confidential. Written consent for use of the information may be required. Some organizations have committees that review and approve research proposals seeking to recruit from their membership. Once approved, the recruitment requests are posted in newsletters and other publications.

ternative was 1.645 at $\alpha = 0.05$. We estimated r_{MZ} to be 0.90 based on preliminary data from 12 MZ twin pairs where the intrapair correlations (under our experimental conditions) were 0.94 for LDL and 0.92 for HDL (84). Under the assumption that $h^2 = 1.0$, r_{DZ} was determined to be 0.45. Substituting these values into the above equation yielded a value for n of 8.55. Similarly, under the assumption that $h^2 = 0.50$, $r_{DZ} = 0.68$ and $n = 15.72$. Therefore, a sample size of 16 MZ and 16 DZ twins was predicted to be adequate to detect 50% heritability of LDL-C, HDL-C, and any other parameters in the protocol given that the assumption $r_{MZ} = 0.90$ is valid.

ETHICAL AND SOCIAL ISSUES IN GENETIC STUDIES OF DIETARY RESPONSE

Participant Recruitment

Target Individuals and Exclusion Criteria

Recruitment strategies for genetic studies of dietary response depend on the specific research questions of the particular study. Experimental designs should include both men and women with adequate representation of minority groups.

Often it may be advisable to conduct separate analyses on men and women if there are fundamental gender-specific differences in the etiology and/or pathophysiology of the parameter(s) of interest. Under special circumstances, single-gender studies may be appropriate to investigate phenotypes influenced by sex hormones, such as the effects of estrogen on the genesis of osteoporosis. Medical history and laboratory screening should be conducted to evaluate the overall health status of potential participants. A variety of general exclusion criteria such as the presence of renal, hepatic, hematologic, and immunologic disorders may be appropriate. Specific exclusion criteria for metabolic studies should include alcohol consumption and use of medications known to alter physiological levels of compounds associated with the phenotype under study.

Verifying Family Relationships

Misspecification of family relationships can be problematic in genetic studies and is of particular concern when twins or sibling pairs are examined. Unreported half-sibling ("half-sib") relationships are often readily evident in nuclear families as departures from Mendelian segregation (the child in question will possess alleles not present in either of the purported parents). However, it may be difficult to determine the actual biological relationships between two individuals believed to be full siblings ("full-sibs") if no additional family members (particularly parents) are available. One method, which can be used with data from genome-wide scans that examine many highly polymorphic markers, is to compare the distributions of alleles for the individuals in question with the distributions of alleles observed for known true full-sibling pairs. Alleles *identical by state* will be found more frequently among true full-sibs than among half-sibs (20).

Zygosity determination is an important issue in twin studies because misclassification of twins will bias the resulting heritability estimates. Zygosity has traditionally been determined by self-description and direct observation of physical similarity (85). Initial screenings of study subjects customarily include queries regarding the degree of physical similarity among siblings (ie, questions about whether they are repeatedly confused by family members and friends, or whether they are considered like "two peas in a pod"; positive answers often suggest monozygosity) (86, 87). Although these methods have been frequently used and found to be fairly reliable (88), questionnaires and self-reports may be inconclusive. A more accurate approach would include verification of zygosity status by molecular genetic techniques. Previous investigations used blood group typings or other serological markers, but with the advent and rapid development of DNA-based "fingerprinting" technologies (reviewed in 89), more robust and reliable approaches are now available.

Informed Consent

Within the scientific community it is generally accepted that adequate informed consent must be obtained when investigators conduct research. This includes informing prospective participants that biological specimens (tissue, blood, saliva, or other bodily fluids that can serve as a source of DNA) will be used for genetic analyses. Informed consent procedures use easily understood language to disclose detailed information regarding: the nature and objectives of the research project, potential risks and anticipated benefits that may result from participation, future contact for additional information, the extent to which confidentiality of all research data including genetic results will be maintained, and procedures that will be implemented to minimize inadvertent release of personal information (90, 91).

Participants are told that they have the right to refuse to enroll in the study, as well as the option to withdraw at any time in the future. They are apprised of their right to make specific inquiries about the investigation should they choose to participate. Information is also provided to prospective subjects regarding the conditions for long-term storage of biological samples and potential future use of their DNA in research that may be unrelated to the objectives of the present investigation (92). Informed consent may not be required for retrospective access to residual samples previously collected in conjunction with clinical care, provided the samples are anonymous (lack identifiers) or are anony-

mized (identifiers removed). Once potential participants have been adequately informed, agreements to participate in the research should be strictly voluntary and should be obtained under conditions free of coercion and undue influence. (Note: Other aspects of informed consent and research ethics are discussed in Chapter 5, "Ethical Considerations in Dietary Studies.")

Ethics and Issues of Confidentiality

There is growing public concern regarding the confidentiality of personal medical and genetic information that may be generated as a consequence of participation in research programs. Research records and the identity of program participants must be strictly controlled by the investigators and must remain confidential on publication of research findings. Although ordinary clinical results such as measurements of blood pressure and cholesterol levels are typically provided to each participant (or to his or her personal physician with written permission), genetic findings should not be incorporated into the medical records of participants. Privacy and strict confidentiality of the genetic data are necessary to prevent personal and social stigmatization as well as possible discrimination in insurance or employment (93).

Participants are not usually given the option to receive genetic information about themselves. However, the ability to obtain personal information may be medically beneficial to the participant as well as his/her family. The benefit occurs because individuals who know that they have a genetic predisposition to disease may choose to make beneficial lifestyle changes (selecting a more healthful diet, increasing physical activity, discontinuing tobacco and alcohol use) or to seek preventive treatments that may decrease their risk of developing symptoms. Conversely, such information may lead to ethical dilemmas and difficult personal or reproductive decisions. Personal genetic information should therefore be presented by a certified genetic health care professional or genetic counselor who can educate the subjects as to the benefits and limitations of molecular diagnostic tests and provide counsel regarding therapeutic options or personal issues.

CONCLUSION

The effects of genetic variation on individual response to dietary change often are of interest in nutrition studies, even if this is not the primary focus of the investigation. Consideration of appropriate and specific genetic effects is likely to enhance the study overall and may strengthen or corroborate the main conclusions. Interactions may be detected between changes in metabolic parameters and genetic variables, which then may provide insight into the interpretation of discrepant outcomes. Even in large family- or population-based dietary studies that do not examine genetic factors, it is of paramount importance to properly collect and store biological samples (blood samples or buccal swabs) that may serve as a source of DNA for future retrospective examinations of gene-nutrient interactions. Likewise it is vital to obtain proper informed consent that will allow for possible future genetic research.

Novel candidate genes for a variety of complex phenotypes and human diseases are likely to emerge as the Human Genome Project advances and methods for mapping and characterizing genes become more refined. Because most dietary response phenotypes appear to be influenced by multiple genes (each with a relatively small effect) that may interact with other genes and/or the environment, continuing developments in genome technology and statistical methods of analysis will aid our ability to decipher the complexities of dietary response in humans.

GLOSSARY OF TERMS

Alleles: alternate forms of a gene or genetic locus that differ in DNA sequence. Such differences may or may not affect the function of the RNA or protein product.

Candidate genes: genes believed to influence the expression of complex phenotypes because of known biological and/or physiological properties of their products.

Genome-wide scan: scans used to localize genes contributing to complex diseases by analyzing many highly polymorphic DNA markers spaced at approximately regular intervals throughout the genome. Statistical (linkage) analyses are then used to identify one or more chromosomal regions in which susceptibility genes are believed to reside.

Genotype: the genetic constitution of an organism. The term is often used to refer to the identity of the two alleles at a specific gene or genetic locus.

Heritability (h^2): for a quantitative trait, the proportion of the total phenotypic variation that is attributable to genetic factors. Heritability in the broad sense represents the degree to which a trait is genetically determined; heritability in the narrow sense is the degree to which a trait is transmitted from parents to offspring.

Identity by state (IBS): alleles are considered to be identical by state if they appear to be identical (for example, alleles at microsatellite markers may appear to be the same size and hence inferred to be identical). Conversely, alleles are identical by descent (IBD) if they are descended from the same allele in an ancestral generation. For linkage analyses, IBD information is more informative than IBS.

Linkage analysis: linkage between a genetic marker and a disease susceptibility gene is detected when specific forms (alleles) of the marker and the gene are inherited together (cosegregate) more often than would be expected by chance and is caused by the close proximity of the marker and the gene on a chromosome.

Linkage disequilibrium: the nonrandom transmission from parents to offspring of alleles from genes that are located on the same chromosome. Alleles at tightly linked (located close together) loci are often inherited together; therefore linkage disequilibrium is useful for identifying regions of the genome that historically have been inherited as a linkage group and may identify the approximate location of genes that contribute to disease.

Oligonucleotide ligation assay (OLA): a gel-free assay normally used to characterize known biallelic polymorphisms in a large population. Oligonucleotides (short synthetic fragments of DNA) that are specific to each form of the DNA sequence (each allele) at a particular genetic locus are used to determine the allelic composition of that locus in a large number of individuals.

Phenotype: the observable physical appearance or other properties of an organism that are primarily determined by the genotype but may be influenced by the environment.

Polymerase chain reaction (PCR): a method that has revolutionized the fields of genetics and molecular biology because it can be used to make many copies of (amplify) a particular region of DNA that can then be used in a number of molecular biology applications.

Restriction fragment length polymorphism (RFLP): a genetic marker based on DNA fragments that differ in length due to the presence or absence of specific sequences (restriction sites) that are recognized by certain enzymes. A restriction enzyme will cut the DNA if its recognition sequence is intact but will be unable to cut the DNA if the restriction site has been altered by a mutation (Figure 4–2).

Segregation analysis: analysis whose objective is to explain the inheritance pattern of a particular trait in families by inferring the number of genes influencing the trait, the relative contribution of these genes to the observed phenotype, frequencies of the "normal" and "disease-associated" alleles, and the proportion of individuals with a given genotype that will exhibit the expected phenotype under specific environmental conditions (penetrance).

Transmission disequilibrium test (TDT): a method used to test for linkage between a genetic marker and a complex phenotype when an association between the phenotype and a genetic variant at the marker has previously been detected. The TDT examines the transmission of the disease-associated allele from a heterozygous parent to an affected child. A particular allele in linkage disequilibrium with the disease susceptibility allele will be transmitted more frequently to affected children than would be expected if all alleles were transmitted randomly.

REFERENCES

1. Clarke SD, Abraham S. Gene expression: nutrient control of pre- and posttranscriptional events. *FASEB J.* 1992;6:3146–3152.
2. Kuczmarski RJ, Flegal KM, Campbell SM, Johnson CL. Increasing prevalence of overweight among US adults. The National Health and Nutrition Examination Surveys, 1960 to 1991. *JAMA.* 1994;272:205–211.
3. Manson JE, Colditz GA, Stampfer MJ, Willett WC, Rosner B, Monson RR, Speizer FE, Hennekens CH. A

prospective study of obesity and risk of coronary heart disease in women. *N Engl J Med.* 1990;322:882–889.

4. Kissebah AH, Freedman DS, Peiris AN. Health risks of obesity. *Med Clin North Am.* 1989;73:111–138.

5. Després JP, Moorjani S, Lupien PJ, Tremblay A, Nadeau A, Bouchard C. Regional distribution of body fat, plasma lipoproteins, and cardiovascular disease. *Arteriosclerosis.* 1990;10:497–511.

6. Johnson D, Prud'homme D, Després JP, Nadeau A, Tremblay A, Bouchard C. Relation of abdominal obesity to hyperinsulinemia and high blood pressure in men. *Int J Obes Relat Metab Disord.* 1992;16:881–890.

7. Bouchard C, Rice T, Lemieux S, Després J-P, Pérusse L, Rao DC. Major gene for abdominal visceral fat area in the Québec Family Study. *Int J Obes Relat Metab Disord.* 1996;20:420–427.

8. Rice T, Pérusse L, Bouchard C, Rao DC. Familial clustering of abdominal visceral fat and total fat mass: the Quebec Family Study. *Obes Res.* 1996;4:253–261.

9. Bouchard C, Tremblay A, Després JP, Nadeau A, Lupien PJ, Thériault G, Dussault J, Moorjani S, Pinault S, Fournier G. The response to long-term overfeeding in identical twins. *N Engl J Med.* 1990;322:1477–1482.

10. Chagnon YC, Pérusse L, Bouchard C. The human obesity gene map: the 1997 update. *Obes Res.* 1998;6:76–92.

11. Chagnon YC, Pérusse L, Bouchard C. Familial aggregation of obesity, candidate genes, and quantitative trait loci. *Curr Opin Lipidol.* 1997;8:205–211.

12. Postma DS, Meyers DA. Approaches to family studies of asthma. In: Liggett SB, Meyers DA, eds. *The Genetics of Asthma.* New York, NY: Marcel Dekker, Inc; 1996:443–453.

13. Feinleib M, Garrison RJ, Fabsitz R, Christian JC, Hrubec Z, Borhani NO, Kannel WB, Rosenman R, Schwartz JT, Wagner JO. The NHLBI twin study of cardiovascular disease risk factors: methodology and summary of results. *Am J Epidemiol.* 1977;106:284–295.

14. Austin MA, Newman B, Selby JV, Edwards K, Mayer EJ, Krauss RM. Genetics of LDL subclass phenotypes in women twins: concordance, heritability, and commingling analysis. *Arterioscler Thromb.* 1993;13:687–695.

15. Duffy DL. Twin studies in medical research. *Lancet.* 1993;341:1418–1419.

16. Phillips DI. Twin studies in medical research: can they tell us whether diseases are genetically determined? *Lancet.* 1993;341:1008–1009.

17. Khoury MJ, Beaty TH, Cohen BH. *Fundamentals of Genetic Epidemiology.* Cambridge, UK: Cambridge University Press; 1993.

18. Lusis AJ. Genetic factors affecting blood lipoproteins: the candidate gene approach. *J Lipid Res.* 1988;29:397–429.

19. Hajjar DP, Nicholson AC. Atherosclerosis: an understanding of the cellular and molecular basis of the disease promises new approaches for its treatment in the near future. *Am Scientist.* 1995;83:460–467.

20. Hanis CL, Boerwinkle E, Chakraborty R, Ellsworth DL, Concannon P, Stirling B, Morrison VA, Wapelhorst B, Spielman RS, Gogolin-Ewens KJ, Shephard JM, Williams SR, Risch N, Hinds D, Iwasaki N, Ogata M, Omori Y, Petzold C, Rietzsch H, Schröder H-E, Schulze J, Cox NJ, Menzel S, Boriraj VV, Chen X, Lim LR, Lindner T, Mereu LE, Wang Y-Q, Xiang K, Yamagata K, Yang Y, Bell GI. A genome-wide search for human non-insulin-dependent (type 2) diabetes genes reveals a major susceptibility locus on chromosome 2. *Nat Genet.* 1996;13:161–166.

21. Nichols WC, Koller DL, Slovis B, Foroud T, Terry VH, Arnold ND, Siemieniak DR, Wheeler L, Phillips JA 3rd, Newman JH, Conneally PM, Ginsburg D, Loyd JE. Localization of the gene for familial primary pulmonary hypertension to chromosome 2q31–32. *Nat Genet.* 1997;15:277–280.

22. Ott J. *Analysis of Human Genetic Linkage.* Baltimore, Md: Johns Hopkins University Press; 1991.

23. Weeks DE, Lange K. The affected-pedigree-member method of linkage analysis. *Am J Hum Genet.* 1988;42:315–326.

24. Amos CI. Robust variance-components approach for assessing genetic linkage in pedigrees. *Am J Hum Genet.* 1994;54:535–543.

25. Risch N, Zhang H. Extreme discordant sib pairs for mapping quantitative trait loci in humans. *Science.* 1995;268:1584–1589.

26. Landegren U, ed. *Laboratory Protocols for Mutation Detection.* Oxford, UK: Oxford University Press; 1996.

27. Hixson JE, Vernier DT. Restriction isotyping of human apolipoprotein E by gene amplification and cleavage with *Hha* I. *J Lipid Res.* 1990;31:545–548.

28. Frosst P, Blom HJ, Milos R, Goyette P, Sheppard CA, Matthews RG, Boers GJH, den Heijer M, Kluijtmans LAJ, van den Heuvel LP, Rozen R. A candidate genetic risk factor for vascular disease: a common mutation in methylenetetrahydrofolate reductase. *Nat Genet.* 1995;10:111–113.

29. Nickerson DA, Kaiser R, Lappin S, Stewart J, Hood L, Landegren U. Automated DNA diagnostics using an ELISA-based oligonucleotide ligation assay. *Proc Natl Acad Sci USA.* 1990;87:8923–8927.

30. Nikiforov TT, Rendle RB, Goelet P, Rogers YH, Kotewicz ML, Anderson S, Trainor GL, Knapp MR. Genetic bit analysis: a solid phase method for typing single nucleotide polymorphisms. *Nucleic Acids Res.* 1994;22:4167–4175.

31. Hacia JG, Brody LC, Chee MS, Fodor SPA, Collins FS. Detection of heterozygous mutations in *BRCA1* using high-density oligonucleotide arrays and two-colour fluorescence analysis. *Nat Genet.* 1996;14:441–447.

32. Woolley AT, Sensabaugh GF, Mathies RA. High-speed DNA genotyping using microfabricated capillary array electrophoresis chips. *Anal Chem.* 1997;69:2181–2186.

33. Spielman RS, McGinnis RE, Ewens WJ. Transmission test for linkage disequilibrium: the insulin gene region and insulin-dependent diabetes mellitus (IDDM). *Am J Hum Genet.* 1993;52:506–516.

34. Thomson G. Mapping disease genes: family-based association studies. *Am J Hum Genet.* 1995;57:487–498.

35. Clarkson TB, Lofland HB Jr, Bullock BC, Goodman HO. Genetic control of plasma cholesterol: studies on squirrel monkeys. *Arch Pathol.* 1971;92:37–45.

36. McGill HC Jr, Kushwaha RS. Individuality of lipemic responses to diet. *Can J Cardiol.* 1995;11 (suppl G): 15G-27G.

37. Kushwaha RS, McGill HC Jr. Mechanisms controlling lipemic responses to dietary lipids. *World Rev Nutr Diet.* 1997;80:82–125.

38. Poorman JA, Buck RA, Smith SA, Overturf ML, Loose-Mitchell DS. Bile acid excretion and cholesterol 7 α-hydroxylase expression in hypercholesterolemia-resistant rabbits. *J Lipid Res.* 1993;34:1675–1685.

39. Kushwaha RS, Guntupalli B, Rice KS, Carey KD, McGill HC Jr. Effect of dietary cholesterol and fat on the expression of hepatic sterol 27-hydroxylase and other hepatic cholesterol-responsive genes in baboons (*Papio* species). *Arterioscler Thromb Vasc Biol.* 1995;15:1404–1411.

40. Rudel L, Deckelman C, Wilson M, Scobey M, Anderson R. Dietary cholesterol and downregulation of cholesterol 7 α-hydroxylase and cholesterol absorption in African green monkeys. *J Clin Invest.* 1994;93:2463–2472.

41. Jacobs DR Jr, Anderson JT, Hannan P, Keys A, Blackburn H. Variability in individual serum cholesterol response to change in diet. *Arteriosclerosis.* 1983;3:349–356.

42. Keys A, Anderson JT, Grande F. Serum cholesterol response to changes in the diet. III: differences among individuals. *Metabolism.* 1965;14:766–775.

43. Mistry P, Miller NE, Laker M, Hazzard WR, Lewis B. Individual variation in the effects of dietary cholesterol on plasma lipoproteins and cellular cholesterol homeostasis in man: studies of low-density lipoprotein receptor activity and 3-hydroxy-3-methylglutaryl coenzyme A reductase activity in blood mononuclear cells. *J Clin Invest.* 1981;67:493–502.

44. Beynen AC, Katan MB. Reproducibility of the variations between humans in the response of serum cholesterol to cessation of egg consumption. *Atherosclerosis.* 1985;57:19–31.

45. McNamara DJ, Kolb R, Parker TS, Batwin H, Samuel P, Brown CD, Ahrens EH Jr. Heterogeneity of cholesterol homeostasis in man: response to changes in dietary fat quality and cholesterol quantity. *J Clin Invest.* 1987;79: 1729–1739.

46. Zanni EE, Zannis VI, Blum CB, Herbert PN, Breslow JL. Effect of egg cholesterol and dietary fats on plasma lipids, lipoproteins, and apoproteins of normal women consuming natural diets. *J Lipid Res.* 1987;28:518–527.

47. Martin LJ, Connelly PW, Nancoo D, Wood N, Zhang ZJ, Maguire G, Quinet E, Tall AR, Marcel YL, McPherson R. Cholesteryl ester transfer protein and high-density lipoprotein responses to cholesterol feeding in men: relationship to apolipoprotein E genotype. *J Lipid Res.* 1993;34:437–446.

48. Katan MB, Beynen AC. Characteristics of human hypo- and hyperresponders to dietary cholesterol. *Am J Epidemiol.* 1987;125:387–399.

49. Nestel PJ, Poyser A. Changes in cholesterol synthesis and excretion when cholesterol intake is increased. *Metabolism.* 1976;25:1591–1599.

50. Miettinen TA, Kesaniemi YA. Cholesterol absorption: regulation of cholesterol synthesis and elimination and within-population variations of serum cholesterol levels. *Am J Clin Nutr.* 1989;49:629–635.

51. Denke MA, Grundy SM. Individual responses to a cholesterol-lowering diet in 50 men with moderate hypercholesterolemia. *Arch Intern Med.* 1994;154:317–325.

52. Dietschy JM, Turley SD, Spady DK. Role of liver in the maintenance of cholesterol and low-density lipoprotein homeostasis in different animal species, including humans. *J Lipid Res.* 1993;34:1637–1659.

53. Ellsworth DL, Hallman DM, Boerwinkle E. Impact of the human genome project on epidemiologic research. *Epidemiol Rev.* 1997;19:3–13.

54. Menzel H-J, Kladetzky R-G, Assmann G. Apolipoprotein E polymorphism and coronary artery disease. *Arteriosclerosis.* 1983;3:310–315.

55. Kuusi T, Nieminen MS, Ehnholm C, Yki-Järvinen H, Valle M, Nikkilä EA, Taskinen M-R. Apoprotein E polymorphism and coronary artery disease: increased prevalence of apolipoprotein E-4 in angiographically verified coronary patients. *Arteriosclerosis.* 1989;9: 237–241.

56. Hixson JE. Pathobiological Determinants of Atherosclerosis in Youth Research Group. Apolipoprotein E polymorphisms affect atherosclerosis in young males. *Arterioscler Thromb.* 1991;11:1237–1244.

57. Mahley RW. Apolipoprotein E: cholesterol transport protein with expanding role in cell biology. *Science.* 1988;240:622–630.

58. Sing CF, Davignon J. Role of the apolipoprotein E polymorphism in determining normal plasma lipid and lipoprotein variation. *Am J Hum Genet.* 1985;37:268–285.

59. Gregg RE, Zech LA, Schaefer EJ, Stark D, Wilson D, Brewer HB Jr. Abnormal *in vivo* metabolism of apolipoprotein E_4 in humans. *J Clin Invest.* 1986;78:815–821.

60. Sharrett AR, Patsch W, Sorlie PD, Heiss G, Bond MG, Davis CE. Associations of lipoprotein cholesterols, apolipoproteins A-I and B, and triglycerides with carotid atherosclerosis and coronary heart disease. *Arterioscler Thromb.* 1994;14:1098–1104.

61. Wilson PW, Myers RH, Larson MG, Ordovas JM, Wolf PA, Schaefer EJ. Apolipoprotein E alleles, dyslipidemia,

and coronary heart disease: the Framingham Offspring Study. *JAMA.* 1994;272:1666–1671.

62. Boerwinkle E, Utermann G. Simultaneous effects of the apolipoprotein E polymorphism on apolipoprotein E, apolipoprotein B, and cholesterol metabolism. *Am J Hum Genet.* 1988;42:104–112.

63. Davignon J, Gregg RE, Sing CF. Apolipoprotein E polymorphism and atherosclerosis. *Arteriosclerosis.* 1988;8:1–21.

64. Manttari M, Koskinen P, Ehnholm C, Huttunen JK, Manninen V. Apolipoprotein E polymorphism influences the serum cholesterol response to dietary intervention. *Metabolism.* 1991;40:217–221.

65. Gylling H, Miettinen TA. Cholesterol absorption and synthesis related to low-density lipoprotein metabolism during varying cholesterol intake in men with different apoE phenotypes. *J Lipid Res.* 1992;33:1361–1371.

66. Lopez-Miranda J, Ordovas JM, Mata P, Lichtenstein AH, Clevidence B, Judd JT, Schaefer EJ. Effect of apolipoprotein E phenotype on diet-induced lowering of plasma low-density lipoprotein cholesterol. *J Lipid Res.* 1994;35:1965–1975.

67. Kesaniemi YA, Ehnholm C, Miettinen TA. Intestinal cholesterol absorption efficiency in man is related to apoprotein E phenotype. *J Clin Invest.* 1987;80:578–581.

68. Lefevre M, Ginsberg HN, Kris-Etherton PM, Elmer PJ, Stewart PW, Ershow A, Pearson TA, Roheim PS, Ramakrishnan R, Derr J, Gordon DJ, Reed R. ApoE genotype does not predict lipid response to changes in dietary saturated fatty acids in a heterogeneous normolipidemic population: the DELTA Research Group: Dietary Effects on Lipoproteins and Thrombogenic Activity. *Aterioscler Thromb Vasc Biol.* 1997;17(11):2914–2923.

69. Friedlander Y, Berry EM, Eisenberg S, Stein Y, Leitersdorf E. Plasma lipids and lipoproteins response to a dietary challenge: analysis of four candidate genes. *Clin Genet.* 1995;47:1–12.

70. Zambon D, Ros E, Casals E, Sanllehy C, Bertomeu A, Campero I. Effect of apolipoprotein E polymorphism on the serum lipid response to a hypolipidemic diet rich in monounsaturated fatty acids in patients with hypercholesterolemia and combined hyperlipidemia. *Am J Clin Nutr.* 1995;61:141–148.

71. Lohse P, Kindt MR, Rader DJ, Brewer HB Jr. Genetic polymorphism of human plasma apolipoprotein A-IV is due to nucleotide substitutions in the apolipoprotein A-IV gene. *J Biol Chem.* 1990;265:10061–10064.

72. Menzel HJ, Sigurdsson G, Boerwinkle E, Schrangl-Will S, Dieplinger H, Utermann G. Frequency and effect of human apolipoprotein A-IV polymorphism on lipid and lipoprotein levels in an Icelandic population. *Hum Genet.* 1990;84:344–346.

73. McCombs RJ, Marcadis DE, Ellis J, Weinberg RB. Attenuated hypercholesterolemic response to a high-cholesterol diet in subjects heterozygous for the apoli-poprotein A-IV-2 allele. *N Engl J Med.* 1994;331:706–710.

74. Law A, Wallis SC, Powell LM, Pease RJ, Brunt H, Priestley LM, Knott TJ, Scott J, Altman DG, Miller GJ, Rajput J, Miller NE. Common DNA polymorphism within coding sequence of apolipoprotein B gene associated with altered lipid levels. *Lancet.* 1986;1:1301–1303.

75. Rajput-Williams J, Knott TJ, Wallis SC, Sweetnam P, Yarnell J, Cox N, Bell GI, Miller NE, Scott J. Variation of apolipoprotein-B gene is associated with obesity, high blood cholesterol levels, and increased risk of coronary heart disease. *Lancet.* 1988;2:1442–1446.

76. Demant T, Houlston RS, Caslake MJ, Series JJ, Shepherd J, Packard CJ, Humphries SE. Catabolic rate of low density lipoprotein is influenced by variation in the apolipoprotein B gene. *J Clin Invest.* 1988;82:797–802.

77. Corsini A, Fantappie S, Granata A, Bernini F, Catapano AL, Fumagalli R, Romano L, Romano C. Binding-defective low-density lipoprotein in family with hypercholesterolemia. *Lancet.* 1989;1:623.

78. Fisher RM, Mailly F, Peacock RE, Hamsten A, Seed M, Yudkin JS, Beisiegel U, Feussner G, Miller G, Humphries SE, Talmud PJ. Interaction of the lipoprotein lipase asparagine 291 → serine mutation with body mass index determines elevated plasma triacylglycerol concentrations: a study in hyperlipidemic subjects, myocardial infarction survivors, and healthy adults. *J Lipid Res.* 1995;36:2104–2112.

79. McGue M, Rao DC, Iselius L, Russell JM. Resolution of genetic and cultural inheritance in twin families by path analysis: application to HDL-cholesterol. *Am J Hum Genet.* 1985;37:998–1014.

80. Austin MA, King M-C, Bawol RD, Hulley SB, Friedman GD. Risk factors for coronary heart disease in adult female twins. Genetic heritability and shared environmental influences. *Am J Epidemiol.* 1987;125:308–318.

81. De Oliveira e Silva ER, Arnberg R, Seidman CE. Environmental and genetic considerations in plasma lipoprotein levels in identical twins. *Clin Res.* 1992;40:140A.

82. Wade J, Milner J, and Krondl M. Evidence for a physiological regulation of food selection and nutrient intake in twins. *Am J Clin Nutr.* 1981;34:143–147.

83. Kleinbaum DG, Kupper LL. *Applied Regression Analysis and Other Multivariable Methods.* North Situate, Mass: Duxbury Press; 1978.

84. De Oliveira e Silva ER, Brinton EA, Cundey KB, Breslow JL. Heritability of HDL turnover parameters. *Circulation.* 1991;84(supp. II):339.

85. Nichols RC, Bilbro WC Jr. The diagnosis of twin zygosity. *Acta Genet Stat Med.* 1966;16:265–275.

86. Carmelli D, Swan GE, Robinette D, Fabsitz RR. Heritability of substance use in the NAS-NRC Twin Registry. *Acta Genet Med Gemellol (Roma).* 1990;39:91–98.

87. Lykken DT, Bouchard TJ Jr, McGue M, Tellegen A. The Minnesota Twin Family Registry: some initial findings. *Acta Genet Med Gemellol (Roma)*. 1990;39:35–70.

88. Cohen DJ, Dibble E, Grawe JM, Pollin W. Reliably separating identical from fraternal twins. *Arch Gen Psychiatry*. 1975;32:1371–1375.

89. Alford RL, Caskey CT. DNA analysis in forensics, disease and animal/plant identification. *Curr Opin Biotechnol*. 1994;5:29–33.

90. Clayton EW, Steinberg KK, Khoury MJ, Thomson E, Andrews L, Kahn MJE, Kopelman LM, Weiss JO. Informed consent for genetic research on stored tissue samples. *JAMA*. 1995;274:1786–1792.

91. The American Society of Human Genetics. ASHG report: statement on informed consent for genetic research. *Am J Hum Genet*. 1996;59:471–474.

92. Knoppers BM, Laberge CM. Research and stored tissues: persons as sources, samples as persons? *JAMA*. 1995;274:1806–1807.

93. Durfy SJ. Ethics and the Human Genome Project. *Arch Pathol Lab Med*. 1993;117:466–469.

94. McGuire RE, Daiger SP, Green ED. Localization and characterization of the human ADP-ribosylation factor 5 (ARF5) gene. *Genomics*. 1997;41:481–484.

PART 2

Human Factors

CHAPTER 5

ETHICAL CONSIDERATIONS IN DIETARY STUDIES

PHYLLIS E. BOWEN, PHD, RD; AND EVA OBARZANEK, PHD, MPH, RD

The principal investigator and coinvestigators are responsible for the welfare of participants and staff before and during the study, and for a limited time after its completion. This is the guiding principle for all plans and decisions concerning the design and conduct of human studies so that they are ethical and safe. Institutional safeguards and professionalism work together to ensure that studies involving human subjects are ethical and safe, that informed consent is obtained, that data collection and reporting of results follow approved written guidelines (eg, the protocol), that participant confidentiality and privacy are strictly maintained, and that conflicts of interest are avoided. The primary institutional structure supporting these efforts is the institutional review board (IRB). The IRB is the authorized body having oversight over study protocols and other aspects of human research activity, and gives assurances to funding agencies and other parties that research involving humans complies with federal regulations for the protection of human research subjects.

    Professional organizations support ethical conduct by developing and promoting codes of ethics to their members. Safety monitoring committees and external bodies such as data and safety monitoring boards may also be used, mainly in large studies or studies in which the well-being of human subjects must be safeguarded.

Issues of ethics and safety can arise at any step of a human feeding study. By anticipating and developing plans and procedures in advance, unethical situations can be avoided. (Note: Many of the considerations outlined in this chapter will not apply to all studies in all research settings.)

PLANNING THE STUDY

Study Design

When researchers design a study, it is generally desirable to maximize the difference in independent variables to ensure that the study will detect an effect, but the magnitude of the difference often must be tempered in human studies to protect the welfare of study participants. In contrast to animal studies, which may be designed to produce an unhealthy outcome (eg, a deficiency or excess of dietary components), human studies should leave the study participants in no worse health than when they entered the study. Study designs that could produce a potentially adverse biochemical or physiological effect should also offer the participants a post-study corrective period. For example, in a 6-month research study conducted on obese women, the design required participants to maintain their body weights. Because obesity is a health risk, the obese women were required to obtain permission from their physicians to remain obese for that 6-month period. Immediately following the study, these women were provided with weight-reduction counseling (1). In addition, if the correction is included in the research design, more can be learned about the effect being studied.

Three main factors related to participant burden and research risk should be considered when investigators design a study: (1) invasiveness of the specific procedures, (2) malaise, and (3) excessive burden caused by too many measurements, activities, or restrictions.

During the planning phase, investigators must carefully consider the need for invasive procedures and particularly the amount of blood that will be collected. Because studies are expensive, there is a tendency to assess as many outcome variables as possible, which may require drawing a large amount of blood. Although this issue is carefully reviewed by IRBs, it is the investigator's responsibility in planning a study to be even more fastidious than the IRB requirements demand. Investigators often find it difficult, however, to truly appreciate the invasiveness of a procedure purely through "thinking." It thus is wise (when feasible) for investigators to experience the contemplated procedures and also the entire measurement protocol. This helps in making modifications that not only preserve participant well-being but also aid in recruitment and in encouragement of participants once the study has started. Investigators who can honestly say that they have gone through the procedures and have found them tolerable will engender trust and protocol adherence.

In addition to experiencing and understanding the degree of invasiveness, the primary investigator who goes through the entire measurement protocol can also experience the potential overall malaise produced by the procedures. For example, investigators participated in a pilot study designed to assess the absorption and metabolism of β-carotene (2). A small butterfly needle was inserted into a vein in the hand and, after each blood draw, a small amount of heparin-saline solution was injected to keep the blood from clotting in the line (ie, a heparin lock). Blood was taken for 8 hourly draws but the investigators went on with day-to-day work. Although the investigators found the procedures to be quite tolerable that day, the next day they all experienced a small degree of malaise (ie, they were able to work but were not their most productive). In this example, the question of ethics is: how many times in the course of a study must a study participant experience malaise? Investigators who are aware of this effect can make every effort to minimize these occurrences and can point out to potential participants that they may experience days or times of reduced productivity and vitality. When students are participants, it is important to be aware of when they need to be performing at their best (ie, during examinations) and avoid scheduling such collections at those times.

When planning studies, investigators must be aware of the total participant burden. It is easy to make increasing requests of participants either as part of the original study plan or as interesting issues arise during the course of the study. These requests may seem fairly benign on an individual basis; for example, asking subjects to fill out a daily activity sheet, weigh themselves each day and plot their weight, mark down how many snacks they consumed, and fill out a form for each take-out meal. Many of these demands may not be specified in the original informed consent document but are involved in the day-to-day quality control of the study. The sum of the requests, however, can produce an overwhelming participant burden. Symptoms of burden appear as partial responses, sloppy forms, forgetting about forms, and need for constant reminding by staff. It sets up an unhappy study atmosphere for both the participants and the staff, who often are not the ones who decided to manage the study by "filling out forms." The burden to the participant can be minimized by eliminating all but the most necessary data collection and management forms and by having the staff take up as much of this burden as possible. If extra forms are required, the investigator must explain this to all the participants and may need to obtain their consent to the additions.

Principal Investigators

Some investigators avoid human studies in the belief that only physicians should be principally responsible for the welfare of participants. However, many of the classical nutrition studies of healthy individuals have been led by investigators with other doctoral degrees (ie, PhDs). In clinical studies involving patients who suffer from a specific disease, principal investigators may need to be physicians because of the chance that study conditions will compromise the health of the participants. Alternatively, physicians may be named as coinvestigators and directly participate in the study, or they may be named as consultants and provide advice as needed. Regardless of medical background, the principal investigator must be willing to take full responsibility for the welfare of the participants. The main organizational structure that provides principal investigators with guidance and oversight is the IRB. Other organizational structures include safety monitoring committees, independent data and safety monitoring boards, and professional organizations' codes of ethics.

Institutional Review Boards

Each institution, whether hospital, clinic, university, or other research organization, must have its own IRB to review each study protocol and the language of the informed consent document for the propriety of the approach, the physical and psychological safety issues, and the possible risks and benefits to participants. No recruitment of participants or advertisement of the study may commence before IRB approval is obtained. Studies may require the participation of more than one institution. For example, university-based investigators and graduate students may be conducting the study, but one of the measurements or procedures must be carried out in a hospital or clinic facility. IRB approval is usually necessary from both institutions, which often means filling out two completely different sets of forms. Requests for funding from federal sources, trade organizations, or foundations also require IRB approval of protocols before the study is funded.

In order to meet deadlines for grant applications, institutions with experience in grant applications may issue a "pending IRB" document once the application has been submitted to the IRB committee.

In this situation it is anticipated that the investigator's IRB application will be approved during the time period that the grant proposal is under review by the funding agency. This permits the review process to go forward, but funds are withheld until the agency receives documented proof of final IRB approval.

IRBs vary in their operating procedures, in the forms they require, and in the time it takes to grant approval. IRBs also vary in their willingness to allow research studies of various types. It is worthwhile for researchers to learn, in advance, the usual concerns of IRBs and to address them in the protocol. Because IRBs may meet monthly, a month should be allowed for approval and another period of time allowed to answer any questions or concerns of the IRB. Such concerns and requests for changes often relate to the informed consent documents.

In the federal government the Office for Protection from Research Risks (OPRR) is an administrative unit within the Department of Health and Human Services (DHHS). OPPR is organizationally located at the Office of the Director, National Institutes of Health (NIH). The main responsibility of the OPPR is to implement DHHS Regulations for the Protection of Human Subjects (45 CFR 46) and to provide guidance on ethical issues in biomedical or behavioral research (3). In order for human research to be funded by NIH, the research institution must provide written assurance of compliance with DHHS regulations. In addition, the principal investigator must provide evidence that the proposed research has been approved by his or her institution's IRB.

Other Oversight Committees and Guidelines

Oversight committees and professional guidelines assist principal investigators in planning and conducting studies that are ethical and safe.

Safety Monitoring Committee

To ensure the impartial monitoring of participant welfare, longer human studies can benefit from the expertise of a safety monitoring committee. If the principal investigator is not a physician, it is important for the committee to be partially composed of physicians with training appropriate to the evaluation of health effects that study participants might experience. Committees composed of two to four physicians, at least one of whom is actively engaged in research,

can effectively oversee the ethical and safe conduct of a study. This committee may or may not be the same as the oversight committee that may be required for IRB approval of the study.

The chairman of the safety monitoring committee should be empowered to call meetings of the committee at any time with or without the attendance of the study investigators. The major objectives of an oversight or safety monitoring committee are to: (1) review the study protocol for ethical issues and safety, including policies for referrals to health care providers; (2) review the health status of prospective participants in order to protect their interests with regard to participation in the study; and (3) be "on call" for questions concerning ethics and safety during the study.

Investigators can facilitate the performance of the safety monitoring committee by appointing the committee early enough so that substantive protocol changes can be made if necessary. The safety monitoring committee reviews written procedures that specify under what conditions participants should be referred to their own physician or other health care provider for evaluation. The safety monitoring committee also may help evaluate the health status of prospective participants. The principal investigator can assist the committee in this process by providing physical examination information, laboratory values, and screening information about each of the potential participants, and pointing out any particular concerns.

It is rare for all potential participants to have all laboratory values within the normal range, and sometimes other issues arise. When participants are older or have a particular disorder, such as high blood pressure or raised serum cholesterol concentrations, usually a decision must be made about whether the study protocol will in any way jeopardize the potential participants' well-being. In order to have this information available for the safety monitoring committee, investigators should plan for an adequate recruitment and screening period. The more exclusion criteria there are, the greater the difficulty of recruitment and screening. The safety monitoring committee provides an important restraint against the tendency to justify the acceptance of participants into the study in order to meet recruitment goals, especially when finding eligible participants is difficult.

The safety monitoring committee is also helpful in providing advice concerning decisions that must be made during the study. For example, four months into a study to assess the lipid response of premenopausal women to the American Heart Association Diet (30% of energy from total fat, with a polyunsaturated to saturated fat ratio of 1.0) a participant suffered a gall bladder attack and had her gall bladder removed. She was sure that the diet had caused her attack and demanded that investigators pay the hospital expenses, which were not included in the tight budget for the study. The safety monitoring committee decided that the diet was highly unlikely to be the cause of her attack. The informed consent document, which was signed by this participant, clearly stated that the investigators or the university could not be held responsible for health problems not related to study participation, so she was not paid for hospital costs. It would have been difficult to come to this decision without the committee's involvement. The committee also recommended that for future studies investigators screen out all potential participants who could not document their health insurance coverage. However, this could cause the loss of a large pool of participants, greatly limiting the generalizability of the findings and restricting equal access to the benefits of research.

Data and Safety Monitoring Boards

For larger studies, especially multicenter ones, formal and independent data and safety monitoring boards may be appointed, often by the funding agency, to serve as an oversight committee. To guard against conflicts of interest, the members of this board should generally not be affiliated with the institutions of any of the investigators.

The role of the data and safety monitoring board is to monitor, review, and assess the progress of the study. The data and safety monitoring board has access to unblinded outcome data during the study and has the responsibility to ensure that participants are not exposed to unreasonable or unnecessary research risks. Toward this aim, the data and safety monitoring board may recommend early termination of a study if the data suggest significant adverse risk to study participants or if the research questions and objectives appear to have been answered and therefore participants should not continue to be exposed to risk. The data and safety monitoring board also monitors recruitment progress and reviews the quality of the data.

Professional Code of Ethics

Professional associations support ethical conduct by developing and enforcing codes of ethics relevant to their professions. For dietitians, the relevant code of ethics is The American Dietetic Association Code of Ethics for the Profession of Dietetics (4), which sets forth professional principles and standards of conduct. The code is important for guidance of professional activity and strengthens the credibility and integrity of the profession.

Obtaining IRB Approval

Informed Consent

Under the 1974 Federal Act for Research with Human Subjects (5), the concept of informed consent was developed as a guiding principal for the ethical conduct of human research. Since then, commissions have been established and regulations revised and/or expanded (3, 6). The main principle of the act was that potential study participants were free to consent to study participation as long as they were informed of all the study requirements, risks, and benefits.

Certain groups were identified as less able to give informed consent. Among these were children, the mentally ill or retarded persons, and prisoners. These classes of individuals can participate in research studies if a legal guardian gives informed consent for their participation. (Students may also fall into this category if the situation is coercive, such as when study participation is required to obtain a passing grade.) Although the original policy legally applied only to federally funded research, many states have enacted their own statutes.

To implement this policy, study participants are required to sign an informed consent document that clearly describes the requirements of the study in language that can be easily understood. The study participant must sign the document before entering the study.

Each institution has different requirements for the format of the official informed consent document, but the basic intention among documents is similar. The document must describe, in detail and in language that the prospective participant can understand, all that will be expected of him or her in the research project. For complex protocols such as a feeding study, the day-to-day expectations for study management (such as filling out a daily well-being form, taking shoes off and being weighed each day, signing a log book for take-out meals, attending to meal serving times, and scheduling of appointments for measurements) cannot be explained in a concise enough fashion for the informed consent document. All the particulars of a study need not be included in this document but should be orally explained (sometimes with the help of written materials) to potential participants at one or more meetings. In this case the informed consent document would concisely describe the basic requirements of the study. Exhibit 5–1 provides an example of an informed consent document.

It is useful to make a checklist of handouts, descriptions, and caveats for the study manager or recruitment interviewer to discuss with the participants. Because the study manager talks to a number of potential participants over a period of time, the checklist for each participant is checked off as each item is discussed, and the participant signs this checklist to assert that each item has indeed been described to his or her satisfaction. Exhibit 5–2 is an example of such a checklist. Note that the checklist can be used to document whether participants have seen these criteria. Participants are given a copy of the checklist along with their informed consent document.

Informed consent documents must always state that the participant, being a volunteer, has the right to withdraw from the study without fear of any retribution and that withdrawal will not affect the participant's standard medical care. However, it may also be important to note in the informed consent document that the participant may be terminated from the study. Such a step becomes necessary if a participant displays abusive or highly emotional behavior, which may occur in feeding studies because of the combination of highly restrictive protocol requirements and a lengthy study period. Criteria that specify behaviors that would precipitate participant termination are listed in Exhibit 5–3. This form can be incorporated into the informed consent documents or presented to participants after they are enrolled.

EXHIBIT 5-1

Example of Informed Consent Document for Adults

UNIVERSITY OF ILLINOIS AT CHICAGO
INSTITUTIONAL REVIEW BOARD
ADULT CONSENT FOR PARTICIPATION IN AN EXPERIMENTAL PROJECT

Please complete the following statements in the first person and in lay language.

1. I, _____, state that I am _____ years of age and I wish to participate in a program of medical research being conducted by: _____ (investigator).

2. The purpose of the research is: to determine the effects of dietary modification consistent with the recommendations in the American Heart Association Phase Diets (AHA Diet), namely reduced total fat and cholesterol intake along with altered polyunsaturated fatty acid (PUFA) to saturated fatty acid (SFA) ratio, on various lipid parameters, nonlipid atherogenic parameters, and other parameters that may be influenced by such dietary measures. The effects of dietary soluble fibers will also be explored.

3. The experimental procedures are:

   a. Consume only the foods provided in the Metabolic Unit (two regimens: high-fat (40%) diet for one month and low-fat (20% or 30%) diet for next months) over a period of 6 months. In case of a need, packed meals will be given to eat outside the site. The study runs from January through June. The major holiday during this time is Easter. We will make arrangements for you to take packed meals for this day or Passover or other special holidays. It will not be possible for you to leave the campus for more than 1 day at a time. This means that spring break and the remainder of the month of June after classes are finished must be spent on campus.

   b. Provide blood samples at regular intervals as specified below: 2.7 oz on days 22, 29, 67, 141, and 169 during the 6-month study period; 1.34 oz on days 1, 85 and 113 during the 6-month study period; .34 oz on the eighth and eighteenth days of each menstrual period during the study; 1.9 oz on a day in the fourth week and again in the twenty-fourth week for the post-prandial testing.

   c. Provide adipose tissue biopsy samples on days 29 and 169 of the study period (a physician will take these samples).

   d. Subject to underwater weighing once in the fourth and again in the twenty-fourth week.

   e. Provide complete fecal and urine collections from day 20 through 24, day 50 through 56, and again from day 129 through 133.

   f. Keep records of physical activity for 5 days during the months of January, April, and June.

4. The personal risks involved are (if none, so state): Essentially, none. The diets are those advocated by the American Heart Association, National Cancer Institute; and Dietary Guidelines for Americans. No adverse effect is expected. A small bruise as a result of pricking for blood drawing or adipose tissue biopsy may be evident for a while. Trained phlebotomists and physicians will be performing these tasks; hence bruising will be minimal. Participation in a diet study may be very stressful because of change in lifestyle. These stresses have been discussed with me in this interview.

5. I understand that I will receive standard medical care, if required, even if I do not participate in this study. Alternative procedure and therapy that might benefit me personally are: Not applicable because all are healthy adults.

5. I understand and accept the following research related costs (this refers to costs which are beyond those required for my normal diagnostic and treatment purposes). If no additional research costs are to be paid by the employee/ volunteer state NONE.

   NONE

7. I understand that I will be paid $5/day (168 days = $840 in installments: $100 to be paid after each of the following sessions of blood drawing—days 28, 56, 84, 112, and 140 (total $500). The remaining $340 will be paid on day 168. These payments will be made in compensation for the time and attention I give the project.

Continued

EXHIBIT 5-1

8. COMPENSATION STATEMENT (Check appropriate statement).

    ☐ I understand that in the event of physical injury resulting from this research there is no compensation and/or payment for medical treatment from the University of Illinois at Chicago for such injury except as may be required of the University by law.

    ☐ I understand that in the event of physical injury resulting from this research, compensation and/or medical treatment may be available from _____ Corporation (who is sponsoring this research). I understand that if I believe that I am eligible for compensation or medical treatment, I may contact:

Name_____

Address_____

_____

Phone of sponsoring company _____

    However, there is no compensation and/or payment for medical treatment from the University of Illinois at Chicago for such injury except as may be required of the university by law.

9. ADULT CONSENT (a. Will apply unless b. Is completed).

    a. I acknowledge that I have been informed that this procedure is not involved in my treatment and is not intended to benefit my personal health.

    b. I acknowledge that I have been informed that this procedure is also designed to assist in maintaining or improving my personal health and will benefit me personally in the following way:

_____

    I acknowledge that _____ (investigator) has explained to me the risks involved and the need for the research; has informed me that I may withdraw from participation at any time and has offered to answer any inquiries that I may make concerning the procedures to be followed. I freely and voluntarily consent to my participation in this project.

I UNDERSTAND THAT I MAY KEEP A COPY OF THIS CONSENT FORM FOR MY OWN INFORMATION.

X_____   _____   _____
    Employee Volunteer signature   Date   (Type Name)

X_____   _____   _____
    Investigator signature   Date   (Type Name)

X_____   _____   _____
    Witness of Explanation signature   Date   (Type Name)

Thus, in addition to the informed consent document, a list of criteria for participant termination and a checklist that serves to document the oral explanation given to a participant may be submitted to the IRB for review to help prevent potentially adverse situations. Having an on-call psychologist or a trained counselor not connected with the study and requesting funding for psychological services in grant applications may be useful. (Also see Chapter 7, "Managing Participants and Maximizing Compliance.")

An emerging complex issue in research ethics involves informed consent for future analyses of blood or other tissues for measurements not yet identified, which often include genes and genetic markers. Unless otherwise noted, informed consent typically must be obtained for new measurements that were not specifically identified in the original informed consent document. Informed consent for genetic studies is currently a highly sensitive area and policies and guidelines for informed consent are currently being developed. (Also see Chapter 4, "Genetic Effects in Human Dietary Studies.")

Informed Consent for Dependent Groups

The basic assumption for informed consent documents is that the participant is literate or is a guardian representing the participant. Participants who are vision-impaired or functionally illiterate can be accommodated by having a study staff member read the forms and help fill them out. The document can be translated for participants who do not read English fluently. In studies with children age 5 years or older, it is advisable to include a line for their signature as well as

EXHIBIT 5-2

Women's Lipid Study: Interviewer Checklist

Name of Participant _____

    _____ 1. Explanation of study benefits and handout given.
    _____ 2. Explanation of study dietary rules and handout given.
    _____ 3. Explanation of study schedule and handouts given.
    _____ 4. Menu copies given.
    _____ 5. Explanation of procedures and handout given.
    _____ 6. Weight maintenance agreement signed.
    _____ 7. Orientation rules explained and food take-out policy explained.
    _____ 8. Consent form given.
    _____ 9. Consent form signed and returned.
    _____ 10. Appointment for physical examination made.
    _____ 11. Medical and family history forms completed.
    _____ 12. Three-day food record forms given.
    _____ 13. Criteria for termination reviewed.
    _____ 14. Stress due to study participation discussed.

Comments: _____

_____

_____

Participant Signature _____

Interviewer Signature _____ Date _____

---

that of their guardian. (Refer also to Chapter 9, "Children as Participants in Feeding Studies.")

Ancillary Measurements and IRB Approval

The investigator may want to add variables or otherwise modify the protocol after IRB approval. Any new measurements—for example, extra blood draws—or any additional major requirements that impinge on participant time usually must be submitted to the IRB for approval. These approvals can be obtained in two ways. If the original informed consent document has already been signed, the new measurements or requirements must be described in an appendix (which must also be signed). Otherwise, a new (revised) informed consent document must be developed and signed. In general, changes in protocol that are not substantive are quickly approved by the IRB staff without the requirement of a meeting of the full IRB.

STUDY RECRUITMENT AND SCREENING

Advertising the Study

It might be assumed that few ethical issues arise once a research study has obtained IRB approval. However, new issues can arise from recruitment and screening activities. Consider a protocol to study individuals with high serum cholesterol or high blood pressure. One approach to recruiting is to advertise free cholesterol or blood pressure testing with no further information and then invite those who meet the study criteria to participate in the research study.

This approach, however, may present ethical concerns. Presumably those responding to the free tests were concerned about their cholesterol or blood pressure and had no knowledge about being considered for participation in a research study. To be suddenly confronted with the request places them in the situation of responding without due consideration at a time when they are vulnerable. By straightforwardly advertising the study and the type of participants needed for the study, the investigators not only receive responses from those genuinely interested in research participation but also save effort in scheduling and screening many individuals who would not be interested in study participation. In addition, the investigator can obtain advice on ethical considerations raised by the content of the study advertisements and recruitment brochures by submitting them to the IRB for review. (Also refer to Chapter 6, "Recruiting and Screening of Study Participants.")

Explaining the Study to Prospective Participants

Because informed consent is the foundation of the ethical conduct of research involving humans, it is mandatory that participants receive a full and truthful description of all that

EXHIBIT 5-3

Women's Lipid Study Criteria for Termination of Study Participants

1. Repeated altercations with staff members, investigators, or other study participants.
2. Missing two days of meals (consecutively or not) without calling.
3. Not reporting weight honestly.
4. Not reporting unfinished food or nonstudy food consumed.
5. Unauthorized entrance into participant or staff files or staff offices.
6. Not reporting for small or big blood draws or postprandial lipid response study and not informing the staff in advance if there is a schedule conflict.
7. Violent behavior or abusive language.
8. Calling or visiting staff at home. (Investigators' home phone numbers are available to participants for use in emergencies.)
9. Harassment or threatening the safety of staff members, investigators or participants.
10. Refusing to eat study food.
11. Inability or unwillingness to provide samples according to study protocol.
12. Nonadherence to study protocol.

The investigators reserve the right to terminate study participation of any participant at any time for any reason for the benefit of the research study being conducted.

---

the study entails. A common issue is whether the purpose of the study should be disclosed to the participant, because knowing the purpose may influence the outcome of the study. Many IRB committees require a general statement of study purpose in the informed consent document. Disclosing the general purpose of the study and its possible importance to society is an important ethical issue and can also encourage adherence when the burden of a long study is particularly heavy. Participants have often referred to this importance as a reason for continuing in a study despite its restrictiveness. The specific measurements and what they mean need not be discussed in detail during the study if participant knowledge would bias the results of the study.

The study staff is responsible for explaining the study requirements, informing the participants of what they will be expected to do, and helping participants understand the ramifications of the requirements. For example, the requirement of eating all meals at the study site except for allowed take-out meals means that participants may experience: (1) loss of time and money required for traveling back and forth from the study site; (2) reduced family and social contact because mealtime is an important socialization time for family and friends; (3) for students, difficulty in getting their dormitory meal contract waived for the period of the study; and (4) interference with class field trips, vacations, scientific meetings, home emergencies, and leisure activities.

Potential participants are unlikely to have thought through all these consequences. They need to be raised with each candidate. A full discussion at the outset can help reduce early study dropouts because we have found that the conflict of study requirements with lifestyle is a major cause of dropouts.

When investigators are working with children, it is important to find inventive ways to describe what will be expected of them. One way to evaluate their understanding is to ask them to explain what they will be doing in the study.

(Refer to Chapter 9, "Children as Participants in Feeding Studies.")

Screening

Screening is usually focused on obtaining study participants who qualify according to the eligibility criteria, which are inclusions and exclusions set by the study protocol. These guidelines should be objectively and rigidly followed in order to define the study population sample, the characteristics of which are guided by the research question. (Chapter 6, "Recruitment and Screening of Study Participants," explores recruitment in detail.)

Some eligibility criteria are related to safety issues. It may be insufficient to ask a participant if she is pregnant; some facilities screen premenopausal women for pregnancy. Additional screening procedures may be necessary to ensure the safety of children, pregnant women, the older individuals, and particular groups of patients. Screening for HIV and hepatitis B infections is, in some cases, justifiable to protect the participant whose health might be further impaired by the study. However, IRBs may expressly prohibit screening for HIV and hepatitis B because the testing can be considered an invasion of the participant's privacy.

As noted previously, there are often potential participants with a few abnormal laboratory values who otherwise meet all the eligible criteria. What is the ethical and scientific approach for these variances from protocol requirements? This is where the safety monitoring committee's advice is invaluable. One common problem, for example, is posed by women with low hemoglobin levels. In some instances, safety monitoring committees have recommended remedial measures such as iron supplementation with provisional acceptance into the study if blood hemoglobin levels reach a particular value by the first day of the study. Because there are usually a few low laboratory values caused by laboratory error, physiological fluctuations, and chance, a second blood test is advisable to substantiate the values in question.

Whether or not they qualify for the study, screenees should be notified of abnormal laboratory values and encouraged to see their physician or other health care provider. The screenees also should be told that the abnormal value is not a diagnosis but rather a possible problem.

In addition, it is important to screen potential participants for ability to participate because screenees often do not understand the ramifications of participation. It is human nature to commit to more than a person can reasonably accomplish. This requires sensitive inquiries concerning the distance a screenee must travel, means of transportation to the study site, family responsibilities, work schedules, and impending trips and vacations. Screenees can be ethically excluded from study participation because their circumstances would overly burden them.

Many IRB-approved eligibility exclusion criteria can include a phrase such as "unlikely in the opinion of investigators to be able to complete the study," which is a nonspecific default explanation for such decisions. Although some participants can carry out the study requirements despite difficult circumstances, the investigators are still responsible for excluding from participation those screenees whose life circumstances are not consistent with the rigors of study participation. The investigators may be in a better position to make that decision than the screenee. Because some callers responding to advertisements for study participation may believe that they have been discriminated against and were denied what they considered a constitutional right to participate, study staff handling these inquiry calls should be warned that they may have to deal with angry individuals who do not meet eligibility criteria.

STUDY MANAGEMENT: OBLIGATIONS TO PARTICIPANTS AND STAFF

Study Participants

During a study, many issues may come up that require ethical decisions. When these issues are anticipated, provisions and decisions can be made in advance that are more likely to be ethical and yet consistent with the scientific progress of the study. Despite the best planning, new issues may arise, and it is important for the investigator to hold weekly staff meetings and be available to make responsible decisions on the spot. A lack of timely action can cause ethical problems in the long run.

Illnesses

Most informed consent documents clearly indicate that the study investigators and research institution are not responsible for health care costs incurred independent of the study. However, study staff are obliged to know about and inves-

tigate each illness to make sure that it is not connected with study participation, as potential participants may not be covered by health insurance. Alternative means of health care should be provided if participants without health insurance are accepted into a study. Participants who do not have a regular physician or health care provider should be provided with names of health care providers who would see them if the need arose. Because of the need to be informed of illnesses, it is a common practice in feeding studies to have participants fill out a daily form concerning health and medication that is checked by the study manager.

In some instances it is not clear whether a health change is the consequence of study participation. If a participant is constipated, it may be unclear whether the change of diet or some other health problem caused the constipation. Should the study pick up the cost of the health care provider's fees and any medication that might be prescribed? Some investigators would view this as a valid claim on the study and pay the fees; others would not.

Medications

The standard approach toward medications for feeding studies is to disallow the use of any medication during the course of the study and clearly state this as part of the study protocol. This may work relatively well for short-term studies, but studies lasting several months may encounter participants needing to take antibiotics, aspirin, antacids, or other medications. Ethically, the health of the participant takes precedence over study protocol.

One approach is to know when the participant is seeing a physician or health care provider and (with the participant's written permission) to have the provider call the investigator during the appointment to discuss the best medication—ideally, one that satisfies the needs of the participant and the science of the study. Another approach is to provide participants with a list of specific medications or groups of medication that either are allowable or that must be avoided, and the times in the study they must be avoided (eg, medication taken up to 3 weeks before the next blood draw may be permissible).

Handling Life Events

In studies lasting several months, a participant may have a death in the family or some other life event that requires out-of-state travel. The participant will be emotionally distraught and may declare that he or she "must leave town immediately for at least a week." Study investigators are put in an ethical dilemma: do they try to talk the study participant out of going through guilt and obligation to the study or do they tolerate nonadherence to the protocol? If investigators have thought out possible alternatives beforehand, they are in a better position to describe a number of options and their consequences, which allows the participant to decide which is the most appropriate course of action. Investigators must know how many days a participant could leave each study (with packed food and food advice) and whether there are certain times during the study that are less crucial. Very long periods of absence may mean study termination for that participant.

Emotional Problems and Stress

On occasion participants appear to be under great stress, usually because they have taken on too much. Although there are steps that can accommodate these participants, it may be more cost effective to arrange one or more appointments with a counselor (psychologist) not connected with the study but familiar with the study protocol. These visits are paid from study funds. Issues of whether study termination is appropriate and how to approach the stresses in the participant's life can be dealt with independently of study considerations.

When researchers work with children, close communication with parents is essential. Children generally "act out" their stresses rather than communicate them verbally.

Terminating Participants from the Study

The most common reason that participants may wish to drop out of a study is their inability to adhere to the study requirements. These participants typically will miss appointments and meal times or will eat nonstudy food. These participants do not necessarily request to terminate their participation. In some feeding trials, investigators do not terminate these participants in order to follow "intention-to-treat" data analysis guidelines established for the study. The investigators encourage the participants to continue with data collection, even if they are nonadherent to the research diet. In other studies, termination may be considered, and usually the study manager and investigators observe the problem and suggest to these participants that continuance in the study may be against their own best interests.

Laboratory Values That May Indicate Illness

Generally, biological samples are taken through the course of the study and study variables are assessed quickly enough that results become available while participants are still in the study. What is the ethical response to laboratory values that become abnormal during the course of the study? If the study is a double-blind clinical trial there is generally one investigator who prepares the data and presents them to the safety monitoring committee to assess. Generally, feeding studies are too short to produce enough data for this mechanism to be practical in informing participants of the abnormal values.

What is more likely to happen is that study staff making the assessments will note the abnormal value (eg, an extremely high blood pressure, blood glucose, or liver enzyme value) and bring this to the attention of the study investigators. The investigators are ethically obligated to investigate the accuracy of the measurement and its health implications, examine whether there is any connection to the study intervention, refer the participant to his or her health care provider, and determine whether the participant must be terminated from the study. Phone conversations with individual members of the safety monitoring committee can be helpful under such circumstances. Ideally, the study protocol will stipulate the conditions that warrant referral to a physician or other health care provider, as well as other ameliorative actions that can be taken (for example, providing iron supplements to individuals who develop low hemoglobin and hematocrit during the study) should be stated in the protocol prior to the start of the study.

The Semi-adherent Participant

The study manager should be attuned to the signs of nonadherence. There could be one or two participants who consume all their meals and adhere to other study protocol requirements but find it difficult to deny themselves nonstudy foods. Despite an atmosphere of nonjudgment and honesty, these participants may not report their nonadherence. The nonadherence may become known to the study staff, who must then confront the participant with the problem.

It is important to educate study staff on an appropriate and ethical approach. Participants can be ethically approached by describing the facts that are known and asked whether they want to continue their participation. If the participant wishes to continue in the study, the study manager or other investigator has a basis for identifying the personal impediments to adherence and working with the participant to address them. What if the participant denies consuming nonstudy food on a continuing basis? If evidence is insufficient, if the participant has worked out specific approaches to solving the problem, or if continued participation is valuable, it may be worthwhile to continue to work with the participant while observing his or her activities. Psychological counseling may also be useful.

However, if reasons for termination have been clearly stipulated at the beginning of the study, investigators are under no ethical obligation to retain the participant in the study.

Payment for Participation

The protocol requirements and the personal disruptions of daily life are so great in most controlled feeding studies that recognition of this disruption through financial remuneration is an important symbolic and ethical act. Some payment schedules reflect the amount of money that participants personally might have to expend on a daily basis for study adherence (parking fees, public transportation costs, occasional baby sitting) plus an additional amount for undergoing the rigors of the study. This per diem rate can be used to calculate the overall participant payment. The free food offered by the study also has a monetary value.

Even if the limits of funding were not a consideration, however, it is unwise to set payments at the level that would substitute for employment. Study participation can be motivated by the financial reward, among other things. Larger financial awards may attract participants that are in greater need of that money, which means that they are less free to leave the study, and investigators are placed in a more difficult position in terminating their participation. This creates a great pressure for participants to remain in the study and may be considered coercive. Residential vs free-living feeding studies in which participants are free to continue their daily pursuits and sleep at home require different approaches to the timing of payments and the amount paid.

IRBs may specify rules for participant payments. Some IRBs prohibit withholding all payment until study completion; others may dislike large final (balloon) payments at a study's completion because they feel such payments constitute possible coercion of the participant to remain in the study. Others require prorated payments, especially if the amount of remuneration is large. Many investigators pay participants as the study progresses, with a small balloon payment at the end as an incentive to complete the study. Payments also can be linked to the collection of biological samples. For example, payment can be scheduled to follow a monthly blood draw. A small bonus can be an appropriate incentive for not taking out more than a set number of meals during the entire study.

All of these financial incentives are considered ethical as long as they are clearly spelled out at the beginning of the study, well-documented, and consistently applied. Policies concerning payment must be made clear to the participants from the beginning.

Another ethical concern is the promptness of the receipt of the payments. Some institutions have bureaucracies that make it extremely difficult to pay participants promptly. It is advisable to work with the institution's payment personnel well in advance of the study to expedite payment to participants.

When investigators are working with children, appropriate toys and savings bonds are a good incentive and ensure that the reward truly belongs to the child rather than their guardian.

Ensuring Meals Are Wholesome

Investigators are ethically responsible for providing participants nutritious, wholesome food. Local health departments have food safety guidelines, which should be followed rigorously even by a feeding facility not subject to official inspections. Quality assurance procedures should be in place to guarantee that food is stored, cooked, and held at the proper temperature, that dishes and utensils are properly cleaned, and that pests are adequately controlled. If gastrointestinal symptoms arise in several participants, it is the responsibility of the investigators to ascertain whether the food supplied may be the source of the trouble.

Additional Procedures and Measurements

In the course of the study, opportunities present possibilities for additional procedures or measurements. The participants' involvement should be on a voluntary basis, without compromising ongoing activities, and only after IRB approval for the addition.

Privacy and Confidentiality of Participant Materials

Investigators should plan for allowing privacy for participants when required, for example, during physical examinations or personal questions. In addition, because a great deal of cooperation among participants and staff is required in these studies, diet staff and participants cannot help but know the participants' names and identification numbers. Although anonymity is out of the question, confidentiality can be preserved.

All materials should be stored by identification number, not by name, and files should be kept locked because there are a great number of people coming and going during the course of the study day. Staff access to participant information should be limited, with someone in authority granting that access. Likewise, computer access to data files should be limited to authorized staff. Use of passwords facilitates this process. Jokes about individual participant measurements should be avoided by staff and discouraged for participants. Staff and participants should be reminded to avoid speaking about individual participants to friends and colleagues during or after the study.

Study Staff

Feeding studies place inordinate demands on research unit personnel. The principal investigator has a dual obligation to the staff: first, to ensure that they conduct themselves in an ethical and professional manner; and second, to be responsible for their well-being during the study.

Ethical Scientific Conduct and Conflict of Interest

Study investigators and staff must follow ethical conduct guidelines when interacting with prospective participants during screening, and then must continue to do so throughout the study. All eligibility criteria and procedures for randomization (if the study is a randomized trial) must be meticulously observed by staff. If recruitment is slower than anticipated, there may be a temptation to enroll participants who may not quite meet all the eligibility criteria. However, staff should execute all of the recruitment and measurement procedures exactly according to the protocol.

Study data must be recorded according to specific established procedures. If any recorded data must be changed, the documentation for these changes should indicate the date, the reason, and the names of all responsible staff members. If problems with the protocol make it difficult to carry out recruitment or implementation of other study procedures, the problems must be brought to the attention of the principal investigator. The study leadership is also responsible for making any necessary changes to the protocol—including changes to eligibility criteria. Depending on the scope of the changes, appropriate bodies, such as the IRB, safety monitoring committee, or data and safety monitoring board, may need to be informed of these changes. Finally, principal investigators need to be cognizant of conflict of interest or the appearance of conflict of interest. Conflict of interest may arise if the principal investigator has financial ties to commercial entities that are likely to be affected by the outcome of the study. Not all conflicts have a financial basis, however. For example, researchers may have an emotional investment in the results of the study, such that they would prefer certain outcomes to others; this could influence the conduct of the protocol or bias the interpretation of results.

Requests to Participate

Faculty and graduate students are commonly accepted as participants as long as they are independent of the activities of the study (eg, they not working on a thesis that depends on the outcome of the study). However, staff of the research unit are not truly free to refuse to participate; therefore, requests for their participation are unethical under any circumstance. In addition, staff participation could lead to unintentional situations that may raise questions concerning the validity and integrity of the study, such as breaking the blind or finding out the results of primary outcome measurements before the study is over. It is therefore best not to allow staff to participate in a study, even if they request to volunteer.

Long Work Hours

Studies may be underfunded, resulting in inadequate staffing for the amount of work to be done. Study managers and graduate students are likely to bear the brunt of this situation. Investigators are responsible for ensuring that staff are not overwhelmed. Staff should be told what to expect and that they are responsible for their own well-being. This means that they must take care of themselves and communicate their needs for extra help or time.

Because of their dedication, staff members may work too long and see no other immediate solution, whereas study directors generally have a broader picture and access to other resources. This means that at least one investigator should be in frequent contact with staff so that communication is an active and ongoing process.

Handling Biohazardous Materials

Feeding studies may require collection of blood, urine, feces, or other tissues from study participants. Staff who handle these materials should be trained to know and actively carry out procedures for protection from HIV, hepatitis, and other infections. Gloves, masks, glasses, and lab coats should be worn when appropriate, and investigators should make sure these procedures are carried out.

Many institutions mandate regular blood testing for HIV and hepatitis, and also immunize staff and graduate students working with biohazardous materials against hepatitis B. Academic departments generally pay the costs. Surveillance and protection are advisable whether mandated or not.

Hiring and Firing

Each institution has rules for personnel of various classes, and the rules need to be understood and followed. Kitchen staff pose the greatest problem because some may be part-time employees and a study of any size needs sufficient staff time to cover sickness, vacations, and other times off. Student labor can also be problematic, particularly during times of exams and vacations. Many facilities successfully employ part-time personnel from the surrounding community. Occasionally a staff worker must be terminated for sound reasons such as theft. Termination is ethically easier with clear, written guidelines of what behavior is expected and what constitutes a firing offense. (Also see Chapter 20, "Staffing Needs for Research Diet Studies.")

STUDY TERMINATION

Premature Termination

The issue of stopping a feeding study midcourse does not usually come up because such studies are usually relatively short-term. Long-term clinical trials, especially drug trials, are ethically required to consider circumstances under which a study should be called to a halt. This charge is given to an external data and safety monitoring board. The main reasons for terminating a trial prematurely are: (1) unexpected adverse side effects; or (2) the efficacy of the treatment being tested has been proven so that it is no longer ethical to deny the experimental treatment to participants in the control group. The reasons to terminate a relatively short-term feeding study are less clear-cut, but the possibilities should be thought out ahead of time and these consequences delineated. Examples might include: severe gastrointestinal effects caused by the inclusion of large amounts of a particular dietary fiber in the feeding trial; a rise in fasting blood sugar in diabetic participants; a dramatic rise in prostaglandin levels caused by a digestive irritant; or the development of skin rashes in a significant proportion of participants.

What kind of change would be grounds for stopping the study early? What proportion of participants would have to exhibit the symptom? If these issues are thought out ahead of time, the most ethical decision is easier to make.

When a study is prematurely terminated, the investigators are responsible for returning participants to their original health status. Often simply terminating the study is adequate, but participants' health should be followed to make sure symptoms have disappeared.

Planned Study Termination

Exit interviews are commonly conducted with the participants after they have completed the study. The goal of the interview is to assess adherence to the protocol and to ensure that participants leave the study satisfied that their rights have been respected. Individuals may be given their study data at that time because one of the primary motivations for study participation is increased knowledge about oneself. It is advisable to remain available to participants after the study is terminated and respond to their calls and requests promptly.

One of the ethical problems that investigators frequently encounter is that of fulfilling promises; any promises made to participants before or during the study must be kept when the project is terminated. This is often more difficult than expected because resources are generally exhausted and there are no funds to keep sufficient staff employed. Therefore, it is important to limit promises to those that can definitely be fulfilled. These might include providing weight loss and other diet counseling, the overall results of the study, and other generally available information.

REPORTING STUDY RESULTS

Confidentiality for study participants must be maintained. When researchers give presentations about the study, it is tempting to use photographs of study participants engaged in the activities of protocol. These cannot be used without a signed release from the study participants pictured. Also, only identification numbers are attached to samples and data. Feeding studies often attract post hoc investigations by investigators and graduate students not originally engaged in the study. These subsequent investigators may be less sensitive to the issue of confidentiality and must be reminded of ethical behavior with respect to confidentiality. Of course, any presentation or scientific paper should present group data and disguise even the original identification number if an individual participant is singled out for discussion.

Because many people contribute to the conduct of a feeding study, the issue of who should be listed as authors on scientific papers and presentations can become a source of contention. It is best to work out these issues before the study begins. There appears to be little agreement about the inclusion of study staff as authors. A major ethical concern is the tendency of investigators to *include* as authors technicians who have performed some of the biochemical analyses but *exclude* dietitians who have had major responsibility for the development and delivery of the diets that form the independent variables of the study. Another tendency among investigators performing post hoc analyses is the failure to credit the investigators who have overseen the conduct of the study. It is important that the principal investigator provide strong leadership to ensure that individuals having a substantial contribution to the study are honored with authorship or at least acknowledgment for their contributions. There are suggested guidelines for assigning authorship and order of authorship (7, 8), which may help to resolve some of these emotionally charged situations.

CONCLUSION

Ethical considerations and the safety of participants are an overriding concern in human research studies. Principal in-

vestigators are responsible for the ethics and safety of a study, and their efforts are assisted by organizational structures. The IRB is the primary organizational structure that provides guidance to investigators and assurances to funding agencies that the research protocol is ethical and safe for participants. Safety monitoring committees and external data and safety monitoring boards also may be used to advise investigators in the planning and designing of the study and later in monitoring safety, recruitment, data quality, and overall study progress. Professional organizations also support ethical conduct through development of a code of ethics for their professions.

In planning a study, principal investigators must be aware of participant burden when developing data collection procedures, including the degree of invasiveness and the frequency of collection. After the study protocol is developed, investigators must seek IRB approval for the protocol. An accurate, instructive, well-written informed consent document is key to conducting an ethical study and receiving IRB approval.

Issues of ethics and safety arise throughout the study: during recruitment and screening, during the course of the study, and at the conclusion of the research. Advertisements for recruitment must be ethical, and comprehensive explanation of the study to potential participants is essential so that informed consent is truly informed. During screening and during the course of the study, procedures concerning notification and referral to other health care providers should be in place. These are activated if laboratory values are outside established norms or when clinical measurements exceed thresholds for which standard treatment guidelines exist. During the course of the study, principal investigators must make sure policies regarding participant illnesses, medication needs, life events, and stress are ethical. Ethically based policies must also be in place for nonadherent participants or for terminating participants from the study. Monetary incentives must not be perceived as coercive. Particularly important in feeding studies is the attention paid to quality control of the foodservice and assurance of safe and wholesome meals. Strict confidentiality and privacy must be maintained throughout the study, and conflicts of interest must be avoided. Principal investigators also bear some responsibility for the well-being of their staff.

After the conclusion of a study, whether terminated prematurely or as planned, all promises made to the participants must be kept, and study results must be reported in ways that maintain the confidentiality of the participants. Ethical issues regarding authorship of papers must also be carefully considered.

Planning, conducting, and concluding an ethical, safe study of high scientific merit with human subjects requires safeguards, assurances, and continual oversight, but also provides the ability to answer important research questions. Thus, ethically conducted human feeding studies are extremely rewarding, as the information they generate provides the scientific basis for promoting better health for individuals and the general public.

REFERENCES

1. Cole TG, Bowen PE, Schmeisser D, et al. Differential reduction of plasma cholesterol by the AHA Phase 3 diet in moderately hypercholesterolemic, premenopausal women with differing body mass index. *Am J Clin Nutr.* 1992;55:385–394.

2. Mobarhan S, Bowen PE, Anderson B, et al. Effects of beta-carotene repletion on beta-carotene absorption, lipid peroxidation, and neutrophil superoxide formation in young men. *Nutr Cancer.* 1990;14:195–206.

3. *Code of Federal Regulations.* Title 45 CFR Part 46, Protection of Human Subjects, Rev. June 18, 1991.

4. American Dietetic Association. Code of Ethics for the Profession of Dietetics. *J Am Diet Assoc.* 1988;88:1592–1596.

5. The National Research Act. Pub L No 93–348 (1974).

6. The National Commission for the Protection of Human Subjects of Biomedical and Behavioral Research. *The Belmont Report: Ethical Principles and Guidelines for the Protection of Human Subjects of Research.* Bethesda, Md: Office for Protection from Research Risks Reports, National Institutes of Health, Public Health Service, Department of Health and Human Services; 1979.

7. Winston RB. A suggested procedure for determining order of authorship in research publications. *J Counseling Dev.* 1985;63:515–518.

8. International Committee of Medical Journal Editors. Uniform requirements for manuscripts submitted to biomedical journals. *N Engl J Med.* 1991;324:424–428.

CHAPTER 6

Recruitment and Screening of Study Participants

Penny M. Kris-Etherton, PhD, RD; Vikkie A. Mustad, PhD; and
Alice H. Lichtenstein, DSc

Experienced investigators have long recognized the importance of well-planned recruitment and screening activities for a successful clinical study. It is surprising, therefore, that the literature in this area is so recent. Studies formally began in the 1980s with the recruitment and screening activities and procedures of the Lipid Research Clinics Coronary Primary Prevention Trial (LRC-CPPT). Prior to this time, many new investigators learned about recruiting and screening subjects either by word-of-mouth from experienced investigators or by conducting their own studies. Many actually assumed that recruitment and screening would be effortless and free of problems (1).

The LRC-CPPT study has provided a wealth of information about how to recruit and screen participants successfully for large clinical trials. Many of these approaches are applicable to smaller studies as well. An important legacy of the LRC-CPPT is that it demonstrated the importance of developing recruitment plans and screening strategies and allocating adequate resources for them. Standardized recruitment and screening procedures are now part of the protocol for many different types of clinical studies (2), including well-controlled feeding studies. This chapter discusses issues and strategies needed to meet recruitment goals.

Recruitment

The major goal of recruitment is to enroll the required number of eligible participants necessary for the study within a projected time line with the resources available (3). Careful planning, a well-trained staff, good communication among the staff as well as with potential study participants, flexibility, and contingency plans are critically important. Close attention to all aspects of recruitment will help launch the research project successfully. This will help keep staff and participant morale high from the start, which is key for sustaining interest and participation throughout the study.

A detailed recruitment plan includes realistic short- and long-term goals; carefully defined recruitment strategies with consideration given to the effort required for the number of participants needed for the study; and adequate resources including funding, staff, space, and time. The eligibility criteria for participation in the study must be defined and screening procedures must be in place before the study begins. Eligibility criteria, recruitment, and screening are all linked. The success of the study depends on how effectively eligibility criteria are defined and how well recruitment and screening activities are planned and carried out.

Eligibility Criteria and Screening

The eligibility criteria are guided by the research questions and objectives and essentially define the study population. A study population can be broadly or narrowly defined based on eligibility criteria. For example, a study may be designed to examine the effects of diet on a selected outcome variable in women. Specific eligibility criteria would identify a subgroup of women on the basis of factors such as age, body weight, menopausal status, smoking status, alcohol consumption, or vitamin and mineral supplement usage. Eligibility criteria help to control for factors that may confound the interpretation of the results.

However, a general caution for investigators is that, although there is decreased variability in the study population when a larger number of eligibility criteria are used, the results are less generalizable to the general population. For example, in Protocol 1 of the Dietary Effects on Lipoproteins and Thrombogenic Activity (DELTA) study, the effects of diet on lipoprotein and hemostatic endpoints of interest were studied in healthy, adult, Caucasian and African-American men and women. In Protocol 2, subjects were dyslipidemic and/or insulin resistant. Thus, the results of the first study are generalizable to essentially the entire healthy, adult US population, whereas the results of the second study are applicable to a much smaller group, approximately 25% of adults. Both, however, address significant clinical issues that are relevant to different population groups. (See Chapter 25, "The Multicenter Approach to Human Feeding Studies," for more information on the DELTA program.)

Eligibility criteria affect the resources required to screen participants adequately. Broadly defined eligibility criteria generally require fewer resources for screening than eligibility criteria that are narrowly defined. It is relatively simple to recruit potential participants for a study if the eligibility criteria are just for women of all ages. In contrast, considerably more resources (time, staff, space, and specialized equipment) are required to recruit participants for a study designed to examine the effects of an experimental diet on selected outcome variables of, for example, Native American men from one tribe, between the ages of 20 and 30 years, with body mass indexes (BMIs) of 27 to 32, a sedentary activity level, and an abnormal glucose tolerance test. More resources are needed principally because there is a smaller pool of potential participants and because many volunteers would have to be screened, measurements of BMI and physical activity would have to be obtained, and results of a laboratory test would be required. Thus, when planning a study, investigators must consider fully the resources needed to recruit and screen an adequate number of individuals to answer the research question of interest.

Sometimes eligibility is determined in a certain order during a series of screening visits. For cost-effectiveness, easily ascertained information is obtained first, like age or past history of disease, to screen out early in the process individuals who are obviously ineligible. Also, because of measurement error and regression to the mean (see Chapter 2, "Statistical Aspects of Controlled Diet Studies"), eligibility criteria for primary outcome measures may be broader at the earlier stages of screening and narrower at the later stages to minimize excluding potential participants who are indeed eligible.

In some instances, it may become necessary to revise eligibility criteria and, in so doing, the research question may become modified. In the example of Native American men just cited, the age range and BMI of the study participants could be less restrictive; however, this may affect the research objectives. Eliminating the glucose tolerance criteria would simplify screening considerably but would also markedly change the research question.

Sometimes eligibility criteria may be redefined during the study based on the recruitment experience. For example, if recruitment difficulties are encountered (eg, an inadequate number of participants is recruited within the expected time line), it may become necessary to relax or reduce some of the exclusion criteria. Should recruitment proceed more easily than expected, then the exclusion criteria actually can become more restrictive. Both of these situations occur sometimes. In the Multiple Risk Factor Intervention Trial (MRFIT), the age criteria were more broadly defined, whereas the blood pressure criteria initially defined to classify men as hypertensive were made more exclusive simply because a greater than expected number of potential participants were found to be eligible (4).

If recruitment difficulties occur, the alternatives to redefining the eligibility criteria are to delay the starting date of the study and allocate more time and resources to recruit the required number of participants. This option, however, is not without potentially serious ramifications, such as

- Losing the interest of participants recruited early on.
- Possibly not meeting the proposed objectives of the funded research because of less funds and less time available for the implementation of the study.
- Loss of staff morale.

Commonly used eligibility criteria for many feeding studies and comments about their use are listed in Table 6–1. There are many eligibility criteria to consider. Although these may seem easy to apply in most studies, in practice considerable thought and discussion must be given to the

TABLE 6-1

Common Eligibility Criteria for Well-Controlled Feeding Studies

Inclusion/Exclusion Criteria	Comment
Demographic Criteria	
Gender	Including only one gender controls for the effects of sex; including both genders enables comparisons to be made between sexes.
Age	Narrow age criteria reduce variability but also increase recruitment efforts and reduce generalizability. Including different age groups permits determination of age effects. Chronological age may differ from biological age. For example, some women are postmenopausal at age 45; others at 55.
Race and ethnicity	Race and ethnic groups usually are heterogeneous and difficult to define. Usually obtained by self-report.
Anthropometric Criteria	
Height, weight, body mass index, adiposity, % of ideal weight	Ideal body weight is difficult to define. Strict upper-limit criteria can eliminate many potential participants especially in older age or some ethnic groups. May be appropriate to also establish lower weight limit and exclude for underweight.
Length of time stable weight has been maintained	Recent (must be defined) weight gain or loss (amount gained or lost also must be defined) may be a confounding variable.
Biochemical Criteria	
Various indexes of health status such as albumin, creatinine, liver enzymes, thyroid-stimulating hormone	Helps identify individuals with coexisting diseases and conditions who should not participate in this study.
Indexes of nutritional status such as protein, iron, calcium, zinc levels	The research question will determine the use of biochemical indexes. For example, to study the effect of iron status on heme iron absorption, hemoglobin, hematocrit, and transferrin measurements would be important for stratifying participants according to iron status or adjusting for iron status.
Plasma Lipid Concentrations	
Total cholesterol, low-density lipoprotein cholesterol, high-density lipoprotein cholesterol, triglycerides	Cut points for dyslipidemia are used to define the study population or are based on ethical considerations to exclude dyslipidemic individuals who need treatment and should not be subjected to a control condition. Cut points can be established on the basis of percentiles (using NHANES or LRC data) or national recommendations. Using absolute value cut points will influence the age of participants who are eligible because total cholesterol and low-density lipoprotein cholesterol increase with age. A narrow range will increase recruitment efforts. A wide range permits evaluation of the effects of baseline lipids on outcome variables. Most individuals with a total cholesterol level between the 10th and 90th percentile are responsive to diet.
Dietary Criteria	
Habitual diet and eating practices	Investigators should assess whether prospective participants will adhere to the experimental diet. Food allergies and food avoidances including vegetarianism not compatible with the experimental diet are the basis for exclusion, as are other atypical eating practices. Potential participants following a prescribed therapeutic diet or other special diet (eg, for weight loss) usually are ineligible.
Nutritional supplement use	Usually an excessive nutrient supplement intake and even intake of a multivitamin supplement that meets the RDA is contraindicated if the potential participant is unwilling to discontinue use during the study.

Continued

TABLE 6-1

Inclusion/Exclusion Criteria	Comment
Dietary Criteria (continued)	
Alcohol consumption	In addition to assessing average weekly consumption, it is important to examine binge drinking habits and history of alcoholism. During the study, for participants who meet the alcohol eligibility criteria, consumption practices should not change.
Caffeine consumption	It often is necessary to permit consumption of caffeinated beverages in moderation especially for long-term feeding studies to facilitate recruitment.
Smoking Criteria	
Use of tobacco	Eligibility criteria related to tobacco products must be defined. If a potential participant is a former smoker, criteria for smoking cessation period must be defined.
Physical Activity Criteria	
Physical activity Occupational and leisure time activity	Considerations include type, intensity, frequency, and duration of physical activity. Long-term and seasonal exercise practices should be assessed to ensure that they are compatible with the study protocol.
Medical History Criteria	
History of diseases and conditions	Diseases and conditions that will adversely affect the outcome variables or adherence to the study protocol should be identified. Examples to consider include cancer, diabetes, hypertension, renal disease, major gastrointestinal diseases, and mental illness.
Medication Criteria	
Use of prescription and nonprescription drugs	Potential participants who take any medications or substances that will affect the outcome variables of the study should be excluded. Examples of commonly used medications to consider include antihypertensive and lipid-lowering drugs, oral hypoglycemic agents, antidepressive drugs, oral contraceptive agents, hormone replacement agents, antibiotics, steroidal compounds, and allergy medications. Nonprescription drugs such as aspirin antihistamines, laxatives, and antacids should be considered.
Attitude Criteria	
Willingness to adhere to the experimental diet(s) and protocol	A means of assessing willingness to participate is important. Even one participant with a poor attitude is a risk to the study. Many can become dropouts, adversely influence staff morale, or cause other participants to leave the study.
Other Criteria	
Expectation of not being away	Investigators should determine whether potential participants have plans to relocate or be away (eg, for vacation or a business trip).
Pregnancy	Because of the effects of pregnancy and lactation on the metabolism of various nutrients, it is advisable to control for these conditions. Conversely, there may be concerns related to safety of experimental regimens during pregnancy or lactation. Knowledge of exact stage of pregnancy and lactation is needed when these are specific areas of interest.

cutoff points appropriate for each criterion for every study. Sometimes the population distributions for variables of interest are not current or available, which necessitates making some decisions arbitrarily.

Despite careful attention to defining eligibility criteria, investigators should understand that study participants who meet these eligibility criteria may be different from individuals who do not volunteer for a research study (5). This is a philosophical issue of some interest, but it is not amenable to being tested, and the scientific·importance of this observation is not known. Nonetheless, researchers should be aware of a possible limitation in the generalizability of their findings to groups that are similar to the study participants.

Planning and Monitoring Recruitment

Successful recruitment of a sufficient number of participants requires considerable planning. A well-defined and organized recruitment effort must include a realistic time line, including time allowed for institutional review board (IRB) approval of recruitment materials and consent form, consideration of staffing needs, an itemized budget, advertising strategies and approaches, and a monitoring system. Important considerations for each of these components of the research plan are described in this discussion.

Institutional Review Board's Role in Recruitment

Investigators must avoid any recruitment tactic that might be perceived as coercing individuals to participate in the study. The IRB must be assured no coercion is involved in recruiting study subjects. IRBs may also have oversight of the recruitment effort. Consequently, the IRB is mandated to approve all recruitment activities and advertisements that investigators propose to use in their study. At institutions where IRBs do not have this authority, the IRBs nonetheless play an important role in reviewing the planned recruitment effort to ensure that it is appropriate, highly professional, and has the utmost regard for the rights of the participants. (Also see Chapter 5, "Ethical Considerations in Dietary Studies.")

Time Needed for Recruitment

The time frame for achieving the recruitment goals must be clearly defined. Recruitment must be initiated far enough in advance of the study start date to elicit a response to advertising and to complete the screening activities. Estimating a realistic time frame depends on understanding factors that influence recruitment. In general, the difficulty of recruiting for a study depends on its complexity. A demanding study for which the selection criteria are restrictive requires more time and effort than less intensive studies with broadly defined eligibility criteria. Factors that affect the recruitment process include the number of participants needed, the study's inclusion and exclusion criteria, and the density of the target population in the community:

Recruitment plan considerations
Time allotment
Staff
Budget
Recruitment strategies
Recruitment monitoring

Factors that affect the rate of recruitment
Study-related issues:
    Number of participants
    Inclusion and exclusion criteria
    Density of target population in community
Participant-related issues:
    Study design and requirements
    Length of participation and time commitments
    Perceived benefits
        Remuneration
        Health benefits
        Good of society and altruism

Factors that directly influence the potential participant—such as study requirements, time commitment, and compensation—also affect the ease of participant recruitment. A prudent philosophy is to overestimate the time needed for recruitment and to have a variety of strategies in place to ensure recruitment goals. Usually the amount of time estimated for meeting recruitment goals is overly optimistic. For a long-term study of dietary fat and blood cholesterol concentrations (6), 4 months were required to recruit 30 male students. One month was spent planning the recruitment strategies, making contacts, and designing the advertising campaign, and 3 months were spent recruiting participants.

Recruitment efforts for another study with a similar design did not require a long planning phase, and only 2 months were needed to recruit 30 participants. For a less complex study, 2 weeks were ample to recruit 6 participants for a small, 1-month pilot study. Personal experience will also help define the amount of time needed for recruitment.

An overly long recruitment effort can not only increase the cost of the study but also cause individuals recruited early to lose interest before the study begins. Maintaining close contact with potential participants throughout recruitment as well as staggering screening efforts are recommended so that individuals recruited early on will not have a long wait from initial contact to acceptance into or exclusion from the study.

Depending on the effectiveness of the recruitment strategies, a large initial response can be expected during the 2 to 3 days after the advertising campaign begins. The response rate should be monitored weekly, and alternative methods should be available and easily implemented if necessary to meet recruitment goals within the prescribed amount of time. Suggestions for alternative strategies are discussed later in Recruitment Strategies.

Staffing Needs

Recruitment can require a large and specialized staff. The staff must be well trained and able to maintain a professional, friendly, and composed attitude when they interact with the potential participants. For larger studies, a recruitment coordinator is needed to organize recruitment strategies and manage staff and paperwork. Support staff may be full-time staff members of the research team whose duties are shifted during the different phases of the study. Likewise, newly hired staff can assume other responsibilities during the study after recruitment is over. Temporary personnel (eg, people to answer telephone calls) are also important.

Approximately one to one-and-a-half full-time personnel are needed to carry out a recruitment effort for a controlled feeding study with about 30 participants. For a smaller study with fewer participants or simpler eligibility requirements, one half-time position may be sufficient for recruitment activities. In addition to actual recruitment (ie, advertising and telephone or in-person contacts designed to attract potential participants), screening activities that require further gathering of information through measurements and questionnaires require additional staff time.

Budget Considerations

The costs of recruitment can be large depending on the number of people to be screened, the advertising methods used, and the number of staff needed to carry out recruitment. Estimates of costs for various recruitment methods and the associated staff hours are listed in Table 6-2 (6, 7). These estimates are based on recruitment costs in rural central Pennsylvania; however, costs vary by geographic location.

Other factors that contribute to the costs of recruitment include extra telephone lines for telephone interviews, printing costs for screening questionnaires, and laboratory analyses for biomedical screening tests. These costs can be considerable, depending on the complexity of the screening criteria. For smaller studies and studies recruiting college students, simple placement of fliers in mailboxes or small ads in the local or campus newspaper may be sufficient and are considerably less costly than recruitment activities required for larger studies or for studies requiring a diverse population.

Monitoring Recruitment

Careful record keeping is extremely important during recruitment to keep track of recruitment progress, and perhaps even more importantly, to document that the eligibility criteria are met. For small studies involving fewer than 10 subjects in which 1 person manages the entire recruitment and screening process, monitoring and record keeping can be fairly simple and performed either manually or with the use of a simple computer database or spreadsheet program. However, this task can become overwhelming when investigators are recruiting for a large study or when several categories of participants must be managed through a series of screening visits. In addition, enlisting new recruits, scheduling of telephone interviews, face-to-face appointments, laboratory tests and other measurements, and evaluating eligibility data must be effectively coordinated to efficiently use resources and meet the recruitment deadline.

During the first DELTA study, each of the four field centers had recruitment goals for African-American and Caucasian subjects in the following categories: males younger than 40 years; males older than 40 years; premenopausal females; postmenopausal females. The field centers, which often had several staff members involved in recruitment and screening, had to quickly identify and differentiate between new contacts and the participants who were going through each phase of screening. A computerized system was developed in which each new contact was assigned an identification number that was entered into a database. This database subsequently provided staff members with current information about the status of each participant. The system also facilitated monitoring the recruitment progress to identify when each category was filled (and thus recruitment for that group could end) and which category needed more intensive recruitment efforts. With recruitment monitoring and analysis of the yields for each screening step, investigators can plan how many people need to be screened and estimate when recruitment activities may be halted.

Another use of the monitoring database is in enabling the research center to maintain essential information from interested volunteers, who perhaps are ineligible for the cur-

TABLE 6-2

Recruitment Costs for Feeding Studies Conducted by the Authors (6, 7)

Strategies	Cost/Item	Total Staff Hours
Mailing (1,000 letters)	$0.60	20
Fliers (100)	$0.05	5
Telephone calls (100)	(local)	20
Recruitment meetings (10)	Staff salary	40
Ads		
Newspaper (per ad)	$25–$150	1–2
Television (15 seconds)	$50	1–2
Radio (15 seconds)	$0 (public service)	1–2

rent study but who may be eligible for future studies. The system can be adapted so that mailing and telephone lists can be generated from a list of potential participants, thus aiding recruitment for future studies.

Recruitment Strategies

The goal of recruitment is to attract potential participants into the study. Using different methods to advertise the study will facilitate recruitment. Common recruitment advertising venues include newspaper, television and radio, work sites, fliers and posters, letters, mass mailings, health fairs and community screenings, telephone solicitation, word-of-mouth, and physician referrals. The choice of recruitment methods varies with the number of participants needed, budget considerations, and participant needs. Using multiple methods to advertise the study will facilitate recruiting enough participants into the study.

In addition to having a wide-reaching distribution and high visibility, advertising enhances the study's credibility and acceptability within the target population, factors that are important determinants of volunteerism (5). The advantages and disadvantages of various recruitment methods are summarized in Table 6–3. Table 6–4 rates the effectiveness of common recruitment methods experienced by several research centers (see references 7–20 for descriptions of these studies).

Newspaper Advertising

An ad in a local newspaper is a common and effective form of recruiting participants (21). Content and location are important considerations in placing newspaper advertisements.

Advertising Content

Consider the target population and requirements of the study during advertisement design. An effective advertisement provides enough information to generate interest as well as to discourage ineligible individuals. A brief, concise description of the study should be included, as well as several key inclusion and exclusion criteria.

Exhibit 6–1 illustrates how newspaper advertisements can be used as a screening tool. The first advertisement (A) does not provide sufficient information and many ineligible individuals may call for more information, flooding the phone lines and wasting time and money. The second advertisement (B) provides some important selection criteria (ie, those for nonsmoking males, requirements for blood samples) that will screen out many ineligible individuals and those not willing to give blood. In addition, individuals interested in losing weight will not be eligible. Including in the advertising the requirement to maintain weight during the study is important in screening out a large number of persons who want to lose weight. Ad B also lists some incentives (ie, all food provided plus some financial compensation) that could encourage interested individuals to call for more information. The affiliation of the study with the local university enhances its legitimacy and may encourage potential participants to respond.

Advertising Placement

Most newspapers allow the designation of a particular section in which the ad should appear. For example, in a study targeting male college students conducted at Pennsylvania State University, ads drawing the greatest response were

TABLE 6-3

Advantages and Disadvantages of the Various Recruitment Methods

Method	Example	Advantage(s)	Disadvantage(s)
Newspaper	Large ads in specific sections. Smaller ads in classifieds	Reaches a wide audience Inexpensive (small ads)	Can be costly (large ads)
Radio and television	Public service announcements	Reaches a wide audience	Can be costly
Mass mailings	Letter describing study sent to target population. Addresses from registrar, directories, other organizational memberships	Letters can be personalized	Labor-intensive Can be costly
Flyers, posters	Posted in high visibility areas	Inexpensive	Usually insufficient when used alone
Physician referrals	Physician describes study to patient	Targeted population	Slow rate of referrals
Word-of-mouth and networking	Presentations to clubs or individuals	Inexpensive Targeted population	Yield small
Recruitment meetings	Potential participants attend informational meeting	Personal contact Large audience	Requires participant effort
Telephone solicitation	Individuals are called, study is described	Personal contact	Labor intensive

TABLE 6-4

Effectiveness of Common Recruitment Methods for Feeding Studies[1]

	Pennsylvania State University[2]	Tufts University[3]	Columbia University[4]	University of Minnesota[5]
Newspaper	1	1	—	1
Mailings	2[6]	—	1[7]	2
Word of Mouth	3	3	3	3
Flyers/Posters	4	—	2[8]	—
Radio	—	4	—	—
Other: (television, physician referrals, articles, unknown)	5	2	—	—

[1]Not all methods used by each group. Rated on a scale from 1 to 5 (Most Effective = 1; Least Effective = 5).
[2]Information provided by Vikkie Mustad, PhD; see reference 7.
[3]Information provided by Alice Lichtenstein, ScD; see references 8–14.
[4]Information provided by Maliha Siddiqui, MS, MPH, and Wahida Karmally, MS, RD, CDE; see references 15, 16.
[5]Information provided by Peggy Martini, PhD, and Joanne Slavin, PhD; see references 17–20.
[6]Letters sent to all age-eligible students.
[7]Letters to incoming medical school students were included with admission materials with letters of recommendation from the College Dean.
[8]Flyers placed in student post mailboxes and posted in communal locations.

large (5″ × 7″) copy ads located in the highly visible sports sections of the university publication. Smaller, less expensive ads placed in the classified, personal, and help wanted sections were less successful. Designating a specific section for the ad is more expensive, but an ad with low visibility can slow recruitment efforts. It may be worthwhile to discuss placement of the ad with an advertising editor.

Radio and Television Advertising

Advertising on radio and television may be the best way to target a large number of participants in a short period of time; however, it is not commonly used because of its expense. A low-cost alternative to more formal advertising is to use public service announcements on local radio or cable television stations. A major drawback to these advertisements is the limited time (less than 15-second spots) as well as lack

of control over when the message is aired (ie, possibly at a time when the audience is small). Thus, radio and television may be best used in conjunction with other media promotions (ie, newspaper ads).

News Stories

An alternative and free method of advertising results from a news story, featured by the local newspaper, television station, or radio news. Nutrition and health science news topics are regular features in most local papers and some radio and television news programs. News stories that describe human research are excellent advertisements for any upcoming studies. For example, a short press release about the DELTA study evoked such interest that it led to local and national television, radio, and newspaper stories.

EXHIBIT 6-1

Sample Advertisements Used to Recruit Subjects into a Well-controlled Feeding Study

A

Healthy men needed for diet study.
Call J. Smith, 555-1212 for more information.

B

NUTRITION STUDY
– Healthy, nonsmoking men (25–50 years)
  needed for study of diet and blood cholesterol.

- All food provided by University's Nutrition Department.
- Must maintain weight.
- Must be able to provide blood samples.
- Some financial compensation.

For more information, call J. Smith, PhD, at 555-1212.

Newsletters

Many workplaces routinely publish an in-house newsletter or newspaper that can be an effective means of advertising the study. Professional, civic, and special-interest groups and clubs publish newsletters regularly that are distributed locally. This is a particularly good way of targeting special groups of interest for the study. Employers may also have a space on employees' pay stubs for comments or news and may allow the study to be advertised this way.

Physician Referrals

Recruitment of participants with metabolic disorders or medical conditions (eg, diabetes or hyperlipidemia) can be carried out through physicians' offices, hospitals, or clinics. Access to a patient population that can be contacted quickly can facilitate meeting recruitment goals within the projected time line. Alternatively, patients are given information about the study during a regular visit, in which case the recruitment effort will require more time. The major advantage of recruiting through referrals is the reliable identification of the target population. Another advantage is the perceived credibility of the study by potential participants because of their physicians' support of it.

To maintain the confidentiality of the medical information, investigators do not ask physicians directly to supply the names of patients. Rather the physician's office is provided, at the study's expense, with materials to send to the patients. Labor costs are also covered by the study.

Fliers and Posters

In general, fliers and posted advertisements work best to supplement other recruitment efforts. Location is an important determinant of the effectiveness of posted advertisements, and those that are seen by individuals many times per day work best to reinforce continually the need for study participants. Posters in a medical clinic or physician's waiting room generally are more effective than those posted in a storefront window. Posters hung in the workplace can reinforce the employer's support of the study. Posters should include tear-off slips with the name and phone number of the contact person.

Mass Mailings and Electronic Communications

Although the yield—that is, the number of participants randomized per hundred mailings sent—from mass mailings is low, the number of mailings is large, usually many tens of thousands. Thus, mass mailings have been found to be an effective method of recruitment, particularly in some large-scale studies (22). An advantage of advertising by mass mailings is that most of the pertinent information about the study can be included in a single letter. Mailing lists can be generated randomly, by zip code region, from employers' club registries, from state motor vehicle bureaus, and from university registrars. These lists can be used to target seg-ments of the population. Using official letterhead for the return address also can ensure that the envelope will be opened and not considered junk mail.

A major drawback is that mailings can be fairly expensive in terms of postage and staff time. However, mailing services can be contracted to stuff envelopes and address envelopes.

Electronic mail (e-mail) and bulletin boards (Web sites) are relatively new forms of communication with promising potential for recruiting certain population groups efficiently and inexpensively. For example, all incoming students at some universities are required to have a personal computer. E-mail frequently is used by the faculty and administrators to communicate with students. Likewise, researchers can advertise a study widely using e-mail and the Internet. However, at this time individuals must have a computer to use e-mail or to access the Internet.

Future technologies, such as interactive television, will also make electronic information more accessible. Thus far, recruitment experience through electronic mail has not been widely reported.

Personal Contacts

Word-of-mouth and networking for recruitment are often adequate for acquiring participants in small studies, but larger recruitment efforts require other strategies or a combination of methods. Such strategies may also include word-of-mouth and networking. Word-of-mouth recruitment can be effective, especially if done by former participants or by those who are considering participating in an ongoing study (eg, to create a buddy system). Personal contacts with directors of local organizations tap into a pool of potential volunteers. Enlisting the aid of instructors or group leaders to make announcements prior to college or adult education classes or local meetings is another way to advertise the study. Networking with other experienced researchers also provides access to another pool of volunteers.

Recruitment Meetings

An efficient method of recruiting and simultaneously screening a large number of individuals is to hold recruitment meetings. Interested individuals are invited in the advertisement to attend one of several meetings, held at different dates and times, at which they can learn more about the study (ie, its purpose, general design, time commitments, attendance requirements, and key criteria for participation). Individuals are invited to leave at any time throughout the meeting if they are no longer interested.

At the conclusion of the meeting the attendees are given an opportunity to ask any questions in private. Interested individuals also can be given an opportunity to schedule a formal screening visit or instructed to call back if they need time to consider their participation.

The location of this meeting may be an important consideration. A neighborhood community center, church, or school auditorium may be a convenient location for studies seeking participants within the community. For studies conducted on the Pennsylvania State University campus, holding recruitment meetings in the dining room and giving interested individuals an opportunity to tour the facility was found to be ideal. Not only did this approach allow potential participants to visualize their involvement in the study but it also eased some of their apprehensions.

Recruiting Special Populations

The National Institutes of Health (NIH) has established guidelines for the inclusion of women and minorities and their subpopulations in its funded research with human subjects (23). Updates to these guidelines are released periodically and should be reviewed before submission of any grant application. Federal funding agencies now require that all proposals and applications with human subjects must include women and minority groups to improve gender and race representation in clinical trials. Such requirements target understudied groups that are disproportionately affected by certain diseases or disorders. To comply with these guidelines, special recruitment efforts are necessary.

The initial step in recruiting special populations is to identify rich pools of potential participants. A valuable resource for identifying potential target groups is census data. Information on population census data, cross-classified by age, race, and gender, can be obtained for any county or township from the Bureau of the Census. Summary books of "General Population and Housing Characteristics" are prepared for each state for each decennial census by the Bureau of the Census, US Department of Commerce. This documentation is generally available in the reference section of a university library and can be requested by contacting Customer Services, Bureau of the Census, Washington DC 20233, telephone (301) 763–4100. Some states also have regional census offices.

Once target groups of interest have been identified, the most appropriate recruitment strategies can be implemented. Strategies for recruiting minorities, women, older adults, and other groups are discussed next. (Recruitment of children is discussed in Chapter 9, "Children as Participants in Feeding Studies.")

Minorities

One way to establish and promote multiethnic contacts is to develop and maintain ongoing relationships with minority organizations and professional associations at the worksite and within the community. Enlisting the aid of churches and networking through church programs are effective ways in which to recruit minorities in the community. Effective presentation programs concentrated within these organizations also can initiate positive word-of-mouth publicity.

A key factor in recruiting minority populations is having a liaison or recruiters of similar ethnicity and socioeconomic background to allay concerns about cultural or ethnic bias.

If necessary, special bicultural and bilingual liaisons and recruiters should be hired. In special cases, it may be necessary for the liaison or recruiter to make personal contact in the families' homes for successful recruitment. Such an approach may be especially helpful in Hispanic communities, in which the support of the male head of household may be the major determinant for participation of family members in research studies.

Women

Women within the community can be targeted through service organizations, religious institutions, parent-teacher associations, women's organizations and volunteer clubs, and health clubs. College women can be targeted through sororities, women's dormitories, or through other programs (eg, nursing, dietetics) that enroll a large proportion of women. Pregnant and lactating women can be targeted through obstetricians' offices; Lamaze classes; La Leche groups; or government-sponsored Special Supplemental Nutrition Program for Women, Infants, and Children (WIC) programs. Women with children living at home are more difficult to recruit because of family and household responsibilities. Similar difficulties are also encountered with older women whose husbands are retired and at home.

Women with career responsibilities can be difficult to recruit because of time constraints. Programs that minimize the time imposed on these potential participants are most effective. For example, women may be more interested in studies that provide incentives designed to save time (eg, precooked meals that are delivered and research sites providing child care services). In the DELTA study, some women did not want to participate in the study if their significant other was not also eligible. In some instances, meals have been provided for spouses and children when difficulties were encountered in recruiting women.

Older Adults

Recruitment of older individuals for research can be a difficult task. Poor health, mental confusion, fatigue, sensory impairment, and lack of transportation are problems commonly encountered (24). Although these obstacles can be overcome to some extent if a rich pool of healthy older individuals has been identified, a substantially larger number of interested potential participants may be required to yield one participant who meets the eligibility criteria and is enrolled in the study.

Individuals who do not perceive a direct health benefit from participation are less motivated to participate in the study (Mustad and Kris-Etherton, unpublished observation). Additionally, attrition due to illness means that more older individuals must be recruited into longer-term studies in order to ensure adequate sample size (25).

A personalized approach to recruitment has been shown to be effective with older individuals (25). Personal letters sent to retired individuals (eg, mailing lists obtained from university or employer's records or from the American Association for Retired Persons) also have been effectively to recruit older individuals for studies. Letters and newsletter articles that describe the study and its staff in particular, with pictures if possible, also are ideal for this population (26).

A personal presentation conducted by a staff member to groups of older individuals is a popular recruitment strategy at senior centers, community meal sites, churches, and retirement residence communities (27). The recruiter should have experience dealing with older adults because personal contact and extensive interviews will be helpful in alleviating fears and concerns about any adverse health effects of the study. Older individuals need time to think about participating in the study without feeling pressured. Close contact between the staff and participant during the recruitment and screening is essential to successful recruitment of older individuals.

Patients

Research with individuals who have medical conditions or metabolic abnormalities (eg, diabetes, hypercholesterolemia, or arthritis) can present special recruitment problems. Identification of these groups can be simplified by recruiting through physicians' offices or medical clinics (see the earlier discussion under Physician Referrals) or patient support groups. National registries (eg, cancer registries) also can be used to identify individuals with a specific or rare condition. A recruitment effort that is combined with free medical screening (eg, cholesterol assessment at the local mall) is also a way to identify these individuals, but must be done in ways that avoid coercion. (See Chapter 5, "Ethical Considerations in Dietary Studies.")

Other Considerations

Factors that Motivate Individuals to Participate in Feeding Studies

Understanding the factors that motivate individuals to participate in feeding studies will facilitate choosing appropriate recruitment strategies. Sounder (25) provides a detailed report of motivators of older individuals gathered during several years of recruiting subjects for aging and dementia studies. Sounder found that motivators were: altruism (opportunity to help others), need for personal contact, curiosity of a novel experience, hope for a personal health benefit, and interest in scientific involvement. Our experience in conducting studies of diet and heart disease risk factors suggests that most younger (<40 years) participants are motivated by financial reasons (free food, reduced grocery bills, financial compensation) and the convenience of having food prepared and served. Middle-aged and older people appear to be less motivated by the financial benefits of study participation but have a greater interest in personal health benefits and their own results. Participation in studies that have no obvious or immediate health benefit in this group may require more intensive approaches to recruitment.

Modifying Recruitment Efforts

Recruitment progress should be monitored in a timely fashion (eg, weekly), and when recruitment goals are not met, alternative recruitment strategies must be implemented. Different advertising strategies or multiple strategies should be used. Modification of the exclusion criteria (eg, age restrictions) may be considered to expand the participant pool; however, this should be done so as not to compromise the study's research question. Another strategy is to offer incentives to encourage individuals to participate in recruitment (see the discussion under Incentives). A final option is to extend the recruitment period; however, this should be considered last because it could increase study costs, inconvenience participants already recruited, and compromise staff morale.

In multicenter studies, one center that has been more successful with recruitment can make up for a recruitment shortage at another center. However, it is important for the final distribution of all study populations to be evenly divided among the field centers to eliminate possible geographical bias.

Incentives

Incentives are used to stimulate interest in the study and to encourage potential participants to participate in the screening activities. Examples of appropriate incentives include blood test results, diet assessments, medical exams, coffee mugs, T-shirts, calendars, movie tickets, and gift certificates. Incentives should not be so attractive that they give the impression of coercion; they are only offered to encourage individuals to participate in screening. Moreover, they should not be inappropriately generous prior to study enrollment such that individuals go through screening but have no intention of becoming a participant in the study. Also, IRBs often assess the appropriateness of incentives as part of their human subjects review of research protocols.

Incentives can be useful to encourage individuals to participate in recruitment and screening activities during the initial phases of the study. The most cost-effective incentives are those that are combined with the screening process. Incentives also can be offered to encourage enrolled participants to recruit other potential participants. These incentives can include small monetary incentives in addition to those already mentioned. Any incentives that are provided for participant screening should be appropriate and offered to promote genuine interest in the study.

"Professional" or Repeat Volunteers

Some individuals keep volunteering for many studies because of financial incentives, social reasons, concern about their health, a strong sense of altruism, or other reasons. Investigators should consider whether potential participants' prior enrollment in other studies would compromise the results of the proposed investigation. As a matter of routine, investigators should ask recruits about prior participation in research studies.

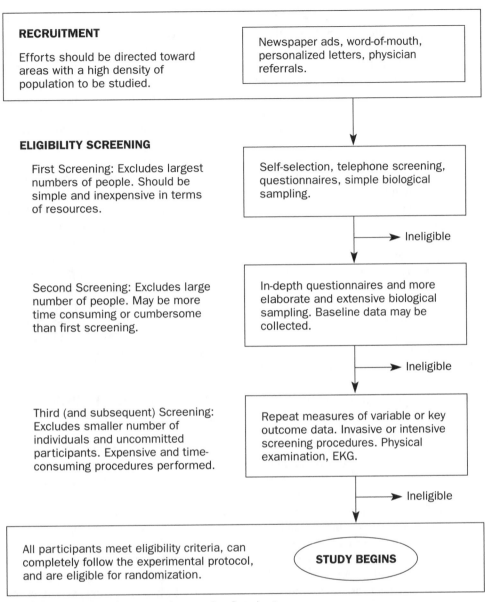

FIGURE 6-1.   Recruitment and screening flowchart.

SCREENING

The goal of screening is to recruit the best possible participants into the study. Although this activity can require considerable time and effort, it is well worth the investment because participant retention is enhanced. Experienced staff frequently can identify individuals who likely will not complete the study or adhere to the study protocol. This will reduce the participant dropout rate, enhance compliance, and improve the research environment for participants and staff.

The screening process must be carefully planned. Information is collected during screening not only to establish the eligibility of potential participants and assess (often subjectively) their ability to adhere to all aspects of the study protocol, but also to collect baseline data as well as other data of interest. Enthusiastic and inexperienced investigators may attempt to collect too much data at this time. This can

be a disincentive for potential participants to participate in the study, can unnecessarily increase the workload of the staff, and can waste time and resources.

A general rule is to collect only data that will be analyzed or used. Experienced investigators appreciate that some data may be important for interpreting the results of the study or planning future research directions. Therefore, data should be collected prudently.

Screening Visits

Most typically, screening proceeds in a step-wise fashion (Figure 6–1). The eligibility criteria will, in practice, be used to screen potential participants. Many interested individuals will be screened out simply because they do not meet the eligibility criteria listed in the recruitment materials and advertisements. For potential participants who meet the initial screening criteria, further screening then can be scheduled. Initial screening may involve a telephone interview or rapid collection of various simple laboratory measurements, such as a blood total cholesterol level, hemoglobin level, blood pressure, or a brief dietary assessment about dietary intake and food practices.

Some of these measurements can be made at a health fair, in a shopping mall, or supermarket. Another initial screening approach can be carried out in a primary health care provider's office followed by the referral of a potential participant to the study staff. This referral is based on the eligibility criteria and information from the patient's chart.

In some instances initial screening can be done without directly contacting the potential participant. If the first screening contact is a telephone interview, an interested potential participant could subsequently receive various forms in the mail to complete and return. Forms that might be given to a potential participant in this manner are a food record, physical activity record, family history questionnaire, and body weight log. This information then could be mailed to the investigator or hand-delivered at the next screening visit or other scheduled visit. Thus, this early stage of screening actually often requires little contact between screenee and staff.

The next screening visit involves more intensive or invasive data collection. A potential participant may have height, weight, skinfold thickness, and blood pressure measurements taken, and blood may be collected. Some measurements made earlier may be repeated and verified. Information about a potential participant's diet is often collected during screening. In addition to the 24-hour dietary recall—which can be obtained by a telephone interview—or a food record, information should be collected about food patterns and behaviors (eg, whether they are atypical or inappropriate for participation in the study, and whether they are highly variable), and food avoidances. Potential participants can be shown menus of the experimental diet to assess whether they think they can follow it.

Whenever possible, more than one screening visit should be required so that major variables that determine eligibility—especially if those variables are also primary endpoints of the study—can be thoroughly assessed. For example, a second visit for repeat blood cholesterol or blood pressure measurement would be used to establish the accuracy of the first measurement, especially if eligibility criteria define the limits for blood cholesterol or blood pressure levels of the study participants. Because of regression to the mean (see Chapter 2, "Statistical Aspects of Controlled Diet Studies") the extra effort to obtain at least a second measurement will result in a higher likelihood that the study participants are truly within the range of eligibility limits when the study begins. Sometimes biological samples that are collected at this second visit (eg, blood and urine) are analyzed at a later time for certain parameters should the potential participant meet all other eligibility criteria. This reduces assay costs and simplifies screening efforts.

A third screening is frequently required. For many parameters, it is necessary to collect more than 2 repeated measurements. For example, at least 3 blood pressure measurements are required to diagnose hypertension and 3 triglyceride measurements are recommended to diagnose hypertriglyceridemia. If there is considerable variation in these 3 measurements, another might be warranted. Another reason for a third screening visit is to carry out more sophisticated measurements. Examples include hormone measurements, lipoprotein analyses, and body composition determinations from hydrostatic weighing.

Finally, more extensive screening procedures, if needed, can be done. These might include a complete medical exam, a treadmill test, various invasive procedures such as a cardiac catheterization, a sigmoidoscopy, or a tissue biopsy. During this visit, potential participants may be interviewed by a behavioral scientist or asked to complete a personality assessment questionnaire to determine their suitability for participating in the study. Because of the time required and cost of these more extensive procedures, they are only done if necessary and only during the latter stages of screening after the majority of ineligible individuals have been already screened out—usually just before the study begins.

Eligibility Criteria Issues During Screening

To avoid confusion and minimize wasted effort during the screening process, clear cut criteria regarding medical issues should be detailed prior to the initiation of the screening process. These criteria are usually formalized in the consent form and reviewed and approved by the institutional review board (IRB). (Also see Chapter 5, "Ethical Considerations in Dietary Studies.")

Every effort should be made to be as specific as possible in order to anticipate as many permutations or individual scenarios as possible. However, it is inevitable that gray areas will arise. Whereas use of medications may be the basis for exclusion, questions always arise about allergy medications, aspirin, and antacids. If a volunteer is identified as having an elevated thyroid-stimulating hormone level during screening and thyroid hormone replacement is initiated, investigators must decide whether the volunteer is still eligible to participate in the study. The medical officer for the study can review individual situations and make decisions about the suitability of a potential participant for a particular study.

Frequently during screening some persons are identified with high levels of blood pressure, blood glucose, or plasma cholesterol. These individuals should be referred to their physician. In addition to ensuring that a referral procedure is in place and followed, investigators must assume responsibility for the safety of potential subjects during screening. Those who require immediate medical attention must be informed immediately of their condition. A listing of medical clinics in the surrounding area could be made available to individuals who do not have a personal physician, medical insurance, or adequate resources for medical care.

Common strategies for collecting screening information are described in Table 6–5. Although not inclusive, the table provides a representative listing of frequently collected screening data. Methods used to collect this information also are presented. Several screening instruments used for different feeding studies conducted by the authors are included in Exhibits 6–2 through 6–4.

It is critical during the screening process to assess the ability of the potential volunteer to understand and follow directions. This is particularly important for outpatient studies that require specimen collections, reporting to the study center in the fasted state at certain intervals, or the use of some type of self-administered supplements. An individual's response to the screening process is a valuable way to assess important qualities for compliance with the experimental protocol. These include adherence to all aspects of the screening protocol, for example, attending all scheduled sessions, being prepared as required, completing all assessments, and having a positive attitude.

Usually, if potential participants do not carry out their responsibilities related to the screening process, it is unlikely they will comply with all aspects of the study protocol. Therefore, noncompliance during the screening process can be the basis for excluding an individual from the study.

Estimating Screening Pool Size

As discussed throughout this chapter, the major determinant of the difficulty or ease of recruiting subjects depends on the number of participants needed, the restrictiveness of the eligibility criteria, and the participant burden based on the complexity of the study. Table 6–6 shows response, screening, and recruitment yields for well-controlled diet studies having different participant characteristics and study designs.

For example, the studies conducted at Pennsylvania State University (7), Tufts University (8–14), and Columbia University (15, 16) focused primarily on effects of dietary fatty acids and cholesterol on plasma lipids and lipoproteins and required that free-living participants consume prepared diets in a metabolic study setting. The examples from University of Minnesota are from studies in which participants repeatedly self-selected experimental diets and were instructed to incorporate daily fiber and flax seed supplements (17–20).

The number of respondents that is encountered during the recruitment period is greatly influenced by the overall participant burden based on the study requirements as well as by the methods used to advertise the study. The data included in Table 6–6 give a general overview of the effort involved in recruiting participants for different studies. As Table 6–6 illustrates, younger men and medical students of both sexes appear to be relatively easier to recruit into feeding studies (~2–3 respondents screened for each participant randomized into the study) than either younger women (9 screened: 1 randomized) or healthy middle-aged and older men and women (~6–22 screened: 1 randomized). The latter groups often require a larger number of initial respondents in order to meet the recruitment goals, usually as a result of

TABLE 6-5

Strategies for Collecting Screening Information

Criteria	Methods
Demographics	• Questionnaire, self-administered, or interviewer-administered
Anthropometrics	• Direct measurement • Obtained from participant's medical record • Self-reported with or without interviewer assistance
Biochemical data	• Direct measurement • Obtained from participant's medical records
Diet	• Multiple 24-hour recalls • Food records • Food frequency questionnaire (self- or interviewer-administered) to query about supplement use, food allergies and avoidances, special dietary practices and needs, and alcohol and caffeine consumption practices • Ask prospective participant to review test diet menus to assess willingness to adhere to the controlled diet
Smoking habits	• Questionnaire including information about active and passive exposure • Saliva or blood for cotinine or breath CO_2 to verify questionnaire
Physical activity	• Questionnaire • Activity monitoring device
Medical history	• Questionnaire • Participant's medical record
Attitude	• Interview • Follow-through on screening protocol

EXHIBIT 6-2

Medical Questionnaire[1]

Name:_____

    Address:_____

            _____

            _____

    Phone number (Daytime):_____ (Evening):_____
    Date of Birth:_____ Age:_____

Smoking:

    Do you smoke cigarettes at present? Yes ( ) No ( )
    Did you quit in the last year? Yes ( ) No ( )
    If yes, how many cigarettes did you smoke per day?_____

Alcohol:

    Do you drink alcoholic beverages? Yes ( ) No ( )
    If ''yes,'' which of the following do you drink?
    Beer_____ Wine_____ Mixed drinks_____
    How much do you drink in one week?
    Beer_____ Wine_____ Mixed drinks_____

Medications:

Are you currently taking any medications or treatments? Yes ( ) No ( )
If ''yes,'' list all below:

_____

_____

_____

Medical Problems:

Do you have, or have you had, any of the following? Please indicate the dates, frequency, and seriousness of the condition.

	Yes	No	Dates/Frequency/Seriousness
Nausea	_____	_____	_____
Vomiting	_____	_____	_____
Diarrhea	_____	_____	_____
Constipation	_____	_____	_____
Ulcer-peptic	_____	_____	_____
Irritable Bowel Syndrome	_____	_____	_____
Colitis	_____	_____	_____

Other medical conditions (such as high blood pressure or diabetes):

_____

_____

_____

Continued

EXHIBIT 6-2   *(continued)*

Family History:

Please indicate if any of the following family members has or had a history of heart disease, high blood pressure, hyperlipidemia, overweight, stroke, diabetes, liver disease, etc:

Relationship	Living		Deceased	
	Age	Ailments	Age	Ailments
Paternal Grandfather	_____	_____	_____	_____
Paternal Grandmother	_____	_____	_____	_____
Maternal Grandfather	_____	_____	_____	_____
Maternal Grandmother	_____	_____	_____	_____
Father	_____	_____	_____	_____
Mother	_____	_____	_____	_____
Brothers	_____	_____	_____	_____
Sisters	_____	_____	_____	_____

[1]This form can be used as a screening form and set up to exclude potential subjects if they do not meet the established medical history criteria. In addition, it can be set up to collect screening data.

a greater number of exclusions because of confounding co-morbidities.

In general, the greatest number of potential participants is excluded during the initial screening phase. Exclusion during this phase is often through the participant not meeting the major eligibility criteria or through participant self-exclusion, either because of the study's restrictions and other conflicts, or aversion to the study's protocol (eg, blood draws, fecal collections). Of those who pass through the initial screening visits, subsequent exclusion of potential participants is usually the result of failure to pass the eligibility criteria measured at the last screening visit, which tend to be more invasive or have time-consuming measurements.

Specific Issues in Selecting Participants for Feeding Studies

Study Disclosure

For the protection of human subjects, IRBs require that informed consent be obtained prior to participation in any aspect of screening. As discussed in Chapter 5, "Ethical Considerations in Dietary Studies," it is essential for the potential participant to understand fully what is expected during screening, as well as during the study. Adequate time and resources must be allocated to this aspect of the study. Screening activities can be useful in helping potential participants understand their responsibilities during the study. Full disclosure of the benefits of the study revealed during screening include incentives to participate as well as the realities of participation (eg, inconveniences, boredom with the diet, potential risks).

Psychosocial Factors

Habitual Lifestyle

Involvement in a feeding study will necessarily interfere with participants' habitual lifestyle relative to food preparation and eating behavior. In addition to collecting information about a potential participant's habitual diet, investigators also should collect information about food practices and behavior. This can be done during an interview with a screenee or by a questionnaire that is either interviewer- or self-administered. Examples of questions that are typically asked are as follows:

- Do potential participants usually eat at home or out?
- If they dine at home, do they eat with other members of the household?
- Are potential participants the main food preparers at home? If so, how will study participation influence the rest of the household unit?
- Has participation in the study been addressed with other members of the household?
- If the potential participants usually eat out, does this involve other people? Would the pattern of social interaction and support system be altered by the lack of this activity? Is there a substitute activity for social interaction?

EXHIBIT 6-3

Nutrition History[1]

Name:_____ Today's Date:_____

Measured Height:_____   Measured Weight:_____

Have you recently gained or lost weight: Yes (   ) No (   )
If yes, how much?_____ gained (   ) lost (   )

How long have you been at your present weight?_____

Do you follow any strict restriction in your diet? Yes (   ) No (   )
If yes, list what they are:_____

Do you have any food dislikes? Yes (   ) No (   ) (Examples: fish, vegetables, beans, etc)

_____

Do you have any food intolerances? Yes (   ) No (   ) (Examples: milk, spices, etc)

_____

Do you have any food allergies? Yes (   ) No (   ) (Examples: wheat, shellfish, milk, berries, nuts, etc)

_____

Do you take any vitamins or nutritional supplements? Yes (   ) No (   )

If yes, what kind, and how often?_____

Do you have any problems chewing or swallowing? Yes (   ) No (   )

Are your bowels (check one): Normal (   ) Constipated (   ) Diarrhetic (   )

Do you eat regularly? Yes (   ) No (   )

How many meals a day do you eat?_____

Where are most of your meals prepared?_____

How often do you eat in restaurants?_____

Do you think your diet is nutritionally well-balanced?_____

[1]This form can be used as a screening form and set up to exclude potential subjects if they do not meet the established nutrition history criteria. In addition, it can be set up to collect screening data.

A similar, but more intensive evaluation needs to be made if the protocol involves an inpatient feeding protocol.

Interaction Patterns with Staff and Other Participants

Protocols that involve extensive staff interaction are, for example, studies that involve inpatient protocols, frequent study-related visits, or overnight stays. Important points on which to evaluate the subject include the ability to adapt to small changes in the routine or in personnel, any tendency to be manipulative of rules, or evidence of attempts to manipulate or be divisive of staff.

Protocols that involve extensive participant interaction would be, for example, those that involve sharing one or more common meals. A participant who has a tendency to complain about the screening process, especially to other potential participants, may continue to complain and create problems during the study.

Food- and Diet-Related Issues

Food Preferences

In most well-controlled feeding studies there are essentially no food choices. When potential participants review the test diet menus and express concern about the inclusion of specific foods categories or food allergies, subsequent problems are likely. Thus, it is important to identify these problems early in the screening phase. The degree to which the study protocol can allow substitutions must be predetermined and the potential participant must understand these boundaries. Numerous requests for minor changes may be an important predictor of future problems.

Habitual Dietary Practices and Patterns

A comprehensive screening process should include a discussion of various dietary practices and patterns that involve restriction of foods and food combinations entirely or during

EXHIBIT 6-4

Physical Activity Questionnaire[1]

1. Do you train for a competitive sport(s)?

_____ Yes
_____ No

2. If you live greater than ½ mile from campus, do you regularly bike or walk?

_____ Yes
_____ No

3. List physical activities you regularly engage in.

Type of Activity: _____

Frequency: Number of times per week or month you engage in the activity: _____
Duration: How long do you engage in the activity (in minutes or hours)? _____
Intensity:

_____ Low (slow movement with occasional breaks)
_____ Moderate (brisk, steady movement)
_____ High (rapid, continuous movement)

How long has this physical exercise been a part of your normal routine (ie, weeks, months, years)? _____

Type of Activity: _____

Frequency: Number of times per week or month you engage in the activity: _____
Duration: How long do you engage in the activity (in minutes or hours)? _____
Intensity:

_____ Low (slow movement with occasional breaks)
_____ Moderate (brisk, steady movement)
_____ High (rapid, continuous movement)

How long has this physical exercise been a part of your normal routine (ie, weeks, months, years)? _____

COMMENTS:

[1] This form can be used as a screening form and set up to exclude potential subjects if they do not meet the established physical activity history criteria. In addition, it can be set up to collect screening data.

certain periods. This includes religious practices. The ability to participate in a study depends on the specific issues raised.

Facilities at Home for Storing and Heating Food

Requirements for safe storage and warming of the participant's packed meals at home should be discussed. The ability to understand food storage safety should be one of the selection criteria for participants, and adequate refrigeration space at their home is fundamental to this issue.

Accommodating Special Needs

Long-term feeding studies that require subjects to commit to the protocol for extended periods of time must address

the reality that subjects will have conflicts that may interfere with the study's protocol. Occasional work-related travel, schedule conflicts, transportation problems, and family responsibilities are common situations that may interfere with the complete adherence of an otherwise outstanding participant.

If the conflict does not interfere with the study protocol, important questions to ask are: How much effort is required? and, How much can be spent accommodating special needs? Data from subjects who have participated in the study for a long period of time are especially valuable, as are those in a group with a small number of participants. In some studies, meals for an ineligible spouse have been provided in order to collect data from a participant who would not participate

TABLE 6-6

Screening and Enrollment Rates for Well-Controlled Feeding Studies with Different Designs and Populations[1]

	Pennsylvania State University[2]	Tufts University[3]			Columbia University[4]	University of Minnesota[5]	
	Healthy Men (21–35 yr)	Healthy Men (≥40 yr) and Postmenopausal Women[6]			Male & Female Medical Students (~25–30 yr)	Healthy Young Women	Healthy Young Men
Length of entire study	14 wk	30 wk	30 wk	55 wk	27 wk	7 mo	9 wk
Number of individuals:							
Initial response	350	666	578	220	150	NA[7]	NA
Screened	125	203	315	114	90	200	40
Randomized into study	51	17	14	19	39	23	20
Screened: Randomized ratio	3:1	12:1	22:1	6:1	3:1	9:1	2:1
Time for recruitment and screening	8 wk	4–6 wk			4–6 wk	4–6 wk	

[1]For methods of recruitment, see Table 6–5.
[2]Information provided by Vikkie Mustad, PhD; see reference 7.
[3]Information provided by Alice Lichtenstein, ScD; see references 8–14.
[4]Information provided by Maliha Siddiqui, MS, MPH, and Wahida Karmally, MS, RD; see references 15, 16.
[5]Information provided by Peggy Martini, PhD, and Joanne Slavin, PhD; see references 17–20.
[6]Data reported for 3 different studies using a similar participant population for 30 or 55 weeks.
[7]NA = not available.

alone. Studies also have provided reimbursement for parking and transportation for participants who could or would not participate otherwise.

The ramifications of each special request must be considered carefully in terms of how it affects other participants' expectations and additional requests to accommodate special needs. Sometimes it is not possible to accommodate the special needs of participants. The expense, time, and inconvenience incurred to accommodate any special need must be balanced by extra time needed for recruitment and screening of additional participants.

PILOT STUDIES

Once the recruitment and screening procedures have been developed, they then can be pilot-tested and "debugged." Even for small studies, a pilot study to test recruitment and screening procedures can help to identify and resolve potentially significant problems before the actual study begins. A pilot study also is an efficient and effective staff training activity that helps prepare competent and experienced members of the research team. A pilot study, therefore, enables investigators to assess the adequacy of the recruitment plan, revise it as indicated, and train staff to conduct recruitment and screening activities. It is well worth the time and effort, even if conducted on a small scale, to ensure that the study can begin on schedule.

Pilot studies sometimes are conducted to demonstrate to a funding agency that the investigative team can recruit the study population described in a grant application. These pilot data provide convincing evidence that the research question

and protocol will be carried out as planned and not modified because of an inability to recruit the proposed populations.

CONCLUSION

This chapter describes important components of recruitment strategies and screening procedures for well-controlled feeding studies. The scope of the recruitment and screening effort depends principally on the sample size and complexity of the study, which in turn depend on the research question.

It is important that eligibility criteria be defined carefully. Screening is essential for determining potential participants' suitability for a study. This process includes establishing whether they meet the eligibility criteria and also whether they are likely to comply with the experimental protocol. Screening usually is conducted in a series of visits, and increasingly more comprehensive procedures are conducted in the later stages.

It is important for investigators to advertise the study effectively so that the recruitment goals are met. Using different methods to advertise the study will facilitate recruiting enough subjects into the study. The choice of advertising strategies depends on many factors, including number of subjects needed, size of the eligible participant pool, requirements of the study, budget, and other factors. Researchers should also develop a contingency plan in case initial strategies do not yield enough recruits.

A well-thought-out plan is essential to avoid recruitment shortfalls, reduce recruitment costs, and prevent cost and time overruns. A realistic time line, an adequate and well-managed staff, and an appropriate budget that can accommodate unexpected events and problems are necessary to plan a good recruitment effort that can be implemented successfully.

REFERENCES

1. The Lipid Research Clinics Program. Participant recruitment to the Coronary Primary Prevention Trial. *J Chron Dis.* 1983;36:451–465.
2. Lovato LC, Hill K, Hertert S, et al. Recruitment for controlled clinical trials: literature summary and annotated bibliography. *Contr Clin Trials.* 1997;18:328–352.
3. Agras WS, Marshall GD, Kraemer HC. Planning recruitment. *Circulation.* 1982;66(Suppl):S54–S78.
4. Multiple Risk Factor Intervention Trial. Risk factor changes and mortality results. *JAMA.* 1982;248:1465–1477.
5. Rosenthal R, Rosnow RL, eds. *Artifacts in Behavioral Research.* New York, NY: Academic Press; 1969.
6. Kris-Etherton PM, Derr J, Mitchell DC, et al. The role of fatty acid saturation on plasma lipids, lipoproteins, and apolipoproteins: I. Effects of whole food diets high in cocoa butter, olive oil, soybean oil, dairy butter, and milk chocolate on the plasma lipids of young men. *Metabolism.* 1993;42:121–129.
7. Kris-Etherton PM, Derr JA, Mustad VA, et al. Effects of a milk chocolate bar per day substituted for a high-carbohydrate snack in young men on an NCEP/AHA Step 1 Diet. *Am J Clin Nutr.* 1994;60(Suppl):1037S–1042S.
8. Lichtenstein AH, Ausman LM, Carrasco W, et al. Rice bran oil consumption and plasma lipid levels in moderately hypercholesterolemic humans. *Arterioscler Thromb Vasc Biol.* 1994;14:549–556.
9. Lichtenstein AH, Ausman L, Carrasco W, et al. Hydrogenation impairs the hypolipidemic effect of corn oil in humans. *Arterioscler Thromb Vasc Biol.* 1993;13:154–161.
10. Lichtenstein AH, Ausman LM, Carrasco W, et al. Short-term consumption of a low-fat diet has a positive impact on plasma lipid concentrations only when accompanied by weight loss. *Arterioscler Thromb Vasc Biol.* 1994;14:1751–1760.
11. Schaefer EJ, Lichtenstein AH, Lamon-Fava S, et al. Efficacy of National Cholesterol Education Program Step 2 diet in normolipidemic and hypercholesterolemic middle aged and elderly men and women. *Arterioscler Thromb Vasc Biol.* 1995;15:1079–1085.
12. Meydani SN, Lichtenstein AH, Cornwall S, et al. Immunological effects of National Cholesterol Education Panel Step 2 diets with and without fish-derived n-3 fatty acid enrichment. *J Clin Invest.* 1993;92:105–113.
13. Schaefer EJ, Lichtenstein AH, Lamon-Fava S, et al. Comparative effects of National Cholesterol Education Program Step 2 diets relatively high or relatively low in fish-derived fatty acids on plasma lipoproteins in middle aged and elderly subjects. *Am J Clin Nutr.* 1996;63:234–241.
14. Lichtenstein AH, Ausman LM, Carrasco W, et al. Hypercholesterolemic effect of dietary cholesterol in diets enriched in polyunsaturated and saturated fat. Dietary cholesterol, fat saturation, and plasma lipids. *Arterioscler Thromb Vasc Biol.* 1994;14:168–175.
15. Ginsberg HN, Karmally W, Siddiqui M, et al. Dose-response of effects of dietary cholesterol on fasting and post-prandial lipids and lipoprotein metabolism in young healthy men. *Arterioscler Thromb Vasc Biol.* 1994;14:576–586.
16. Ginsberg HN, Karmally W, Siddiqui M, et al. Increases in dietary cholesterol are associated with modest increases in both LDL and HDL cholesterol in healthy young women. *Arterioscler Thromb Vasc Biol.* 1995;15:169–178.
17. Lampe JW, Wetsch R, Thompson RO, et al. Gastrointestinal effects of sugarbeet fiber and wheat bran in healthy men. *Eur J Clin Nutr.* 1993;47:543–548.
18. Phipps WR, Martini MC, Lampe JW, et al. Effects of flax seed ingestion on the menstrual cycle. *J Clin Metab.* 1993;77:1215–1219.
19. Lampe JW, Martini MC, Kurzer MS, et al. Urinary lignan and isoflavonoid excretion in premenopausal women consuming flaxseed powder. *Am J Clin Nutr.* 1994;60:122–128.
20. Kurzer MS, Lampe JW, Martini MC, et al. Fecal lignan and isoflavonoid excretion in premenopausal women consuming flaxseed powder. *Cancer Epidemiol Biomarker Prev.* 1995;4:353–358.
21. Levenkron JC, Farquhar JW. Recruitment using mass media strategies. *Circulation.* 1982;66:32–46.
22. Hollis JF, Satterfield S, Smith F, et al. Recruitment for phase II of the Trials of Hypertension Prevention: effective strategies and predictors of randomization. *Ann Epidemiol.* 1995;5:140–148.
23. Department of Health and Human Services, National Institutes of Health. NIH Guidelines on the Inclusion of Women and Minorities as Subjects in Clinical Research. *Federal Register.* 1994;59:11146–11151.
24. Camp CJ, West R, Poon LW. Recruitment practices for research in gerontology. *Special Research Methods for Gerontology.* Amityville, NY: Baywood Publishing Company, Inc; 1989:163.
25. Sounder JE. The consumer approach to recruitment of elder subjects. *Nurs Res.* 1992;41:314–316.
26. Nystrom KM, Forman WB, Holdsworth MT. Clinical research trials: evaluation of a recruitment strategy for healthy elders. *J Clin Res Pharmacoepidemiol.* 1992;6:293–301.
27. Lipitz LA, Pluchino FC, Wright SM. Biomedical research in the nursing home: methodological issues and subject recruitment results. *J Am Geriatr Soc.* 1987;35:629–634.

CHAPTER 7

MANAGING PARTICIPANTS AND MAXIMIZING COMPLIANCE

ALICE H. LICHTENSTEIN, DSc; T. ELAINE PREWITT, DrPH, RD;
HELEN RASMUSSEN, MS, RD, FADA; AND CARLA R. HEISER, MS, RD

Managing participants to minimize dropouts and maximize dietary compliance (adherence) is an art as well as a science (1). This chapter addresses specific areas that impinge on initiating and executing a study protocol involving human participants. The concepts discussed are based on years of experience from a wide variety of studies conducted by the authors. This experience is seldom described in the research literature. The topics that are discussed include study initiation, implementation and orientation (staff and participants), study management, maintenance of morale, and close-out and discharge.

PARTICIPANT SELECTION

Participant selection is one of the most critical factors related to managing study participants with the intent of maximizing dietary adherence and minimizing dropouts. (Also see Chapter 6, "Recruitment and Screening of Study Participants.") Because a comprehensive participant selection protocol frequently requires more than one screening visit, the willingness and ability of a potential participant to comply with this process is itself a good indicator of subsequent compliance in the study. Potential study participants need to be well informed with respect to what is involved and expected of them so that they understand their commitments and can make an informed judgment about whether these commitments can be met. Likewise, the investigator needs to make an independent assessment of the likelihood that a potential participant can in fact complete the study in accordance with the protocol.

The ultimate decision whether a potential participant will be included in a particular study depends on the judgment of both the participant and investigator. A comprehensive evaluation of the potential participant can minimize the management demands necessary during the actual study period.

STUDY INITIATION

The initiation stage or run-in period of a new protocol may well be the most critical period of the investigation. A smooth start to a study can maximize efficiency and create a positive framework within which both staff and participants can operate. Alternatively, unnecessary ambiguity, confusion, or the burden of unnecessary data collection early in a study can undermine working relationships among participants and staff, the consequences of which may resurface throughout the study period.

Investigators

A number of responsibilities must be borne by the person taking primary responsibility for actually supervising the study. If these duties are divided among individuals, a detailed plan should be in place for delineating specific responsibilities well ahead of study implementation. This will help to ensure that all necessary groundwork is accomplished in a timely manner and that staff and participants know the person who can resolve specific issues and provide clarification or direction.

For many areas, failure to plan well can create small discrepancies that may be difficult to reconcile as the study progresses. Alternatively, some areas, such as diet, are of such a pervasive, repetitive, and immediate nature that all staff should be prepared to field basic questions and be aware of when to defer them.

Institutional Review Board (IRB)

The management schedule must allow enough time to make alterations in accordance with institutional review board (IRB) requests and obtain final approval from the IRB before the study is scheduled to begin. This can add several months to the time line. The consent forms should be as detailed as possible and include the expectations of both the investigators and participants as well as any restrictions placed on the participants. (See Chapter 5, "Ethical Considerations in Dietary Studies.")

Written Materials, Scheduling, and Flow Sheets

Prior to the initiation of a protocol, a staff meeting should be held to review the protocol (which should be a written document) and its implementation in detail. It is important for the principal investigator and all staff involved in the study to attend. At this meeting the responsibilities of each staff member should be defined and discussed thoroughly, as should the day-by-day study procedures and tests. Additionally, all written procedures, instructions, and educational materials should be reviewed in their final form.

The complexity of the study and the number of staff people involved will dictate the level of complexity of procedures, instructions, and flow sheets provided to the staff and participants. The advantage of providing separate written procedures to both the staff and participants is that the staff material can be more detailed and customized without risk of confusion. A disadvantage to this approach is the increased risk of ambiguity. Slight wording differences may eventually cause confusion.

However, unless the study is relatively short in duration and has a simple schedule, having separate materials for staff and participants is preferable. Useful differences in the instructions and schedules provided the staff and participants are as follows.

Participant materials should be more specific with respect to their roles and responsibilities in language that is appropriate to their educational level. Clearly indicated and highlighted should be such issues as the day the participant is scheduled to come into the research center fasting or days that the participant is responsible for urine collections. Wording should be set at about a high school level. The format of materials designed for the participants is frequently dictated by the characteristics of the specific group. For example, schedules designed for elderly participants should have relatively large print and be printed on heavy paper that is easy to grip. Instructions for studies involving groups whose primary language is not English should be provided in their native tongue. Translating materials properly requires translating into the common vernacular of the participant's language. There should also be a subsequent "back translation" into English to assure the investigators that the translation conveys the message and associated nuances accurately.

Staff materials should stress days that necessitate reminder calls to the participants about fasting or specific containers to be used for multiple blood samples or urine collections. Any material provided to the participants should be available and on file for the staff, even if the staff material is an expanded version of the participants' information.

The Study Diet

All staff in contact with the participants must understand all the procedures involved in the dietary aspect of the study because questions will arise. The participants will assume that anyone associated with the study will be able to address their queries. Although it is perfectly acceptable to refer answers or decisions to the appropriate staff member, the more quickly an issue is resolved, the happier the participant will be. A detailed discussion of developing, producing, and delivering research diets is provided in Chapters 10–13.

Staff Protocol Meeting

Before the study begins, staff should meet to review all written materials in their final form, clarify any ambiguities that are perceived, and consider potential problems and strategies for solving them (see Study Management). At this time all staff members should thoroughly review their subject area with the rest of the staff. As before, these meetings should involve as many staff as possible so that a consistent approach is maintained throughout the study period. Optimally, a pilot test of the protocol should be made. Any investment in time and labor will most likely be offset by the avoidance of problems once the full protocol is initiated.

Study Implementation

Because a large number of staff frequently are involved in bringing a study to completion it is important for clear policies and procedures to be communicated orally and in writing. A convenient technique for this is a formal orientation to the study. The orientation provides an opportunity for both reflection on the written material and discussion about implementation protocols so that the procedures are fine-tuned prior to the start of the study. As with most projects, a clear and unambiguous initiation phase to the study protocol can "set the stage" for the entire study.

Orientation for Staff

A well-thought-out, comprehensive orientation is crucial to ensure that staff adhere to the study protocol and that study operations proceed smoothly. In addition to providing uniform training and information, the orientation process defines rules, expectations, and standards of performance. Critical during the staff orientation is a review of the overall study. This review would include a brief description of reasons the study is being conducted, its specific objectives, the characteristics of the participants, data collection activities, time frames, and other procedures.

Also important to clarify are such issues as job responsibilities, administrative organization, and channels of communication. Clearly written descriptions of tasks to be performed and standards of acceptable performance should be presented. Staff orientation procedures are summarized in Table 7–1.

Additional orientation meetings may be scheduled after this general orientation for specific groups of staff. For example, staff involved in food preparation should receive an in-depth orientation on issues pertaining to the study diet. Special emphasis would be placed on diet specifications; specific foods and menu cycle; food preparation and service; rules regarding food substitutions, if any; quality control procedures; and a review of food handling and sanitation standards.

In addition to orientation meetings, regular staff meetings provide a forum for timely resolution of problems. Information on study progress can be shared and staff contributions toward accomplishing study goals can be recognized. Meetings also allow for an ongoing assessment of quality control and efficiency of operations on a regular basis. It is important to keep in mind that inconsistent answers from different staff members will lead participants to conclude that the study is not well managed. This leads to a sense of insecurity and loss of respect for the investigators with attendant consequences for adherence and retention.

Orientation for Participants

It is important from the outset that participants have a clear understanding of their roles and responsibilities, as well as the benefits they will realize as a result of their participation in the study. Participants should be aware of the nature and extent of the changes and constraints in lifestyle that will result from study participation. Orientation topics that are specifically important to the participants are discussed here.

Study Overview

The study overview comprises a description of study objectives, conduct of the study, testing procedures, data collection, and frequency of data collection.

Study Diet

If possible, a copy of the study menus should be provided prior to the study so that participants are aware of the foods they will be served. Policies regarding the number of meals per day to be eaten at the facility, missed meals, study food items not eaten, and nonstudy food eaten require extensive discussion and should be provided in oral and written form. Rules regarding the frequency and number of off-site meals

TABLE 7-1

Staff Orientation

Area	Major Points
Study overview	Purpose of the study Specific objectives Characteristics of participants Details of data to be collected Time lines Procedures
Organizational structure	General descriptions of job responsibilities Administrative organization Channels of communication
Job description	Clearly written descriptions of tasks Standards of acceptable performance

(eg, total number permitted) and procedures for obtaining food in emergency situations also require discussion.

Problems and uncertainties related to dietary infractions are major concerns in well-controlled diet studies. Thus, areas in which the participant has flexibility or "freedom in food choice" need particular emphasis. Providing a discretionary snack that meets study specifications or a list of allowable snacks can be helpful in reducing the likelihood of eating nonstudy foods or discarding food provided. Staff should provide a specific list of any "free foods," such as diet soft drinks, tea or coffee, mineral water, tap water, condiments, and hard candy, that participants may consume. It is important to be specific and absolutely clear in instructions to avoid confusion for the participants. Levels of knowledge vary greatly, and nothing is obvious. If there are limits to the use of free foods, staff should be even more specific, eg, "You can have two 12-ounce diet, caffeine-free colas a day, and one 12-ounce mineral water per day."

Staff should include a "packing list" of food items on the bag or cooler as part of quality control procedures for packed meals. This checklist reduces errors of omission for the staff when putting together several take-out meals, and the list identifies for the participants the food items and when they are to be consumed.

Staff should give clear, written directions for safe storage and reheating of foods. Again, staff should not take anything for granted; participants' levels of knowledge on food safety and sanitation vary widely. Instructions must list a phone number and contact person to call for questions or emergency situations. Include a preweighed paper towel in a resealable plastic bag for collecting spills and instruct subjects to collect any spilled food and secure it in the plastic bag so that it can be weighed. Also, participants should learn that they are to return any food or beverage not eaten and report any illness immediately.

Some research units have meals delivered by a staff member or by courier directly to participants. However, most units require participants to come to the facility to pick up their food. A contact person is essential in order to answer questions and solve problems such as, "My son ate my lunch," "I dropped the cheese and the dog ate it," "I spilled the apple juice on the meatloaf," or "My car broke down, and I can't come today to pick up my food." A staff member or courier can be sent to deliver the replacement food.

Data Collection Policies and Schedules

An atmosphere that fosters a trusting relationship between the staff and participants is important in supporting the data collection process. Such a relationship can contribute to smooth study operations and promote participant compliance and accurate self-reporting of deviations from the study protocol. The nature of the data to be collected (ie, what, how, and when) must be clearly described. It is helpful in this regard to distribute a data collection calendar listing such information.

Participants also need to understand the importance of reporting lifestyle changes (ie, exercise patterns) to appro-

priate staff. They need to know which behaviors should not be undertaken during the study (ie, smoking, alcohol). Finally, policies regarding special circumstances and criteria for termination from the study should be reiterated. At this point the study coordinator should meet with each participant to ensure that the orientation material has been read and understood and the informed consent signed. A checklist can be used to ensure that all essential information has been discussed during the orientation.

STUDY MANAGEMENT

Managing a study can be challenging. It can frequently become a balancing act between maintaining the integrity of the study and trying to keep all parties happy. Once a study begins, only rarely does management entail sitting back and hearing how well things are going. Anticipating potential trouble areas and planning strategies to deal with them can be a valuable and efficient use of time.

Managing Conflicts or Problems

Clear lines of responsibility need be established for the management of participants to ensure that problems get handled quickly, efficiently, and without confusion of the participant or manipulation of the staff. The following are general guidelines. The specifics are determined by the number of staff involved and the predetermined role of each. Problems or conflicts raised by a participant to the staff or investigator should be directed to the appropriate staff person. Immediate action should be taken to avoid any "domino effect" with the other participants.

Flexibility within the constraints of the protocol is very helpful. All encounters should be documented and the resolution reported to all staff coming in contact with the participant. The decision should be communicated to the participant by a mutually agreed-upon staff member. A respect for delineated roles is critical to this system.

Participants' Requests for Changes or Modifications

Participants are likely to have difficulties complying with even the best-thought-out and most detailed protocols. The first step in resolving problems without compromising adherence to the protocol is for the staff person first contacted to refer the issue to the colleague responsible for that aspect of the study. For example, a participant may ask the nurse taking his blood pressure whether milk from an evening meal can be shifted to midmorning because he really misses a traditional morning milk and tea break. This issue should be brought to the dietitian, who would determine whether this request could be accommodated within the confines of the protocol. Another participant may request that the principal investigator change the days she comes in for blood sampling. This issue should be referred to the person responsible for scheduling, even though the requested change may not breach the study protocol and the principal investigator would like to personally accommodate the participant and foster a positive relationship. In the vast majority of such cases the request can be accommodated with no problem, but, occasionally, the schedule change cannot be made because it would overburden the workload of either the phlebotomist or laboratory for a given day. Sometimes, however, the participant has first requested the change from the appropriate person, been turned down, and then decided to try an alternative means of achieving his or her goals.

Getting first a "yes" from the principal investigator and then a "no" when the conflict is discovered can lead to an awkward situation for all involved. A situation of this sort can undermine working relationships among staff and the participant as well as among staff members. The only way to avoid this is for all staff to respect the predetermined roles of their colleagues and to always defer questions or requests to the appropriate person (2).

Resolution of Minor Conflicts

When studies are carefully planned, they typically proceed smoothly and minor changes as requested by participants can be accommodated. However, regardless of how well thought out and meticulously executed a protocol is, questions, misunderstandings, and special requests will occur. If clear lines of responsibility are defined and adhered to, a satisfactory resolution can be reached without the participant dropping out of the study. However, if an issue is raised and the outcome is unsatisfactory to the participant or staff, the principal investigator will have to resolve it. Under most circumstances the ultimate decision will be acceptable to all parties involved, especially when the rules are clearly detailed at the beginning of the study.

Examples of minor conflicts are given here. A participant was under the impression that when he had blood draws scheduled for 2 consecutive days he could choose the more convenient day. A week prior to the dates he committed himself to another activity for 1 of the 2 days. The situation was communicated to the staff 2 days prior to the first scheduled blood draw during a review of the schedule with the participant. An explanation concerning the necessity of obtaining 2 *consecutive* blood samples and shifting the inconvenient date forward or backward solved the problem.

In another case, a participant's work schedule was changed without warning in midstudy. Although the dietary department could accommodate different meal pickup and/ or consumption times, the participant for this study could not come in for the collection of fasting blood samples in the morning. She did not want to drop out of the study and did not understand why, if she were willing to fast all day, the fasting sample could not be taken in the evening, especially because she knew that staff would be available to collect the sample at that time. At this point it was necessary

for staff to clarify that although the now agitated participant did not perceive a problem in compliance, the effects of circadian rhythms precluded the proposed change. The manager suggested that the fasting blood samples be collected on a nonwork day if the laboratories involved could accommodate this schedule change.

Mediating Issues Among Participants

Situations arise where one participant perceives that another participant is making inappropriate comments or breaching the protocol and feels compelled to inform a staff person. For example, Participant A continually complained about the packaging of the food prepared for take-out. Participant B did not perceive a problem and did not like to hear the continual complaining. Participant B requested some intervention but did not want to be identified as the person bringing the issue to the attention of the investigator.

Another example might be the witnessing of Participant C hiding a disliked food in a napkin and disposing of it. Similarly, Participant C might boast that he never eats a certain food and there is no way the investigators can find out.

It is important to address such issues when they occur; failure or perceived failure to do so undermines the morale of the other participants. If a staff member is present and mingling with the participants at a mealtime, he or she will frequently overhear conversations and be able to resolve conflicts readily. Possibly asking, in the presence of others, how things are going or how the new food wrap is working out can adequately redress the problem. Issues pertaining to bragging about nonconsumption of food are far more difficult to verify and address. A casual private interview with the purported offending participant could rectify the situation by allowing him or her to bring up a specific problem or by providing the extra attention the participant sought.

Investigators must keep in mind, especially for long-term diet studies, that participants surrender a tremendous amount of control over everyday life during diet studies. This lack of control can manifest itself in many ways. For example, participants might revert to surprisingly childlike behavior such as blatantly testing limits. Awareness of this possible hidden resentment when investigators deal with staff-participant or participant-participant problems can help focus the issue. Planning can help to resolve such issues in a manner that saves face for the participant and fosters strict adherence to the protocol.

Areas of Flexibility

It is important to remain as flexible as possible, especially when the study is relatively long and restrictive. However, to advertise this policy up front is probably not advisable. Handling specific issues with participants on a case-by-case basis in a confidential manner is probably the wisest approach. Even the appearance of willingness to accommodate a small schedule or food change may make the difference between a participant completing a study or not. In some situations if a request cannot be accommodated, an alternative can be proposed that creates good will with the participant and conveys the willingness of the staff to treat the participant as an individual and not just a number.

Although inconvenient, it is not unreasonable for participants to request small changes in their diets to accommodate personal preferences, especially if participants will consume the diet for a long period of time. In an ideal situation, sample menus are available in advance. This enables the participant to note a food or food combination he or she feels is totally unacceptable, and the issue can be resolved in advance. For example, Participant X does not normally eat broccoli but felt that, if it meant participation in the study, she could. After the first week, however, Participant X felt she could no longer consume broccoli and wanted to switch to string beans. In some studies, such a switch would not present a problem with respect to the study protocol. Should the change be made? If possible, yes, without question. However, although this solution appears relatively straightforward, the following ramifications occur:

- Participant Y now has seen the switch made for Participant X and also wants "one small change."
- Participant Z heard that Participant X was able to switch a food, and he requested to switch an orange for orange juice because he hates to peel oranges. In this case, the substitution could not be made because the fiber content of the diet was being controlled. An apple might be an acceptable substitute.

In another scenario, carrot sticks were incorporated into the menu. Because of her denture problems, carrots were difficult for one of the participants to chew. Incorporating grated carrots into a salad solved what could have potentially turned into an embarrassing situation. The ultimate resolution would be dictated by the specific protocol. Incorporating a limited number of food choices into the menus from the outset is an alternative approach that may serve to avoid a large number of requests for changes as a study progresses.

Voluntary Premature Terminations (Dropouts)

What can be done to keep participants from deciding to stop participating in a protocol before the study ends? A thorough screening process as discussed in Chapter 6, "Recruitment and Screening of Study Participants," will probably contribute the most to minimizing the dropout rate by avoiding enrollment of participants who will find the protocol too difficult to comply with. However, unavoidable situations do occur, especially during studies of relatively long duration.

If a participant indicates that he or she has decided to terminate participation in a study, all efforts should be made to meet with the participant immediately. Without any attempt or appearance of an attempt to coerce the participant, the reason for termination should be discussed. At this point it will most likely become clear whether there is a way to avoid losing the participant midstudy or whether the situation is unresolvable. Keeping in mind that it is legally and ethically within the rights of a participant at any time and for any reason to terminate participation in the study, the meeting should end on a positive note. An offer should likewise be made to follow up with any data that would normally be provided to the remaining participants once the protocol is completed. Queries by other participants about why the person terminated should be addressed with as few details as possible. This protects the departing participant's privacy unless he or she gives specific instructions for this information to be divulged. Experience indicates that in most cases, the other participants are aware of the situation, sometimes before the staff know anything about it.

Involuntary Premature Termination

It may become necessary to terminate a participant who wishes to remain in the study. Clear criteria for involuntary termination should be incorporated into the consent form. (See Chapter 5, "Ethical Considerations in Dietary Studies.") Whenever possible, a warning should first be given both verbally and in writing that failure to adhere to the policies and procedures will result in involuntary termination if the protocol allows for such an action. This is not always possible, as in the case of unexplained absence.

In one example of noncompliance, a participant continually returns uneaten food although it was clearly stated at the onset that a criterion of the study was total food consumption. The investigator should confront the participant and provide the participant with a written summary of the discussion. Possible solutions might include spreading food consumption out over the entire day. The issue and a summary of the meeting should also be discussed at a staff meeting to make all the staff aware of the situation and determine whether there is an underlying problem that can be addressed. If after a specified period of time the participant continues to breach the protocol, the investigator should inform the participant that his participation in the study is being terminated. This information should be communicated immediately to all staff involved. Once the decision is made, it should be final. Similar to instances of voluntary termination, queries by other participants as to why the person terminated should be addressed with as few details as possible.

Handling Emergency Situations

It is difficult to predict why, when, and how emergency situations will arise. With regard to the staff, it is important not to configure a management plan in which one person is "indispensable," regardless of how tempting or efficient this is. With regard to the participants, it is important to keep in mind that when an emergency does arise the overall aim is to avoid having a situation that causes a participant to drop out. Dropouts are disappointing to the investigators, lower the morale of the remaining participants, and obviously have adverse consequences for the study. It is therefore helpful to have a variety of strategies in place to cope with various situations, to anticipate as many permutations of calamities as possible, and, most importantly, to be creative. Some planning suggestions are to create:

- Extra cycle of frozen and nonperishable foods stored by the participant.
- Rules for making substitutions for perishable items.
- Written instructions concerning substitutions.
- Emergency meal delivery systems.

MAINTAINING MORALE AMONG PARTICIPANTS

The participants' morale will wax and wane for reasons unrelated and related to the protocol. Factors pertaining to this area are outside the scope of this discussion. However, certain situations frequently occur within the context of experimental protocols that have been found to affect the morale of participants as a group and, occasionally, as individuals. Most of these issues have already been dealt with in other sections of this chapter.

Briefly, careful attention must be paid to the characteristics of potential participants during the screening process, with emphasis on the ability of the participant to follow directions and comply with requests. The tendency of a potential participant to complain about routine requests is important to note. Although these minor complaints can be handled by staff on a one-to-one basis, discussion with fellow participants can serve to lower the morale of the entire group. It can be unsettling to all the participants if the investigators keep changing the study schedules or protocols. Optimally, studies will be designed to have a run-in period; very large studies can allow a few participants to "pilot" the materials and diet prior to the start of the full-scale study. Unfortunately, these optimal situations may not always be possible.

MORALE-BUILDING STRATEGIES

Factors that have a positive effect on morale, no matter how small, can result in big improvements in the quality of the data. Conversely, factors that have a negative effect on morale can undermine protocol adherence, increase the risk of participant dropout, and compromise the study's results. Ongoing communication with participants is necessary to remain aware of situations that potentially threaten morale.

Special incentives can be a valuable asset in building morale and supporting adherence to protocol. These can include gifts (tokens, gift certificates, flowers, or magazines) or special events. In the latter case, a little creativity can turn routine meal service into a festive occasion such as a "special evening out," for which participants bring a guest to dinner. The meal might be served by staff in special attire and include entertainment and changes in decor. Other suggestions to boost morale and promote enthusiasm and commitment of participants include:

- Partial payment of the honorarium at each period of data collection.
- A get-acquainted event during the early stages of the study, followed by periodic social events or holiday celebrations that include family and friends.
- Availability of a participant suggestion box with timely, prompt responses to individual complaints and concerns.
- Special attention to the atmosphere and environment. The provision of a pleasant environment builds morale, particularly if the facility provides a "home away from home" atmosphere. The availability of magazines, newspaper, TVs, VCRs, and other amenities are important fringe benefits for the participant.
- A common channel for disseminating information, answering questions, and responding to comments. Regular newsletters and communiques can be valuable in providing information about study progress and can build a sense of cohesion through human interest features.

STUDY CLOSE-OUT, DISCHARGE, AND FOLLOW-UP

An exit interview should be conducted with each participant at the end of the study. The purpose of the interview is to allow participants an opportunity to freely discuss feelings about the study and the degree to which they actually adhered to the protocol. Dietary infractions, including their nature and frequency, should be discussed in detail and documented in terms of when they occurred. Alternatively, information on dietary infractions can be obtained by an anonymous questionnaire.

Providing individual results can enhance participants' motivation to participate in the exit interview. Additionally, an individual or group follow-up session at the end of the study (eg, topics selected by participants) helps to show the investigators' commitment to addressing diet-related concerns and questions of participants in a broader context than the study per se. An offer to provide individualized nutrition counseling or diet plans (ie, for weight loss or cholesterol reduction) at the end of the study is also helpful. An example of an exit interview for an inpatient feeding study aimed at lowering blood cholesterol is given in Exhibit 7–1. The questions can be modified to be appropriate for studies using other types of diets.

ASSESSING AND FOSTERING DIETARY COMPLIANCE

One of the primary questions of conducting feeding studies is whether the participant really ate only and all the food and

EXHIBIT 7-1

Sample Exit Interview for an Inpatient Feeding Study

Name_____ Date_____

During the diet study, there may have been things that you were hesitant to report or record. This is natural. Now that the study is over, it is important that we know about these things to have accurate information in assessing the effectiveness of the study. Please answer the following questions as honestly as possible.

1. What motivated you to join this study?
2. Do you feel you still want to follow a cholesterol-lowering diet? Why or why not?
3. When specifically were the most difficult times to follow the study diet and why?
4. What could we have done to help you during these "difficult times"?
5. Please tell us what you liked about the study. What did you dislike?
6. Please tell us how we could have improved the study.
7. Personally, what do you feel you gained from the study?
8. Did you eat any nonstudy food or drink nonstudy beverages or alcohol during the study period that you did not report or record? If so please try to remember what you consumed, how much, and how often. Please record below.

Food Eaten	Average Portion	Number of Times Eaten		
		Daily	Weekly	Monthly

9. What caused you to consume nonstudy items if you did so?
10. How could we have helped you prevent this?
11. Did you eat all the food we provided during the study? If you did not eat all the study foods, please record below.

Food Not Eaten	Average Portion Not Eaten	Number of Times Not Eaten		
		Daily	Weekly	Monthly

12. If you did not eat all of the food provided, why do you think this happened?
13. What could we have done to help you prevent this?
14. Did you notice any changes in your physical health or feeling of well-being during the study period, compared to before the study began? If so, what changes did you notice? Please be specific.
15. Are there any other comments you would like to make?

TABLE 7-2

Screening Information Used in Planning for Maximal Compliance

Factor	Interview Information	Participant Management Planning
Personal health	Participant has poor dentition or arthritis in his or her hands.	Cut up or shred food items. Substitute soft foods for hard-to-chew items. Send food home in easy-to-open containers.
Psychosocial	Participant is out of work and needs to be at job interviews sporadically. This also can apply to students with variable schedules (ie, medical students with unpredictable ward rotation requirements).	Give participant clear instructions about when data are to be collected and when his or her presence at the research facility is required. Do not enroll participant until daily routines are predictable.
Diet/Nutrition	Participant will be required to drink a large amount of milk at each meal. Participant admits to not liking milk but is not sure why.	Have participant try a certain specified amount of milk at home and report on the results. Acceptance into the study is contingent on these results.
	The study prohibits consumption of caffeine-containing foods.	If participant is sensitive, try going without caffeine for a specified period of time to be "weaned" from caffeine prior to study.

drink that was provided. The verification of this information is difficult; however, there are some techniques, both objective and subjective, of assessing adherence that can be used in the research setting. Additionally, methods can be built into each study that can directly optimize a participant's performance.

Objective Methods

A detailed discussion of the objective techniques used for assessing dietary adherence is included in Chapter 24, "Biological Sample Collection and Markers of Dietary Compliance." To date, no one single biochemical marker, urine test, or serum level of a nutrient can predict with 100% accuracy whether an individual ate only the food and drink provided. The measurements that do exist all have limitations and are only useful within a narrow context or as a measure of group adherence. For this reason, although less precise, subjective measures of assessing dietary adherence have been found to be helpful.

Subjective Methods

Selecting appropriate participants is the cornerstone of a well-controlled study. This selection should be done in a team approach, with input from all the staff involved with study implementation. Techniques for screening research participants are discussed in Chapter 6, "Recruitment and Screening of Study Participants"; however, careful investigation on this point cannot be stressed enough. Screening the study participants carefully with respect to personal and psychosocial health, dietary habits, and nutritional status helps in the initial assessment of participant selection. These findings should be factored into a study orientation and edu-

cation program tailored specifically to the population chosen. Table 7–2 shows how screening can be conducted within this framework and provides ideas for individualizing a research protocol to accommodate participants' circumstances.

Compliance checks that can be standardized for each study are outlined here.

Meal- and Food-Related Methods

Checklists

Participants should be provided with a copy of their menu plan as a quality control check. When the participant receives his or her tray, the food can be checked against the menu. This method of checking for all food provided is also imperative for take-out meals when the participant is free living. Dietary employees use it to verify that the take-out meal bags were packed with all necessary food items. For hungry participants who arrive home without the dinner entree, study adherence may not seem to be of primary importance, particularly if they have to travel quite a distance to the research center. Experience suggests that the participants do compare their food to the list and readily point out inconsistencies.

Meal checklists can also be used for the participant to check off and initial all food consumed. Checklists can be collected at each visit for outpatients or after each meal for residents. Additional questions can be added to these meal lists, such as whether anything was eaten in addition to the menu items, or which free foods were consumed. This is important both for assessing compliance and for total nutrient intake records. An example of a meal checklist is provided in Chapter 18, "Documentation, Record Keeping, and Recipes." Computer-generated checklists are described in Chapter 3, "Computer Applications in Controlled Diet Studies."

Tray Checks

A tray-check procedure should be part of every research unit's meal delivery routine. The participant's meal tray should be checked for completeness prior to serving and for uneaten foods after the tray is returned after the meal. If the food is not completely consumed, the participant should be called back to finish the food. If for some reason the participant cannot finish the food, the food should be weighed and recorded, consumed at the next meal, or replaced. This deviation should always be noted in the participant's record, along with the reason for not finishing the food. This is a way of not only assessing compliance but also of determining whether the foods are acceptable or if the study design is realistic. For example, a participant in an inpatient study returned her food to the dish room and retired to her living quarters. The diet technician who was checking the lunch tray noticed that she did not consume all of her sandwich. The participant was called back to finish it and responded that she was very uncomfortable because she had undergone an experimental procedure early that morning that didn't end until 10:00 a.m. She had eaten a late breakfast and then was expected to consume the full lunch tray at 12:00 p.m. She felt she could not finish the sandwich.

This example describes a problem distinct from the participant's not consuming all of her study diet. It is a flag to the study coordinators to reassess the meals that are provided on testing days. It needs to be determined whether the participant must consume all of the food on those days. If so, the food should be rearranged in a different way, such as spreading out the breakfast items over lunch, dinner, and snack to make the participant more comfortable. Additionally, a participant should be encouraged to voice his or her discomfort rather than being placed in a position of compromising his or her performance on the research study.

Food Containers Returned

For outpatient studies, sending food home in returnable containers can be a method of documenting food consumed. However, just as counting pills is no guarantee that the participant took the medication, neither is returning food containers an indication that the individual ate the food. The message conveyed through this effort is the interest that the investigators take in encouraging compliance, which is then communicated to participants by having them complete this exercise. An added benefit to returning food containers is that they can be reused or recycled, cutting down on the research budget and waste.

Regular Interviews

It is important to meet with participants to review the diet and ascertain whether there are problems with any of the food items. Making food substitutions or modifications can be beneficial. Discussing or graphically illustrating what may look like compliance problems, such as unexpected weight fluctuations when they take out meals or go away for the weekend, helps to inform participants that the study personnel are aware of these inconsistencies. Participants also should be questioned directly about whether they ate anything other than their experimental diet. Elderly participants may need these interviews to remind them of study guidelines if they are not residing at the research unit. Likewise, young participants may need to have "pep talks" if they are anticipating a problem socializing with their friends.

Role-playing exercises in which the participant is placed in a position of being tempted by a friend not to adhere to the diet can help participants withstand events such as sit-down dinners, weddings, and cocktail parties.

"Gut Feeling"

Research study personnel can often sense when a participant is being evasive or uncomfortable about participation in a study. If a participant feels he or she cannot forthrightly speak with the investigator or cannot discuss issues about the study that create discomfort, he or she may give other signals that he or she cannot comply with this research study. For example, if something on the diet is unpleasant or the study procedures result in feelings of discomfort, the participant may simply avoid eating the food and rationalize the nonadherence. If a participant's complaints about a study protocol are numerous enough, the individual generally finds a way to withdraw. This is one of the reasons that direct communication at regular intervals is important. It is difficult to assess whether a participant really is complying with the protocol without any direct two-way communication.

Involvement of Family and "Significant Others"

Long-term studies requiring resident living and separation from family members can frequently impose undue stress on both the participant and the family. On the other hand, eating a controlled research diet while living with people eating an uncontrolled diet can present many temptations and opportunities for food sharing or extra food consumption. It is suggested that, at the time of screening, this burden be outlined thoroughly to the potential participant, so that he or she can discuss the study diet and routine at length with family before participating in the study. Food sharing should not be tolerated, nor should the food be prepared (rewarmed or heated) in a different way than the instructions describe. Inviting the participant's housemates to the research center and to review the particulars of the study diet involves them in the study and is a good way of providing extra support to the participant.

For example, a woman was participating in a closely controlled calcium balance study. Because of the length of this study, she participated as a nonresident. She continued to live at home with her husband and came into the research center daily for meal pick-ups. While she was in the middle of the study, her husband called the study dietitian to ask what kind of cake he could serve her on her birthday, which was going to be celebrated with some friends coming over for a surprise dinner. When told that she could not eat any

EXHIBIT 7-2

Example of an Interim Questionnaire for Free-Living Participants in a Well-Controlled Diet Study

Name_____ Date_____

Please answer the following questions about meals and snacks. The information that you provide will be used to improve diets for future studies.

1. What is your favorite meal(s)?

2. What meal(s) do you like least?

3. How do you handle less favored meals?

4. If you are adding foods from the "What to Choose When I'm Definitely Going to Have a Snack List," please list types and amounts of foods added.

5. What are the types and amounts of foods deleted per week? List them here and indicate rationale.

6. How often do you take a free day or use free meals?

7. What kinds and amounts of foods do you substitute for unused jams?

8. Do you have additional ideas for meals or snacks?

9. Do you have additional comments, suggestions, or criticisms?

cake, he decided it would be an unfair temptation to present her with one and asked for alternatives. The dietitian suggested that he make a dinner for the invited guests that resembled the study meal she would eat that night (chicken, rice, and green beans). There was some food allowable as a dessert within the diet study guidelines (jelly beans and soft drinks). This family support was an extra bonus for maximizing dietary compliance for this woman.

Team Approach

Other areas within the study may require the participants to collect data for which they may exhibit noncompliant behavior. Examples include not completing a 24-hour urine or stool collection, not keeping appointments, or forgetting to fast for blood draws. This could be reason to suspect that the participant is not adhering to the protocol at all. Keeping an active communication with the nursing department or the clinical labs that process the participant's specimens is important. If a participant keeps forgetting appointments, often has discrepant pill counts, or overtly does not complete a task required on a protocol, this undesirable conduct must be discussed immediately as a team.

Knowing of such behavior early on in the protocol may necessitate participant dismissal but can save precious resources. This team approach also is important in lending support and credibility when a participant is being counseled to withdraw from the study (see Involuntary Premature Termination).

EVALUATION OF THE RESEARCH STUDY

An effective method of eliciting participant feedback and gauging protocol adherence is to employ interim and exit questionnaires. These tools are designed to assess participants' perceived compliance and to register suggestions or complaints. Additionally, staff perceptions can be compared to participants' perceptions.

In response to interim questionnaires, some suggestions may be appropriate for immediate implementation whereas others, which would substantially alter the study, may be implemented in subsequent studies. Comments from interim questionnaires can be used to develop a menu cycle composed of favorite meals from a number of studies and to provide for specific food substitutions where appropriate.

Interim questionnaires may identify specific participants who need counseling or specific topics that need to be discussed or clarified. Comments in response to interim questionnaires can be summarized in a newsletter and distributed to all study participants. For example, it can be valuable for a participant to see that his least favorite meal is someone else's favorite meal. An example of an interim questionnaire used in a diet study aimed at lowering blood cholesterol is given in Exhibit 7–2. This questionnaire can be modified to be appropriate for other types of diet studies.

Participants may find it easier to be frank when answering questions on exit questionnaires as compared to interim questionnaires, and candid answers should be encouraged. Explaining that information from exit questionnaires is used to improve future studies also encourages honest responses. An example, which can be modified for other types of diet studies, is given in Exhibit 7–3.

CONCLUSION

Managing participants to maximize dietary adherence and minimize dropouts is crucial to the success of a study and is accomplished through careful planning. Participant selection

EXHIBIT 7-3

Example of an Exit Questionnaire for Free-Living Participants in a Diet Study

Name_____ Date_____

During the diet study there may have been infractions or misunderstandings that you were hesitant to report or record. This is natural. However, it is important that we know about these occurrences to accurately assess the effectiveness of the study diets and to make appropriate changes for future studies. Please provide frank answers to the questions that follow.

1. What initially motivated you to participate in the diet study?

2. How do you feel about following a low-fat, low-cholesterol diet in the future?

3. Describe new food choices or nutrition strategies you have acquired as a result of study involvement.

4. When was it most difficult to follow the study diet? Why?

5. What could have been done to help you through the rough times?

6. Describe the strengths of this study.

7. Describe what you did not like and how we could have improved the study.

8. List the points that you feel would be important to tell your successors.

9. What have you gained from study involvement?

10. Describe your compliance with entrees, breakfast, and snack foods. Overall, on a scale of 0 to 10, rate how well you followed the study guidelines. (A score of 0 indicates least compliant and a score of 10 indicates most compliant.)

11. Describe any nonstudy foods, beverages, or alcohol consumed during the study period that you did not report or record. Please indicate type of food, amount, and frequency eaten.

12. If you did consume nonstudy foods, what may have caused you to choose nonstudy items?

13. How could we have anticipated the need or desire to include additional foods?

14. Describe the amount of study foods, including entrees, breakfast or snack items and beverages not consumed. Indicate percent of portions not eaten and the frequency with which this occurred.

15. If you did not consume all study foods or beverages, what caused this to happen?

16. What could we have done to prevent this?

17. Describe changes in your physical health or feeling of well being during the first 6 weeks of the study, compared to before enrollment.

18. Describe changes in your physical health or well-being during the low-fat intervention phases, the last 24 weeks of the study, compared to before enrollment.

19. List any medications (prescription or over-the-counter medications) taken that were not listed on your daily reports. Indicate dosage and frequency used.

20. Describe any illnesses or accidents subsequent to starting the diet study.

21. Would you participate in this study (or one like it) again?

procedures are critical for recruiting individuals who are likely to adhere to the study protocol. The process of participant management occurs throughout the study and even before the study actually begins. The principal investigator has the primary and ultimate responsibility for managing study participants. Management of the study staff is also important to the ability to successfully manage study participants. Staff must be trained to follow the protocol and study procedures. Effective means of communication among staff, including regular meetings, are essential.

Providing information to participants, including a clear understanding of their responsibilities, is a key component of participant management. Clearly written study materials that include instructions and procedures assist this process.

Managing and resolving problems and conflicts require good understanding of the study purpose and protocol, knowledge of human behavior, and common sense. Flexibility appropriately applied provides the means for managing difficult situations. Planning for commonly occurring contingencies prior to the start of the study is usually helpful. Assessing dietary adherence is useful for the interpretation of study results as well as for planning for the next study. Strategies should be developed to boost morale for both the participants and the study staff. Finally, maintaining good relations with study participants at the end of the study is important and requires careful planning, including procedures for study close-out, for providing information about their individual results, and for conducting an exit interview whereby the participant evaluates the experience of being a participant. Thus, throughout the entire study, careful planning is key to managing participants.

REFERENCES

1. Spilker B. Methods of assessing and improving patient compliance in clinical trials. In: Spilker B, ed. *Guide to Clinical Trials.* New York, NY: Raven Press; 1991.
2. Davis MS. Variations in patients' compliance with doctors' advice: an empirical analysis of patterns of communication. *Am J Pub Health.* 1968;58:274–288.

CHAPTER 8

WOMEN AS PARTICIPANTS IN CONTROLLED DIET STUDIES

JANE E. STEGNER, MS, RD; AND ABBY G. ERSHOW, ScD, RD

Historically most medical research has been conducted using male subjects. Women have often been excluded from clinical studies for many reasons, including protection from risk to a potential fetus or nursing infant, lower rates of the disease under study, and possible confounding from menstrual cycle variations. Also, cost constraints have discouraged gender-specific data analyses, which require larger sample sizes to obtain sufficient statistical power in each subgroup.

Results of research on men, however, cannot always be extrapolated directly to women. For example, important differences in drug metabolism or the natural history of disease can occur in women because of hormonal changes associated with the menstrual cycle or menopause. These natural biological events can affect many physiological systems and can complicate study design and interpretation, but they are important characteristics of the recipients of the resulting health care. Recent guidelines of the National Institutes of Health mandate inclusion of women in health research unless there are compelling arguments to the contrary (1). If there is evidence of significant gender differences in response, the research design and sample size must be able to answer the research question separately for each gender. In this way, research findings will apply to both men and women, and all persons can benefit.

This chapter addresses female hormone status and other related issues in the specific context of well-controlled feeding studies.

The ovarian cycle, methods of identifying the phases, oral contraceptives, menopause, and hormone replacement therapy are reviewed. Dietary issues and effects of the menstrual cycle on physiological systems that influence the results of nutrition research are discussed. Approaches are also presented for improving research design, data collection and analysis, recruitment strategies, and subject management. (Readers wishing to obtain a more comprehensive, general overview can consult DA Krummel and PM Kris-Etherton, eds, *Nutrition in Women's Health,* Gaithersburg, Md: Aspen Publishers, Inc; 1996.)

HORMONAL STATUS: MENARCHE TO MENOPAUSE

Normal Menstrual Cycle

The onset of menstrual cycles, *menarche,* typically occurs at 12 years to 13 years of age; the normal range extends from 8 years to 18 years (Table 8–1). Menarche is one step in the process of puberty, which can span several years (2–4). Although young girls and adolescents are seldom enrolled in controlled diet studies, investigators should consider whether menarche represents a possible confounding factor in study design.

The normal menstrual cycle is a complex interaction of hypothalamic, pituitary, and ovarian endocrinology (5–8).

TABLE 8-1

Reproductive States in Women

State	Typical Age Range[1] (yr)	Menstrual Cycles	Other Characteristics
Prepuberty	0–12	None	Physically immature (Tanner Stage 1)
Puberty	8–18	Irregular; anovulatory at first	Physical maturation (Tanner Stages 2–4) Peak height velocity precedes menarche Menarche: menses begin
Childbearing potential	12–50	Regular	Physically mature (Tanner Stage 5) Pregnancy; Lactation Infertility; Amenorrhea (primary, secondary) Contraceptive use
Menopause: Perimenopausal	45–55	Irregular; still ovulatory	Endogenous hormone levels reach new ''set'' points Multiple physical and other changes (''climacteric'') Hormone replacement therapy
Menopause: Postmenopausal	45 + (average 52)	None	Natural menopause Surgical menopause (with/without oophorectomy) Hormone replacement therapy

[1]Age ranges overlap to indicate the range of normal biological variation.
Sources: Gerhard I, Heinrich U. Puberty and its disorders. In: Runnebaum B, Rabe T, eds, *Gynecological Endocrinology and Reproductive Medicine,* Vol 1, *Gynecological Endocrinology,* New York, NY: Springer-Verlag; 1994. Jones RE, *Human Reproductive Biology,* 2nd ed, New York, NY: Academic Press; 1997.

Under hypothalamic control, the anterior pituitary produces two main gonadotropins, follicle-stimulating hormone (FSH) and luteinizing hormone (LH), and other hormones that affect the cycle to a lesser degree. The ovaries produce the sex steroids, estrogen (estradiol) and progesterone.

The normal cycle averages 28 days in length, with ovulation occurring between the 13th day and 15th day when the cycle is numbered from the first day of menses (Figure 8–1a). The cycle can vary within and among women from 25 to 32 days in length. Cycles of less than 21 days or greater than 35 days may not represent normal ovulation.

The cycle can be divided broadly into two major phases: follicular and luteal. The follicular phase begins with the onset of menstruation, which is really the culmination of the preceding cycle. During the early follicular phase, all serum hormone levels are low (Figure 8–1b). Then estrogen begins to rise, stimulating FSH production and the maturation of an ovum (egg follicle). Rising estrogen levels stimulate LH production, and both LH and FSH rise abruptly. On release of these pituitary hormones, estrogen levels drop sharply. The peak of LH and FSH marks the end of the follicular phase and the beginning of the luteal phase. Within 1 day of the peak, ovulation occurs; the ovum is released from the ovary. Estrogen begins to rise again and progesterone increases to maximum about 5 to 7 days after ovulation. Estrogen and progesterone levels decline toward baseline during the late luteal phase and menstruation begins as the lining of the endometrium is sloughed.

Documenting the occurrence of ovulation can be important in studies of specific cycle phases. Some authors divide the cycle into four phases: menstrual, follicular, ovulatory, and luteal. Cycles within an individual woman can be classified as ovulatory or anovulatory or as having a short luteal phase (ie, lasting fewer than 10 days) (9).

Chronological age can also affect menstrual cycle parameters in actively cycling women. Older premenopausal women (37–45 yr) have been found to have higher serum gonadotrophin (LH and FSH) levels, lower follicular phase length, later ovulation, and increased endometrial thickness compared with younger women (21–25 yr) (10).

Cessation of menses is almost always the first sign of pregnancy, although a small proportion of women continue to bleed periodically. After delivery there is considerable variation in the time before regular ovulatory cycles resume. This interval generally is longer in lactating women.

Methods of Phase Identification

Many of the techniques for monitoring reproductive function and detecting ovulation were originally developed for treating infertility, but they also have facilitated the study of

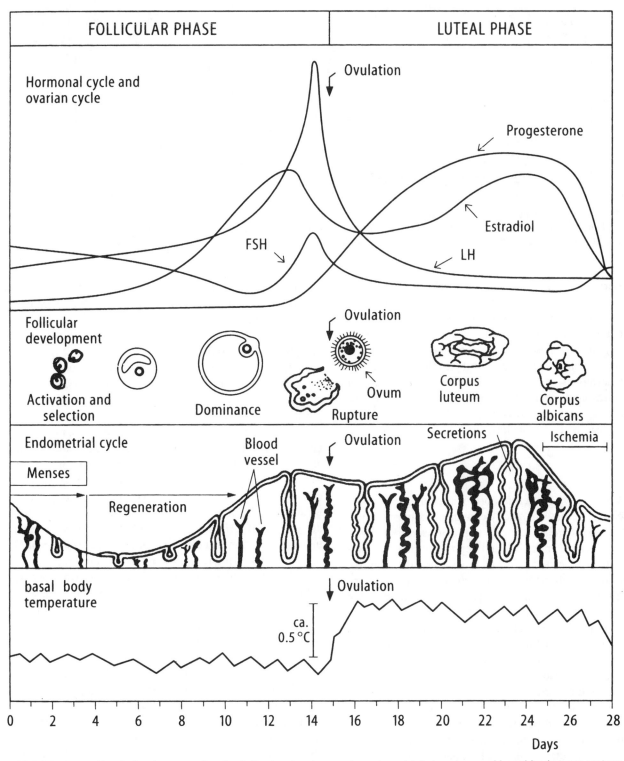

FIGURE 8–1a.   Circulating hormone levels, follicular development, endometrial changes, and basal body temperature during the menstrual cycle. Reprinted with permission from: Weinbauer GF, Nieschlag E, Hormonal regulation of reproductive organs. In: Greger R, Windhorst U, eds, *Comprehensive Human Physiology*, Vol 2, New York, NY: Springer-Verlag; 1996:2243.

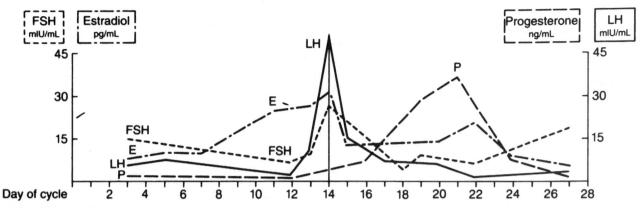

FIGURE 8-1b.   Concentrations of circulating hormones during the menstrual cycle. Reprinted with permission from Grunwald K, Rabe T, Keisel L, Runnebaum B, Physiology of the menstrual cycle. In: Runnebaum B, Rabe T, eds, *Gynecological Endocrinology and Reproductive Medicine,* Vol 1, *Gynecological Endocrinology,* New York, NY: Springer-Verlag; 1994:132.

normal hormone status and menstrual cycle phases. Identifying specific phases of the menstrual cycle enables investigators to evaluate outcome variables as they relate to hormone fluctuation and to synchronize sample collection with the corresponding phase. Currently available methods for monitoring the phases and stages of the cycle include direct assay of hormones or their metabolites in serum, urine, or saliva; ultrasound; and observation of the physiological changes that occur in response to hormonal changes (menses, basal body temperature, and cervical mucus consistency) (11, 12).

Serum

Many of the assays for serum hormone levels are accurate and reliable, and they are readily conducted in most clinical laboratories. Researchers considering their use should evaluate the accuracy, precision, and reproducibility of commercial kits or other analytical methods when planning the study protocol. Laboratory quality control procedures appropriate for clinical practice and patient treatment may not be sufficiently stringent for research purposes. The monitoring techniques discussed here can be employed to identify the days most crucial for analysis of serum levels if pinpointing stages of the cycle is of interest. However, daily blood sampling is seldom done because of the high cost of analysis and the burden on participants.

The phases of the ovulatory cycle generally are documented using serum progesterone levels, which are usually less than 1 ng/mL in the follicular phase and rise to above 10 ng/mL in the luteal phase. Values above 5 ng/mL generally indicate that the subject is in the luteal phase of an ovulatory cycle (13).

Urine

Daily urine sampling is feasible for research studies, and new technologies make kit assays practical (14, 15). Regularly timed daily urine specimens can be assayed for metabolites of steroid hormones. Urinary hormone levels have less diurnal variation than serum levels and do not reflect the

pulsatile secretion rate of some hormones. This can be an advantage over serum sampling if average levels are of interest, but peaks may be missed. The sample usually is the first void of the day; results are normalized to the urinary creatinine concentration.

During the luteal phase, urinary levels of pregnanediol, a metabolite of progesterone, reach 4 to 6 ng per 24-hour collection. Values above 2 ng per 24 hours indicate the luteal phase of an ovulatory cycle (10).

In-home ovulation prediction kits contain a monoclonal antibody specific for LH. An enzyme-linked immunosorbant assay reaction (ELISA) elicits a color change proportional to the level of LH in the urine. If baseline observations are established before ovulation is expected, the LH surge will be apparent. Testing for 10 consecutive days is sufficient to detect 95% of LH surges. Strict adherence to the manufacturer's instructions is necessary for accurate results. Samples can be stored in the refrigerator for later analysis, if necessary, but the analysis must be done at room temperature. Samples should be collected at the same time each day, with beverages restricted 1 or 2 hours immediately preceding collection so the urine is not too dilute. The various commercially available kits differ in details such as: cost, the number of days the kit can be used, the length of time for the color change to stabilize, the time of day the urine sample is collected, and the length of time between a positive result and the occurrence of ovulation. Examples of such kits include: First Response Ovulation Predictor Test, Carter-Wallace, Inc; Answer Ovulation Test Kit, Carter-Wallace, Inc; and pharmaceutical house generic brands. (Examples are provided for information purposes only and do not represent endorsements by either The American Dietetic Association or the National Heart, Lung, and Blood Institute.)

Saliva

Unconjugated steroid hormones diffuse freely and appear in saliva in small amounts proportional to serum levels (16, 17). Salivary steroids are 0.5% to 2% that of serum (18). Concentrations are not affected by the rate of saliva production, but any bleeding in the mouth will greatly increase steroid levels in the saliva.

Daily sampling of saliva is feasible in the context of research protocols. Two to 5 ml of fasting saliva is needed for the assay, which is relatively simple and inexpensive (19, 20). Specimens should be collected as participants arise, before they eat, or brush or floss their teeth. Citric acid applied to the tongue will increase saliva flow without affecting the assays (12). Samples can be stored in the home freezer for 1 month and are stable for 6 months at $-20°C$. Testing the saliva samples for hemoglobin or another marker of bleeding gums would allow contaminated samples to be discarded.

Ultrasound

Ultrasound can be used to observe the physiological changes in the ovaries and uterus during the menstrual cycle (21). During the follicular phase the size of the dominant follicle and the thickness of the endometrium correlate with the serum levels of estradiol (see Figure 8–1a). At ovulation the dominant follicle will typically have a maximum diameter of 20 mm to 23 mm, ranging from 14 mm to 29 mm. This coincides with the LH peak. Ultrasound can document ovulation and differentiate the cycle phases; endometrial thickness reaches a peak during the luteal phase. High cost and potential discomfort to the subject must be taken into account when investigators design protocols requiring ultrasound evaluations.

Menstrual Calendars

The appearance of the menses is the most commonly used parameter for determining the phases of the menstrual cycle. To control for hormone cycling, many research studies use the phase immediately following menses (ie, early follicular phase), when the hormone levels are low and steady. This period lasts about 6 days before estrogen begins to increase, but there is much variation within and among women. Phases can be identified retrospectively by counting back 14 days from the menses to determine the approximate day of ovulation. There is less variation within and among women in length of the luteal phase. For women with regular cycles, these methods can effectively approximate the hormone cycle. However, ovulation is a more critical event than menstruation in terms of hormonal surges and changes that affect metabolic parameters.

The menstrual calendar is a convenient and inexpensive means of collecting necessary data. It is easily incorporated into many types of study protocols. (An example is provided in Exhibit 8–1.)

Basal Body Temperature

Measurement of basal body temperature (BBT) can be used to identify ovulation and demarcate follicular and luteal phases (see Figure 8–1a and Figure 8–2). A rise in BBT occurs from 2 days before to 3 days after the LH peak and is a reliable indicator that ovulation has occurred (22, 23). Least-squares methods of analyzing BBT data yield good

correlations with LH concentration and can generate detailed data on menstrual cycle type (normal ovulatory, short luteal phase, or anovulatory) and luteal phase length (24).

BBT is a simple method of monitoring the menstrual cycle. It is well accepted by subjects, is noninvasive, and is inexpensive. However, the method relies on the subjects to monitor and record temperatures accurately. Mercury thermometers are fragile, take 3 to 5 minutes to register an accurate temperature, and are easily misread. The temperature must be taken on awakening, before participants arise. At this time of day, body temperatures are approximately $1.0°C$ $(1.5°F)$ lower than usual. Oral, vaginal, or rectal temperatures can be used, but the same site must be used consistently. Irregular sleep and emotional stress can invalidate the measurements. (An example of a BBT chart is provided in Figure 8–2.)

Computerized electronic devices combine the BBT and the calendar methods of identifying the fertile and infertile periods of the menstrual cycle (21). This eliminates the need for subjects to read and record temperatures. The general operation of these devices follows a similar pattern. The Bioself 110 (Bioself Distribution SA, 7 Avenue de Thorex, 1226, Geneva, Switzerland) is an example of such a device. (This example is provided for information purposes only and does not represent an endorsement by either The American Dietetic Association or the National Heart, Lung, and Blood Institute.) The user inputs the start of each menses by pushing a button. During the first month of use the program assumes a 28-day cycle. In subsequent months the program becomes increasingly more accurate for the individual user. The microprocessor subtracts 18 days from the length of the shortest cycle recorded and, with a steady red light, indicates this day as the beginning of the fertile period (late follicular phase). A display such as a flashing red light indicates the expected ovulatory phase. After the temperature rise following ovulation, another display (such as a green light) indicates the luteal phase. If ovulation does not occur during this cycle, and the temperature does not rise, the ovulatory phase display persists until the onset of menses is indicated by the user. The memory stores the temperatures and the displays each day for 2–3 months and the cycle lengths for 6 months. The devices can be programmed to accept temperature measurement at restricted times of the day, thus promoting a consistent daily time that the BBT is measured. Twenty-four hours after the last reading, the device emits a reminder tone signal. Data usually can be retrieved in graphic form, permitting review of the temperature charts and cycle lengths. Identification of the ovulatory period using electronic calendars correlates strongly with the ultrasound documentation of maximum follicular diameter (25) and the serum LH peak (26). The technology for such devices is improving rapidly and can be expected to yield modifications that would be useful in the research setting.

Cervical Mucus

Klaus (27) described monitoring of cervical mucus, used extensively in fertility and contraception techniques. The

EXHIBIT 8-1

Example of a Menstrual Calendar[1]
DELTA
Menstrual Calendar

Subject number:_____   Usual cycle length:_____days

On the calendar below put an X in the block corresponding to the first day of your period (first day of bleeding). Check (√) each day that bleeding continues enough to require a pad or tampon. Turn in this calendar to study personnel at your last blood drawing.

SEPTEMBER						
SUN	**MON**	**TUES**	**WED**	**THU**	**FRI**	**SAT**
26	27	28	29	30		

OCTOBER						
SUN	**MON**	**TUES**	**WED**	**THU**	**FRI**	**SAT**
					1	2
3	4	5	6	7	8	9
10	11	12	13	14	15	16
17	18	19	20	21	22	23
24	25	26	27	28	29	30
31						

NOVEMBER						
SUN	**MON**	**TUES**	**WED**	**THU**	**FRI**	**SAT**
	1	2	3	4	5	6
7	8	9	10	11	12	13
14	15	16	17	18	19	20

Note any *abnormalities* in your periods during the 8 weeks of the diet study with a √.

		Period[2]		
		1	**2**	**3**
Start date	Earlier than usual	_____	_____	_____
	Later than usual	_____	_____	_____
Cramps	Worse than usual	_____	_____	_____
	Not as bad as usual	_____	_____	_____
Premenstrual	More severe than usual	_____	_____	_____
Syndrome (PMS)[3]	Less severe than usual	_____	_____	_____

[1] Adapted from *Manual of Operations for the DELTA Program* (74).

[2] Most women will have only 2 periods during the diet study. However, 3 columns are provided because occasionally someone may have 3 periods within this time.

[3] PMS is a constellation of symptoms that usually occurs 7–10 days before menstruation and that disappears with the start of the new cycle. Physical symptoms include bloating, breast swelling, pelvic pain, headache, ankle swelling, and bowel changes. Psychological symptoms include irritability, aggressiveness, anxiety, tension, and changes of libido.

Days of the cycle

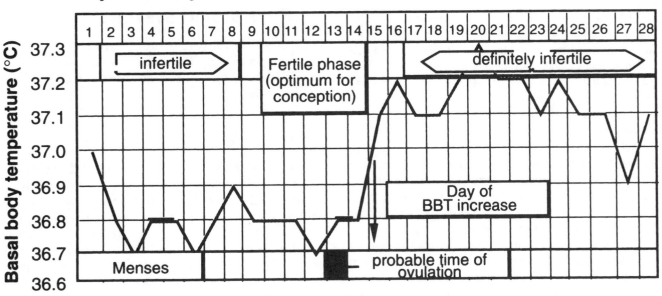

FIGURE 8-2. BBT chart for determining the time of ovulation. Reprinted with permission from Rabe T, Runnebaum B, Contraception. In: Runnebaum B, Rabe T, eds, *Gynecological Endocrinology and Reproductive Medicine*, Vol 1, *Gynecological Endocrinology*, New York, NY: Springer-Verlag; 1994:405.

mucus is a hydrogel of two components: one of high and one of low viscosity. The proportions of these components vary directly with hormone changes. "Type E" (estrogenic) mucus is thin, slippery, and acellular; it is in high proportion before and at ovulation, correlating with the LH surge in response to estrogen. "Type G" (gestagenic) mucus is thick, sticky, and dense; it occurs after ovulation in response to progesterone.

Subjects can be taught to identify the onset of mucus production and the changes in consistency. These techniques could be applied to research studies to identify ovulatory cycles and the phases accurately.

Steroidal Contraceptive Medications

Ninety percent of women at risk of pregnancy use some form of contraception. About 28% use steroidal contraceptives (28). These act to inhibit ovulation by negative feedback on LH and FSH so that the ovum does not develop. Steroidal contraceptives also render the cervical mucus and the endometrium less supportive of fertilization and pregnancy.

Three major classifications of oral contraceptives (OC) contain both estrogen and progestin: (1) *monophasic,* with a constant amount of the two hormones in each tablet; (2) *biphasic,* with a constant amount of estrogen but with progestin lower for the first 10 days and higher in the last 11 days; (3) *triphasic,* with constant or varied levels of estrogen and varied progestin. The purpose of varying the hormone levels is to mimic the natural cycle. Recently, oral contraceptives that contain only progestin have become available.

Not all contraceptive drugs are taken by mouth. Long-acting steroidal contraceptive systems that deliver proges-

togens continuously over an extended period of time are also in use. They include injectable depot formation; subcutaneous polymer implant; vaginal rings; medicated intrauterine devices; and injectable polymeric formulations (29).

Steroidal contraceptive use, which usually represents OC use, must be examined in light of protocol criteria to determine whether it is a potential confounding factor or effect modifier. Use is not a problem for some studies but is highly problematic for others. A problem situation develops if the steroidal contraceptive has direct biological effects on the study outcome variables, if the contraceptive modulates the influence of diet on the outcome variables, or both. If it is necessary or desirable to enroll steroidal contraceptive users in the study, confounding can be minimized through crossover designs or random balanced assignment of users and nonusers to treatment groups.

Menopause and Hormone Replacement Therapy

Menopause is the permanent cessation of menstrual cycles (Table 8–1). It occurs typically between ages 45 and 55 years, with small percentages of women experiencing menopause before 45 or after 55 years of age (3). As natural menopause approaches, cycling becomes irregular, then ceases—a process that can take months or years. During this time a decline in estrogen and an increase in FSH occur. For several years before cycles decrease, ovarian estradiol and progesterone production diminishes. This decreases the negative feedback inhibition on the hypothalamic pituitary system, and FSH levels gradually rise. The ovarian follicles become increasingly refractory to elevated concentrations of FSH.

Postmenopausal ovarian estrogen production is minimal. The adrenal androgens, especially androstenedione, can be converted in adipose tissue to estrogens; the degree of adiposity correlates with the amount of conversion. The ovaries continue to produce testosterone and androstenedione at or near premenopausal levels. The change in estrogen:testosterone hormone ratios may lead to increased facial hair and other masculinized characteristics.

Relatively large numbers of women undergo surgical menopause following hysterectomy procedures. Depending on medical considerations the ovaries may either be removed (oophorectomy) or left intact. Ovarian function then may be sustained as before but may in some cases decline more rapidly than normally would be expected.

The acute drop in serum estrogen levels from natural menopause or surgical oophorectomy can cause instability of the hypothalamic thermoregulatory set-point, leading to vasomotor flushes or "hot flashes." During a hot flash cutaneous blood flow and skin temperature increase; core body temperature falls. Blood pressure remains stable. Plasma LH rises to peak at about 12 minutes after onset of the flush. These flushes can interfere with sleep and contribute to irritability, reduced concentration, and impaired memory. It is not known how these events—either through physiologic mechanisms or by affecting compliance—might confound a study that includes perimenopausal women.

For some (but not all) protocols, confounding from these issues and from shifting hormonal levels will render the perimenopausal age range unsuitable for recruitment. In this case investigators are advised to recruit participants who are clearly pre- or postmenopausal as determined by blood FSH levels or by questionnaire (ie, about the number of months or years since last menstrual period).

An increasing number of women who reach menopause choose to take hormone replacement therapy, either to treat direct symptoms of menopause or to retain the health benefits of estrogen. Many different hormone preparations are available. If the formulation contains both estrogen and progestin, menstrual cycles will continue in a woman who retains an intact uterus, but ovulation does not occur.

Chronological age, menopausal age, hormonal status, and hormone replacement are factors that may affect disease risk factors and response to diet. All of these need to be carefully considered in the design and implementation of research studies. Potential study participants can be categorized according to whether the menopause was natural or surgical (oophorectomy); whether hormones are replaced; and whether the hormones are provided as estrogen alone or with progestin (30), for how long, and by what routes of administration (31). How menopause and replacement hormones affect risk of chronic disease (such as cancer, heart disease, and osteoporosis) has become a high research priority now that greater numbers of women are living 30 years or more after the menopause (32, 33).

Effects of the Menstrual Cycle on Physiologic Systems

Many physiological systems are affected by the hormonal cycle and menopause. This section presents some interesting examples, many of which are pertinent to well-controlled feeding studies.

Lipids

Serum cholesterol levels appear to be affected by the menstrual cycle. Total cholesterol is approximately 10% higher in the follicular phase, especially close to ovulation, than in the menstrual and luteal phases (34–36). Cholesterol is a substrate for steroid synthesis, and it is biologically plausible that the hormone cycle would affect serum cholesterol levels. The evidence for menstrual cycle effects on serum triglycerides is inconclusive (37, 38).

Serum low-density lipoprotein cholesterol and triglycerides rise with declining sex hormones after menopause, and high density lipoproteins fall, independently of age and other factors (39). Unopposed estrogen replacement is the optimal treatment for maintaining serum lipids at premenopausal levels, but combined estrogen/progestin replacement also is highly effective (39).

Blood Pressure

Systolic blood pressure is higher in the luteal phase, with a gradual increase until the day of menstruation. Thereafter, blood pressure drops sharply and remains low through the follicular phase. Variability among women is wide (40, 41). Conflicting results between studies may be caused by hormonal changes that do not directly affect blood pressure but instead affect response to stress. For example, mental stress tests applied to normally menstruating women caused greater increases in heart rate and systolic and diastolic blood pressure during the luteal phase than in the follicular phase (42). Without applied mental stress, no differences were observed between the phases. This suggests it is reaction to stress, not blood pressure per se, that varies with the menstrual cycle.

Regensteiner et al (43) found that hormone replacement therapy (HRT) as combined estrogen and progestin maintained blood pressure at premenopausal levels, whereas lack of HRT or estrogen alone could not prevent the rise in blood pressure frequently seen in postmenopausal women. The relationship of dietary calcium and blood pressure also may be different in pre- vs postmenopausal women (44).

Sodium Balance

Urinary sodium balance may fluctuate during the luteal phase because the progesterone surge at ovulation can interfere with the action of aldosterone on the renal tubules, causing net sodium loss. Aldosterone levels may increase in response to the interference, whereas the progesterone levels are declining. This leads to sodium retention and low urine sodium levels (45).

Caffeine Clearance

Caffeine clearance may differ between the phases of the cycle. Lane et al found an 11% reduction in caffeine clearance during the luteal phase (46). As clearance had a negative correlation with estrogen levels, it may also be reduced in persons taking estrogen replacement or oral contraceptives. This difference is not enough to cause caffeine intoxication but may affect the results of metabolic studies.

Fluid Balance

Some women complain of "bloating" (a feeling of swelling) premenstrually, but weight gain does not necessarily accompany this complaint, suggesting a shift of fluids between compartments. Oian et al, studying transcapillary fluid dynamics, found a reduction of the plasma and interstitial colloid osmotic pressures in the luteal phase, which may be from simple dilution and reduction in total body protein mass (47). Changes in the metabolism of plasma proteins during the menstrual cycle may account for this observation, because there was no external loss of plasma protein. Mechanisms are as yet unknown.

Vokes et al (48) demonstrated that osmotic thresholds for thirst and vasopressin secretion decreased during the luteal phase. Plasma sodium also dropped 2 mEq/L during the luteal phase. These changes were small but statistically significant. Therefore, a true shift may occur in the setting of the osmoregulatory system between follicular and luteal phases.

Energy Expenditure, Energy Intake, and Eating Patterns

Several investigators (49–52) have reported increased energy expenditure during the luteal phase compared to the follicular phase. In particular, Webb reported a mean increase of 9% in daily energy expenditure in the luteal phase (49). Intraindividual variation was also greatest in the luteal phase. Bisdee observed a consistent pattern of 7% maximum increase in 24-hour energy expenditure in the late luteal phase and lowest expenditure in the late follicular phase (ie, immediately before preovulation) (50).

Spontaneous food intake also may vary across the menstrual cycle and between monthly cycles. Protocols requiring information on typical dietary patterns may thus require multiple dietary assessments during each phase for an accurate picture of overall intake. Several outpatient studies of food intake across the menstrual cycle have reported energy in-

take during the luteal phase that was higher by 100 or 200 calories per day (53, 54). In contrast, a study that confined subjects to a metabolic unit and controlled for activity found no significant changes in energy intake over the menstrual cycle (55). Food intake was monitored inconspicuously, but the inpatient setting may have diminished spontaneous intake. An increased intake of sucrose—in the form of candy, chocolate, and soft drinks—was observed in the luteal phase. Fluid intake, as food water and beverages, increased during the luteal phase, and urine volume was correspondingly higher; dry weight of foods was equal.

Gastrointestinal Function

Study results of the menstrual cycle's effects on gastrointestinal function are conflicting (56–59). Some report slower mean transit time in the luteal phase, whereas others find no difference with phases of the cycle. Subjects eating a controlled diet had increased starch absorption, decreased breath hydrogen, and decreased stool weight (dry and wet) in the luteal phase. No effects have been found of the cycle phases on gastrin, somatostatin, oxytocin, and gastric inhibitory polypeptide (60). Cholecystokinin, however, is higher in the luteal phase (61). Its expected effects, such as increased gallbladder contractility, increased gut motility, and increased satiety, are counteracted by progesterone, which also has high levels during the luteal phase. This competition may contribute to the inconsistent results reported.

DESIGN ISSUES FOR STUDIES ENROLLING WOMEN

Common Problems

Much of the data obtained on the effects of the menstrual cycle on physiological systems are derived as adjuncts to other studies, and confounding variables are often not adequately controlled. Diet is seldom controlled, even in studies of serum lipids, blood pressure, or fluid dynamics. Activity is not always controlled in studies of energy intake; stresses are not controlled in studies of blood pressure. Techniques and procedures for sample collection, such as fasted or fed state, should be (but often are not) standardized. Sample size in many studies may be too small to identify significant effects of the hormone changes. Therefore, study results may have large variability as a result of uncontrolled factors that could potentially modify the outcome variable and may lead to inconsistent conclusions about menstrual cycle effects.

Many studies lack clear definition and objective identification of the phases of the menstrual cycle. Many rely on the subjects' self-report of the appearance of menstruation to number the days of the cycle and identify the phases. Investigators use different methods of numbering the days and identifying the phases of the cycle, making it difficult to compare studies. Some professionals count forward from menstruation and designate the phases by convention. Some count backward to identify ovulation, using population averages for the length of the luteal phase. If the phases are not clearly identified in endocrinological terms, the timing of the hormonal changes and phases may not be precisely identified. The occurrence of folliculogenesis and ovulation should be confirmed if nonovulatory cycles are to be excluded from the analysis. Some otherwise well-characterized studies report data from only one cycle per subject. Investigators may not be blinded as to the phase of the subject.

In many studies that have attempted to control for the menstrual cycle, the follicular phase has been used exclusively because the hormone levels are steady and low. This may simplify study design but may obscure significant physiological effects that occur with the hormonal surges of ovulation and the luteal phase. Also, the length of the follicular phase varies more within and between women than does the luteal phase. To accurately study the effects of the hormonal cycle on physiological systems, the phases must be correctly identified and all phases should be studied.

Also to be considered in the design of research protocols, especially when cycle phase or hormonal status are outcome variables, are personal lifestyle factors, physiological characteristics, or environmental factors that can affect the cycle and contribute to unpredictability and to intra- and interpersonal variability, such as the following:

- Strenuous activity, inadequate nutrient intake, and mental and emotional stresses can alter the individual woman's cycle.
- Inadequate caloric intake, acute or long-term, attenuates hormonal rises and can prevent ovulation. Unnaturally low levels of body fat in women can prevent ovulation secondary to low hormone levels.
- Extreme physical exercise, with or without adequate energy intake, will prevent ovulation and disrupt the cycle (62). Modest exercise has not been shown to have this effect.
- Seasonal changes in the amount of daylight can also affect the cycle, especially in the far northern latitudes. Some women may experience ovarian hormone suppression during the dark photoperiod of autumn to spring.

The effects of vegetarian diets on menstrual cycle parameters and fertility, although of high interest, are not well understood. Pirke et al (63) reported that women who followed a vegetarian diet had an increased incidence of anovulatory cycles, with lower luteal-phase serum estrogen and progesterone levels compared to omnivorous women. Other investigators, however, found that behavioral factors associated with restrained eating habits, rather than vegetarianism per se, were related to menstrual irregularities (24). Different dietary levels of soy products, which contain estrogen-like compounds, also may confound the results of many studies on vegetarians (64). More well-controlled research is needed on this topic.

Improving Study Design

Statistical Power and Sample Size

When designers create the study protocol, a decision must be made whether a separate measure of the outcome effect is to be made in each status group (eg, males, females; males, premenopausal females, postmenopausal females; postmenopausal females with and without hormones) or whether data from all the groups will be combined for a single estimate of the effect. This may have enormous impact on statistical power and related sample size. If it is not necessary to make separate estimates, data from all subjects can be combined. To make separate estimates, sample size will roughly increase according to the number of groups. To be able to make a comparison of the effects in response to diet among the different groups, even more subjects must be enrolled.

Many studies will not have adequate power to actually compare the magnitude of response in men vs women. Rather there may instead be enough power to make separate statements of magnitude of response in men and in women. (Also see Chapter 2, "Statistical Aspects of Controlled Diet Studies.")

Hormonal and reproductive status can be considered as sources of between-subject or within-subject variation. Corresponding adjustments must be made in study design, statistical power calculations, data analysis procedures, and reporting of data.

The ovarian cycle contributes to within-subject variation, as phases change during a cycle and as cycles vary within the same woman, and also to between-subject variation among women. These sources of variation can be addressed at both the design and the analysis stages of the study. To control for cycle phase, the study's start date and specimen collection schedule may have to be tailored to each individual and may have to be kept flexible according to the events of each individual cycle (this may not be practical for larger studies).

The average cycle length of 28 days can be a useful consideration when investigators design studies and plan sample collections. Taking multiple outcome samples can control for within-cycle variation, and observations of cycle phase can be linked to other study results. For studies with relatively large numbers of participants, or for short-term studies (<1 month), it may be appropriate to assume that the subjects are evenly distributed across the phases of the cycle. This likely will control for the potential confounding because the diet intervention will be randomly started at different points in the subjects' cycles. Or, by monitoring and recording the cycle events during the study, this issue can be dealt with later during data analysis.

When a potentially important source of between-subject variation is known at the outset of a study, there are several ways to use the information to avoid confounding. Preferably, subjects can be classified according to status, and treatments then randomized for each status group. This will ensure that each treatment group contains a similar proportion of subjects from each status group. For example, if there are three diet treatment groups, randomization would place premenopausal and postmenopausal women into each diet group in numbers reflecting their proportions in the group as a whole. Alternatively, the study can be designed to recruit specific proportions of subjects in each status group. This process sometimes is referred to as *filling cells.* In either case, sample size calculations are used to determine the number of subjects required to provide sufficient statistical power to make separate estimates of each group's response to diet. If separate estimates cannot be made, data from all subjects are pooled to make a single estimate and then analyzed using statistical procedures that can "adjust for" status, ie, they incorporate weighting factors that reflect the proportions of subjects in each group.

In crossover designs, in which each subject receives all treatments and results are analyzed as within-subject comparisons, controlling for cycle phase becomes imperative. Results can be confounded if the endpoints from the different treatments are obtained in different phases of the cycle (eg, if Diet 1 endpoints were collected only during the luteal phase, and Diet 2 endpoints only during the follicular phase). By collecting endpoint data for each diet phase throughout the entire menstrual cycle, the investigator can detect the overall effect of diet without confounding. The same data will also allow the investigator to evaluate the effect of diet at each phase of the cycle (64, 65).

In parallel-arm protocols, in which subjects are randomized to one of multiple treatments, confounding can occur if many of the Group A subjects happen to be in, say, luteal phase, whereas many of the Group B subjects happen to be in follicular phase. If endpoint data are collected over the course of the entire cycle, or if cycle phase is at least monitored throughout the study, appropriate data analysis techniques can adjust for cycle phase during evaluation of the dietary treatment effects.

Data Collection and Analysis

The approximately 4-week length of the typical menstrual cycle should be considered when designing the collection of samples and data for study endpoints. If investigators expect that the menstrual cycle is likely to exert relatively strong effects on study results, it may be desirable to collect multiple endpoint samples or make multiple observations throughout the course of the cycle. Menstrual calendars or other data needed for staging the cycle are collected at the same time. It may be feasible to collect endpoint samples once weekly over a 4-week time period. The cycle phase for each subject can in this way be characterized adequately and then linked to the other study results.

For other studies, it will be necessary to take samples for endpoint measurements at precisely defined times of the cycle, such as Day 0. It also might be possible to collect endpoint samples at planned intervals, such as once per week during the last 4 weeks of an 8-week diet period, and use

hormone levels or menstrual calendars to make a judgment about cycle phase. Few studies will have the financial resources to collect daily blood samples for hormone determinations, and subjects might become averse to repeated phlebotomies. Thus, a less intensive approach that yields adequate precision, albeit with slightly greater error (ovulation day (± 2 days instead of within a single day), may have advantages for many studies.

Data obtained to define cycle phase throughout the course of endpoint sample collection usually are formed into categorical or collapsed variables that lend themselves to stratified data analyses. For example, the information from a daily menstrual calendar (a sequence of categorical data points: menstruating yes/no) is often used to yield another categorical variable (such as menstrual phase: follicular or luteal). Blood hormone levels, although originally collected as continuous variables, also are often used in this way.

It is usually better, however, to take advantage of analysis techniques that incorporate "uncollapsed" continuous data without loss of detail. Such data can be included as covariates in multivariate models that adjust for potential confounding of study results by menstrual cycle phase. This approach generally has greater statistical power compared with stratified analyses, provided the data are in suitable form.

The sophisticated techniques that statisticians apply to circadian rhythm analyses (ie, patterns of diurnal and seasonal variations) also are suitable for analyses of the menstrual cycle per se (65, 66). Cyclic trigonometric models such as sine and cosine curves can be fitted to hormonal data and other continuous distributions, provided there are enough data points. This type of analysis might be useful, for example, in evaluating within-subject variation after stabilization on a constant diet. As mentioned earlier, least-squares methods can be turned to the analysis of basal body temperature data (24).

When menstrual cycle parameters are primary dependent outcome variables, the results are reported in the usual fashion with descriptive statistics. A good example is found in Cassidy et al (64). Direct dietary effects on the menstrual cycle, such as changes in phase length, hormone levels, and cycle length, can be assessed this way. Also, when researchers are studying the effects of exercise or light, for example, on the menstrual cycle, constant metabolic diets can be used to control for dietary confounding.

WOMEN AS STUDY PARTICIPANTS

Recruitment

Classification of women by hormone status must be unambiguous. Assigning a subject to the wrong category or having a subject change categories leads to loss of statistical power and errors in data interpretation, particularly if the investigator wishes to elucidate differences among groups. Appropriate advertisements and recruiting materials, along with rigorously defined and carefully applied selection criteria, help the investigator to avoid recruiting subjects at risk for changing their hormonal status (such as entering menopause) during the study. The hormonal and reproductive status of women seeking to participate in a feeding study must be assessed in a systematic fashion directly linked to the study protocol. The numbers of subjects needed in a particular enrollment category and the exclusion criteria must be established as part of the study design.

For example, few investigators would enroll pregnant women unless the research question was specifically directed to them. Other investigators might seek to enroll a specific number of postmenopausal women but would not recruit those taking estrogens. Some protocols might require premenopausal females willing to keep detailed menstrual diaries but must exclude users of oral contraceptives.

Preliminary assessment of status is generally carried out using screening questionnaires administered over the telephone or during a clinic visit. Questions generally address whether the woman is pregnant or considering pregnancy; is lactating; has recently delivered a child or otherwise ended a pregnancy; is still menstruating or has attained natural or surgical menopause; and is taking oral contraceptives or postmenopausal hormonal preparations. For this last group, it is helpful to have the subject bring their pill packets with them to the clinic or to have various sample kinds of pill packets on hand at the clinic for identification to document accurately which formulation each woman is taking. Examples of screening questionnaires are found in Exhibit 8–2.

Eating disorders are particularly common among women (67) and should be screened for at the outset. Many people respond to recruiting advertisements for controlled feeding studies with the hope that they will lose weight. Unless weight loss is a planned study outcome, recruiters must be explicit that entry weight will be maintained. Screening questions about whether the prospective participant has had large weight fluctuations or has been dieting to lose weight will help the study team to identify individuals with these concerns.

Protection from Research Risks

Inclusion of women in research studies may require special considerations for informed consent statements and other institutional clearances. For example, women with regular menstrual cycles are more prone to anemia. This leads to higher dietary iron requirements but also puts a limit on the total volume of blood that can be drawn during the course of study.

Informed consent statements usually include commitments concerning participants' intention not to become pregnant and to inform the investigator immediately if pregnancy is suspected. Pregnancy testing may be necessary both initially and also periodically throughout the study if there is any potential risk to a developing fetus. Nutrition research generally does not usually pose risks to a fetus, but pregnancy may affect compliance with the protocol and confound interpretation of the study outcome parameters. If use of OC is an exclusion criterion, other reliable forms of birth control, such as tubal ligation, monogamous relationship with vasectomized partner, same-sex partner, or celibacy, are usually discussed with the subject before participant enrollment.

Well-controlled feeding studies occasionally are specifically conducted with pregnant or lactating subjects. Usually such studies are conducted to answer specific biologic questions about nutrient metabolism during these physiologic states. Under these circumstances, it is likely that the institutional review board (IRB) approving the protocol will require extra attention to safety issues and informed consent procedures. For example, use of radioactive isotopes is contraindicated in pregnant or lactating women unless specifically justified for these populations. Otherwise, enrolling a small number of pregnant or lactating women in a study addressing more general questions will introduce excessive variability into the study population. (See also Chapter 5, "Ethical Considerations in Feeding Studies.")

Participant Management Issues

Monitoring the menstrual cycle may be a new idea for many women recruited into studies. The activities may seem strange to them, especially if the study is not investigating a gynecologic topic. Education about the cycle and the importance of the data to the study is necessary to obtain good compliance, especially if self-monitoring procedures are being used. Privacy and confidentiality, as always, are of utmost importance. The clinic site must have an area with adequate privacy for reviewing menstrual calendars with subjects. Confidence and ease of the staff in discussing self-monitoring techniques in a straightforward manner will make the subjects more comfortable. The subjects should be emphatically reminded that monitoring the cycle does not, in itself, constitute contraception.

Financial reimbursement, even if small, helps to communicate the seriousness of the study and improves compliance and retention. An additional stipend for those women subjects who are monitoring their cycles is justifiable, especially to compensate for the burden of blood draws and the extra work required for recording the data.

Studying subjects in a specific phase of the cycle requires flexibility on the part of the staff and the facility. The subjects' schedules must be accommodated. If the subjects make telephone calls to give the investigators the results of self-monitoring techniques, it is helpful to establish codes so that subjects can call in the presence of others without being explicit. Usually communication between female staff and female subjects works best.

Halbreich et al (68) describe recruiting techniques for studies of menstrual cycle per se that can be used in studies to control for phase. A telephone checklist of inclusion and exclusion criteria can save time by avoiding unnecessary

EXHIBIT 8-2

Examples of Screening Questionnaires for Hormonal Status[1]

EXAMPLE 1: TELEPHONE SCREENING QUESTIONNAIRE FOR PREGNANCY AND LACTATION

WOMEN BORN AFTER 1953 ONLY
37. Are you pregnant or planning to become pregnant within the next year?   YES   NO
38. Are you breast-feeding?   YES   NO
39. Have you had a baby within the last 6 months?   YES   NO
If the answer to either question 37, or 38, or 39 is YES, then the applicant has become ineligible. If so, terminate the interview and complete questions 12 and 13.

EXAMPLE 2: CLINIC VISIT SCREENING QUESTIONNAIRE FOR HORMONAL STATUS

WOMEN ONLY
27a. Are you currently taking an oral contraceptive?   YES   NO
b. If YES to 27a, are you planning to stop?   YES   NO
c. If NO to 27a, are you planning to start?   YES   NO
[Circle the letter preceding the response.]
28. What is your current menstrual status?
R Regular (normal) [go to question 30]
I Irregular [go to question 29a]
N Not menstruating [go to question 29c]
29. If you are menstruating irregularly, what is the reason?
A Undergoing menopause
B Other (describe): _____
30. If you are not menstruating, what is the reason?
_____ Natural menopause
_____ Hysterectomy
_____ Medication stopped period
_____ Other (describe): _____
31. When did you have your last period?
A Less than 2 months ago
B 2 months to 6 months ago
C 6 months to 1 year ago
D 1 year but less than 3 years ago
E At least 3 years ago
32. a. Are you taking or have you ever taken estrogen? [Estrogen or female hormones for hot flashes or symptoms of menopause]   YES   NO
b. If YES to 31a, are you currently taking estrogen?   YES   NO
c. If NO to 31a, do you plan to start taking estrogen?   YES   NO
Resume asking questions of all applicants.

[1]Adapted from *Manual of Operations for the DELTA Program* (74).

screening appointments, but face-to-face contact is required to establish and build rapport. Continued contact by a specific staff member and generation of a "group" feeling among the subjects improves recruitment, compliance, and retention. Detailed screening procedures that correctly classify subjects are worthwhile.

As mentioned earlier, serious eating disorders and excessive concerns about body weight are prevalent in the general population of US women (67). Good screening questionnaires and interviews will likely eliminate individuals with clinical-grade eating disorders. Milder forms of these problems, however, may surface during the protocol, affecting compliance and ability to complete the study. For example, female participants may be more concerned than are males during the study about body weight fluctuations, energy content and cognitive attributes of study foods, and minor gastrointestinal and other physical side effects of the research diet. Investigators should be prepared to identify and address these issues appropriately.

The collection of biological samples for study endpoints may be affected by reproductive status or menstrual cycle phase. For example, as mentioned earlier, the total volume of blood that can be drawn from premenopausal women may be constrained by risk of anemia. Another example is that of urine collection; contamination by menstrual blood may affect some assays and special collection procedures may be needed.

Planning Research Diets

For studies enrolling both males and females, nutritional adequacy is always a primary consideration, but there generally are no major gender effects on diet planning. However, investigators must recognize that smaller women and older women, particularly after menopause, may have fairly low energy needs. B-vitamin requirements, such as thiamin, riboflavin, and niacin, are tied closely to lean body mass and more broadly to energy intake and are not especially difficult to provide.

It can be difficult, however, to achieve nutrient goals for dietary components that are needed as absolute total daily levels rather than relative amounts (ie, per 1,000 kcal). For example, a fiber allowance of 15 g/day is difficult to achieve on a 1,500 kcal diet; iron, zinc, and folate present a similar challenge. This reflects the generally higher nutrient density diets that women need. The Food and Nutrition Board has acknowledged that women have different nutritional needs at different life stages (69–71): women require less iron after menopause and more folate during pregnancy, for example. Reaching the new calcium goals of 1,000–1,500 mg/day (72) can be particularly problematic, depending on study design and the particulars of the research diet; fortified foods, such as calcium-supplemented orange juice, may be necessary.

Fixed nutrient levels specified by study design can be difficult to provide when the study participants have a large range of energy needs. In the DELTA studies that enrolled males and females consuming 1,500–3,000 kcal/day, a single level of total daily cholesterol (300 mg/day) was provided to all subjects regardless of calorie intake by adding egg yolk powder in varying amounts to each calorie level (73, 74). Otherwise, if all foods had been increased or decreased in proportional increments, the higher calorie diets would have contained far more cholesterol.

If pregnant or lactating women are enrolled in controlled feeding studies, researchers are ethically obligated to ensure that the diets meet their increased nutrient needs. Folate and mineral requirements are especially elevated (69). Menus should not include foods generally known to be unappealing to pregnant women, who are prone to taste and smell aversions. For lactating women, menus should be reviewed for foods that might be considered to predispose the infant to colic (eg, cabbage) or which might make the milk taste unpleasant to the infant (eg, garlic).

CONCLUSION

Controlled diet studies provide the most fundamental way to obtain data on nutrient requirements for women of all ages. By eliminating some potential sources of confounding, controlled feeding studies can also be a good way to clarify various aspects of female reproductive biology. Moreover, even if there is no major expected effect on study outcome variables, accounting for hormone status and the menstrual cycle in the study design may enhance the precision of the research. By paying more attention to protocol design, data collection techniques, hormonal status definition, and data analysis, the quality of research conducted with female subjects can be greatly improved. The research techniques for addressing these points are feasible and often inexpensive and should serve to promote the inclusion of women in nearly all study protocols.

REFERENCES

1. NIH Guidelines for Inclusion of Women and Minorities as Subjects in Clinical Research. (FR 59 14508–14513) March 28, 1994. *NIH Guide to Grants and Contracts.* 1994;23;11, March 18.
2. Stone SC, Rosen GF. Physiology of puberty. In: Speroff L, Simpson JL, Sciarra JJ, eds. *Gynecology and Obstetrics.* Vol 5. Philadelphia, Pa: JB Lippincott Co; 1994:1–7.
3. Gerhard I, Heinrich U. Puberty and its disorders. In: Runnebaum B, Rabe T, eds. *Gynecological Endocrinology and Reproductive Medicine.* Vol 1. *Gynecological Endocrinology.* New York, NY: Springer-Verlag; 1994.
4. Jones RE. *Human Reproductive Biology.* 2nd ed. New York, NY: Academic Press; 1997.
5. Ferin M, Jewelewicz R, Warren M. The menstrual cycle. In: *Physiology, Reproductive Disorders, and Infertility.* New York, NY: Oxford University Press; 1993.

6. Weinbauer GF, Nieschlag E. Hormonal regulation of reproductive organs. In: Greger R, Windhorst U, eds. *Comprehensive Human Physiology*. Vol 2. New York, NY: Springer-Verlag; 1996.

7. Grunwald K, Rabe T, Keisel L, Runnebaum B. Physiology of the menstrual cycle. In: Runnebaum B, Rabe T, eds. *Gynecological Endocrinology and Reproductive Medicine*. Vol 1. *Gynecological Endocrinology*. New York, NY: Springer-Verlag; 1994.

8. *Ovarian Endocrinology*. Oxford, UK: Blackwell Scientific Publications; 1991.

9. Barr SI, Janelle KC, Prior JC. Energy intakes are higher during the luteal phase of ovulatory menstrual cycles. *Am J Clin Nutr.* 1995;61:39–43.

10. Fitzgerald CT, Seif MW, Lillick SR, Elstein M. Age-related changes in the female reproductive cycle. *Br J Obstet Gynaecol.* 1994;101(3):229–233.

11. Moghissi KS. Ovulation detection. *Reprod Endocrin.* 1992;21 :39–55.

12. Vermesh M, Kletzky OA, Davajan V, et al. Monitoring techniques to predict and detect ovulation. *Fertil Steril.* 1987;47:259–264.

13. Moghissi KS. How to document ovulation. In: Speroff L, Simpson JL, Sciarra JJ, eds. *Gynecology and Obstetrics*. Vol 5. Philadelphia: JB Lippincott Co; 1994. Chapter 54.

14. Wilcox AJ, Baird DD, Weinberg CR, et al. The use of biochemical assays in epidemiologic studies of reproduction. *Environ Health Perspect.* 1987;75:29–35.

15. Kesner JS, Krieg EF Jr, Knech EA, et al. Power analyses and immunoassays for measuring reproductive hormones in urine to assess female reproductive potential in field studies. *Scand J Work Environ Health.* 1992;18 (suppl 2):33–36.

16. Zorn JR, McDonough PG, Nessman CY, Janssens Y, Cedard L. Salivary progesterone as an index of the luteal function. *Fertil Steril.* 1984;41:248–253.

17. Vining RF, McGinley RA, Symons RG. Hormones in saliva: mode of entry and consequent implications for clinical interpretation. *Clin Chem.* 1983;29:1752–1756.

18. Sufi SB, Donaldson A, Gandy SC, et al. Multicenter evaluation of assays for estradiol and progesterone in saliva. *Clin Chem.* 1985;31:101–103.

19. Tallon DF, Gosling JP, Buckley PM, et al. Direct solid phase enzyme immunoassay of progesterone in saliva. *Clin Chem.* 1984;30:1507.

20. Walker RF, Read GF, Riad-Fahmy D. Radioimmunoassay of progesterone in saliva: application to the assessment of ovarian function. *Clin Chem.* 1979;25:2030–2033.

21. Bakos O, Lundvist O, Wide L, et al. Ultrasonographical and hormonal description of the normal ovulatory menstrual cycle. *Acta Obstet Gynecol Scand.* 1994;73:790–796.

22. Rabe T, Runnebaum B. Contraception. In: Runnebaum B, Rabe T, eds. *Gynecological Endocrinology and Reproductive Medicine*. Vol 1. *Gynecological Endocrinology*. New York, NY: Springer-Verlag; 1994.

23. Martinez AR, van Hooff MHA, Schoute E, et al. The reliability, acceptability, and applications of basal body temperature (BBT) records in the diagnosis and treatment of infertility. *Eur J Obstet Gyn Reprod Biol.* 1992;47:121–127.

24. Barr SI, Janell KC, Prior JC. Vegetarian vs nonvegetarian diets, dietary restraint, and subclinical ovulatory disturbances: prospective 6-month study. *Am J Clin Nutr.* 1994;60:887–894.

25. Ismail M, Arshat H, Pulcrano J, et al. An evaluation of the Bioself 110 fertility indicator. *Contraception.* 1989;39:53–71.

26. Flynn A, Pulcrano J, Royston P, et al. An evaluation of the Bioself 110 electronic fertility indicator. *Contraception.* 1991;44:125–139.

27. Klaus H. Natural family planning: a review. *Obstet Gynecol Survey.* 1982;37:128–150.

28. Shoupe D. Steroidal contraception: clinical aspects. In: Zatuchni GI, Steege JF, Sciarra JJ, eds. *Gynecology and Obstetrics*. Vol 6. Philadelphia, Pa: JB Lippincott Co; 1994. Chapter 21.

29. Beck LR, Pope VZ. Long-acting steroidal contraceptive systems. In: Zatuchni GI, Steege JF, Sciarra JJ, eds. *Gynecology and Obstetrics*. Vol 6. Philadelphia, Pa: JB Lippincott Co; 1994. Chapter 22.

30. Nabulsi AA, Folsom AR, White A, et al. Association of hormone-replacement therapy with various cardiovascular risk factors in postmenopausal women. *N Engl J Med.* 1993;328:1069–1075.

31. Sessions DR, Kelly AC, Jewelewicz R. Current concepts in estrogen replacement therapy in the menopause. *Fertil Steril.* 1993;59:277–284.

32. Barrett-Connor E. Epidemiology and the menopause: a global overview. *Int J Fert Menopause Studies.* 1993;38 (suppl 1):6–14.

33. Ravnikar VA. Diet, exercise, and lifestyle in preparation for menopause. *Obstet Gynecol Clin North Am.* 1993;20(2):365–378.

34. Lussier-Cacan S, Xhignesse M, Desmarais JL, et al. Cyclic fluctuations in human serum lipid and apolipoprotein levels during the normal menstrual cycle: comparison with changes occurring during oral contraceptive therapy. *Metabolism.* 1991;40:849–854.

35. Jones DY, Judd JT, Taylor PR, et al. Menstrual cycle effect on plasma lipids. *Metabolism.* 1988;37:1–2.

36. Berlin E, Judd JT, Nair PP, et al. Dietary fat and hormonal influences on lipoprotein fluidity and composition in premenopausal women. *Atherosclerosis.* 1991;86:95–110.

37. Heiling VJ, Jensen MD. Free fatty acid metabolism in the follicular and luteal phases of the menstrual cycle. *J Clin Endocrine Metab.* 1992;74: 806–810.

38. Wendler D, Michel E, Kastner P, et al. Menstrual cycle exhibits no effect on postprandial lipemia. *Horm Metab Res.* 1992;24:580–581.

39. PEPI Trial Writing Group. Effects of estrogen or estrogen/progestin regimens on heart disease risk factors in postmenopausal women. *JAMA.* 1995;273(3):199–208.

40. Kelleher C, Joyce C, Kelly G, et al. Blood pressure alters during the normal menstrual cycle. *Br J Obstet Gynecol.* 1986;93:523–526.

41. Greenberg G, Imeson JD, Thompson SG, et al. Blood pressure and the menstrual cycle. *Br J Obstet Gynecol.* 1985;92:1010–1014.

42. Jern C, Manhem K, Eriksson E, et al. Hemostatic responses to mental stress during the menstrual cycle. *Thromb Haemost.* 1991;66(5):614–618.

43. Regensteiner JG, Hiatt WR, Byyny RL, et al. Short-term effects of estrogen and progestin on blood pressure of normotensive postmenopausal women. *J Clin Pharm Ther.* 1991;31:543–548.

44. Van Beresteijn EC, Riedstra M, van der Wel A, et al. Habitual dietary calcium intake and blood pressure change around the menopause: a longitudinal study. *Int J Epidemiol.* 1992;21:683–689.

45. Landau RL, Lugibihl K. Inhibition of the sodium-retaining influence of aldosterone by progesterone. *J Clin Endocrinol.* 1958;18:1237–1245.

46. Lane JD, Steege JF, Rupp SL, et al. Menstrual cycle effects on caffeine elimination in the human female. *Eur J Clin Pharmacol.* 1992;43:543–546.

47. Oian P, Tollan A, Fadnes HO, et al. Transcapillary fluid dynamics during the menstrual cycle. *Am J Obstet Gynecol.* 1987;156:952–955.

48. Vokes TJ, Weiss NM, Schreiber J, et al. Osmoregulation of thirst and vasopressin during normal menstrual cycle. *Am J Physiol.* 1988;254:R641–R647.

49. Webb P. 24-hour energy expenditure and the menstrual cycle. *Am J Clin Nutr.* 1986;44:614–619.

50. Bisdee JT, James WP, Shaw MA. Changes in energy expenditure during the menstrual cycle. *Br J Nutr.* 1989;61:187–199.

51. Bisdee JT, Garlick PJ, James WP. Metabolic changes during the menstrual cycle. *Br J Nutr.* 1989;61:641–650.

52. Solomon SJ, Kurzer MS, Calloway DH. Menstrual cycle and basal metabolic rate in women. *Am J Clin Nutr.* 1982;36:611–616.

53. Lissner L, Stevens J, Levitsky DA, et al. Variation in energy intake during the menstrual cycle: implications for food-intake research. *Am J Clin Nutr.* 1988;48:956–962.

54. Gong EJ, Garrel D, Callow DH. Menstrual cycle and voluntary food intake. *Am J Clin Nutr.* 1989;49:252–258.

55. Fong AKH, Kretsch MJ. Changes in dietary intake, urinary nitrogen, and urinary volume across the menstrual cycle. *Am J Clin Nutr.* 1993;57:43–46.

56. Hinds JP, Stoney B, Wald A. Does gender or the menstrual cycle affect colonic transit? *Am J Gastroenterol.* 1989;84:123–126.

57. Wald A, Van Thiel DH, Hiechstetter L, et al. Gastrointestinal transit: the effect of the menstrual cycle. *Gastroenterology.* 1981;80:1497–1500.

58. McBurney MI. Starch malabsorption and stool excretion are influenced by the menstrual cycle in women consuming low-fibre Western diets. *Scand J Gastroenterol.* 1991;26:880–886.

59. Kamm MA, Farthing MJG, Lennard-Jones JE. Bowel function and transit rate during the menstrual cycle. *Gut.* 1989;30:605–608.

60. Uvnas-Moberg K, Sjogren C, Westlin L, et al. Plasma levels of gastrin, somatostatin, VIP, insulin, and oxytocin during the menstrual cycle in women (with and without oral contraceptives). *Acta Obstet Gynecol Scand.* 1989;68:165–169.

61. Frick G, Bremrne K, Sjogren C, et al. Plasma levels of cholecystokinin and gastrin during the menstrual cycle and pregnancy. *Acta Obstet Gynecol Scand.* 1990;69:317–320.

62. Ronkainen H, Pakarinen A, Kirkinen P, et al. Physical exercise-induced changes and season-associated differences in the pituitary-ovarian function of runners and joggers. *J Clin Endocrinol Metab.* 1985;60:416.

63. Pirke KM, Schweiger U, Laessle R, et al. Dieting influences the menstrual cycle: vegetarian versus nonvegetarian diet. *Fertil Steril.* 1986;46:1083.

64. Cassidy A, Bingham S, Setchell KDR. Biological effects of a diet of soy protein rich in isoflavones on the menstrual cycle of premenopausal women. *Am J Clin Nutr.* 1994;60:333–40.

65. Reed RG, Kris-Etherton PM, Stewart P, Pearson TA. Cyclic variability of plasma lipids, lipoproteins, and thrombotic factors in premenopausal women. FASEB Journal. 1996;10(3):A507.

66. Mustad V, Derr J, Channa Reddy CC, Pearson TA, Kris-Etherton PM. Seasonal variation in parameters related to coronary heart disease risk in young men. *Atherosclerosis.* 1996;126:117–129.

67. McDuffie JR, Kirkley BG. Eating disorders. In: Krummel DA, Kris Etherton PM, eds. *Nutrition in Women's Health.* Gaithersburg, Md: Aspen Publishers Inc; 1996.

68. Halbreich U, Bakhai Y, Bacon KB, et al. Screening and selection process for studies of menstrually-related changes. *J Psychiatr Res.* 1989;23:65–72.

69. Food and Nutrition Board, National Research Council. *Recommended Dietary Allowances.* 10th ed. Washington, DC: National Academy Press; 1989.

70. Food and Nutrition Board, National Research Council. *Dietary Reference Intakes: Calcium, Phosphorus, Magnesium, Vitamin D, and Fluoride.* Washington, DC: National Academy Press; 1998.

71. Food and Nutrition Board, National Research Council. *Dietary Reference Intakes: Thiamin, Riboflavin, Niacin, Vitamin B6, Folate, Vitamin B12, Pantothenic Acid, Biotin, and Choline.* Washington, DC: National Academy Press; 1998.

72. *Optimal Calcium Intake.* NIH Consensus Conference Report, Vol 12, No 4, June 6–8, 1994. Office of Medical Application of Research, National Institutes of Health, Bethesda, MD 20892.

73. Dennis BH, Champagne C, Ershow A, Karmally W, Kris-Etherton PM, Phillips K, Stewart KK, Stewart PW, Van Heel N, Wang C-H, Windhauser M, Wood AF. Diet design for a multicenter controlled feeding trial: The DELTA Program. *J Am Diet Assoc.* 1998;98:766–776.

74. DELTA Investigators. *Manual of Operations for the DELTA Program (Dietary Effects on Lipoproteins and Thrombogenic Activity), Second Protocol.* 1993. (Available from Department of Biostatistics, Collaborative Studies Coordinating Center, University of North Carolina, 137 E Franklin St, Chapel Hill, NC 27514–4145.)

CHAPTER 9

CHILDREN AS PARTICIPANTS IN FEEDING STUDIES

MADELEINE SIGMAN-GRANT, PhD, RD; MARY ANN TILLEY KIDD, MS, RD; AND
ABBY G. ERSHOW, ScD, RD

THE NEED FOR STUDIES IN CHILDREN

There are many unanswered questions about the dietary needs of children, specifically regarding nutrient requirements and physiologic responses to dietary components. For example, the Dietary Reference Intakes and other dietary guidelines for children are based on extrapolations and calculations from those established for adults (1–3). Data generated by research on children would be far more suitable for answering these questions. Feeding studies that include children also can lend insight into age-related differences in response to diet; data resulting from such studies are needed to determine the appropriate age for instituting preventive dietary guidance. In addition, studies that enroll not just children but also their close relatives can be useful in clarifying genetic influences on response to diet. (See Chapter 4, "Genetic Effects in Human Dietary Studies.")

Enrollment of children in well-controlled feeding studies poses unique challenges to the investigator and to the participating families. Controlled feeding studies can be performed fairly easily during early life when the infant is solely bottle-fed (4, 5). Studies of older children's food consumption are more difficult, however, and typically have relied on one of two primary approaches: either supplying test foods on an ad libitum basis along with recording daily food intake (6–8), or collecting intake data solely through use of dietary records (9). Little has been published about the logistics of conducting feeding studies with children, but it is clear that the biological, psychological, and social factors associated with growth and development will be superimposed on the usual challenges encountered with adult subjects participating in such studies. Investigators thus must be prepared to develop innovative approaches to ensure meeting the scientific needs of the study.

A variety of research settings can be considered in planning feeding studies for children. Occasionally inpatient settings will be appropriate, necessary, and feasible; these offer the highest level of control, but this approach is expensive and not representative of the child's usual environment. Outpatient studies are the more likely option, in which children are provided with their food for consumption on-site or off-site but are otherwise free to pursue their usual schedule and activities. Such studies can also enroll other family members (parents, siblings) if doing so provides an effective means of testing the hypothesis. Residential group settings such as camps and boarding schools also can be considered if the enrollment criteria for the study are relatively broad; such settings would likely provide large numbers of children within specific age and gender groups. Special programs for children with particular health conditions (such as obesity or diabetes) might prove an effective setting for some studies.

The inclusion of children in research studies can be expected to increase in the future. This notion is grounded in a recognition that children have not benefited from many advances in medical research because they have not been included as study participants in a sufficient variety of protocols. Acknowledging this situation, the National Institutes of Health (NIH) recently initiated a new policy requiring that all of its supported research studies involving human subjects consider whether children (in this case, defined as up to 21 years old) can appropriately be enrolled as study participants (10). Although there will continue to be studies that solely enroll children, it is likely that many investigators will instead be adding children to studies originally designed for adults.

These investigators thus must expect to make child-appropriate adaptations of study designs, protocols, management techniques, and outcome measurements. Researchers also will be called on to provide expanded ethical protections; for example, the informed consent procedures used for adults are not adequate for children, who cannot reasonably be expected to have an adult understanding of the consequences of involvement in research. (More information about this evolving issue can be obtained through the NIH Web site: http:\\www.nih.gov.)

This chapter will present a brief overview of the factors that investigators should consider in designing feeding studies with children. We will draw on our own recent experience as part of the Dietary Effects on Lipoproteins and Thrombogenic Activity (DELTA) program, a multicenter controlled feeding study in adults that examined the effects of dietary fat modifications on plasma lipoproteins and thrombogenic factors. (Also see Chapter 25, "The Multicenter Approach to Human Feeding Studies.") The DELTA study diets were whole-food diets with modified total fat and fatty acid composition; the desired nutrient goals were achieved by using specially prepared fat blends and baked goods in addition to other readily available foods (11).

We wished to develop the methodology for enrolling families and their children in controlled feeding protocols at our institution, so we took advantage of the DELTA program to conduct a feasibility study, the Family Feeding Study (FFS) (12). The FFS had a two-part prefeeding phase as well as a feeding phase. The first part of the prefeeding phase of the FFS enrolled 25 children aged 6 years to 10 years, who participated in focus groups to identify food preferences. The results were used to modify the original menus fed to the adult participants in the main protocol of the DELTA study. The second part of the prefeeding phase recruited 60 children aged 6 years to 10 years to do hedonic preference testing of several menu items from the modified DELTA research diets. Finally, in the feeding phase, 6 children from 3 families participated in a controlled diet study comprising two 7-week diet periods separated by one 7-week break.

BEHAVIORAL CONSIDERATIONS

Psychosocial Development

According to models developed by Piaget and Erikson (13–15), children progress through five main phases of cognitive and psychosocial development (Table 9-1). These phases affect the act of feeding as well as food selection (16, 17). To be successful, research designs and study protocols must be matched to the children's stage of intellectual, moral, emotional, and social development while meeting nutritional needs. This concept is illustrated in Table 9-1, which shows

the linkage between various aspects of feeding studies and Piaget's and Erikson's developmental stages. The table indicates the issues an investigator must consider in designing a protocol appropriate to the age group under study; areas of potential difficulty also are highlighted. If there is flexibility in selecting the age group, investigators can choose which challenges they wish to undertake and which ones they wish to avoid.

As mentioned earlier, in the FFS we chose to work with children aged 6 to 10 years, avoiding the challenges of including preschool-age children and adolescents. However, the youngest child in our study (age 6 years) proved to be the most difficult to work with. Insight into her behavior regarding food preferences and actual food consumption was gained by considering cognitive development theories (see Table 9-1). Although she agreed to adhere to the study diet, she may not truly have understood why she was being asked to consume specific foods. Often, she returned her high-fiber cereal, resulting in a fiber intake well below study goals. A 6-year-old also is likely to separate foods into polarized classes of "like" or "dislike" and thus may be unwilling to try foods she has classified as "don't like." Once she decided she disliked a food, she was unwilling to try any modification made to that food. Her reluctance limited available study foods.

On the other hand, our 8- to 10-year-old participants were more cooperative. Children at this age begin to think logically, are industrious, and strive for feelings of accomplishment. The older children likely had a firmer understanding of the reasons for participating in the study and consequently had a greater "need" to comply.

Although adults can conceptualize beyond personal needs to see the potential good of participation in research, children are essentially egocentric. This means that most decisions about participation and cooperation are generally made through filters of "me first" until adolescence is complete (about age 20 years). Consequently, an investigator cannot guarantee consistent dietary adherence through use of verbal reasoning or rationalization. For example, children in a feeding study who do not understand the need to eat every last bit of food on their plates may resist all adult attempts to get them to eat it all. To the children, it is an issue of whether they are in control or whether an adult is telling them what to do.

School-age children, anxious to please the investigator or their parents, may not be truthful about what they did or did not eat. Investigators should recognize that this is not an issue of dishonesty and noncompliance in the adult sense; it is merely a manifestation of the child's stage of moral development. In the child's mind, it may be far better to be dishonest if one gains immediate approval rather than to be honest and receive severe reprimands. Indeed, in our study, despite an apparent strong rapport between investigator and subjects, several children would only reveal consumption of nonstudy foods when their parent was out of the room. This conflict can be disturbing to children. One child, who even-

TABLE 9-1

Developmental Characteristics of Children That Are Pertinent to Feeding Studies

Age Range[1]	Cognitive Stages (Piaget)	Psychological Stages (Erickson)	Physical Considerations
0–2 yr	*Sensorimotor period.* Learning occurs through the interaction of senses and environment, and through manipulation of objects.	*Stage I: Basic trust vs mistrust.* Development of a predominantly unconscious but reasonable trustfulness as far as others are concerned, and a simple sense of trustworthiness as far as oneself is concerned.	Limited motor skills Limited food choices (variety, texture, flavor) Easy to collect urine and feces Difficult to obtain venous blood Rapid growth
1–4 yr	*Preconceptual period.* Classification by a single feature (eg, size). No concern for contradictions. Rapid language development.	*Stage II: Autonomy vs shame and doubt.* Child becomes more dependent and independent at the same time. As the muscle system matures, child has the consequent ability and felt inability to coordinate a number of highly conflicting action patterns. Development of self-control without loss of self-esteem. Recognition of existence as a person.	Erratic appetite (varies with growth and activity) Initiates self-feeding Practices fine-motor skills Food choices limited by texture Increased exposure to potential illness (child care, preschool) Slowed growth rate
3–8 yr	*Intuitive thought period.* Intuitive reasoning based on perception rather than logical inference. Imaginative play.	*Stage III: Initiative vs guilt.* Development of conscience. Advanced language and locomotion permits expansion of imagination, which can lead to fear of what child has dreamed and thought. Child feels guilt for thoughts as well as deeds.	Appetite affected by growth, illness, activity, fatigue Begins to lose teeth Exposure to illness (child care, school)
7–12 yr[2]	*Concrete operations period.* Develops logical cause-and-effect thought. Reasoning becomes rational. Learns to organize, classify, and generalize.	*Stage IV: Mastery and industry vs inferiority.* Child wants to be constructive and wins recognition by producing things and completing work. Industry involves doing things with others. Child can develop sense of inadequacy and inferiority.	Weight gain ~7 lb/yr Prepubertal and pubertal changes begin Fat deposition begins for both boys and girls Rapid growth begins for girls and for some boys Permanent dentition completed
11–20 yr[2]	*Formal operations period.* Comprehension of abstract concepts. Formation of "ideas".	*Stage V: Ego identity vs role confusion.* Accrued confidence in one's abilities (ego). Child realizes that his or her own way of mastering experiences is a successful variant of the way others master experience (this often displaces strong previous doubt).	Pubertal changes occur Rapid growth for boys Growth rate slows for girls

[1]Source: Inhelder B, Piaget J (13); Erikson EH (14); Lucas B (15).
[1]Age ranges are approximate. Overlapping age ranges reflect differences in Piaget's and Erickson's definition of developmental stages.
[2]The biological and behavioral changes of preadolescence and adolescence do not occur at the same time, at the same rate, or in the same amount for all children. Thorough individual evaluations must be conducted to determine the developmental stage of each child.

tually terminated participation, sobbed as she revealed consumption of nonstudy candy.

Food Choices: Acceptance and Preference

Two major issues need to be considered before and during the study to ensure children will eat the required food. First, children need to demonstrate acceptance of the foods. Then, investigators must make arrangements so that the child can consume the foods as needed in school and at after-school activities. Investigators usually can adjust the study food to make it more acceptable while still maintaining the required dietary composition. Accommodating environmental and social needs, however, usually leads to the research team having less direct supervision of the participants and less control over the study diet.

Acceptance, which is the degree to which a child likes a particular food (18), differs from *preference,* which is the liking of one food relative to another (19). Children's food choices can be influenced by simply being given the food ("mere exposure"), by the number of times they are served the food (frequency of exposure), by the manner (context) in which food is presented, by the behaviors of family and nonfamily members, and by the environment in which the food is eaten (20–24). Although the taste and texture of many foods are acceptable to children, some foods are preferred to a higher degree than others (Table 9-2). Alternatively, when asked to choose (in a preference test), children may select one food over another while not liking (accepting) either food.

For the most part, each child must be evaluated for his or her own preferences. Parents should not be asked to evaluate the food preferences of their children (25, 26). Even when staff are talking with an individual child, they must take care to distinguish between preference and acceptance. For example, the child may state a preference for pears over peaches but may only accept pears canned in heavy syrup.

Before the study begins, it is important to arrange for each child to taste each of the menu items at least once and preferably several times. This process should include any specialty items produced by the research kitchen (9, 12, 27). Such a step is helpful for several reasons. First, as mentioned earlier, food preferences are specific to the individual and not always predictable. In addition, it may be difficult to describe the items so that children fully understand what each food is and can state whether they will consume the food. Even if every measure is taken to ensure acceptance of study foods, the children's preferences might change as the study progresses. For example, a turkey casserole that was highly acceptable at the start of our study was not accepted at all by the end of the study. Adults are capable of taking a relatively stoic attitude (they "grin and bear it"); children will eat less of the food or refuse it altogether.

Finally, children are influenced, both positively and negatively, by the likes and dislikes of their peers. This can work to the advantage of the research team, or it can have devastating consequences on their ability to offer variety in the study menu.

It may be unrealistic to expect to develop a lengthy study diet for children in which each participant accepts all foods in prescribed amounts, so that the continual adjustment of foods can be avoided. Therefore, when working with children, researchers should be prepared to adapt menus and recipes on an individual basis. To accomplish this, investigators

TABLE 9-2

Overall Favorite Foods and Favorite Snack Foods of 25 Focus Group Participants 7 Years to 11 Years Old[1]

Favorite Foods	Percentage of Responses
Overall Foods (20 Responses)	
Pizza	40
Spaghetti	10
Macaroni and cheese	10
Mashed potatoes	10
Oodles of Noodles® soup	5
Grilled cheese sandwich	5
Shrimp and rice	5
Baked chicken	5
Tacos	5
Chocolate bars	5
Snack Foods (73 Responses)	
Pizza, all types	26
Granola	16
Fruit	11
Candy	9
Popcorn	8
Potato chips	7
Ice cream	7
Soft pretzels	4
French fries	3
Low-fat granola bars	3
Peanuts	1
Jello®	1
Dry cereal	1

[1]Data from Tilley MA (12).

TABLE 9-3

Adaptation of Adult Menus for Use with Children[1,2,3,4]

Meal	Day 1 Adult	Day 1 Child	Day 2 Adult	Day 2 Child	Day 3 Adult	Day 3 Child
Breakfast	Orange juice Three-grain cereal White bread Margarine Jelly Whole milk	Same	Tangerines Raisin Bran® White bread Margarine Skim milk	Same	Orange juice Cheerios® English muffin Margarine Jelly 2% milk	Same
Lunch	Turkey on white bread Mayonnaise Lettuce salad Olive oil Peaches Ginger cookie	Chicken breast on hoagie roll Miracle Whip® Dinner roll Jelly Pineapple Pretzels	Shrimp pasta salad French roll Oatmeal cookie[4]	Turkey on white bread Miracle Whip® Peaches Ginger cookie	Chicken salad White bread Lettuce Tomato Pineapple[4]	Turkey breast on hoagie roll Miracle Whip® Pears Oatmeal cookie
Dinner	Sirloin tips with gravy Corn kernels Lettuce salad with tomato and carrots Dinner roll Butter Applesauce	Same except: No tomato in salad	Chicken jambalaya Spinach salad with green onion French roll Fruit cocktail	Broiled chicken Green beans Lettuce salad (no green onion in salad) French roll Fruit cocktail	Pork chops Spaghetti Green peas Lettuce salad with green pepper and tomato Dinner roll Rolled oat macaroon	Same, except: No tomato in salad[4]
Snack	Snack mix: peanuts, raisins, and pretzels	Same	Pudding Vanilla wafers	Same	Low-fat yogurt	Same

should plan to have at least one researcher and one cook devoted solely to working with the children on a daily basis. In addition, all cooks and kitchen staff must be flexible and the nutrient database must be extremely accurate. Investigators must carefully weigh the advantages of group needs vs individual requests. If allowable, flexibility for some foods should be considered (eg, a peach for a pear) or peanut butter for peanuts. However, if the study requires all children to eat exactly the same foods, once a food is eliminated for one child, it has to be eliminated for all children. This may create tension between individual children and between families while seriously reducing the variety of study foods.

PLANNING RESEARCH DIET PROTOCOLS FOR CHILDREN

Beyond the specific research hypothesis, investigators must consider each of the following factors in designing a feeding study protocol for children:

- Safety and ethical considerations
- Nutrient requirements and dietary adequacy
- Physical growth
- Recruitment
- Exclusion criteria
- Screening
- Length of study periods
- Menu and recipe development
- Amounts of food
- Method of monitoring food intake
- Production considerations
- Dining environment
- Incentives and rewards
- Study outcomes, sometimes referred to as endpoint measurements (9, 12, 27)

If the study also includes adults, the menus and recipes may require modification to meet the needs of children (see Table 9-3).

Safety and Ethical Considerations

Investigators must carefully justify any feeding study with children. Research organizations have internal committees, usually termed institutional review boards (IRBs), which are

TABLE 9-3

Continued

Meal	Day 4		Day 5		Day 6	
	Adult	Child	Adult	Child	Adult	Child
Breakfast	Orange juice Bran flakes White bread Margarine Jelly Skim milk	Same	Apple juice Cheerios® English muffin Margarine Jelly 2% milk	Same	Orange juice Corn Flakes® Blueberry muffin Margarine Skim milk	Same except: Blueberry muffin replaced by Applesauce muffin
Lunch	Sliced beef round on onion bun Macaroni salad Peaches[4]	Chicken breast on white bread Lettuce Miracle Whip® Pineapple	Pork stir-fry White rice Rolled oat macaroon	Sliced beef round on onion bun Pretzels Roll Jelly Peaches	Chili Raw carrots Corn chips Dinner roll Jello	Chicken breast on hoagie roll Rolled oat macaroon Carrot sticks Tangerines
Dinner	Turkey almond casserole Green beans Lettuce and tomato salad Dinner roll Ginger cookie	Same except: No tomato in salad[4]	Breaded chicken Pasta with tomato sauce Lettuce and tomato salad Dinner roll Margarine Pears	Same except: Chicken replaced with pork No tomato in salad[4]	Lemon sage chicken Broccoli Dinner roll Margarine Rice pilaf Pineapple	Chili Raw Carrots Broccoli Dinner roll Margarine Rice pilaf Corn chips[4]
Snack	Snack mix: peanuts, raisins, and pretzels	Same	Low-fat yogurt	Same	Brownie	Same

[1] Based on studies with 6-year-old to 10-year-old children as described in Tilley MA (12) and Tilley MA, et al. (27).

[2] The Child Lunch reflects the Adult Lunch from previous day (when foods were made and distributed).

[3] Children were allowed additional snacks by either saving parts of lunch or dinner for later consumption or by eating foods from a preapproved list.

[4] The children disliked eating the composed salads (macaroni salad, shrimp pasta salad, and chicken salad) that were used as vehicles for oils and egg yolk powder in the Adult Lunch menus. Instead the oils and egg yolk from these recipes were added to the Child Dinner menus on the same or following day.

legally mandated to review all research protocols that will enroll human subjects; the research cannot proceed without approval from the IRB. (Also see Chapter 5, "Ethical Considerations in Dietary Studies.") Primary concerns are safety and prevention of needless pain and suffering. Investigators must be able to present a thoughtful summary of why the research is necessary, whether the same information could be obtained without inclusion of children, and why inclusion of children is appropriate given the goals of the study.

Parents or legal guardians have the formal responsibility for signing the informed consent documents on behalf of legal minors. These documents should be prepared with the intention of providing the clearest possible explanation of the protocol, its associated risks for the children, and the responsibilities of those who decide to participate. Investigators should also plan to develop informational materials for the children. As mentioned earlier, the younger the children are, the less can they appreciate the consequences of involvement in research. Nevertheless, children who are potential participants deserve to receive an age-appropriate description of the study.

To minimize the likelihood of problems and reassure the IRB, investigators should prepare a written protocol for monitoring safety. This protocol should include procedures for documentation of baseline (prestudy) and during-study data, and also should include "trigger" points indicating when it may be appropriate to refer the child to a pediatrician. (It would be prudent to engage the expert advice of a pediatrician during the development of this protocol; a consulting pediatrician experienced in biomedical research might be an appropriate choice as the project medical officer.)

Prominent concerns for children enrolled in research protocols include protection from undue physical or psychological discomfort. In the context of a feeding study, it is relatively easy to imagine the possibility of physical discomfort stemming from hunger (eg, due to delayed mealtimes or a diet with insufficient calories), or from biological sample collection (eg, due to phlebotomy). Many of the potential physical hazards or health risks for children engaged in feeding studies also are predictable and are similar to those faced by adults who participate in such research. Such risks include those associated with invasive sampling or measuring procedures and allergic reactions to study food (described later).

The possibility of nutritional inadequacy is higher with children because of their higher nutrient density needs. The inadequacy can manifest itself through effects on physical growth and maturation. A thorough description of plans for preventing potential growth problems will help address concerns. For example, to accommodate the expected rate of linear growth during the time frame of the study, investigators must describe their plans for ensuring that the children's needs for energy (and other nutrients) are met, and for evaluating whether the protocol has had any negative impact on growth.

Food allergies and intolerances are common problems with unique implications for feeding studies. Allergies are mediated through the immunologic system; nonallergic intolerances are caused by pharmacologic effects (such as foods with high histamine content) or metabolic factors (such as lactase deficiency) (28). Because both allergy and intolerance can evoke unpleasant or even dangerous symptoms, it is imperative that the screening phase of a feeding study eliminate any person who is likely to react adversely to study foods. The foods most often causing serious allergic reactions are milk, eggs, fish, shellfish, peanuts, tree nuts, soybeans, and wheat, but unexpected cross-reactions with other foods also can occur in susceptible individuals (28). For studies with children, investigators must plan to interview the parent or guardian in detail about any past or current allergies and intolerances; some do not persist as the child matures, but it is advisable to err on the side of caution if there is uncertainty about whether a food sensitivity has resolved. Once the initial screening is over, the parents or guardians of eligible participants should make a final check of all menus for potential high-risk foods.

Psychological constraints imposed by research protocols are less obvious but nevertheless could have undesirable effects on behavior or self-image. Researchers must be thoughtful in anticipating such constraints because they are not well-characterized and will vary among children as well as among studies. Difficulties could arise from protocol features such as strict timing of meals, coercion from adults (parents or research team members) to adhere to the protocol, and social isolation or feelings of being "different" from other children (for example, not being able to eat certain foods in settings outside the study). Some children might misconstrue the reason for their enrollment in the study, thinking it is because something is "wrong" with them. The possibility of time lost from school, and the consequences of such lost time, should also be considered. Certain behavioral traits, such as extreme shyness or a very slow rate of eating, may make it inappropriate to enroll particular children in a protocol. Researchers should discuss the child's potential behavioral reactions to the protocol with the parents during the recruitment phase.

Nutrient Requirements and Dietary Adequacy

Nutrient requirements for children must be met as carefully as possible throughout the study. There are several sets of guidelines available to assist in planning menus and checking the calculated diets for adequacy of nutrient content. The Dietary Guidelines for Americans (3) suggests the number of daily servings of various food groups that can be expected to provide an adequate intake of most nutrients. The content of specific nutrients, however, should be evaluated by comparison with either the recently published Dietary Reference Intakes (DRI) (1, 29, 30) or the Recommended Dietary Allowances (RDA) (2). The DRI provide recommendations for intake of calcium, phosphorus, magnesium, vitamin D, fluoride, B vitamins, and choline. The RDA provide recommendations for other nutrients, notably energy, protein, and certain minerals (iron, zinc, iodine, and selenium) and vitamins (A, C, E, and K).

Researchers planning diets for individual study participants should note that the DRI and RDA use different age groupings for recommended levels of intake (DRI:

- DRI groups males (M) and females (F) jointly for ages 0 year to 0.5 year, 0.5 year to 1 year, 1 year to 3 years, and 4 years to 8 years.
- DRI groups M and F separately for ages 9 years to 13 years and 14 years to 18 years.
- RDA groups M and F jointly for ages 0 year to 0.5 year, 0.5 year to 1 year, 1 year to 3 years, 4 years to 6 years, and 7 years to 10 years.
- RDA groups M and F separately for ages 11 years to 14 years and 15 years to 18 years.

Energy

Caloric adequacy is the planner's first consideration in designing menus for a feeding study. Basic estimates of energy requirements can be made according to the RDA (2). (Note: As of this time the DRI do not address energy requirements [1].) Recommended levels of energy intake for children are based on the same general algorithms as those described later in this book (see Chapter 17, "Energy Needs and Weight Maintenance in Controlled Feeding Studies"), but the levels have been adjusted to account for children's higher activity levels (typically 1.7 to 2.0 × Resting Energy Expenditure) and constantly maturing body composition (2). Expressed on a body weight basis (ie, kcal/kg), energy needs are similar in boys and girls up through age 10 years; during puberty and adolescence, girls' lower activity level and lower percentage of lean muscle mass make their energy needs approximately 10% to 15% lower than those of boys of the same age (2).

The problem of insufficient calories often is easily identified (ie, it is "self-advertising") because the child is hungry and says so. (Shy or quiet children may not articulate this need as clearly). To prevent hunger related to altered meal-times, flexibly timed snacks can be designed as part of the meal plan. Investigators can reduce the likelihood of insufficient energy intake by providing a slight overage of food through use of unit foods and snacks and allow the child to eat to repletion. Intake is then estimated by measuring the difference between provided food and consumed food. Caloric excess also usually corrects itself within a few days because the children will not eat food they do not need.

Carefully allowing access to food to meet energy needs throughout the study should prevent any negative impact on growth. This can be accomplished by using unit foods specifically designed to both supply energy and to reflect the diet composition being tested. The initial energy levels that are provided for each subject can be determined with the use of 3-day intake records prior to study initiation and validated during the run-in period. Energy levels during the study are manipulated by participants through unlimited access to acceptable unit foods and confirmed by measuring body weight on a continuing and frequent basis throughout the study.

Other Nutrients

The adequacy of protein or micronutrient intake cannot be detected through the immediate symptom of hunger. Menus should be checked for their percent of the recommended intake as either the DRI or RDA (described earlier). The purpose is to guard against deficiencies for all nutrients and to protect against excesses for a smaller number (such as fat-soluble vitamins).

A typical standard for dietary adequacy is that the diet contain 75% of the recommended intake for that nutrient (100% may not be practical or necessary for every nutrient for every day, especially for short-term studies) (31). It then is possible to calculate each child's likely range of intake and requirement of calories and nutrients; examine the resulting data on the basis of either nutrient density (units nutrient/1,000 kcal) or absolute daily intake; and then evaluate intake against the recommended level (DRI or RDA) expressed in the same units. Physical activity level should be considered in this assessment. Depending on the protocol, it also may be appropriate to monitor for adequacy of protein, vitamin, and mineral status using biochemical markers, provided the protocol permits collection of the needed biological samples.

Physical Growth and Anthropometric Data

Growth Charts

Protocols collecting anthropometric data on children, either as primary endpoints or to monitor safety, should be designed in keeping with published standards for making the measurements and evaluating the results (32). In the United States, these are provided to the public by the National Center

for Health Statistics, an agency of the US Public Health Service (Hyattsville, Md) (Web site http://www.cdc.gov/nchswww). The basic descriptive data have been available for many years in the convenient form of charts that enable measurements for height, weight, weight for height, and head circumference to be graphed against age- and gender-specific population-based percentiles (5th, 10th, 25th, 50th, 75th, 90th, and 95th) "bands" (33).

A new set of NCHS growth charts, available in early 1999, represents the first revision of these important data in over 20 years (34, 35). These charts are based on data pooled from five national surveys conducted between 1963 and 1994 (the first, second, and third National Health and Nutrition Examination Surveys and the second and third National Health Examination Surveys). Two sets of charts provide gender- and age-specific percentile distributions for infants (0 months to 35 months, inclusive) and children (2 years to 19 years, inclusive) for weight, stature, and body mass index (replacing the older weight-for-height measurement); the infant charts also provide head circumference percentiles. The charts represent population-based values for the entire US population, with all ethnic/race groups combined, and will have an expanded set of percentile bands: 3, 5, 10, 25, 50, 75, 90, 95, and 97. (The new growth charts, and information about their use, will be made available at the NCHS Web site: http://www.cdc.gov/nchswww.)

Alternatives to the NCHS growth charts occasionally are needed for some protocols. Some investigators may wish to use race-specific standards (36, 37), although the need for this is a matter of debate. Descriptive data are also available for other measurements, such as skinfold thickness, waist-neck length, and limb circumference (37–41).

Collecting and Evaluating Growth Data during Feeding Protocols

As for any other study measurements, the principles of valid research technique apply to anthropometric data and other means of assessing growth and development. The investigator's ability to detect problems with growth thus requires that sources of variability in these measurements be controlled as much as possible. It is critical that the procotol include procedures for standardizing aspects of data collection such as the measuring devices, participant management procedures (eg, type of clothing worn or time of day measurement is made), and techniques for recording data.

Healthy children gain weight and height over time until they reach full adult size. They may go through periods of stable height and weight, then grow quickly in a "spurt." Weight also fluctuates because of erratic physical activity levels. Some of these fluctuations also reflect measurement errors (on the part of the person making the measurement or in the measuring device) and other inconsistencies (such as differences in shoes or clothing, or whether a meal was recently eaten).

In particular, studies assessing height as an endpoint or as a safety marker must consider that height measurements are sensitive to error because of the effect of small changes in child's stance and posture (or body position for prone measurements of infants).

In the context of feeding studies, growth usually is assessed by measuring height and weight. Head circumference also is typically measured in infants (< 3 years). Occasionally skinfold thickness measurements are needed to evaluate changes in adipose tissue content. Studies involving infants may wish to consider assessing developmental stage according to a standard scale such as the Denver Developmental Screening Test (42). Some long-term studies of adolescents may find it pertinent to assess Tanner stages of sexual maturation (although this scale requires a physical examination and highly personal questions that may be considered intrusive) (43).

Concerns about growth focus on three main areas: the possibility of delayed or reduced growth in height and/or weight; the potential for induction of overweight or obesity; and the chance of delayed or accelerated maturation. Some studies might find it necessary to assess body composition in order to evaluate the nature of observed weight gain or weight loss; that is, they might identify which body compartment is gaining or losing such components as water (ie, there is a possibility of dehydration), muscle, or adipose tissue.

The potential for growth problems is greater for certain study designs. Diets that are high in bulk, have very high or low caloric density, or require unpalatable foods can distort the normal regulation of energy intake. Long-term studies (of several months or longer) must institute more stringent monitoring procedures. Finally, studies enrolling children during rapid growth phases (infants or adolescents) must be alert to potential effects on growth velocity. Written protocols for feeding studies with children should include reference values and cutoff points above or below which further evaluation will occur.

There are no hard-and-fast rules for the frequency of making anthropometric measurements during a growth study with children. The frequency of measurements should be based on the data needs of the protocol, the practicalities of coordinating data collection with other study activities, and the expected rate of growth during the time frame of the study. However, frequent measurements can help establish a predictable routine, which can in turn foster adherence to the protocol. Frequent measurements also provide a means of reassuring the parent or guardian that the child's well-being is safeguarded.

Measurements are made at baseline (before the study begins), periodically throughout the study, and then at the end of the data collection period. Again, it is important to ensure that uniform methodology is used at each time point. Baseline data preferably include several repeated measurements, made approximately 1 week apart. This provides information on within-child variance. Historical data from family or pediatrician's records can also be helpful in characterizing long-term growth patterns that are typical for an individual child.

During the course of the study, unless the protocol requires growth data as endpoints, suggested approximate time frames for monitoring and adherence are: weight 1 or more times each week; height 1 or more times each month. The advice of a statistician should be sought in determining the optimal schedule for anthropometric measurements. For example, an 8- to 9-year-old child gains about 8 lb a year. In a 3-month feeding study, weight should be measured often enough to reliably detect a 2-lb gain (approximately once or twice a month), but investigators might establish a routine for adherence and measurement weight 1 to 3 times a week.

After the data are collected, appropriate descriptive statistics should be generated. The age- and sex-specific percentile value should be determined for each child. In addition, the mean, median, range, and so on of age- and sex-specific percentiles should be calculated for the entire study cohort and for the children assigned to each treatment group.

Growth data also must be analyzed with appropriate statistical techniques. In general, data for the treatment group are analyzed for evaluating study outcomes, and data for the individual are analyzed for monitoring safety. Data can be analyzed as continuous variables (actual measurement results) or as categorical variables (specific percentiles or percentile bands). Data analyses for small studies (n < 20) probably will need to use nonparametric statistical methods. Evaluation of data collected at different time points requires appropriate paired or other repeated measures techniques.

Software packages for graphing data on standard charts provide a convenient means of tracking the growth of individual children and of treatment groups overall (44); also consult the NCHS Web site (http://www.cdc.gov/nchswww). For individual children, it is unlikely that changes will be observed in percentile rankings between successive measurements; short-term alterations of less than 10% to 25% in percentile rank may not be meaningful unless accompanied by other problems. For groups of children, the average percentiles likely will be consistent if all is well.

For some data analyses, it may be necessary to statistically adjust for the height (or weight, or other anthropometric measurements) of the child's biological parents. The adjustment would be made by using the parents' data as a covariate in multiple regression or other analytical procedures. The measurements (which are preferably made directly by the investigators rather than by self-report) can either be used as continuous variables (such as height in inches or centimeters), or they can be collapsed into categorical variables based on population percentiles (such as 25th percentile for height for adults).

Food Intake and Appetite

A critical decision concerns the amount of food served to each child. Controlled feeding studies, by definition, require the ingestion of all study foods presented, with flexibility in adding unit foods to accommodate energy needs. Investigators have two primary ways for defining the amount of food that the subjects eat. The first approach is to insist that the entire amount of premeasured food is eaten daily with adjustments made to maintain a stable weight. This technique can be used with young infants or adults, but in our opinion it is not suitable for children. For children of most ages, the most realistic approach (albeit less accurate) is to serve an excess amount of all foods, allow ad lib eating, and calculate portions eaten by difference. It accommodates growth spurts and illnesses that can undermine carefully calculated energy determinations and eliminates potential conflicts.

Whereas a primary issue with physical development is erratic appetites resulting from fluctuating energy needs, a primary issue in the child's psychosocial development is control. As stated previously, during certain stages of development, children have a strong need to exert control over their environment. Refusal to eat some or all of a particular food may be an expression of that need. Investigators must balance these equally important and often divergent concerns prior to determining how much food should be offered.

In addition, investigators must be flexible in adjusting energy needs. On any given day, the child may not want all the food provided or conversely may want more. Use of free-choice foods, such as diet carbonated beverages or fat-free/sugar-free gelatin desserts, should be considered along with provision of unit foods. If free foods are acceptable, investigators should design the study to allow a range of nutrient intakes, rather than a single target figure. In reality, this may be the only practical study design. Another possibility is to work with a mean weekly goal rather than a daily, or even meal-by-meal, target. This built-in flexibility may serve to diminish the anxieties of both investigators and families as well as to facilitate compliance.

Investigators must be pragmatic about the degree to which they can influence children's appetites. The tools available for addressing this issue are well known to experienced parents: encourage physical activity as appropriate and space the snacks and meals at sufficient intervals to allow hunger to develop. These techniques must of course be applied with discretion and without unduly coercing the child.

Rate of growth, physical activity, amount of sleep, stress, and illness all significantly affect a child's appetite (17). Even the loss of a tooth during the study influences subsequent intake. However, investigators should recognize that for any one child, although energy intakes for each meal can vary greatly from day to day, over a week's time energy intake remains fairly constant (6, 9). In addition, there may be tremendous differences in energy intakes between study subjects of the same age (6). It is imperative for the investigator to maintain close daily contact with each child and not rely solely on anthropometric and dietary intake measurements to monitor physical status.

Time Factors

Studies with children likely will require a longer run-in period than studies involving adults. A longer acclimation period allows researchers to carefully scrutinize subjects and their families to determine their compliance and provides sufficient time for menu and recipe adjustments. The actual experimental feeding periods can proceed for the normal length of time. However, if the experimental period is too short, adequate adjustments and a stabilized regime will not have been established. If the study continues for too long a period, boredom, sudden growth spurts, and noncompliance issues may occur.

Another consideration is to determine how many different diets are actually necessary for the study. Children are more comfortable in a routine. Thus, the fewer dietary changes, the more likely the children will cooperate.

Arrangements for birthdays, holidays, and special events should be planned prior to the study. For example, if Halloween occurs during one of the feeding cycles, it is close to impossible for the children not to eat any candy. Therefore, investigators must work with the families to incorporate a favorite candy into the study menus.

Researchers working with school-age children also must accommodate school and after-school needs. To avoid interfering with these activities, studies can be undertaken in the summer. However, many families are unavailable for long-term studies during this period. We found the children enjoyed carrying study foods to school in customized lunch boxes. During the school year, special arrangements must be made for birthday parties, sports events, and holiday celebrations to ensure the study children will not feel different from their peers. Some teachers willingly accommodate study protocols, whereas others believe it is not their role.

If possible, the study diet should include a variety of free-choice foods, in addition to unit foods, that study children can enjoy within the context of the feeding protocol. If children do ingest foods outside the scope of the study, it is extremely important for investigators to be able to account for these selections and to adjust the experimental diet accordingly so that nutrient goals are met.

Collecting Biological Samples

The endpoint measurements needed to test the research question may influence which age group is selected for study. Ultimately, investigators must ask which measures would be preferable to have and which are absolutely critical. Young children may be terrified of venous blood draws but may accept the more familiar finger prick. Conversely, school age children may have the reverse reaction. Venous blood draws may be acceptable on a monthly basis but not on a weekly basis. The volume of blood collected at any one time, and throughout the study, is contingent on the child's weight and body size. Thus, the younger the child, the less frequent the blood draws and the smaller the collected volume. Acclimating children to the collection procedure and using friendly adults dressed in conventional clothing (ie, no laboratory coats or surgical scrub clothes) may facilitate acceptance of blood draws.

Although they may tolerate an initial blood draw, children may change their minds and not cooperate in subsequent collections. As stated, we experienced this situation with a 6-year-old who had to be dropped from the study after participating for 7 weeks. Therefore, our experience suggests that investigators should anticipate a higher termination rate with children than with adult subjects.

Urine collection protocols also must be appropriate to the age of the participants. Spot urine collections might be more feasible for children who attend school. A 24-hour collection might be better suited for weekends and for preschool-age children who have been toilet trained. Collection of feces and urine is easier with older adolescents.

Some biological samples can be collected with minimal physical burden, pain, or risk. These include hair and nails (for trace element studies) and buccal swabs (for genetic analyses). Even so, some children object strenuously to having their nails or hair trimmed, some parents may be concerned about cosmetic aspects of sample collection, and some infants may not have long enough hair or nails to yield an adequate specimen.

STUDY MANAGEMENT
Recruitment and Screening

Establishing early contacts with recruitment sources is essential. Well before the study begins, investigators should develop relationships with local pediatricians and family practice physicians. This can facilitate securing participating families as well as obtaining informed consent through the IRB because many physicians sit on these boards. For example, we contacted our area's primary pediatric practice 12 months prior to initiation of our projects. The pediatric staff distributed a questionnaire to patients' families. From these questionnaires we were able to gather information on: the level of interest in participation (both in taste tests and in the actual studies); existence of food allergies and intolerances that would preclude inclusion of specific families; the ages of children likely to receive parental permission to participate in a feeding study; the types of foods routinely served to children in our area; and issues of outcome measurements (particularly blood draws). This preliminary information proved invaluable as we established study protocol and design.

Recruiters should include an interview with the child and each family member privately, along with a family group interview. Family dynamics should be carefully observed. An ideal way to incorporate this idea into the study protocol is to gather food intake information using individual and group interviews of the study child(ren) and the parent(s). Following the interviews, evaluation of responses regarding acceptance and preference of critical food items can be made. In addition, information regarding the feeding environment (eg, how families handle mealtime behavior or the offering of desserts) can be obtained. If the recruiter senses any problem at this stage of the study, careful consideration should be given to excluding the family. It is far less expensive and detrimental to the study to exclude the family at this point than to have them terminate participation later.

Intensive screening is required, especially if the study will include all other family members. In our experience, to ensure continual participation by the study children, parents and other siblings should be included in all activities of the feeding study even if these family members do not meet study criteria. The increased costs are offset by savings generated in maintaining subjects in the study. Careful consideration should be given if recruiters sense any ambivalence on the part of either the children or the adults about issues such as food likes and dislikes and endpoint measurements (particularly blood draws). Children older than age 8 should be provided with the same detailed description of the study as the adults, should be given an opportunity to ask questions, and should sign the informed consent form along with the parents. In the case of children who live with a guardian or a single head of household, attempts also should be made to obtain the approval of the nonresidential parent (when feasible and appropriate).

Potential subjects should not be included in the study if they seem to change their minds about accepting crucial food items, if there is resistance to working within the group decision-making process, or if parents keep requesting changes on behalf of their children. A key reason for exclusion is the suspected or proven existence of food allergies or sensitivities that might limit consumption of specific foods or entire food groups. Allergies are commonly found to dairy products, wheat, nuts, peanuts, fish, shellfish, and corn; lactose intolerance is prevalent among many ethnic groups. A note signed by the child's doctor should clarify the presence or absence of food reactions.

Children and their families should be offered incentives to participate. Although monetary incentives are generally given to feeding study participants, parents may not agree to such incentives being given directly to their child. In this case, the parent may receive the monetary compensation or a savings bond may be purchased in the child's name. Whether or not money is given directly to the children, additional incentives are required to maintain interest. Facilitated group discussions should be used to tailor incentives to families. For example, although young children might like some identification with the "special" study, school-aged children might not want that recognition. Suggestions for study incentives include gift certificates to book or toy stores; passes to movie, bowling, or miniature golf establishments; "field trips" to an arcade; and trinkets served with meals (such as rubber spiders for Halloween).

A note of caution: Some parents may use incentives (especially monetary ones) as a threat over their child to control compliance. If the investigator becomes aware of this behavior, the issue should be addressed immediately. Indeed, one child was dropped from our study because she was terrified of the blood draws. She did have the first draws done;

however, on one occasion, the investigator overheard the mother coercing the child to cooperate. The mother had promised the child a new color television if she participated and threatened to withhold this reward if the girl did not permit blood collection. We compensated the family for the child's participation but excluded her from continuing with the study.

Mealtimes in the Research Setting

The dining environment should be designed to appeal to children and foster their involvement with the study. In our dining room, tables were arranged to encourage family interaction. We found, however, that the families came in for dinner at different times because of personal schedules, which limited the between-family interaction we had anticipated. We used coloring books, jigsaw puzzles, games, and selected videotapes to entertain the children prior to and after meals and clinical procedures.

All in all, most of the young subjects got along well enough for the entire dining environment to be congenial, even for those adults participating in a concurrent study. This is an important observation when meals are being provided for spouses and children of participants in an adult feeding study. Nevertheless, not all children developed close friendships during these times. In fact, to our dismay, we found the words "I hate (*name of person*)" written in a coloring book. We believe it was written by a subject who complained that another child was ruining the books by drawing a mark on each page without coloring.

The physical arrangements of the research kitchen and the dining room also may require adaptations. Such remodeling includes appropriate furniture (high chairs, booster seats), feeding utensils (sipper cups, small plates, and implements) and play space with toys; child care supervision; and safety precautions (eg, blocked access to kitchen, rounded table edges, covered electrical outlets, placement of hot food and equipment out of harm's way). In addition, sufficient storage and refrigeration space must be available in order for the study to accommodate individual food requests. If food intake is to be assessed by weighing, leftovers may need to be stored for weighing at more convenient times, requiring additional refrigerator and/or freezer space.

The mealtime behavior of families and children can be complicated. Once study subjects have been selected, the staff and parents must develop discipline techniques acceptable to each family. Although we did not encounter any problems, there may be occasions when staff feel it necessary to convey to the child that a particular behavior is disruptive. Some families will be comfortable with the use of relatively stern tones of voice; others may consider this too severe. If parents feel their child is being treated harshly or unfairly, or think the child is being criticized, they may withdraw from the study.

Besides discipline techniques, feeding strategies should be established. In our study, one parent preferred milk to be served to her daughter following, not during, the meal; this was easily accommodated. Toward the end of the study, a 10-year-old boy began to return his leftover food from lunch squashed. The investigator, rather than confronting him about his obvious displeasure, decided to spend more time with him. He revealed his perception that the investigator was ignoring his needs. The child returned to his normal, cooperative demeanor once the investigator acknowledged him in this way.

Enhancing Compliance

Ensuring intake of the study food requires constant adaptation, and table manners may suffer as a result. In our study, we needed to find ways to incorporate specific oils into daily intake. The menus originally designed for adult participants delivered important dietary fats (oils and egg yolk powder) in the form of baked goods, casseroles, salad dressings, and composed pasta and meat or fish salads. Occasionally a layer of oil would rise to the surface of the food or would settle on the bottom of the serving dish. The adults were willing to drink the extra oil directly from the dish, but we could not depend on the children to do this. Initially, we tried using oils as salad dressings but we quickly found out the children would not always eat salad. We resorted to having the children "mop" up most of the oil with their rolls, although some had been taught not to do this at home.

Many decisions concerning variety and plate presentation are dependent on the kitchen staff. Some staff members enjoy accommodating children's needs and will work with the families. They are willing, for example, to use divided plates to make sure the meat does not touch the potatoes, if that is what the child wishes. Other staff complain about these requests and may not be well suited to work on these projects.

Monitoring food intake is a major issue when food is eaten off-site. It is always difficult for subjects to maintain a balance between encouragement to eat only study foods and honesty in reporting consumption of nonstudy foods. This problem is only enhanced when children are involved. Because detailed records are critical during the data analysis phase, daily recording of food intake should be encouraged. However, daily record keeping by children may be impossible, or at best, inaccurate. Children may not read or write well enough to complete even the simplest form and their oral recall may be unreliable, especially if describing food consumption when a parent is present. Parental recall is not recommended, especially if the parent is not present at every eating occasion. We suggest that children should be interviewed, away from their parent, to increase positive interaction between the investigator and the child and to enhance accuracy. Logs or checklists also can facilitate recalls. Accurately monitoring food intake may be more difficult, however, especially for infants who are breast-fed, have begun to explore their environment with their mouth, or have started self-feeding.

It is also imperative for investigators to be aware of any medications the child is taking on a continuous or sporadic basis both before and during the study. Medications can affect many factors relevant to feeding study protocols, including the biological response to the dietary intervention and the taste of the study food. In addition, medications may represent an uncontrolled source of nutrient intake for target nutrients; children's preparations often are compounded in sweet sugar- and alcohol-containing syrups that can contribute calories to the diet (45). The possible contribution of medications to nutrient intake should be evaluated carefully for protocols requiring stringent dietary control.

An alternative way to improve intake accuracy (albeit tedious, labor-intensive, time-consuming, and expensive) is to weigh foods prior to and after eating. However, children often mix foods together on the plate, making it almost impossible to accurately weigh individual food items (especially oils and table spreads).

Throughout the study, investigators must plan to assess behavior that might be linked to problems with dietary protocol. These can be related to a range of issues, such as hunger from insufficient caloric intake, frustration with unsatisfactory timing of meals, and loss of control over food choice. Behavioral problems impinging on the study can range from lack of energy or interest, sleepiness, tantrums, crankiness, somatic complaints such as stomachache or headache, oppositional behavior, and general malaise.

It is valuable to consider in advance what information would be useful and to devise a plan for collecting it in a systematic fashion. Quantitative information is preferable (how many times last week did child do X, or how often did Y happen?), because it lends itself to comparisons of baseline and during-study results, and the chance of evaluation bias is lower (although seldom eliminated). It might be necessary to refer the family for counseling or to drop the child from the study. However, given the high investment of personnel and resources that each participant represents, it is far better for investigators to develop options that would support retention in the project.

Although it may be impossible to eliminate all problems, we found daily contact between a single researcher and all family members was essential in dealing with these feeding issues. This investigator must be diligent in note taking so that, over the course of the study, a written record is carefully maintained. Building close rapport and trust is essential in working with children. Compliance may be compromised when protocols allow consumption of study foods to occur outside the research environment, but a close rapport can facilitate honest and open disclosures by children of ingestion of nonstudy foods and even of accurate dietary recalls of study foods.

CONCLUSION: ADAPTING RESEARCH DIET PROTOCOLS FOR CHILDREN

Investigators must be cognizant of the wide range of physical and psychosocial behaviors inherent to a feeding study involving children. Compromises are necessary to accommodate inclusion of children. Studies enrolling children as well as adults must expect to adapt the diets to fit the needs of both groups. Children in late adolescence often are willing to eat "adult food," but enrolling preadolescent and younger children likely will require many modifications to the original menu plans. Newly instituted requirements for children's inclusion in federally supported biomedical research will make this exercise a common experience for investigators.

Excessive adjustments to protocol may cause final nutrient intake to differ greatly from study goals, but inflexibility in adapting the protocol may led to increased noncompliance and attrition. For this reason, we strongly suggest investigators use a range of acceptable nutrient values (eg, 28% to 32% energy from fat rather than an exact 30%) or determine an acceptable difference between diet treatments (eg, 5 g difference in fiber intake). Rather than expecting a child to comply with a specific level of intake on a daily basis, it is more realistic to expect and accept a defined level of flexibility in nutrient intake over time. Another approach would be to plan a more extensive set of menus, using food substitution lists and even parallel meals and menus, so that the study goals can be met by offering the child a wider choice of foods having equivalent nutrient content.

REFERENCES

1. Yates AA, Schlicker SA, Suitor CW. Dietary Reference Intakes: the new basis for recommendations for calcium and related nutrients, B vitamins, and choline. *J Am Diet Assoc.* 1998;98:699–706.

2. Food and Nutrition Board. *Recommended Dietary Allowances.* 10th ed. Washington, DC: National Academy of Sciences; 1989.

3. US Department of Agriculture and US Department of Health and Human Services. *Nutrition and Your Health; Dietary Guidelines for Americans.* 3rd ed. Home and Garden Bulletin No 232. Washington, DC: US Department of Agriculture; 1990.

4. Fomon SJ. *Nutrition of Normal Infants.* St Louis, Mo: Mosby-Year Book, Inc; 1993.

5. Butte NF, Smith E O'B, Garza C. Energy utilization of breast-fed and formula-fed infants. *Am J Clin Nutr.* 1990;51:350–358.

6. Birch LL, Johnson SL, Andresen G, Peters JC, Schulte MC. The variability of young children's energy intake. *N Engl J Med.* 1991;324:232–235.

7. Woolraich ML, Lindgren SD, Stumbo PJ, Stegink LD, Appelbaum MI, Kiritsy MC. Effects of diets high in sucrose or aspartame on the behavior and cognitive performance of children. *N Engl J Med.* 1994;330:301–307.

8. Cohn LC, Preud'homme DL, Clijsen S, Klijsen C, Mosca LJ, Deckelbaum RJ, Starc TJ. Assessing dietary compliance of hypercholesterolemic children enrolled in a soy supplemental study. *Top Clin Nutr.* 1994;10:27–32.

9. Shea S, Stein AD, Basch CE, Contento IR, Zybert P. Variability and self-regulation of energy intake in young children in their everyday environment. *Pediatrics.* 1992;90:542–546.

10. National Institutes of Health. *NIH Policy and Guidelines on the Inclusion of Children as Participants in Research Involving Human Subjects.* NIH Guide to Grants and Contracts, National Institutes of Health, Public Health Service, US Department of Health and Human Services, Bethesda, Md; 1998. (http://www.nih.gov/grants/guide/notice-files/not98-024.html, accessed March 6, 1998.)

11. Dennis BH, et al. DELTA manuscript. *J Am Diet Assoc.* 1998;98:766–776.

12. Tilley MA. *Investigation of the Feasibility of Performing a Clinical Feeding Study in Families.* University Park, Penn: Pennsylvania State University; 1995. Masters thesis.

13. Inhelder B, Piaget J. *The Growth of Logical Thinking.* New York, NY: Basic Books, Inc; 1958.

14. Erikson EH. Identity and the life cycle. In: *Psychol Issues* (monograph). Vol 1, no 1. New York, NY: International Universities Press, Inc; 1959.

15. Lucas B. Nutrition and Childhood. In: Krause MV, Mahan LK, eds. *Food, Nutrition and Diet Therapy.* Philadelphia, Penn: WB Saunders Co; 1984.

16. Sigman-Grant M. Feeding preschoolers: balancing nutritional and developmental needs. *Nutr Today.* 1992;27:13–17.

17. Pipes PL, Trahrns CM. *Nutrition in Infancy and Childhood.* 5th ed. Chicago, Ill: Mosby; 1993.

18. Meilgaard MC, Civille GV, Carr BT. *Sensory Evaluation Techniques.* 2nd ed. Boca Raton, Fla: CRC Press, Inc; 1991.

19. American Society for Testing and Materials. *ASTM Standards on Sensory Evaluation of Materials and Products.* Philadelphia, Penn: American Society for Testing and Materials; 1988.

20. Rozin, P. The role of learning in the acquisition of food preferences. In: Shepherd R, ed. *Handbook of the Psychophysiology of Human Eating.* Chichester, UK: Wiley; 1989.

21. Rozin P, Fallon AE. The acquisition of likes and dislikes for foods. In: Solms L, Hall RL, eds. *Criteria of Food Acceptance.* Zurich, Switzerland: Forster; 1981.

22. Birch LL, Johnson SL, Fisher JA. Children's eating: the development of food acceptance patterns. *Young Children.* Jan 1995:71–78.

23. Borah-Giddens J, Falciglia GA. A meta-analysis of the relationship in food preferences between parents and children. *J Nutr Ed.* 1993;25:102–107.

24. Newman J, Taylor A. Effect of a means-end contingency on young children's food preferences. *J Exper Child Psychol.* 1992;64:200–216.

25. Eck LH, Klesges RC, Hanson CL. Recall of a child's intake from one meal: are parents accurate? *J Am Diet Assoc.* 1989;89:784–789.

26. Van Horn LV, Stumbo P, Moag-Stahlberg, A. The dietary intervention study in children (DISC): dietary assessment methods for 8- to 10-year-olds. *J Am Diet Assoc.* 1993;93:1396–403.

27. Tilley MA, Sigman-Grant M, Kris-Etherton PM. Product development for a clinical feeding study using families with children. In: Institute of Food Technologists. *Book of Abstracts, 1994 Annual Meeting,* 1995, p 237 (81B–2). Abstract.

28. Bindslev-Jensen C. ABC of allergies: food allergy. *BMJ.* 1998;316:1299–1302.

29. Food and Nutrition Board. *Dietary Reference Intakes: Thiamin, Riboflavin, Niacin, Vitamin B-6, Pantothenic Acid, Biotin, and Choline.* Washington, DC: Institute of Medicine, National Academy of Sciences; 1998.

30. Food and Nutrition Board. *Dietary Reference Intakes: Calcium, Phosphorus, Magnesium, Vitamin D, and Fluoride.* Washington, DC: Institute of Medicine, National Academy of Sciences; 1998.

31. Gibson RS. *Principles of Nutritional Assessment.* New York, NY: Oxford University Press; 1990.

32. National Center for Health Statistics. *Third National Health and Nutrition Examination Survey (NHANES III) Reference Manuals and Reports.* Centers for Disease Control and Prevention, Public Health Service, US Department of Health and Human Services, Hyattsville, Md; 1996. (CD-ROM; Acrobat.PDF format; includes access software; Adobe Systems, Inc, Acrobat Reader 2.1; available from the National Technical Information Service, Springfield, Va.)

33. Hamill PVV, Drizd TA, Johnson CL, Reed RB, Roche AF, Moore WM. Physical growth: National Center for Health Statistics percentiles. *Am J Clin Nutr.* 1979; 32:607–629. (Available from Ross Laboratories, Columbus, OH 43216.)

34. National Center for Health Statistics. *Executive Summary of the Growth Chart Workshop.* Roche AF, ed. Hyattsville, Md: US Department of Health and Human Services, Public Health Service, Centers for Disease Control and Prevention; 1994.

35. National Center for Health Statistics. *Executive Summary of the Workshop to Consider Secular Trends and Possible Pooling of Data in Relation to the Revision of the NCHS Growth Charts.* Roche AF, ed. Hyattsville, Md: Division of Health Examination Statistics, National Center for Health Statistics, Centers for Disease Control and Prevention, Public Health Service, US Department of Health and Human Services; 1997.

36. Frisancho AR. *Anthropometric Standards for the Assessment of Growth and Nutritional Status.* Ann Arbor, Mich: University of Michigan Press; 1990.

37. National Center for Health Statistics. Anthropometric data and prevalence of overweight for Hispanics: 1982–84. *Vital and Health Statistics Reports,* Series 11, No. 239. Hyattsville, Md: Centers for Disease Control and Prevention, US Department of Health and Human Services; March, 1989. DHHS (PHS) publication 89–1689.

38. National Center for Health Statistics. *Third National Health and Nutrition Examination (NHANES III) Anthropometric Procedures Videotape.* Stock number 017–022–01335–5. Hyattsville, Md: National Center for Health Statistics, Centers for Disease Control and Prevention, Public Health Service, US Department of Health and Human Services; 1996.

39. National Center for Health Statistics. *Third National Health and Nutrition Examination Survey, 1988–94*, Series 11 (Vital and Health Statistics); (Available in ASCII Version 1A or in SETS Version 1.22a from the National Technical Information Service, Springfield, Va). Hyattsville, Md: Centers for Disease Control and Prevention, Public Health Service, US Department of Health and Human Services; 1997.

40. Society of Automotive Engineers. *Anthropometry of US Infants and Children.* Report SP 394, Ages 0–12 years. Warrendale, Penn: SAE; 1975.

41. Society of Automotive Engineers. *Anthropometry of US Infants and Children.* Report SP 450, Ages 0–18 years. 400 Warrendale, Penn: SAE; 1977.

42. Frankenburg WK, Dodds JB. *Denver Developmental Screening Test.* Denver, Colo: University of Colorado Medical Center; 1969.

43. Yanovski JA, Cutler GB. The reproductive axis: pubertal activation. In: Adashi EY, Rock JA, Rosenwaks Z, eds. *Reproductive Endocrinology, Surgery, and Technology,* Vol 1. New York, NY: Lippincott-Raven; 1996.

44. Sullivan KM, Gorstein J. ANTHRO software for calculating pediatric anthropometry. Version 1.01, 10 December 1990. In: Dean AG, Dean JA, Burton Ah, Dicker RC, eds. *EpiInfo, Version 5: A Word Processing, Database, and Statistics Program for Epidemiology on Microcomputers.* Atlanta, Ga: US Department of Health and Human services, Public Health Service, Centers for Disease Control and Prevention, National Center for Chronic Disease Prevention and Health Promotion, Division of Nutrition; 1990.

45. Feldstein TJ. Carbohydrate and alcohol content of 200 oral liquid medications for use in patients receiving ketogenic diets. *Pediatrics.* 1996;97(4):506–511.

Note: The Family Feeding Study described in this chapter was partially supported by a research grant to the Pennsylvania State University from the National Heart, Lung, and Blood Institute, Bethesda, Md (U01-HL-49659). The Dietary Effects on Lipoproteins and Thrombogenic Activity (DELTA) program was funded by the National Heart, Lung, and Blood Institute, National Institutes of Health, Bethesda, Md, through RFA NIH-92-HL-03-H (1992–1997).

PART 3

The Dietary Intervention

CHAPTER 10

PLANNING DIET STUDIES

BEVERLY A. CLEVIDENCE, PhD; ALICE K. H. FONG, EdD, RD; KAREN TODD, MS, RD; LINDA J. BRINKLEY, RD; CARLA R. HEISER, MS, RD; JANIS F. SWAIN, MS, RD; HELEN RASMUSSEN, MS, RD, FADA; RITA TSAY, MS, RD; MARY JOAN OEXMANN, MS, RD; ARLINE D. SALBE, PhD, RD; CYNTHIA SEIDMAN, MS, RD; SUSAN LEARNER BARR, MS, RD; AND ABBY G. ERSHOW, ScD, RD

Many types of diets and food preparation techniques are used in clinical and metabolic investigations. Some diets must be strictly controlled in order to detect small changes in outcome variables. Other diets may provide more flexible eating patterns and acceptable food choices for participants. Each has its place in nutrition research, but each has advantages and disadvantages that must be recognized and evaluated. This chapter describes the various types of research diets and their associated terminology, as well as the many factors that must be considered when study designers plan controlled diet studies.

TYPES OF RESEARCH DIETS

Several classification systems can help to distinguish the types of research diets and dietary techniques that are used for human feeding studies.

General Classification of Research Diets

Formula Diets

Formula diets are composed of basic foods or food components from a limited number of sources. A formula diet, repeated daily without variation for the duration of the study, offers the most rigid control and can be designed to accommodate the study of various nutrients (1). Liquid formula diets have been particularly useful for metabolic balance studies in clinical research. Chapter 14, "Planning and Producing Formula Diets," contains a comprehensive description of formula diets and their application in human feeding studies.

Conventional Food Diets

In contrast to liquid formula diets, mixed diets composed of conventional food products permit a normal fashion of eating and thus are generally more acceptable to study participants. Conventional diets can be served according to several meal plans, as described here.

A *24-hour menu* consists of 3 to 6 meals repeated daily without variation for the duration of the study. Preparing and serving the same diet day after day minimizes fluctuation in nutrient composition, reduces the chance of error, and results in less confusion on the part of laboratory and kitchen staff. Metabolic balance studies usually require this type of diet plan to minimize variability (2). Also, frozen metabolic or constant diets that are provided to outpatients usually use this diet plan. However, the 24-hour menu plan may not be suitable for long-term studies because of its repetitive nature.

A *rotation* or *cycle menu* provides a specified number of daily menus that are repeated in an established sequence for the duration of the study. All of the menus have a similar nutrient content. Different menus have different foods, but each menu (and each food item within the menu) remains the same throughout the study. Menus typically are numbered to indicate the order of rotation through the cycle. To avoid confusion and minimize the chance of error, all participants are fed the same menu (eg, Menu Four) on the same day, regardless of their dietary treatment or when they enter the study. Problems would arise, for example, if there were "rolling entry" into a study (ie, subjects starting the protocol on different dates), and each participant began the study with Menu One.

Ad libitum diets, also called *self-selected, free,* or *habitual diets,* can be used for certain research purposes. The food items and amounts eaten are documented in a food record or food diary. This diet offers subjects the most variety, but it requires more computation time than other meal plans in order to analyze the participants' food records. In some cases participants are asked to weigh each food item to be consumed and to record the data, or the staff can weigh the foods in the kitchen and enter the data immediately into a computer. Duplicate portions of each food item may be collected and a composite of these foods analyzed for nutrients of interest.

Diets Used in Association with Clinical or Diagnostic Tests

Test diets are meals of exact composition that are used to prepare the participant for specific types of diagnostic or research-oriented tests. These meals may be provided in an inpatient or an outpatient setting. One to 3 days' worth of meals may be given to a participant to eat at home prior to coming to the research center for testing. For example, meals of specific carbohydrate content may be served 1 day prior to an oral glucose tolerance test. Other examples of test diets include vanillylmandelic acid excretion tests; 5-hydroxy-indoleacetic acid (5-HIAA) and serotonin restricted diets, fat malabsorption test diets; and high-calcium diets to define calcium intake in screening for hypercalciuria (3). Another test diet, one that has a specific aluminum content and is devoid of citrus, is consumed for 24 hours before deferox-amine infusion, a procedure for indirect measurement of aluminum stores (4). For some tests, a single meal of specific composition is required on the day of the test. For example, one meal of known magnesium content may be necessary for a 1-day study that requires intravenous administration of magnesium followed by collection of blood and urine.

Nutrient levels in test diets are not generally excessive in any given meal. Conversely, *load test meals* contain a specific nutrient(s) that may be excessive in relation to the amount typically consumed at any single meal. However, the load test meal does not have a nutrient amount that would be considered excessive for an entire day's intake. One example is the Fat Tolerance Test Meal, which contains a designated amount of fat (eg, 50 g) and typically a specific fatty acid composition (eg, an enhanced proportion of behenic acid). This load test meal is given at a designated time and blood is collected prior to and following the test meal to determine clearance of plasma chylomicrons. Other examples are the Oxalate Load Test Meal to test oxalate bioavailability in foods (5) and the Calcium Load Test Meal to test calcium absorption in hypercalciuria (6).

The Diet Classification System of St Jeor and Bryan

The degree of control required for a diet study depends on study design, the type of study and its length, the emotional and physiological tolerance of the participants, laboratory and kitchen facilities, and the philosophy of the investigator. As St Jeor and Bryan (7) note, "The investigator and research dietitian should be in agreement about the most efficient and successful way to achieve desired study results."

All too frequently there is confusion regarding the terms used to describe research diets. One of the most problematic, for example, is the tendency to refer to all diets as "metabolic diets." In an attempt to standardize the use of terms and define appropriate controls, St Jeor and Bryan (7) listed five basic types of diets—estimated, weighed, controlled-nutrient, constant, and metabolic balance—used in clinical research studies. These diets were named, described, and classified based on various dietary techniques used for calculation, measurement of diet, food source, water source, preparation procedures, food refusals, and need for laboratory analysis.

Estimated Diets

The *estimated diet* relies on a visual estimation of a subject's food and fluid intake, which is then calculated for individual nutrients. This diet is the easiest to administer because it is closest to the self-selected or free diet. However, it is the least reliable because it estimates the participant's intake from equivalency lists or approximate nutrient values for foods measured in usual household (or hospital) portions. These diets may be planned by the research dietitian but are typically provided from a foodservice system other than the research center's facility (eg, the hospital food service).

Weighed Diets

The *weighed diet* may also be served by the hospital food service; but food portions are weighed as served to the participant, and refuse is reweighed on return to the research kitchen. The difference in intake is then charted and nutrient intake calculated. This type of diet may be useful for macronutrient studies testing effects of protein, fat, or carbohydrate intake.

Controlled-Nutrient Diets

The *controlled-nutrient diet* requires study nutrients to be maintained at a constant level throughout the study. Cooked food items are weighed prior to consumption. If foods are refused, they are weighed when returned, nutrient composition of returned food is calculated, and nutrients are replaced.

Controlled-nutrient diets are more demanding of the dietitian's time because nutrients must be maintained at the same level throughout the study. Accurate calculations of daily menus are required, and food preparation procedures are controlled (but not as strictly as for the constant and metabolic diets). This type of diet may be used for long-term studies requiring a specific diet pattern but not rigidly controlled nutrient intake.

Constant Diets and Metabolic Balance Diets

Constant diets and *metabolic balance diets* are the most rigorous forms of the controlled-nutrient diet. Procedures for diet calculation, food and beverage procurement, food preparation, patient instruction, and verification of nutrient content can be essentially identical for these two types of diets; they are equally demanding of the research kitchen. The distinct terminology indicates the type of research design for which the diets are used. *Metabolic balance diets* are used specifically for one type of research: nutrient balance studies (described later). In contrast, a wide variety of research designs, as well as diagnostic tests, may require a *constant diet,* which achieves constant (ie, minimally variable) nutrient intake through particularly close attention to food sources and preparation techniques.

The metabolic balance diet usually requires that nutrient data correspond with specific time periods (or phases) designated for collecting biological materials. The metabolic balance defines net gain or deficit of a particular nutrient or nutrients. The balance is said to be positive when dietary content exceeds loss in urine and feces and negative if losses in urine and feces exceed dietary intake. For a more detailed discussion, see Chapter 16, "Compartmental Modeling, Stable Isotopes, and Balance Studies."

The fundamental principle involved in the metabolic balance study is that of the "single variable." By controlling all dietary intake and keeping the diet as constant as possible from day to day, any changes in balance may be attributed to the disease, procedure, medication, or nutrient under study. The nutrient content of a metabolic balance diet is assessed from a food composite made by preparing a duplicate portion of the subject's food and beverages for a single day. The reliability of metabolic balance data depends on caloric constancy and weight maintenance, a diet that achieves the desired nutrient composition, a fixed volume of food and fluid intake, stabilization on the diet, accurate urine and fecal collections, and control of physical activity and other stresses. Because of its rigorous demands, metabolic balance studies are best done in the setting of a research center equipped with a research kitchen and an analytical laboratory (8). The study design determines the acceptable level of variability in the research diet and, accordingly, the necessary degree of control and "constancy." For example, some hypotheses

can be tested only when the day-to-day coefficient of variation in nutrient content is very small; other hypotheses can tolerate more oscillation. Therefore, when the study is being planned, the levels of control provided by the different types of research diets should be evaluated and matched to the requirements of the protocol. Investigators may find that the most rigorous levels of control are needed for only short periods of time, and that a constant diet can be first preceded and then followed by a less burdensome, less expensive estimated or weighed diet.

The degree of dietary control depends on specific requirements of the study. Investigators adapt these classifications to accommodate the setting and the nutrient control necessary for the study, frequently combining or overlapping the methods to control intake.

Phase Components of Diet Studies

Results from an experimental diet are often compared to those measured during *a baseline period.* This is typically a period just prior to the dietary treatment during which participants consume their usual (ie, self-selected) diets. Diet records are often taken during the baseline period so that outcome variables measured in association with the baseline period can be related to the habitual diet of the study population. This use of the term *baseline period* should not be confused with the baseline period required by some drug trials, in which the diet is kept constant throughout each of three phases: the "baseline period" (no drug), the "trial period" (drug treatment), and the "off period" (no drug).

A *run-in diet* or *stabilization diet* is an initial diet phase that provides a standardized intake for all participants. With this design, all participants begin intervention from the same diet; and the effects of any one eating style are minimized prior to feeding the experimental diets. The run-in diet is often patterned after current dietary patterns (eg, a typical American diet) or a reference diet (eg, the Step 1 diet of the National Cholesterol Education Program). This period adds another diet dimension for statistical comparison with subsequent feeding periods. (See Chapter 2, "Statistical Aspects of Controlled Diet Studies," and see Chapter 6, "Recruitment and Screening of Study Participants," for a discussion of use of the run-in diet during screening.)

When a response that is measured during one diet period is influenced by the previous diet, there has been a *carryover effect* or *diet order effect.* Preventing carryover effects is commonly accomplished by incorporating *washout periods* between experimental diet periods. Washout periods are nontreatment diet periods used to eliminate or minimize the nutrient carryover effect. Washout diets may be controlled diets that are patterned after the typical American diet, or they may be the participants' self-selected diets. Although washout periods between study diets can be used to reduce carryover effects, they may not be required when diets are randomly assigned and dietary treatments are of sufficient duration. In other words, the diet period must be long enough for changes that had been induced by the previous diet to cease (Table 10-1) and for changes associated with the new diet to take effect. (See Chapter 2, "Statistical Aspects of Controlled Diet Studies.")

Depletion diets and *repletion diets* may be used to determine nutrient requirements or to determine the optimal effective dosage of specific medications. For example, a diet low in magnesium, sodium, and potassium may be required to deplete blood levels of these nutrients in preparation for comparing the effectiveness of three preparations of potassium-magnesium citrate in correcting hydrochlorothiazide induced hypokalemia and hypomagnesemia.

PLANNING CONSIDERATIONS

Whether evaluating the feasibility of an existing protocol or planning a diet study from conception, the research dietitian and the principal investigator should give careful consideration to physical, financial, and human resources as they relate to the number, length, and order of dietary treatments; the range of calorie levels; and the recruitment of participants as inpatients or outpatients. Among the research team members, the dietitian is the best judge of how intricate the feeding phase can be without creating error-prone situations in production and delivery of meals.

Inpatient and Outpatient Settings

Research that has a feeding component can be undertaken in different settings. Residential feeding studies where continuous supervision is possible are most often conducted in hospitals, but boarding schools, convents, and monasteries have also been used. Prisons, although theoretically well-situated for feeding studies, are usually not suitable; compliance is likely to be poor, and the element of coercion cannot be ruled out. (In some states, there is legislation that specifically prevents the enrollment of prisoners in research protocols.)

The advantages and disadvantages of all types of study settings must be carefully considered during protocol development. Balance studies or studies requiring frequent measurements are best conducted on an inpatient basis because it is easy to control exercise, supervise food and fluid intake, collect urine and stool specimens, and carry out timed blood collections. During inpatient studies, subjects have fewer temptations to eat unauthorized foods, often share a spirit of camaraderie with other subjects, and find it advantageous to have everything prepared for them. Investigators can easily verify compliance.

Outpatient studies, on the other hand, are much less expensive to conduct and much less disruptive to the subjects.

TABLE 10-1

Length of Feeding Periods or Washout Periods for Selected Nutrients

Nutrient	Amount per Day	Outcome Variable	Study Population	Study Length	Reference
Calcium	400 mg	Steady state or hypercalciuria	Normal adults	4 d	9
Calcium	400 mg	Intestinal adaptation	Healthy adults	4 wk	9
Calcium	400 mg	Steady state	Adults with osteomalacia, osteoporosis, or hypercalciuria	3 d	10
Calcium	300 mg	Calcium retention and stabilization of PTH and 1,25-$(OH)_2$-D_3	Adult women	2 wk	11
Chromium	<20 µg	Impaired glucose tolerance	Adult men and women	4 wk	12
Chromium	200 µg	Glucose and insulin	Adult men and women	4-8 wk	12, 13
Chromium	250 µg	Blood lipids	Adult men and women	7 mo	14
Fats	<30 en%	Lipoprotein levels	Adults over 40 yr	4 wk[1]	15
Fats	40 en%	Lipoprotein levels	Adult men and women	6 wk[2,3]	16
β-carotene	30 mg	Carotenodermia	Healthy men	25-42 d	17
Fish oils	10 g MaxEPA	Stabilization of platelet and erythrocyte phospholipid fatty acids	Health adults	3 mo	18
Fish oils	5 g fish oil + 1 g 20:5 n-3 + 1 g 22:6 n-3	Persistence of ω-3 fatty acids in erythrocyte membranes after discontinuation of ω-3 fatty acids	Healthy men	>18 wks[4]	19

Rationale or implication:
[1]Plasma lipids, apolipoproteins, and fatty acid patterns stabilized by week 4 and remained constant thereafter through week 24.
[2]Lipoprotein levels continued to change between week 3 and week 6 of feeding.
[3]Double the turnover time of the slowest LDL component, which is about 3 weeks (20, 21).
[4]Longitudinal rather than crossover studies are advised because of the protracted washout periods (>18 wk).

Often the participant pool is larger for outpatient studies because people can go about their lives fairly normally. The nature of the study as such may dictate that outpatient studies are more suitable because people are allowed a "more normal lifestyle." For this reason, the results may also be more generalizable to the population at large.

Present-day research goals do not always require a restrictive inpatient setting. Confinement to a metabolic ward is almost always a major interference with the lifestyle of the research participants; and, for some studies, it is not in the best interest of the research to disrupt the participants' daily activities and social habits. Also, inpatient studies are expensive. The high cost of human feeding studies is increasingly important to funding agencies, which are encouraging scientists to develop more efficient and cost-effective research approaches. One of these approaches is to conduct studies using free-living participants.

Outpatient nutrition studies should be considered when there is no other reason to keep subjects confined to the research unit except to provide a "constant" diet, when the costs of hospitalization or institutional overhead are a consideration, or when the participant is unable to reside on the unit. A combination study is often the ideal; meals are provided on an outpatient basis for most of the study and then an abbreviated inpatient phase is employed for critical data collection or testing procedures.

Outpatient studies are more difficult than inpatient studies to standardize and follow because subjects are living out of the "controlled environment." To ensure compliance, some units require that all subjects eat 2 out of 3 meals per day in the research dining room, 5 to 7 days a week. This gives the participants frequent contact with the research dietitian, dietary staff, nursing staff, investigators, and other subjects and keeps motivation high. (Also see Chapter 7, "Managing Participants and Maximizing Compliance.")

Outpatient studies are labor intensive for the research kitchen staff because meals must be safely packed for transport, storage, and convenient reheating. Specific considerations for planning outpatient studies are listed here:

- If possible, plan a cycle menu of at least 2 to 3 days to give variety. A 1-day menu is common for short studies; however, some variety is best for outpatient studies. Longer menu cycles are generally used with longer outpatient feeding studies (see Length of Menu Cycles and Feeding Periods).
- Select foods and recipes that are easy for the research kitchen to prepare in bulk and store. Foods that are easy to prepare, freeze, store, and reheat and that are acceptable to most people include pasta with sauce (prepare and weigh pasta, sauces, and meat separately), meatloaf, Salisbury steak, hamburger patties with gravy, cookies/cakes/muffins and brownies (frozen brand names may be appropriate), rice, mashed potatoes, baked potatoes, and noodles.
- Use foods that "travel" well; eg, canned and frozen products. Limit the use of fresh produce because of the risk of spoilage.

- Select foods that will be readily available throughout the study. Some foods are seasonal and are available only at a high cost during off-season. For example, although fresh strawberries may be available in the market in November, they will cost too much to comply with many purchasing contracts.
- Use foods that are easy to reheat in the containers in which they are packaged; for example, mixed dishes reheat better than do whole pieces of meat. It may be necessary to purchase microwave ovens for participants who do not have them.
- Use foods that do not require multiple transfers from container to pan to dish. This may result in losses from spills or from food adhering to multiple surfaces.
- Make adjustments to accommodate routines of the various volunteers. Although dinner trays for residents may be delivered at a specified time, it may be necessary for a facility to stay open for a window of time, perhaps 4:30 PM to 6:30 PM, to accommodate work schedules of free-living adults.
- Pack take-out meals in insulated coolers with sealed, refreezable ice packs to keep foods cold during transport. On the other hand, a bag lunch for a salesperson or student may require a thermos to keep stew hot.
- Be sure the participants have adequate refrigerator and/or freezer space to store food and beverages for take-out meals. As a rule, no more than 2 to 3 days' worth of fresh food should be provided at once. Meals, snacks, and beverages for a single day often fill a grocery bag; a 2-day supply fills a large cooler. The ability to understand food storage safety should be one of the selection criteria for participants, and adequate cold storage space is fundamental to this issue.

Estimating energy requirements correctly and maintaining body weights during an outpatient study are crucial to the success of most projects. (See Chapter 17, "Energy Needs and Weight Maintenance in Controlled Diet Studies.") If weight maintenance is important, frequent interaction with the dietitian may be critical. This includes frequent weighing as well as monitoring of exercise patterns, sometimes daily but usually once or twice per week.

Outpatient studies require more detailed participant instruction than when participants are provided all the study food on site. "Free foods" and any limits on these items need to be specified. Clear, written instructions about safe food handling, storage, refrigeration, and reheating of foods should be given along with directions for handling emergency situations.

Multiple Dietary Treatments, Multiple Calorie Levels, and Variety of Food Items

A study providing a common background diet to all participants is easier to conduct than a study with multiple dietary treatments. Extra control measures must be implemented to avoid potential mix-ups when multiple dietary treatments are delivered concurrently. In practice, this may mean that less experienced foodservice workers could be assigned to prepare foods that will be served to all participants regardless of treatment, whereas a reliable and experienced employee might be assigned to prepare or portion foods that are vehicles for those nutrients critical to the study. There are many ways to accurately prepare and deliver multiple treatments, but they all require a high degree of organization and supervision. For example, in some facilities one employee may be assigned the task of portioning and labeling muffins of varying composition (but identical appearance) for four different diets. Another facility may prefer to have different foodservice workers portion and label each type of muffin. In both situations, records should be maintained to identify all individuals involved in the preparation and portioning of each food item so that any procedural error can be traced and corrected.

As the number of individual food items and the complexity of the items increases, more time is necessary to prepare and portion these items. Many facilities find it more efficient and less costly to purchase commercially prepared food items than to produce equivalent items. This option should be investigated within the context of the facility as well as that of the study protocol. When foods must be prepared at the facility, it is advisable to use relatively simple recipes to ensure accuracy in production. Accuracy of delivery can be improved by limiting the number of items to be distributed for a given meal. Errors of omission or duplication are easier to catch during the tray-check process when trays are not cluttered.

Although the amount of work involved in food preparation and distribution would seem to be directly related to the number of study participants being fed at a given time, this relationship is not one of direct proportion. Much of the effort of producing and portioning is in setup and cleanup rather than in cooking and weighing. There is consequently an economy of scale associated with increasing numbers of study participants—to a point. The limit of this economy of scale is reached when the burden of additional participants begins to confuse operations.

The number of participants in a study has an effect on the number of calorie levels that must be used. When each serving of food is weighed individually in proportion to energy requirements, portioning is made more complicated by greater numbers of treatments, participants, and calorie levels. In studies having few participants, the use of individually tailored calorie levels is common; the number of calorie levels to be prepared may equal the number of participants in the study. The energy requirement of each participant is assessed as accurately as possible, and daily menus are prepared to meet these calorie requirements. Typically, the kitchen staff assembles an individualized tray for each participant.

With larger numbers of participants, it is more common to use calorie increments. Menus are prepared at designated calorie levels, typically of 200-kcal to 400-kcal increments; each participant is assigned to the calorie level that most closely matches his or her estimated requirements. Participants' calorie level assignments are then changed, if necessary, to maintain their initial body weights. This method is easily used in conjunction with a modified cafeteria style of foodservice. Participants proceed down the food line selecting designated food items according to their dietary treatment and calorie level.

Menus are typically calculated at an "average" calorie level, then scaled so that each food item is fed in proportion to calorie requirements. This means that food items from the average calorie level are of normal serving sizes. Those at the extreme ends may look unusual; for example, a person eating foods of a low calorie level may receive many food items but less of each item than he or she is accustomed to eating. Serving unusual portions of food is a particular problem when large men and small women are included in the same study. For example, if menus are written so that small women can meet their calcium requirement, then large men may receive quantities of dairy products that they find objectionable.

Some studies have a fixed enrollment date for all volunteers. Others may have a "rolling" or sequential admission, in which the subjects may be engaged in different phases of the study at any given time. The latter strategy facilitates recruiting participants and has the advantage of keeping the number of participants manageable. It poses problems associated with consistency of the dietary treatments across time, however, has the potential to confound the study.

Concurrent Studies

Extra precautions are required when multiple studies are conducted simultaneously in a facility. By coordinating activities and planning for space and equipment needs, conflicts about scarce resources can be avoided. To ensure optimal use of the facility, this extra coordination should take place among the principal investigators of the studies as well as among members of the dietary staff and should occur early in the planning process. In some facilities each study is assigned separate counter space, cooking equipment, refrigerators, freezers, serving areas, and dining areas, and little is shared except equipment. In other facilities, all studies must share all resources. This means that facility-wide quality control measures must be instituted to ensure proper delivery of test foods to the intended subjects.

Tracking expenditures for each study is more complex when more than one study is in process. The dietary staff will most likely purchase food and supplies in common for all ongoing studies and subsequently allocate costs to each study. Although this process makes bookkeeping more difficult, food costs may be lower if requirements for quantity discounts are met by combining orders.

Finally, subject morale can be affected when participants with high and low levels of study "burden" share a single dining facility. It is only natural that participants in differing studies will compare their protocols for degree of effort in relation to benefits.

Length of Menu Cycles and Feeding Periods

The decision to use a long or short menu cycle depends on a number of factors specific to the facility and the study design. However, the length of the study is a major factor in determining the length of the menu cycle. Short-term metabolic balance studies typically use menu cycles of 3 days or less. Long feeding studies generally use longer menu cycles of 1 or 2 weeks to add variety and make the diets more acceptable. The disadvantages of long cycles include the added time in menu preparation, the requirement for more labor in food handling, and a greater variability in nutrient content among menus.

Menu cycles frequently are based on 7 days, as in a 7-day or 14-day menu cycle. An advantage of this system is that certain menus can be tailored to the special requirements of carry-out meals (eg, weekend meals). These menus are often written with convenience and food safety issues in mind. Some dietitians and investigators, however, prefer menu cycles that are based on a number other than seven. This approach has the advantage of avoiding the predictability and boredom that are inherent when menus are standardized to the day of the week (eg, "It must be Tuesday; ham sandwiches for lunch again!")

The length of the feeding periods is selected according to estimates of how much time is needed for the outcome variable of interest to stabilize in response to a change in the nutrient variable of interest. This time period may depend on the level of the nutrient in the diet; the degree of change from the previous diet; the level of other dietary components; and characteristics of the study population, including nutritional status, age, gender, and body composition. Table 10-1 provides general estimates of the typical length of feeding periods for various nutrients and associated outcome measurements. (Note: There is seldom universal agreement on the appropriate length of feeding any particular nutrient for any outcome variable.)

Scheduling Diet Studies

In scheduling diet studies, it is prudent to avoid holidays that might interfere with the normal feeding of participants. In the United States, this generally rules out the time period between Thanksgiving and New Year's Day. For Lent and Passover, it is sometimes possible to calculate appropriate alternate meals that will be acceptable to participants observing these holidays. Local events should be taken into account (eg, Mardi Gras in New Orleans). Dates that are likely to be important to a particular study population should be considered (eg, college breaks in a population of young women).

Seasonal effects are another factor to consider in scheduling diet studies. Nutrients in specific foods can change with the season (an example is the carotenoid and vitamin C content of summer vs winter tomatoes). Outcome variables may be affected by colds and flu, which are common in winter, or by allergies, which are commonly induced in spring and fall by pollen. The summer months are problematic for conducting feeding studies because of changes in physical activity and conflicts with vacations. Unwelcome snow storms may interrupt diet studies at critical points of dietary intake and sample collection. Elderly subjects may be less interested in studies conducted in winter months because of anticipation of poor driving conditions and the safety issues that accompany shortened daylight hours.

Tailoring the Study to the Physical Facility

Architectural plans for a metabolic research kitchen must address a variety of special needs. Ideally, these include cooking facilities that allow for multiple modes of preparation; workstations that are efficient and well equipped for weighing, packaging, and preparing food; storage space for refrigerated, frozen, and dry goods; and dishwashing facilities. Office space, including computer workstations for dietitians and technicians, as well as a dining room for outpatients, may also be included. A setting that provides for all of these needs can successfully accommodate multiple studies and large numbers of subjects consuming complex diets for long periods of time either at the facility or as outpatients.

Rarely, however, is this ideal setting available. Usually the study must be tailored to an existing physical facility. (Also see Chapter 19, "Facilities and Equipment for the Research Kitchen.")

Because space restrictions lead to equipment limitations, frequently only one piece of each type of equipment is available. Consequently, contingency plans must be available at all times to provide for emergency situations such as breakdowns, repairs, and replacement of equipment. Most research kitchens that do on-site cooking should have both a conventional range/oven and a microwave oven. A double-oven household range can provide assurance that if one oven breaks down, the other will still be in working order. If a microwave oven breaks down, the range and oven can provide a method of reheating. A portable hotplate can also serve this purpose. If a dishwasher is out of order, paper supplies should be readily available for meal service. Most institutions are required by their state public health department to meet sanitation codes governing dish washing and do not allow washing dishes by hand without a disinfectant. Alternative refrigeration and freezer space should be identified for emergency food storage when such equipment fails. Ideally, important refrigerators and freezers will be connected to an emergency generator.

To conduct successful feeding studies under circumstances of limited storage space, it may be necessary to study fewer participants at a time, to extend the study over a longer time period, and to offer fewer food choices. As long as sufficient quantities of key food items can be stored for the participant at any given time, intrasubject variability in nutrient intake over long periods of time can be minimized. In addition, chemical analysis of diet composites can provide a measure of variability in nutrient intake across time.

Meals may also be simplified so that only those foods containing key nutrients are kept in storage. Other food items may then be procured as needed. For example, in a study investigating the effects of vitamin C on the incidence of colds, the diet can be designed so that frozen orange juice is the only significant source of vitamin C in the diet. Frozen orange juice would then be purchased in a single lot shipment and would be the only food needing storage for the length of the study. The remainder of the diet, composed of foods low in vitamin C, could be replenished on a regular basis.

Food procurement, preparation, storage, and delivery from another foodservice department within the institution can decrease storage needs and reduce on-site food production. This arrangement can be particularly helpful if cooking facilities and personnel are limited. Under these circumstances diets might be designed around portion-controlled, precooked items that may even be available as frozen entrees and preportioned foods such as juice, cereals, and snacks. It is necessary, however, to evaluate in advance whether the composition and weight of such food items are sufficiently accurate and constant for the purposes of the study.

This approach has been effectively used by McCullough et al (22) in studying electrolyte balance. Inpatients consuming rigorously controlled constant diets were compared to outpatients consuming less exactly controlled diets consisting of manufacturers' preportioned foods and other foods prepared and weighed in the hospital's central food production area. Analyzed diet composition for electrolytes and for 24-hour urine collections showed no statistical difference between the two methods of dietary control.

The number of employees that can effectively and efficiently work in a given work area is likewise governed by the amount of space and equipment available. Simplifying the meals, food selections, and meal rotations can decrease the number of food items that need weighing and preparation. This can decrease personnel requirements. The maximum capacity for the types and numbers of research diets produced should be established in advance. Creative staffing patterns, sometimes extending into the late evening, can address the problems of space limitations and increased production needs. The use of temporary personnel can also effectively meet the study's needs for short periods of time.

The efficiency of a research kitchen is maximized in studies that supply food for home consumption because the meals do not have to be prepared and served three times a day. Food pickups by the participants can be arranged for both morning and afternoon to free up refrigeration space. Once the morning food is picked up, refrigeration space then becomes available for the delivery and storage of food for the afternoon or evening pickups. To use a work schedule of this kind, perishable foods and some precooked foods may need to be procured from another foodservice area and brought to the unit on a meal-by-meal basis. These arrangements can frequently be made through the institution's food services.

Ultimately, the limitations of space, equipment, and personnel within a research kitchen must be addressed individually with emphasis on the ability to maintain accuracy of food preparation and service and continuity of function by a trained staff. Careful consideration of the necessary dietary controls will address most scientific and logistical issues in advance. Often, food preparation procedures can be simplified, resulting in improved efficiency and accuracy. With thoughtful creativity and advance planning, well-controlled feeding studies can be conducted in almost any facility.

Pilot Studies

A *pilot study* is a small-scale study that is conducted to facilitate the successful completion of a full-scale study. The many reasons for conducting pilot studies include: gathering preliminary information prior to committing scarce resources; assessing the feasibility of a feeding regimen; and honing techniques for the analysis, storage, and distribution of foods and samples. Pilot studies also are used to refine protocols as well as to make comparisons and choose among alternative approaches.

It is important that treatments, subject populations, and study conditions used in a pilot study closely parallel those planned for the subsequent, full-scale study. Investigators must resist the tendency to use inadequate dietary control groups or treatments; controls are as essential for interpreting the results of a pilot study as they are for interpreting a full-scale study. In addition, the subjects participating in a pilot study should resemble those who will participate in the subsequent, full-scale study; otherwise, the data gathered may be misleading. For example, procedures and menus planned for a study in elderly individuals should be pilot-tested on persons from that age group, not on young students or middle-aged adults.

For the dietary staff, recipe development is an important aspect of pilot studies. Some recipes that initially appear to be successful may not hold up under the close scrutiny of a pilot study. During recipe development, the food is taste-tested for quality and acceptability with several people eating a whole portion as part of a meal. Tasting a spoonful is often not enough; eating the same amount that the participants are expected to consume can lead to a different evaluation of the food item. Portions of the recipe are stored as the food item will be for the study (refrigerated/frozen) and reheated at a later date to evaluate how these treatments affect appearance and quality of the product. Any changes that are made to the recipe are incorporated, and the evaluation process is repeated.

To test for potential problems associated with scaling for quantity preparation, the recipe is made in amounts that will ultimately be used for the study. All procedures and details of preparing the recipe are documented. The insights of kitchen staff can be tapped to assess the ease of preparation, availability of foodstuffs, and other pertinent considerations.

In preparation for the pilot study, the kitchen staff, nursing staff, laboratory staff, and study coordinator develop study-specific flow sheets, ordering forms, and quality control guidelines. (See Chapter 3, "Computer Applications in Controlled Diet Studies," and Chapter 18, "Documentation, Record Keeping, and Recipes," for examples of forms.) As with a full-scale study, a statistician should be included on the research team.

With these steps completed, the pilot study can begin. At this time, many aspects of the study can be fine-tuned, comments collected, and data gathered. Besides cooking and tasting recipes, serving the food, and checking the composition of menus, many other activities and procedures can be pilot-tested. These include all laboratory analytical techniques, sample processing and storage procedures, record-keeping procedures, forms, interviewing techniques, recruitment strategies, nursing techniques such as blood pressure measurements, and data processing. Pilot studies can be extremely useful, not only because many preliminary discoveries are made at this step, but also because the design, diet plan, or procedures can be ameliorated before sponsors invest effort and money on a larger scale study.

A final evaluation of the pilot study is done at this stage and plans are revised. If enough participants were studied and the outcome variables were measured after a time course similar to the one planned for the major study, data collected during the pilot study may be used by the study's statistician in a power analysis. This calculation can provide valuable data to project the number of participants that will be required for the full-scale study in order to determine statistically significant differences among treatments.

There are many advantages to conducting a pilot study:

- Data collected is likely to predict the success of a full-scale study.
- Rough spots and failures in the recruitment process, in the kitchen, and in the research laboratory can be corrected prior to outlay of major resources.
- New staff members can be trained under less pressure than during the full-scale study.
- Recruitment strategies for subjects can be improved.
- Recipes and menus can be improved based on input from study participants and kitchen staff.
- Sample handling and techniques for laboratory analysis can be evaluated.
- Foods can be composited and chemically analyzed to predict accuracy of nutrient content for the full-scale study.
- The number of persons, the time commitment, and the cost required to carry out the full-scale study are more easily predictable.

- Data from the pilot study can be used in a power calculation to estimate the number of subjects required in the full-scale study.
- Data from pilot studies will often convince a funding agency to support a major study. Data from pilot studies are often publishable.

Estimating the Cost of Diet Studies

Producing research diets is an expensive endeavor—so much so that their cost is a major consideration in the design and implementation of human feeding studies. Injudicious cost-cutting maneuvers, however, can jeopardize the integrity of a study. The research dietitian thus walks a fine line in an effort to contain expenses while committing the resources required to achieve the primary goal of producing high-quality diets of specified composition.

Various feeding patterns have been successfully used in research studies, depending on the level of control required, the facility, and the research question to be addressed. As shown in Table 10-2, studies that require a high degree of dietary control usually are more expensive. Such studies typically require longer hours of facility operation, more supervision of research participants, and more personnel, all adding to the cost of conducting a study. The goal is to provide the degree of dietary control required for a particular research question without spending additional resources when control is not required.

Liquid formula diets probably are the most cost-effective of all the research diets. However, ingredients, even when purchased in large quantities, are still expensive. The food costs for some liquid formula diets may match the food cost of a natural food diet, but the labor cost likely will be much lower. For example, in a typical facility an employee can prepare 80 liters of a single formula each day that supplies 64,000 kcal. This is enough to feed a participant for a month, and there is little waste.

The cost of producing research diets varies among studies and among facilities but is based, in large part, on the complexity of the study, including level of labor; number of meals served and hours of facility operation; the type of diet, including the expense of dietary components; the nature of the measurements made on participants; and payments and other charges associated with enrolling study participants.

Labor

Labor is the major operating expense for most feeding facilities. A major responsibility of the research dietitian is to assess, within the framework of each new study, the skills and the time requirements of each position and to make assignments accordingly. Additional employees frequently are needed for days or hours of peak workload; it can be less expensive to make appropriate use of part-time and overtime labor than to hire additional full-time employees. Some fa-

TABLE 10-2

Direct Relationship between Degree of Dietary Control and Expense of Conducting a Study

Level of Dietary Control	Cost	Features
Highest	Highest	• Metabolic ward • Formula and conventional food diets • All meals supervised • No alcohol • All foods analyzed for selected nutrients (23)
High	High	• Free-living participants • Conventional foods • Two supervised meals Monday–Friday • Lunch and weekend meals packed for take-out • No alcohol • Diet composites analyzed for selected nutrients (24)
Medium	Medium	• Free-living participants • Conventional foods • Two supervised meals Monday–Friday • Two self-selected weekend meals (within guidelines) • Alcohol consumption allowed within limits • Diet composites analyzed for selected nutrients (25)
Medium	Low	• Free-living participants • Self-selected diets • Food records • Fiber-rich cereals prepackaged for home consumption (26)
Low	Lowest	• Free-living participants • Self-selected diets based on flexible, individualized diet plan • Food records • Food frequency questionnaire • Diet counseling (27, 28)

cilities successfully employ students, especially college-level dietetic or foodservice management majors, or secondary school students who are enrolled in work training programs. The personnel department can provide advice about institutional regulations and liabilities regarding the use of students and volunteers in the research kitchen. In some settings the kitchen staff may be hired only in accord with strict union contract rules.

It often is advisable to plan the staffing budget on a year-round basis even if the study participants are actively engaged in the feeding protocol for only part of the year. This recommendation acknowledges the complete time sequence of the research protocol. For example, before the study begins the nutrition staff must be trained and must try out the experimental menus to ensure they meet the study design goals. There is a great deal of preparation work before and between feeding periods. Also, if the investigation comprises a series of studies, it is inefficient to lay off the trained staff and hire new recruits a few months later. Studies are not part of the usual hospital foodservice activity, and highly skilled, well-motivated workers are needed to ensure that the protocols are being followed correctly.

In some facilities, free-living participants perform limited but time-saving functions as part of the study protocol. For example, labor hours are saved by having participants rather than staff members assemble the items required for a take-out lunch: participants can collect their lunch items along with breakfast items as they progress along a cafeteria line, then pack lunch items for take-out. The time required for a staff member to check the accuracy of participants' selections can be considerably less than the time required for a staff member to assemble the trays. This must be done without burdening the participants and without breaking the blinding of the study. (Also see Chapter 20, "Staffing Needs for Research Diet Studies.")

Purchasing Food and Supplies

Food

The research dietitian must view food selection and purchasing within the context of three major goals: (1) to control nutrient content of the diets, (2) to aim for participant compliance, and (3) to follow principles of cost containment within the parameters of the research protocol. This means that food costs will vary considerably among studies, depending on the design. Ingredients for a simple formula diet may cost as little as $5 per day, whereas the components for constructing whole-food diets with specially manufactured ingredients may cost as much as $20 per day. The decision to purchase a brand-name cookie at a higher price than a nonbrand-name counterpart may be justified if it promotes compliance or if nutrients are more consistent among lots. Similarly, a particular brand of reduced-sodium and reduced-fat salad dressing may best suit the requirements of the researcher and the palates of the participants.

To minimize waste and save money, the dietitian must order each food in the quantities needed. This is no simple task, because each food item must be assessed separately considering its rate of use, shelf-life, and stability once opened. Additionally, greater waste is associated with weighed food portions. For example, when a hard roll or bagel is portioned and precisely weighed, a large part may be lost to maintain the aesthetic appeal of the served portion.

Buying in large quantities of single batch lots not only ensures consistency in nutrient composition for the entirety of the study but also has the benefit of discounted prices if the supplier's required minimum order is met. Although purchasing in bulk can be cost-effective, it is not appropriate in all situations. For example, when a recipe calls for 10 g more than is supplied in an institutional pack of tuna, it is cost-effective to stock small cans as well. The amount of storage space available also influences whether items are purchased in bulk. If storage space is limited, additional emphasis will be placed on selecting a food item that is readily available and provides consistency of nutrients across lots.

Buying in bulk is an appropriate method of purchasing ingredients for liquid formula diets. However, special consideration must be given to the shelf stability of the ingredients, including the fat and protein sources, which may deteriorate over time. This is particularly important for dried milk powders and other ingredients that undergo Maillard (browning) reactions and other changes affecting taste.

Storage represents another food-associated cost in diet studies. Bulk dry storage at room temperature requires large amounts of floor space, usually in locked rooms; the institution where the study is conducted may charge for this space. Walk-in refrigerators and freezers may be needed. It also may be necessary to rent space for bulk frozen or refrigerated items in specialty warehouses. These facilities usually are located at a distance from the research center. Beyond the rental fees, additional travel and time costs are incurred when staff go to refrigeration sites to retrieve the food.

In deciding whether to make a food product "from scratch" or to purchase a commercially available product, considerations for controlling nutrient content of diets override principles of cost containment. However, in some cases commercially available foods can be used appropriately and offer a cost savings compared to food and labor expenses incurred with the in-house production of a comparable product.

It is wise to allot funds for food composition analysis both before the study (during validation and pilot phases) and during the conduct of the protocol (monitoring phase). The cost of chemically analyzing a commercially prepared mixed dish such as baked lasagna may be less expensive than the labor involved in preparing the dish. Many commercially prepared mixed dishes are highly standardized and companies typically provide nutrient analysis of the product. (Some food companies are willing to share available nutrient data that is not included on their nutrient data sheets.) However, it is important to determine the variation among portions of commercially prepared dishes; within-batch or among-batch variation may be unacceptably high.

Supplies and Materials

Just a generation ago, the term *paper supplies* referred largely to paper napkins and cups, waxed paper, and aluminum foil. Today supplies include a substantial proportion of Styrofoam, plastic wrap, and other disposable containers and utensils. Although the cost of paper supplies varies among facilities, as rule-of-thumb estimate, the expense of paper supplies is approximately 10% of food costs.

Disposable plastic and paper containers have become a mainstay in the preparation and service of research diets. Frequently, foods are weighed in advance of the study, portioned into high-quality disposable containers, frozen until ready for use, and then assembled on permanent ware for service in the hospital setting or kept in the original container when a packed meal is ordered. Food needing to be reheated prior to service can be microwaved in these same containers if plastic or paper is used.

Although disposable containers are convenient, a high price is paid for their purchase and disposal. Disposing of solid waste will be an increasing concern for foodservice managers as disposal costs accelerate. Studies are needed to document the amount and type of solid waste generated in feeding facilities.

Budget Planning for Research Diet Studies

As earlier discussions make clear, feeding studies create some unique budgetary pressures that other types of research are spared. Although categories vary according to institutional policies, the general categories that must be considered when researchers develop the study budget are:

Personnel (includes salaries, wages, overtime, and fringe benefits)
- Principal investigator
- Coprincipal investigator
- Research dietitian
- Medical officer
- Study coordinator
- Secretary/administrative support
- Cooks
- Foodservice workers
- Nursing support
- Laboratory technicians
- Phlebotomist

Statistician
Consultants
Administrative Expenses
  Travel (out-of-town meetings, local mileage)
  Telephone/other communication
  Publications
  Shipping
  Postage
  Office supplies
  Facilities charges
  Nutrient database software
  Printing and photocopying
Foodservice Expenses
  Food
  Paper goods and disposables
  Kitchen supplies, equipment, and maintenance
  Coolers/cold packs
  Off-site freezer/refrigerator storage
  Laundry, linens, and uniforms
Laboratory Expenses
  Equipment
  Clinical laboratory tests
  Laboratory supplies
  Diet composite analysis
  Service contracts on laboratory equipment
  Blood collection and processing supplies
  Sample storage
Subject Costs
  Subject payment
  Recruitment costs/advertising
  Parking fees/public transportation/local mileage

The exact assignment of these costs to specific categories (for example, is food a "supply" cost or does it fall under "other" costs?) will vary among research centers, depending on factors such as the policies of the funding agency and the budget format preferred by the institution.

The financial structure of studies differs among research centers. For example, the nature of institutional support varies considerably: some investigators may need to request funds for nursing services that elsewhere may be provided without charge. Another highly variable factor is the indirect cost or overhead rate. In some situations this is minimal (ie, 10%), whereas in others it can be high enough (ie, 80%) to effectively double the cost of the project.

Costs may be calculated on a per-study, per-subject, per-meal, or per-annum basis. This basis will vary with the category:

- Small equipment (such as kitchen scales) is usually purchased once at the outset of the study.
- Financial compensation or stipends would be paid in fixed amount to each participant.
- Parking fees may be charged each time the participant drives to the center for a meal.
- Salary support for a principal investigator usually represents a percentage of full-time effort per year.

Although it may seem that costs in all categories would be proportional to the number of participants enrolled, this is not the case. Any study, regardless of size, requires a certain minimal number of staff; increments about this, however, may be irregular. The necessary level of labor for dietetic and kitchen staff is particularly high; it tends to range from 0.2 to 0.5 full-time equivalents (FTE) per participant, depending on the complexity of the protocol. In addition to the nutrition personnel, scientific, medical, statistical, managerial, and laboratory effort is needed; when summed, this effort can vary from 2 FTE to 6 FTE.

Study subjects often receive a stipend or financial compensation for participating in the study. This is a common, but not universal, practice. Some investigators believe that a financial incentive is a disservice to participants because it can pressure them to continue with a study when they prefer to withdraw. This consideration is compounded when payment is partially or fully linked with completing the study. Others believe that the study will be taken more seriously when there is payment involved and that this incentive promotes compliance and willingness to complete long studies. Offering a financial incentive also can broaden the recruitment pool, which is often an important consideration when participants with specific characteristics are being sought. (See Chapter 5, "Ethical Considerations in Dietary Studies," for further discussion of stipends.)

CONCLUSION

Controlled human feeding studies are labor intensive, expensive, and require a great deal of attention to numerous details, but they can yield information that cannot be gained by other types of research. Advance planning for all aspects of human feeding studies can lead to cost savings, greater accuracy in data collection, and a more harmonious setting for study participants as well as dietary and research staff.

REFERENCES

1. Aherns EH Jr. The use of liquid formula diets in metabolic studies: 15 years experience. *Adv Metabol Disord.* 1970;4:297–332.
2. Sampson AG, Sprague RG, Wollaeger EE. Dietary techniques for metabolic balance studies. *J Am Diet Assoc.* 1952;28:912–916.
3. American Dietetic Association. *Handbook of Clinical Dietetics. (Part H) Miscellaneous, Test Diets.* New Haven, Conn: Yale University Press; 1981:H15-H18.
4. Malluche HH, Smith AJ, Abreo K, et al. The use of deferoxamine in the management of aluminum accumulation in bone in patients with renal failure. *N Engl J Med.* 1984;311:140–144.
5. Brinkley LJ, Gregory J, Pak CYC. A further study of oxalate bioavailability in foods. *J Urol.* 1990;144:94–96.
6. Pak CYC, Kaplan RA, Bone H, et al. A simple test for

the diagnosis of absorptive, resorptive, and renal hyper-calciurias. *N Engl J Med.* 1975;292:497–500.

7. St Jeor ST, Bryan GT. Clinical research diets: definition of terms. *J Am Diet Assoc.* 1973;62:47–51.

8. Brinkley L, Pak, CYC. Metabolic balance regimen and nutritional aspects of clinical research. In: Pak CYC, Adams PM, eds. *Techniques of Patient-Oriented Research.* Dallas, Tex: University of Texas Southwestern Medical Center at Dallas; 1992:108–120.

9. Leichsenring JM, Norris LM, Lameson SA, et al. The effect of level of intake on calcium and phosphorus metabolism in college women. *J Nutr.* 1951;45:407–419.

10. Pak CYC, Stewart A, Raskin P, et al. A simple and reliable method for calcium balance using combined period and continuous fecal markers. *Metabolism.* 1980;29:793–796.

11. Dawson-Hughes B, Harris S, Kramich C, et al. Calcium retention and hormone levels on high and after adaptation to low calcium diets in black and white women. *J Bone Miner Res.* 1993;8:779–87.

12. Anderson RA, Polansky MM, Bryden NA, et al. Supplemental-chromium effects on glucose, insulin, glucagon, and urinary chromium losses in subjects consuming controlled low-chromium diets. *Am J Clin Nutr.* 1991;54:909–916.

13. Anderson RA, Polansky MM, Bryden NA, et al. Chromium supplementation of human subjects: effects on glucose, insulin, and lipid variables. *Metabolism.* 1983;32:894–899.

14. Abraham AS, Brooks BA, Eylath U. The effects of chromium supplementation on serum glucose and lipids in patients with and without non-insulin-dependent diabetes. *Metabolism.* 1992;41;768–771.

15. Lichtenstein AH, Millar J, McNamara JR, et al. Long term lipoprotein response to the NCEP Step 2 diet enriched in n-3 fatty acids. *Circulation.* 1990;82:III-475. Abstract.

16. Judd JT, Clevidence BA, Muesing RA, et al. Dietary *trans* fatty acids and plasma lipids and lipoproteins of healthy adult men and women fed a controlled diet. *Am J Clin Nutr.* 1994;59:861–868.

17. Micozzi MS, Brown ED, Taylor PR, et al. Carotenodermia in men with elevated carotenoid intake from foods and β-carotene supplements. *Am J Clin Nutr.* 1988;48:1061–1064.

18. Sanders TAB. Influence of moderate intakes of fish oil on blood lipids. In: Lands WEM, ed. *Proceedings of the AOCS Short Course on Polyunsaturated Fatty Acids and Eicosanoids.* Champaign, Ill: American Oil Chemists' Society; 1987.

19. Brown AJ, Pang E, Roberts D. Persistent changes in the fatty acid composition of erythrocyte membranes after moderate intake of n-3 polyunsaturated fatty acids: study design implications. *Am J Clin Nutr.* 1991;54:668–673.

20. Egusa G, Beltz WF, Grundy SM, et al. Influence of obesity on the metabolism of apolipoprotein B in humans. *J Clin Invest.* 1985;76:596–603.

21. Beltz WF, Kesaniemi A, Howard BV, et al. Development of an integrated model for analysis of the kinetics of apolipoprotein B in plasma very low-density lipoproteins, intermediate-density lipoproteins, and low-density lipoproteins. *J Clin Invest.* 1985;76:575–585.

22. McCullough ML, Swain JF, Malarick C, et al. Feasibility of outpatient electrolyte balance studies. *J Am Coll Nutr.* 1991;10:140–148.

23. Ribaya-Mercado JD, Russell RM, Sahyoun N, et al. Vitamin B-6 requirements of elderly men and women. *J Nutr.* 1991;121:1062–1074.

24. Clevidence BA, Judd JT, Schatzkin A, et al. Plasma lipid and lipoprotein concentrations of men consuming a low-fat, high-fiber diet. *Am J Clin Nutr.* 1992;55:689–694.

25. Barr SL, Ramakrishnam R, Johnson C, et al. Reducing total dietary fat without reducing saturated fatty acids does not significantly lower total plasma cholesterol concentrations in normal males. *Am J Clin Nutr.* 1992;55:675–681.

26. Whyte J, McCarthur R, Topping D, et al. Oat bran lowers plasma cholesterol levels in mildly hypercholesterolemic men. *J Am Diet Assoc.* 1992;92:446–449.

27. Henderson MM, Kushi LH, Thompson DJ, et al. Feasibility of a randomized trial of a low-fat diet for the prevention of breast cancer: dietary compliance in the Women's Health Trial Vanguard Study. *Prev Med.* 1990;19:115–133.

28. Kristal AR, White E, Shattuck AL, et al. Long-term maintenance of a low-fat diet: durability of fat-related dietary habits in the Women's Health Trial. *J Am Diet Assoc.* 1992;92:553–559.

CHAPTER 11

DESIGNING RESEARCH DIETS

BEVERLY A. CLEVIDENCE, PHD; ALICE K. H. FONG, EDD, RD; KAREN TODD, MS, RD; SUSAN E. GEBHARDT, MS; LINDA J. BRINKLEY, RD; CARLA R. HEISER, MS, RD; JANIS F. SWAIN, MS, RD; HELEN RASMUSSEN, MS, RD, FADA; RITA TSAY, MS, RD; MARY JOAN OEXMANN, MS, RD; ARLINE D. SALBE, PHD, RD; CYNTHIA SEIDMAN, MS, RD; SUSAN LEARNER BARR, MS, RD; AND ABBY G. ERSHOW, SCD, RD

DESIGN GOALS, NUTRIENT INTAKE, AND DIETARY GUIDELINES

Research diets are first designed, calculated, and analyzed to ensure that study design goals are met and that intake is adequate for all nutrients other than those being investigated. Each nutrient value in the diet should then be compared against a population goal or standard. The Recommended Dietary Allowances (RDA) (1, 2) are often used as the basis for determining whether intake of nutrients other than the study variable(s) is adequate. RDA are standards for nutrient intake designed to meet the nutrient needs of virtually all healthy individuals in the United States. With the exception of energy, the RDA are established at two standard deviations above the mean requirement of the population and are, therefore, believed to meet or exceed the requirements of about 95% of the population. Most people who consume less than the RDA for a specific nutrient will nevertheless meet their own personal nutrient requirement. However, for practical purposes, a cutoff point, such as two-thirds or three-fourths of the RDA, could be used to judge whether intake for a specific nutrient is adequate.

The Food Nutrition Board, National Academy of Sciences, has developed the Dietary Reference Intakes (DRI) with the intention of providing a comprehensive set of parameters for evaluating dietary adequacy. These parameters include, among others, the RDA. This discussion will refer to the RDA as the basis for assessing adequacy of intake.

When a research diet is deliberately designed to be deficient or low in one or more nutrients, other nutrients in the diet are also likely to be inadequate. Likewise, if a very high-fat or low-energy diet is fed, many nutrients in the diet may fall below 70% RDA. In some cases, it may be difficult to feed a nutrient at the RDA level specified for one sex group. For example, the current RDA for iron is 15 mg/day for adult women (1), a level that is often difficult to meet with foods alone, especially at low calorie levels. To meet the RDA in these situations, either a commercial vitamin or mineral supplement may be fed, or the lacking nutrient can be added directly to the diet. Direct addition is preferable to avoid "overbalance" for intakes of other nutrients. Folate, iron, magnesium, vitamin B-6, and calcium are nutrients particularly likely to need special attention.

Whereas the RDA are useful for assessing adequacy of nutrients in research diets, other types of population dietary goals have been developed to target nutrients of excess. The National Cholesterol Education Program (NCEP) Guidelines (3) are commonly used for comparing fat type and amount to dietary goals (Table 11-1). NCEP nutrition publications for patients and professionals are described at the National Heart, Lung, and Blood Institute Web site (www.nhlbi.nih.gov/nhlbi/nhlbi.htm).

It also can be useful to relate nutrient levels in research diets to the current nutrient intakes of the US population. The Continuing Survey of Food Intakes by Individuals (4), published by the USDA Survey Research Laboratory, reports mean intakes of various nutrients by gender and age and compares current intake levels to the RDA. This publication also has useful information about the percent of individuals consuming foods from various food groups, weight status of the population, frequency of physical activity, and perceived importance of dietary guidance. The Food Survey Research Laboratory home page (www.barc.usda.gov/bhnrc/foodsurvey/home.htm) provides information on new releases of survey data, highlights from the surveys, information about the Survey Discussion Group, and links to other USDA Internet sites related to food and nutrition.

The National Health and Nutrition Examination Surveys (NHANES) also provide population-based estimates of nutrient intake, as well as data about physical characteristics and indicators of health and nutritional status (5). The NHANES surveys are conducted by the National Center for Health Statistics. Reports detailing survey results as well as methodology are available in print and electronic format (6). Three study cycles have been completed (NHANES I-III); the fourth (NHANES IV) began its pilot testing phase in 1998.

DETERMINING NUTRIENT INTAKE

Calories

Energy is provided by fat, carbohydrate, protein, and alcohol. The carbon and hydrogen components of these compounds can be oxidized to carbon dioxide and water. The nitrogen component of protein is not oxidized but is, for the most part, excreted from the body as urea. Gross energy of foods can be measured from the heat released by oxidation of foods in a bomb calorimeter (the heat of combustion). An adjustment to this measure is made for apparent digestibility of foods because some nitrogenous materials, fibers, and other organic matter are lost in the feces. From these measurements, calorie factors have been derived for energy sources for individual and complex foods.

The calorie factors that databases use for protein, fat, and carbohydrate are food-specific, meaning they are adaptations of the traditional Atwater factors commonly used for calculating energy in mixed diets (ie, 4, 9, and 4 kcal/g for protein, fat, and carbohydrate, respectively). The Atwater factors used in the current USDA Nutrient Data Base for Standard Reference (Release 12) (9) (see Exhibit 11-1) and also in the print versions of Agricultural Handbook 8 (10)

TABLE 11-1

Intake of Dietary Components: Recommended and Current Levels

	Recommended Intake[1]	Current Intake[2]
Carbohydrate	50-60 en%	50 en%
Protein	10-20 en%	16 en%
Total fat	<30 en%	33 en%
Saturated fat	<10 en%	11 en%
Polyunsaturated fat	≤10 en%	7 en%
Monounsaturated fat	10-15 en%	13 en%
Cholesterol	<300 mg	212 mg (women)
		334 mg (men)
Dietary fiber	20-30 g	14 g (women)
		19 g (men)
Reference age group	Over age 2 years	Adults

[1]Recommended intakes of fat, carbohydrate, and protein are from Report of the Expert Panel on Population Strategies for Blood Cholesterol Reduction, National Cholesterol Education Program. US Department of Health and Human Services, NIH publication 90-3046, 1990 (3). Recommended intake of dietary fiber is from Butrum et al, 1988 (4).
[2]Source: 1994 Continuing Survey of Food Intakes by Individuals and 1994 Diet and Health Knowledge Survey. Agricultural Research Service, US Department of Agriculture, 1996 (5).

EXHIBIT 11-1

USDA Nutrient Database for Standard Reference, Release 12
available at www.nal.usda.gov/fnic/foodcomp

WHAT IS SR12?
The USDA Nutrient Database for Standard Reference, Release 12 (SR12), is prepared by the Nutrient Data Laboratory of USDA's Agricultural Research Service. It is the major compilation of food composition data in the United States and provides the foundation for most public- and private-sector databases. SR12 contains data about 5,976 food items. Data lists up to 81 nutrients when a complete profile is available for a food item. SR12 supercedes the previously published food composition data in printed sections of Agriculture Handbook No. 8 and SR11-1.

FORMAT
The database is being provided in the two relational formats, ASCII and DBF. There are four principal files: Food Description, Nutrient Data, Gram Weight, and Footnotes. Four support files include: Nutrient Definition, Measure Description, Food Group Description, and Source Code. New information (first provided in SR11) about all foods includes scientific name (where appropriate); factors for calculating protein from nitrogen and calories from protein, fat, and carbohydrate; INFOODS tagnames to identify food components internationally; a source code to indicate whether the value is based on analytical data or is an imputed value; and additional measures for many foods. A series of update files is provided for users who have obtained a copy of SR11-1 and who wish to perform their own updates. An abbreviated flat-file format featuring fewer nutrients is also included; this feature was available previously. Also provided are reports on each food item.

NUTRIENTS

Water	Ash	Vitamin A (IU & RE)
Food energy (kcal and KJ)	Amino acids	Ascorbic acid
Protein	Calcium	Thiamin
Total fat	Iron	Riboflavin
Total saturated fatty acids	Magnesium	Niacin
Total monounsaturated fatty acids	Phosphorus	Pantothenic acid
Total polyunsaturated fatty acids	Potassium	Vitamin B-6
Individual fatty acids	Sodium	Folate
Cholesterol	Zinc	Vitamin B-12
Total dietary fiber	Copper	α-tocopherol
Caffeine	Manganese	Alcohol
Theobromine	Selenium	

CHANGES IN THIS RELEASE
Items that are no longer on the market, such as most beef cuts trimmed to ½-inch fat, have been deleted. Several hundred new items have been added and a number of other items have been updated. Two major changes to nutrients in this release concern folate values and selenium. The revised folate values for enriched grain products and foods containing these products reflect the change in FDA regulations that required the addition of folic acid to selected foods effective January 1, 1998. The nutrient data for selenium for most foods in the database was added in this release.

---

are specific to two decimal places. Because this database forms the core of most other food databases, specific Atwater factors are used in most nutrient calculations. These factors, derived from heat of combustion, are adjusted for available energy (11). Thus, the Atwater factor for carbohydrate for a food containing highly digestible carbohydrate forms is higher than for a food with an equivalent amount of which a large proportion is indigestible.

Energy calculations for recipes (and sometimes menus) can differ substantially when general factors rather than specific factors are applied. Consider, for example, that "energy for whole-grain wheat flour is calculated using the specific factors of 3.59 kilocalories per gram of protein, 8.37 kilocalories per gram of fat, and 3.78 kilocalories per gram of carbohydrate. The result is 339 total kilocalories. Using the general factors of 4, 9, and 4, the estimate would be 362 kilocalories" (12). It is a common experience for novice dietitians to be dismayed to discover that hand-calculated values for a recipe, based on general Atwater factors, do not exactly agree with the values calculated using a food database. This problem is greater for individual foods or when a small number of foods are involved than when averages are for many foods. When general Atwater factors are applied to mixed diets as opposed to individual foods, the differences are generally small, (approximately 1%).

Protein and Nitrogen-to-Protein Conversion Factors

Protein values in databases are derived by assessing the nitrogen content of foods and applying a conversion factor reflecting the mass proportion of nitrogen in the protein molecule. Just as there are general and specific values for caloric values of carbohydrate, protein, and fat, there are also general and specific values for nitrogen-to-protein conversion factors. Although the general conversion factor of 6.25 (based on the assumption that protein contains 16% nitrogen by weight) is appropriate for many research diets, some protocols, such as nitrogen balance studies, should use specific factors. In formula diets where the predominant source of protein comes from eggs, the conversion factor will be 6.25, but when milk is the predominant source of protein, the conversion factor used will be 6.38. The nitrogen-to-protein conversion factors used in current food tables are based largely on data published by Jones (13).

Dietary needs for protein exceed the need for a set amount of nitrogen because there are specific requirements for essential amino acids. The literature on protein quality and on estimating nitrogen and amino acid requirements of humans is extensive and includes a collection of papers by the Committee on Amino Acids, National Academy of Sciences (14). Although typical American diets provide ample high-quality protein, research diets low in total protein content or low in animal protein content should be reviewed for adequate protein quality, particularly if the study participants are growing children, adolescents, or pregnant women.

Fiber

Methodological problems are obstacles to the accurate assessment of food fiber (15). Different chemical methods measure different classes of fiber components. Some databases may contain values for fiber analyzed by an array of methods that are not directly comparable (Table 11-2). Values for crude fiber, which have been reported in food tables in the past, should not be used. Analytical values for total dietary fiber in the current USDA Nutrient Data Base for Standard Reference, Release 12, were determined by the Association of Official Analytical Chemists (AOAC) (Gaithersburg, Md) enzymatic-gravimetric method (9, 16). Although soluble and insoluble fiber values may be more informative for nutritionists, these fiber fractions present particularly difficult analytical barriers and their values differ according to method of analysis. Values for total dietary fiber, soluble fiber, and insoluble fiber have been published for a number of foods (17, 18). Several methods have been approved by AOAC International as the official methods for dietary fiber analysis (16).

Recommendations for fiber intake have been expressed in quantitative values and in qualitative terms, based on servings of fiber-rich foods. The dietary guidelines of the National Cancer Institute recommend that fiber intake in the United States be increased to 20 g/day to 30 g/day from a variety of food sources with an upper limit of 35 g/day (8) (Table 11-1). Guidelines based on food selection advocate the consumption of at least five servings of fruits and vegetables per day and at least six servings of grains and legumes (19).

Alcohol

Alcohol is a source of calories for a substantial proportion of adults. Alcohol yields 7.07 kcal/g when combusted in a bomb calorimeter (11) and 6.93 kcal/g when adjusted for a 98% coefficient of digestibility. For protein, fat, and carbohydrate, the values generated by bomb calorimetry, and adjusted for digestibility, are directly applicable to biological use. That is, replacing one nutrient for another at an equivalent calorie level will produce equivalent effects on body weight. However, alcohol appears to contribute to the body's energy balance in a different manner (20–22). Using alcohol to replace carbohydrate calories may fail to maintain body mass in some individuals (20); and alcohol added to a maintenance diet may not produce the anticipated weight gain (21, 23). Other investigators, however, have found that energy balance is maintained by isoenergetic diets that substitute moderate amounts of alcohol for carbohydrate (23).

Vitamins and Minerals

When investigators formulate research diets for vitamin and mineral content, particular attention must be paid to the possibility of inadequate intake. Cooking losses or gains must be accounted for,[1] and diets must be checked carefully to ensure that intakes will be adequate. For example, smoking increases the need for vitamin C; intake of this vitamin should be 140 mg/day or more if the participants of a research study are smokers (24, 25). Also, it may be difficult to meet the RDA for calcium and iron for women and elderly

---

[1]The Provisional Table on Retention of Nutrients in Food Preparation (April 1984) is available from the Nutrient Data Laboratory of the USDA Beltsville Human Nutrition Research Center and can be downloaded from the Nutrient Data Laboratory home page (http://www.nal.usda.gov/fnic/foodcomp) or bulletin board (301) 734-5078. These retention values are based on the True Retention method:

% True retention = (Nutrient content per g cooked food
$\times$ g food after cooking)
$\div$ (Nutrient content per g raw food
$\times$ g food before cooking) $\times$ 100

(This equation can be found in Murphy EW, Criner PE, Gray BC. Comparisons of methods for calculating retentions of nutrients in cooked foods. *J Agric Food Chem.* 1975;23:1153-1157.)

TABLE 11-2

Total Dietary Fiber Content of a Diet Reference Material Analyzed by Six Different Methods[1]

Method	Total Dietary Fiber (g/100 g dry weight)
Crude fiber	1.4
Neutral detergent fiber	1.8
Englyst[2]	3.6
Theander	5.1
AOAC	5.3
Li	5.6

[1]Diet Reference Material 8431, National Institute of Standards and Technology, Gaithersburg, MD. Table adapted from Li (15).
[2]Differences among the Englyst value and those of Theander, AOAC, and Li are caused mainly by the exclusion of lignin.

people, especially at lower calorie levels (26). Although calcium can be obtained from some vegetables, large quantities would be required to meet the RDA. Dairy products are generally required unless calcium supplements are used. Iron supplements may also be required.

Folate, B-12, B-6, and riboflavin intakes may need to be increased if female participants are taking oral contraceptives (27). Folate nutrition is a problem for elderly subjects also; among this group anemia and subnormal erythrocyte levels are common problems (28, 29). The Food and Drug Administration amended the Standards of Identity for enriched grain products to require the addition of folic acid effective January 1, 1998 (30). This fortification policy has made it easier to design low-energy diets that are adequate in folate.

Another factor hampering the design of diets with specific vitamin content is the inadequacy of nutrient databases. For example, little is known about carotene content of foods, particularly the individual carotenoids. Because of the historical view of carotenoids as mainly precursors of vitamin A, most food composition tables provide vitamin A activity or provitamin A carotenoid content of foods (31, 32) rather than total carotenoid content. For data on individual carotenoid content of foods as well as total carotenoid content, research dietitians can refer to the USDA/NCI Carotenoids Food Composition Database (33) (Version 2, 1998), which can be downloaded from the Nutrient Data Laboratory home page or bulletin board.

It is likely that there will be increased emphasis on the tocopherol and ascorbate content of research diets because these antioxidants appear to protect cells from oxidative damage and because the requirement for vitamin E may depend partly on the dietary vitamin C intake. In preparing for studies that investigate both vitamins C and E, it is essential to have nutrient information on these vitamins for all foods. Values for vitamin E in milligram α-tocopherol equivalents are available for only about 60% of the items in Release 12 of the USDA Nutrient Data Base for Standard Reference (9). The vitamin C information in nutrient databases is relatively complete, but comparability to actual vitamin C values of foods in research diets will be questionable, in large part because of variation in such factors as storage time and cooking conditions for food items.

Improved nutrient database values are also badly needed for trace elements. This problem is highlighted in the case of selenium. Because little is known about the biological function of selenium in humans, more investigations are being conducted in selenium metabolism. Topics of interest include the effects of dietary selenium on selenium metabolism and immune status, selenium dependent metabolic and physiological processes, and utilization of different chemical forms of selenium. The current USDA Standard References database (SR-12) (9) has selenium content for the foods that are the major contributors of selenium in the US diet.[2] Because the selenium content of foods varies significantly throughout the United States depending on soil content, when purchasing food for a study of selenium, it is important to specify clearly the regions where wheat (34) and beef products (where selenium content reflects grain—wheat—intake) will be procured.

Absorption of selenium and other trace elements may be affected by the level of major minerals and other trace minerals in the diet and by the presence of other potentially interfering substances such as phytate and other chelating agents. Final review of the overall diet design and calculated nutrient content will help in identifying these food and nutrient interactions.

Commentary: Quality of Nutrient Data

Although critical to the planning of research diets, accurately analyzed data do not exist for all nutrients and all foods. (See Using a Computer to Design Research Diets and Chapter 3, "Computer Applications in Controlled Diet

---

[2]Provisional tables for sugars (HERR-48, 1987), vitamin D (HNIS/PT-108, 1991), selenium (HNIS/PT-109, 1992), and vitamin K (HNIS/PT-104, 1994) are available from the Nutrient Data laboratory, USDA, 4700 River Road, Riverdale, MD 20737. They can be downloaded from the Nutrient Data Laboratory home page (http://www.nal.usda.gov/fnic/foodcomp) and the Nutrient Data Laboratory bulletin board (301) 734-5078.

Studies.") Also, in developing its nutrient databases, the USDA generally has sought to provide data that can be used to represent national average values. Thus, although estimates for nutrient values have been indispensable for evaluating survey data, they may give a false sense of security concerning the preciseness of data for the purposes of feeding studies.

Both the quality and quantity of available data vary depending on the nutrient component of interest. For many foods, values are imputed or missing for folate, pantothenic acid, and vitamins A and E. Similarly, data may be limited for certain categories of foods. The USDA often publishes these smaller databases in provisional form. Although there is a large body of food composition data for commodities, there are fewer data for manufactured or processed foods. Even for commodity foods with adequate analytical data, the standard error often indicates large variation in the nutrient content.

The seasoned research dietitian is aware of these problems and avoids using food items that have missing values or large standard deviations for nutrients of interest. It is standard practice to print the nutrient breakdown for each food in a menu or recipe and check for missing values (many computer programs flag foods that have missing values for nutrients). Each nutrient database handles this problem differently; in some instances nutrient values are imputed from values of similar foods, but other databases will leave a data cell blank rather than supply an estimated value. Missing data can cause calculated values to be falsely low. Chemical validation of research diets thus is highly desirable. (See Chapter 22, "Validating Diet Composition by Chemical Analysis.")

SELECTING THE FOODS

When developing menus, the research dietitian must translate nutrient goals into specific food items and palatable menus that can be prepared at the study facility and that will be appealing to research participants. This section addresses issues to consider in selecting food items for research studies.

Study Goals and Key Foods

Food items are selected for use in diet studies based, in large part, on the nutrient variables to be studied. In formulating diets, it is helpful to have one list of foods containing minimal amounts of the nutrient of interest and another list of foods containing substantial amounts. Typically, key foods are used as vehicles to deliver nutrients of interest. The ideal key food will allow incorporation of the dietary variable in varying amounts, will facilitate masking of dietary treatments, and will provide optimal palatability. For these reasons, baked products are standard vehicles for dietary fats, although fats can also be added to some entrees and side dishes.

Caloric Distribution and Serving Sizes

During menu planning, it is important to examine the caloric distribution of the diet throughout the day. Compliance is thought to be best when approximately 70% to 80% of the day's calories are distributed among the breakfast, lunch, and dinner meals, and the remaining 20% to 30% is disbursed between the afternoon and evening snacks. However, this caloric distribution may not be practical in research units with limited staff to deliver and monitor food intake several times a day.

Compliance in feeding studies also is enhanced when serving sizes have relatively normal appearance on the plate or tray. When investigators develop the research menu these "household measure" servings must be translated into gram amounts. The USDA Nutrient Data Base for Standard Reference (9, Exhibit 11-1) and most other food tables provide nutrient values based on amounts expressed in two forms: as 100-g edible portions (with information on standard error and number of samples) and as one or more common household measures. Practical information on serving sizes, such as approximate measure and weight, also is given. For example, one small loaf of pita bread (4-in diameter) is equivalent to 28 g; one large pita (6½-in diameter) weighs about 64 g.

Information about typical portion sizes of more than 100 foods is available from a government publication entitled *Foods Commonly Eaten in the United States: Quantities Consumed Per Eating Occasion and in a Day, 1989–91* (35). These data were collected from a survey conducted by the US Department of Agriculture (Continuing Survey of Food Intakes by Individuals). Data for each food item are displayed as both means and percentiles and are tabulated for individuals by gender and age.

It is customary in controlled diet studies to portion each food item according to the caloric needs of the participants. In the most conservative approach to this direct proportional allocation of foods, the quantities are "scaled" for calorie level; each food item is weighed to the nearest gram. This practice sometimes yields awkward portions of foods because gram amounts seldom coincide with whole units of foods such as crackers, muffins, or cookies. For example, a participant assigned exactly 30 g of whole wheat bread might receive one whole slice of bread and an additional small piece of bread. This degree of detail is not always necessary. In many studies it is acceptable to serve bread in units of half or quarter slices. When consistent with study objectives, apples and oranges also may be served in units of half or quarter slices; raw vegetables such as carrot sticks and lettuce can be served as pieces. This allows portioning in normal units and is more aesthetically pleasing to participants.

It is necessary to assess in advance how such changes affect a research diet. Nutrient values should be calculated for any prospective liberalized change at all calorie levels and then compared to nutrient values calculated using the more precise measures.

When investigators plan menus, careful consideration must be given to serving sizes and numbers of food items: quantities must first be estimated for intermediate or average calorie levels, but then the menus must be checked to see what happens at the extremes. As discussed in Chapter 10, "Planning Diet Studies," serving sizes often become distorted from typical sizes as food items are scaled for very high- and low-calorie levels. This becomes particularly apparent in studies with both men and women whose energy requirements may range from 1,600 kcal to 4,400 kcal. In order that men at the highest calorie levels do not receive unreasonably large servings, the number of food items must be increased. For example, instead of a single vegetable at dinner, two or three different vegetables may be required. In a direct proportional allocation system, women at the lowest calorie levels then receive two or three very small servings.

Food Preferences of Participants

When designing menus for a study, the research dietitian must consider common food preferences, intolerances, and allergies. It is essential to screen participants carefully before entry to the study in order to evaluate dietary habits as well as to obtain vital information about whether the participant can and will eat the diet study foods.

Although diets can be designed to closely match nutrient goals, this is of little value if participants will not eat the meals. Food aversions are widespread. (See Chapter 13, "Delivering Research Diets.") It is critical to make clear to potential participants what exceptions can and cannot be made to suit their personal preferences. If this is not done, compliance will suffer. A single intolerance for a food, such as applesauce, often can be accommodated by substituting another pureed fruit. An allergy or intolerance to chocolate, however, would be a strong reason to disqualify a potential participant from entering a study that uses chocolate to provide particular fatty acids. If a food item or recipe is widely disliked in the course of a diet study by a large proportion (over one-fifth) of participants, alternate recipes or uses of the key ingredients should be considered.

In many research facilities it is not feasible to offer food choices, so diets are planned using widely acceptable food items. The disadvantage to this approach is that such meals can be bland. Although few people prefer bland foods, there is no common agreement on how to season foods. Onion, garlic, and green peppers are staple seasonings for many people, but these foods are offensive or cause indigestion for others. Similarly, a product may be too salty for some, yet not salted enough for others. Of the 300 potential participants interviewed for a recent study (36), about one-third reported a strong dislike for certain foods. Among those potential subjects, the most disliked foods in decreasing order were: liver and other organ meats, brussels sprouts, milk, cheese, oatmeal, fish, green pepper, onion, and pork.

A prestudy "buffet" featuring different potential diet study recipes and foods is a convenient and helpful forum in which to realistically assess participants' food preferences. Prospective participants should be encouraged to evaluate and comment about the study foods. Following up on comments and suggestions is a small but important way for the staff to build rapport with the participants and to demonstrate receptiveness to their needs. Recipe testing and meal assessment is traditionally conducted using staff members, but a different perspective is gained from having potential participants evaluate food products and menus.

Special Populations and Ethnic Food Patterns

If younger people such as college or graduate school students are participants, it is important to include daily snacks for consumption during evening study hours. Exam and school vacation schedules must be accommodated as well. Students or others who play team sports may have drastic changes in caloric needs and exercise level during certain seasons (eg, baseball players in spring). Providing calculated, portion-controlled snack packages is an option that students are usually grateful to receive. A useful snack item can be a "unit" snack, which is a muffin, cookie, or other food or combination of foods that have a composition that is identical to the composition of the diet. (See recipes for unit foods in Chapter 18, "Documentation, Record Keeping, and Recipes.") With the exception of the unit snack, it is advisable *not* to include essential diet items in snack packages. For example, in a diet study that focuses on fats, it is better to provide low-fat snacks.

For elderly participants, foods that are "kinder" to artificial dentition, such as applesauce or baked apples instead of raw fruit, are recommended. Also, with the elderly, decreased lactose tolerance may necessitate pretreatment of some foods with the enzyme lactase. (See Chapter 13, "Delivering Research Diets," for a discussion of lactose maldigestion.)

When subjects are children, a more repetitive menu cycle may be indicated in order to ensure compliance. Thus, whereas in an adult study a pasta entree may be served once or twice a week, if it is a well-consumed favorite of child participants, it can be served more often if the study design permits. (Also see Chapter 9, "Children as Participants in Feeding Studies.")

Recruitment of ethnically diverse study populations is an increasingly important feature of human studies. Developing menus acceptable to diverse tastes while meeting study design goals presents a particular challenge. This issue actually has several components: population groups, food patterns and choices, and nutrient data. Investigators must assess exactly which demographic groups are likely to contribute individuals to the participant pool. Sometimes this is related to key hypothesis-testing aspects of the protocol. For example, investigators may wish to study whether response to diet differs significantly between Hispanics and Asians; in this case specific numbers of subjects must be recruited to fill predefined statistical "cells." At other times, recruitment strategies will seek participants in proportion to their numbers in the overall US population; in this case a large array of racial or ethnic subgroups may be represented.

Once the likely demographic composition of the study population is known, food patterns must be considered. They can be another challenge because food preferences may be affected by degree of acculturation (eg, food patterns differ greatly between first-, second-, and third-generation immigrants); yet finer demographic distinctions (eg, there are many Asian countries, and food patterns vary among them), and religious practices within ethnic groups (eg, Moslems and Hindus from India have different dietary habits) exist. However, individuals willing to submit to the rigors of a feeding study may also be willing to subjugate food preferences for the duration of the protocol. Appropriate screening procedures will seek out individuals whose food preferences are sufficiently flexible to accommodate most menu plans.

Researchers designing diets to accommodate ethnic food patterns may be interested in exploring these publications:

- Sanjur D. *Hispanic Food Ways, Nutrition and Health.* Needham Heights, Mass: Allyn and Bacon, Publishers; 1995.
- *The American Dietetic Association Ethnic and Regional Food Practice Series.* Chicago, Ill: American Dietetic Association; Hmong, 1992; Filipino, 1994; Soul & Traditional Southern, 1995; Cajun & Creole, 1996; Indian & Pakistani, 1996; Chinese American, Mexican American, Jewish, Navajo, and Alaska Native, 1998. Northern Plains Indians is being developed.
- Achterberg C, Eissenstat B, Peterson S. Intervention strategies for special groups. In: Kris-Etherton PM, Burns J, eds. *Cardiovascular Nutrition: Strategies for Disease Management and Prevention.* Chicago, Ill: American Dietetic Association; 1997.

Finally, foods chosen to accommodate ethnic preferences must meet the same standards for characterization and consistency in appearance, taste, physical properties, and nutrient content that are applied to all other foods used in assembling a research menu. This consistency may be hard to guarantee in imported foods or those manufactured by small specialty producers. Satisfactory data about nutrient content also is needed, but the great demand for nutrient information for ethnic or foreign foods has exceeded the ability of US databases to provide reliable data on these foods. Users may find data from foreign sources to be helpful. A list of composition tables for foreign foods (37) can be obtained from the International Network of Food Data Systems (INFOODS) (e-mail address: http://www.crop.cri.nz/crop/infoods/infoods.html). INFOODS also supports an Internet discussion group about food composition activities around the world (Food-Comp@Infoods.unu.edu). Subscription requests can be sent to Food-Comp-Request@Infoods.unu

.edu. A food description system, Langual, is useful for linking food items in international databases (38).

Food Substitutions

For the most strictly controlled feeding studies, participants rarely have a choice in food selection. When participants are required to eat only the provided foods, individuals who repeatedly fail to consume a particular food typically are dismissed. Other studies allow limited exchange of food items that are similar in composition (eg, sugar for hard candy) or limited addition of items not carrying nutrients of interest (eg, carrots or celery in a study of dietary fat). This flexibility allows participants some degree of control over their diets without compromising the study.

Some investigators will exclude potential participants who strongly dislike a food to be used in a study (eg, cheese); others will accept the participant and make appropriate substitutions (eg, whole milk to achieve equivalent intakes of type and amount of fat). In some controlled feeding studies, it is common to make allowances for "free meals" or "days off" (39). At these times, substitutions or tradeoffs can be used to ensure that nutrient intake does not stray too far from controlled intakes.

A more liberalized approach to food substitution is often appropriate for long-term intervention studies. For example, one intervention study's goal was not only to study outcome parameters but also to permanently change the eating patterns of the study participants. This might be done, for example, to lower fat intake as a potential protection against breast cancer in an intervention study that spans many years. Participants in such studies might be free-living women who prepare their own food and document food intake through diet records; dietary goals would be tailored to food preferences of the participants to add variety, maintain motivation, improve compliance, and retain participants.

If substitutes are deemed acceptable, the dietitian's role is to ensure correct application of substitutions to achieve the study goals. Exhibits 11-2, 11-3, and 11-4 are examples of substitutions or tradeoffs that have been used in an intervention study (40) to reduce fat intake. Participants are provided with a list of tradeoffs and are responsible for implementing appropriate food substitutes, a strategy that promotes more involvement of participants in the research process. Using tradeoffs adds variety and flexibility for participants without the time-consuming effort of recalculating research menus.

The tradeoffs in Exhibits 11-2 and 11-3 are isocaloric substitutes for nonfat foods containing carbohydrates. (It should be noted that in some studies these specific tradeoffs would not be appropriate because of changes in fiber and antioxidant contents of the tradeoff pairs.) Milk products can be substituted for other dairy combinations containing similar fatty acid compositions (Exhibit 11-4). These substitutions are helpful in alleviating varying degrees of lactose—or, more specifically, milk—intolerance, especially

EXHIBIT 11-2

Carbohydrate Equivalents Used in a Study of Dietary Fats[1,2]

1 packet jam (0.5 oz) = ½ small banana	1 cup orange juice = 3 packets jam
1 slice white bread = ½ white bagel	1 cup cranberry juice = 4 packets jam
1 slice wheat bread = ½ wheat bagel	1 cup apple juice = 3 packets jam
5 oz cola = 4 oz orange juice	12 oz cola = 4 packets jam
4.5 oz root beer = 4 oz orange juice	10 oz Mystic® or fruit-flavored soda = 4 packets jam
2 tsp Coffeemate® = 1 packet jam (less than 1 g fat)	12 oz ginger ale = 3 packets jam
2.5 oz cranberry juice = 4 oz orange juice	3 slices of rye or wheat bread = 70 g pita bread
2.5 oz grape juice = 4 oz orange juice	2 packets of jam = 1 cup cantaloupe, watermelon, or papaya
3.5 oz apple juice = 4 oz orange juice	70 g french bread = 70 g pita bread
¼ cup candy corn = 5 packets jam	2 tsp of white or brown sugar, or honey = 1 packet of jam
1 oz gumdrops = 3 packets jam	1 Matzoh cracker = 3 packets of jam
1 oz hard candy = 3 packets jam	

[1]A variety of substitutions should be encouraged. Tradeoffs are isocaloric but may differ in vitamin C content. Orange juice, in particular, should not be consistently substituted for vitamin C-poor foods in studies where this antioxidant might affect outcome variables.
[2]Quantities of food typically reflect single-serving allotments.

EXHIBIT 11-3

Tradeoffs for Popcorn Used in a Study of Dietary Fats[1,2]

Alternatives for 8 cups of Nonfat Popcorn (choose one):

3 fresh, medium apples (with skin), 2¾″ diameter	7 fresh, medium peaches
4 fresh, medium oranges, 2⅝″ diameter	7 fresh, medium plums (2⅛″ diameter)
2 oz hard pretzels (< 2 g fat/oz)	10 cups of raw broccoli or cauliflower
2.5 fresh, medium pears, 2½″ diameter	1.5 cups cooked, drained, cooled macaroni
2.5 fresh, medium, ripe bananas (8¾″)	2 medium baked potatoes with skin (2¼″ to 3″ diameter)
4 cups frozen strawberries, unsweetened	4 slices wheat bread (4 × 4 × ½″)

[1]The substitutes for popcorn provide the same calories. However, some popcorn tradeoffs provide more fiber than others. Therefore, it is important to choose different substitutes each week for variety and to distribute fiber intake. In particular, do not choose broccoli and cauliflower exclusively.
[2]Quantities of food typically reflect allotments for 1 week.

when lactase-containing products or supplements fail to alleviate gastrointestinal symptoms. (Also see Chapter 13, "Delivering Research Diets.") Egg whites or egg substitutes and foods high in sugar content are combined to balance the amounts of protein and carbohydrate and to maintain calorie levels.

It is more difficult to make tradeoffs among complex foods while maintaining a precise distribution of fatty acids in the diet. A useful approach for maintaining a fatty acid profile is to replace a fat-containing food with a fat source that closely matches the fatty acid pattern of the replaced food. Some examples are: substituting soybean or safflower oil for the polyunsaturated fat content of bean curd (tofu); substituting olive oil for the monounsaturated fat content of almonds or olives; and substituting a selected vegetable oil for nuts or seeds containing the same primary unsaturated fat (eg, walnut oil replacing walnuts). In each case, an oil replaces an equivalent amount of fat in the disliked food.

Making any kind of substitutions for research foods requires instructing participants thoroughly on how to trade off amounts of equivalent items. In addition, follow-up measures to ensure compliance must be performed. Measures may include frequent review of food records by dietitians, telephone interviews with participants, and home visits by nutritionists.

Food substitutions have been used to achieve a high degree of compliance, to encourage meal completion, to heighten awareness of diet requirements, and to educate participants about implementing intervention diets. However, meeting participants' individual food choices is challenging within the strict requirements of research diet studies and, in some research settings, making substitutions is not feasible or practical. In those instances, it is advisable to serve universally acceptable foods.

Staff and Facilities

Menus should be designed to be consistent with the capabilities of the staff and the operation of the facility. Ideally, staffing is scheduled to meet the needs of the protocol. In instances where research facilities overlap with larger, insti-

EXHIBIT 11-4

Milk and Dairy Equivalents Used in a Study of Dietary Fats[1,2]

7.5 cups 1% milk = 4 oz part skim mozzarella cheese
and 8 oz Egg Beaters
and 3 cups orange juice

7.5 cups 1% milk = 2½ cups vanilla yogurt
(3%–4% milk fat: 8 g fat/cup)
and 3 packets jam (0.5 oz ea)
and 12 oz Egg Beaters

7.5 cups 1% milk = 19 oz Egg Beaters
and 1¾ cups orange juice
and 1⅓ cups Breyers® Vanilla Ice Cream
omit 1 packet jam

10 cups 1% milk = 4 oz whole-milk mozzarella cheese
and 18 oz Egg Beaters
and 4 cups orange juice

10 cups of 1% milk = 1¾ cups Breyers Vanilla Ice Cream
and 25 oz Egg Beaters
and 2¼ cups orange juice
omit 1 packet jam

10 cups of 1% milk = 3¼ cups vanilla yogurt
(3%–4% milk fat: 8 g fat/cup)
and 17 oz Egg Beaters
omit 4 packets jam

1 qt 2% milk = 2⅓ cups vanilla yogurt
(3%–4% milk fat: 8 g fat/cup)
and 5 oz Egg Beaters
omit 2¼ cups orange juice

1 qt 2% milk = 2 oz cheddar cheese
and 6 oz Egg Beaters
and 1¾ cups orange juice

1 qt 2% milk = 1⅓ cup Breyers Vanilla Ice Cream
and 10 oz Egg Beaters

2 cups (1 pint) whole milk = 2 oz cheddar cheese
and 2 oz Egg Beaters
and 5½ tsp sugar

2 cups whole milk = ½ cup Haagen Daz® Vanilla Ice Cream
and 5 oz Egg Beaters
and ¾ tsp sugar

11.5 cups whole milk = 2 tsp sugar
and 28 oz Egg Beaters
and 3 cups Haagen Daz Vanilla Ice Cream

11.5 cups whole milk = 10 oz cheddar cheese
and 6 oz Egg Beaters
and 4¾ cups orange juice

1 cup skim milk = 1 cup nonfat frozen yogurt
omit 2 packets jam (0.5 oz ea)

9 oz cheddar cheese = 12 oz whole-milk mozzarella cheese

6 oz cheddar cheese = 8 oz whole-milk mozzarella cheese

6.5 oz cheddar cheese = 9 oz whole-milk mozzarella cheese

---

[1]Tradeoffs are balanced for calories and total fat, including saturated, polyunsaturated, and monounsaturated fats. Units are in household measures to facilitate implementation by study participants. Tradeoffs can be calculated in weight equivalents, but accuracy should be verified prior to use.
[2]Quantities of food typically reflect allotments for 1 week.

tutional facilities (eg, university feeding facilities), it may be necessary to plan the most critical aspects of feeding participants to coincide with optimal staffing times. For example, if lunch is the best staffed and best monitored meal, incorporation of key dietary material should take place at this time to enhance accuracy in meal preparation, consumption, and compliance.

Details Can Make a Difference

The examples given here are intended to draw attention to the importance of vigilance in planning diet studies, whether by eliminating extraneous sources of nutrients or carefully making food choices that enhance the match between the menu and the study goals.

- Calcium chloride is added to low-sodium canned tomatoes.
- The sodium content of "quick-cooking" Cream of Wheat® is higher than in the "instant" or regular-cooking Cream of Wheat.
- Some brands of low-sodium cheese actually have sodium chloride added; therefore, direct, chemical analysis is vital.

- When aluminum containers are used for frozen constant/metabolic diets, the aluminum content of the diet may be increased.
- Low-sodium baking powder used in pancakes or baked products for constant/metabolic diets can increase the aluminum content of those diets.
- In studies in which urinary pH changes are important (eg, whether the acidifying effect of exercise on urine contributes to renal stone formation), it is necessary that the diet have at least 10 mEq acid ash content. An alkaline ash diet can negate the results by alkalinizing the urine. The ash content of the diet is determined by adding the milliequivalent values for calcium, sodium, potassium, and magnesium (alkaline ash) and comparing them to the milliequivalent values for phosphorus, chloride, and sulfur (acid ash). A source of food composition information for chloride and sulfur has been published (41).
- If the crust on low-sodium bread seems to be significantly darker and heavier than the rest of the bread, the sodium content of the crust should be analyzed separately. Some bakeries brush the top of bread with raw egg white prior to baking to hasten the browning process. This practice

slightly increases the sodium content of the crust. If this small variation in sodium content from slice to slice is not acceptable for constant or metabolic diets, crusts can be trimmed off before the bread is weighed.

- Very-low-sodium diets are often low in calcium as well, because most dairy products are typically omitted from these diets. For studies (eg, hypertension studies) that involve changing subjects from a very-low- to a high-sodium diet, the sodium content of the diet should not be increased by increasing the content of dairy products. This may alter calcium intake which, in turn, may influence blood pressure.
- At low calorie levels, it is often difficult to meet the RDA for calcium. In these cases, vegetable sources of calcium may be useful for meeting the RDA (eg, tofu, broccoli, and spinach). Orange juice enriched with calcium is another option.
- Drink mixes such as Kool-Aid® are commonly used in research diets, often to increase calorie intake. The major nutrients of Kool-Aid are vitamin C, calcium, phosphorus, and sugar. A serving supplies about 10% of the RDA for vitamin C. Although the calcium and phosphorus contents of these beverages are low compared to the RDA, these quantities may be important in studies of minerals, particularly when participants receive multiple servings of these drinks (Table 11-3).
- Many cereals are fortified with iron and thus will not be appropriate for low-iron studies. These cereals are useful, however, for meeting the RDA for iron for premenopausal women.
- Dietary supplements (eg, NaCl, KHCO₃, KCl, PEG) can be mixed in water to a specified concentration and weighed amounts served to study participants. This eliminates possible errors of loss that can occur if supplements are administered in powdered form.
- The increasing popularity of baking soda toothpaste warrants a strong warning to dietitians and other investigators who study sodium intake. Baking soda toothpastes often have much higher sodium content than regular formulations, but there also is considerable variation among brands. For protocols requiring strict control of sodium intake, it may be advisable to poll the participants about their preferred brand of toothpaste, analyze these brands for sodium content, and choose the brands that best complement the protocol. Another option is to ask a research pharmacist to compound a dentrifice specifically for use in the study. (See Table 13-1.)

Toothpaste manufacturers' data for 6 brands indicated 19 mg to 87 mg sodium is ingested per episode of brushing. (Swain J. Sodium in toothpaste. Practice Note. *The Digest.* Chicago, Ill: American Dietetic Association; Spring 1993.)

USING A COMPUTER TO DESIGN RESEARCH DIETS

General Considerations for Selecting Database Software

The use of printed food composition tables has been superseded in recent years by microcomputer nutrient database programs. Software vendors provide a variety of programs that calculate nutrient intake. For many of these packages, however, the food composition data will not meet the stringent quality control that is required for research diets.

Although a large number of user-friendly software packages are available, no one software package is ideal for all applications. Too often a nutrient calculation package is chosen on the basis of convenience of use rather than the quality of the data. Research nutritionists should carefully evaluate and test the quality of a nutrient analysis system before applying it to diet studies. The evaluation process should include a dem-

TABLE 11-3

Nutrient Content of Three Flavors of Kool-Aid® Soft Drink Mix[1]

Nutrient	Unit	Grape		Cherry		Lemon-Lime	
		Per 100 g[2]	Per Serving[3]	Per 100 g[2]	Per Serving[3]	Per 100 g[2]	Per Serving[3]
Energy[4]	kcal	211	98	210	98	215	98
Sugars (total)	g	0.5	25	<0.5	25	3.0	25
Vitamin C[5]	mg	1,089	6	1,095	6	1,097	6
Calcium[6]	mg	1,963	11	1,119	6	1,077	6
Phosphorus[6]	mg	870	5	512	3	493	3

[1]Manufacturer's data compiled by Janis Swain, MS, RD, Brigham and Women's Hospital, Boston, Mass.
[2]Dry soft drink mix without sugar.
[3]8 fluid oz of reconstituted beverage as prepared (0.140 oz package, 1 cup sugar, and cold water to make 2 quarts).
[4]The main sources of energy in unsweetened Kool-Aid® powder are citric acid and maltodextrin, carbohydrates that are not classified as sugars. (R. Cutrufelli, USDA Nutrient Data Laboratory, personal communication).
[5]The ascorbic acid content of soft drink powders can vary by twofold or more due to storage, manufacturing changes and other factors. Researchers who must control vitamin C intake should assay each batch directly. (R. Cutrufelli, USDA Nutrient Data Laboratory, personal communication).
[6]May be higher if local sources of water rather than deionized water are used.

onstration of the software facilities by the vendor and use of a demonstration disk or system for a trial period. The algorithms used for calculating the research diet must be clearly documented. In addition, the quality of the nutrient composition database used to calculate the diet must be evaluated. Some database factors worth considering are:

- The origin and nutrient completeness of the database.
- The accuracy of the nutrient information.
- The frequency with which nutrient composition data are updated.
- The number of food items included.
- The strategies used to estimate or impute missing nutrient data.
- The ability to add food items and nutrient values.
- The use of manufacturer's data in the database.
- The ability to create recipes with the existing food composition database files.
- The ability to add a recipe as a new record onto the food composition database.

Other factors to evaluate in a nutritional software package include program flexibility, performance speed, user interface, clarity of support material, completeness of nutrient reports, availability of technical support, and appearance and readability of printouts.

Databases with Software

Since 1976, annual National Nutrient Databank (NND) conferences have been held to address issues surrounding the use of nutrient databases. The organizers of the NND conference also produce a Nutrient Databank Directory (42) describing current commercial database systems. Although the features and contents of more than 50 software and database systems are listed in this directory, the directory makes no attempt to evaluate individual systems. Likewise, this manual makes no attempt to evaluate or endorse individual database programs.

Some programs that are widely used to calculate research diets are:

- CBORD Diet Analyzer (The CBORD Group, 61 Brown Road, Ithaca, NY 14850).
- Minnesota Nutrition Data System (NDS) (University of Minnesota, Nutrition Coordinating Center (NCC), 2221 University Avenue, SE, Ste 310, Minneapolis, MN 55414).
- Food Intake Analysis System (FIAS) (University of Texas, School of Public Health, PO Box 20186, Room W606, Houston, TX 77225).
- MENu Database Planning Software (Pennington Biomedical Research Center, Baton Rouge, LA 70808).
- Nutritionist IV (First Databank, The Hearst Corporation, San Bruno, CA 94066).
- Food Processor (ESHA Research, Salem, OR 97302).
- ProNutra Nutrient Analysis System for Metabolic Studies (Princeton Multimedia Technologies, Princeton, NJ).

For more information about database programs, refer to Chapter 3, "Computer Applications in Controlled Diet Studies." Also, professional journals often publish comparative database studies (43–48) that can provide guidelines in selecting an analysis system suitable for designing research diets.

Developing Computer Programs to Analyze Menus

Many metabolic units have found commercial database programs limiting or too costly to purchase. Thus, some research centers have elected to custom design a computer program to analyze research menus. Several steps are involved in this process before a system is available to calculate research diets.

Selecting a Database Management Program

First, the designer must decide what database management system (DBMS) will be used to store the food composition database. The system should be user friendly so that the nutritionist need not depend on a programmer to maintain the database or produce the programs to calculate the diet menu. Some database management packages that have been successfully used to store a food composition database and to create diet calculation programs are dBASE IV Plus®, Microsoft Access®, and SAS® (Statistical Analysis System).

Features to consider in selecting a DBMS include: What version of DOS (desktop operating system) or Microsoft Windows® is needed to operate this system? Is this a relational database management system (RDMS)? Will the system be able to handle meta-data (data about data)? Is the system interactive? Does it have pull-down menus? Is there a file linking capability? Are there entry windows? How many fields can one record contain? How many records can a file hold? Is there an automatic validation of field entry against a look-up file? Can the system provide graphical reports?

Selecting a Food Composition Database

Besides selecting a DBMS, one must select an appropriate food composition database to be the primary file in the calculation program. Most research facilities and database developers use the USDA Nutrient Data Base for Standard Reference in their microcomputer diet calculation programs (9, Exhibit 11-1). This continually updated database incorporates all revisions to Agriculture Handbook No. 8 and now supersedes the earlier print versions (10). Like Handbook 8, the data on this database are expressed per 100 grams of the edible portion of the food item. Included in the Standard Reference is a file that provides a description of the field arrangements for items on the records and a list of food descriptions and item numbers. The food descriptions and item numbers may serve as an online coding source or can be used to generate a paper copy for an in-house coding manual.

The database files for Standard Reference can be downloaded from the Nutrient Data Laboratory of the Beltsville Human Nutrition Research Center, US Department of Agriculture (http://www.nal.usda.gov/fnic/foodcomp). The complete version of Standard Reference is now available only in relational format (a change initiated with Release 11).

Checking Hardware Support Capabilities

After selecting a DBMS and an appropriate food composition database, the designer must calculate the amount of computer memory needed to support the DBMS and the food composition database files. Enough memory must be allotted for data processing and for file storage. In addition, older microcomputers should have math coprocessors to facilitate mathematical calculations. In some cases, hardware will need to be upgraded to support the DBMS and the food composition database. (For details on hardware and computer memory refer to Chapter 3, "Computer Applications in Controlled Diet Studies.")

Converting Food Composition Information into a DBMS File

Generally, in order to associate the food composition information file with the selected DBMS, the food composition files must be converted into files recognizable by the DBMS program. This conversion can be done by importing the food composition information into the DBMS, then saving the food composition information as a file or files with the configurations given by the DBMS.

Creating a Menu

Developing a menu for diet calculation can be done in two ways: a semiautomated method or an online automated method.

In the semiautomated method, the research nutritionist must first create a handwritten food list (Exhibit 11-5). Next, using a coding manual, the nutritionist selects the appropriate food code numbers for each of the menu item on the food list. Then, after a diet file is created, the following information is manually entered into a database management file: food description, food code number, meal sequence, menu day, and food amount. The file is saved after the last item on the food list is entered.

Although some research nutritionists prefer to design a diet by first listing on paper the foods to serve in a menu, it is more convenient to use an online automated method. The menu list is created by directly selecting foods for the menu from an online coding file. To do this, the designer must create a "diet list" file containing variable names such as food description and code number. Then, the designer must have ready a "coding" file that contains a complete list of food descriptions and code numbers for the foods stored in the "food composition" file. Next, using a file linking or multisegment approach, the diet list file and the coding file in the DBMS are simultaneously opened. To select foods from the coding file, the user scans through the foods in the coding file, selects the foods to be included into the diet list file by highlighting or flagging each food record needed, then duplicating the selected food items found in the coding file for the diet list file (Figure 11-1). Once the diet list is created, it can be modified to include information such as intake amounts for each food, meal sequence, and menu day.

Calculating Nutrient Composition

To calculate the nutrient composition of the proposed diet, the diet list file and the food composition file must be merged. The food code numbers on the diet list file are used to link each food to its corresponding nutrients in the food composition file. A diet calculation program can be written such that each code number in the diet list file is matched with the same code number in the food composition file (Figure 11-2). This type of match-up process is referred to as a *relational system*. For quality assurance, after the match-up process, the matched foods must be checked for entry and match-up accuracy.

When all the foods on the menu are linked with their corresponding nutrients, the computer can be programmed to perform an array of calculations. To generate a specific nutrient value for a specific amount of food fed, the proposed food amount from the diet list file must be multiplied with the nutrient values of that food (Table 11-4). To present nutrient intake information as a whole day's intake, the computer can be programmed to sum the values of one nutrient from all foods in the whole day's menu (Table 11-5). Depending on the needs, the calculation program can be written to give information that describes the nutritional values of the menu in a variety of formats. For example, a nutrient summary report can provide nutrient information on a per food item (Table 11-4), per day (Table 11-5), or per meal (Table 11-6) basis. The nutrient summary report also can provide intake statistics (Table 11-7), a review of nutrient deficiencies or excesses (as percent RDA), and an accounting of the frequency of missing nutrient values in a diet (Table 11-8).

Recipes used in research diets can be calculated and stored as records in the food composition file. As new studies are planned, one may adapt these existing recipes, which is more efficient than developing new recipes. Unlike the nutrient summation program, calculating a recipe may involve linking three or more files because of cooking losses/yields and nutrient retention problems (Figure 11-3). For example, if there are three files involved in a recipe calculation program, one of the files is a primary food composition file, whereas the other files are a "nutrient retention" file and a "moisture/fat gain/loss" file. A nutrient retention file should contain factors used to calculate the nutrient retention of vitamins and minerals after cooking. The CD-ROMs for the 1994 and 1996 Continuing Surveys of Food Intakes for In-

EXHIBIT 11-5

Food List for Computer Entry

Description of Diet: _____ Study Number: _____

Food Code	Food Description	Portion Size	Mealtime	Menu Day

dividuals contain a relational file based on an electronic version of the Provisional Table on Retention of Nutrients.

In a recipe, the amounts of vitamins and minerals retained in cooking will vary depending on the method of cooking, the length of cooking time, and the kind of preparation and treatment given to the food before cooking (49). It would be erroneous to calculate a recipe without applying a nutrient retention method in the calculation program. Data describing percentage of moisture or fat gain/loss are also important in recipe calculations. Most ingredients in a recipe are uncooked items that become part of a mixed dish. Without applying moisture and fat gain/loss factors, the actual dish served may be more or less nutrient-dense than the calculated recipe. Depending on the amount served, there may be great differences between calculated nutrient levels and true intake levels.

Comparison with Target Goals

Although the computer can facilitate the mathematical calculation of a research diet, producing a diet that provides nutrients at specified levels is no easy task. Even with the computer performing most of the calculations, planning a research diet is largely a trial-and-error process. After menu items are transformed into nutrient information via nutrient calculation and summary programs, nutrient levels of each menu must be compared with the target goals. Generally, it takes several diet modifications and computer runs before a satisfactory menu is produced. For more complex diet designs, the diet manipulation and calculation process can take days of work.

Although there is no easy way to make the comparison between the calculated results and the target goals, the com-

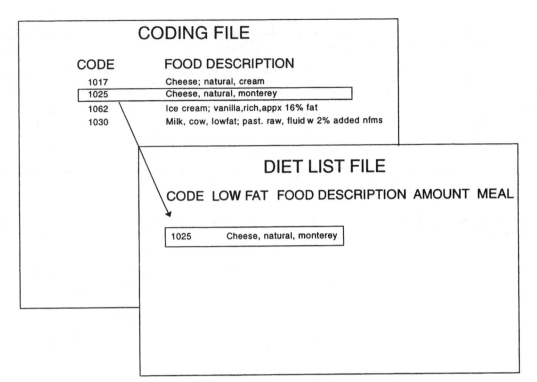

FIGURE 11-1.   Selecting foods from coding file to create the diet list file.

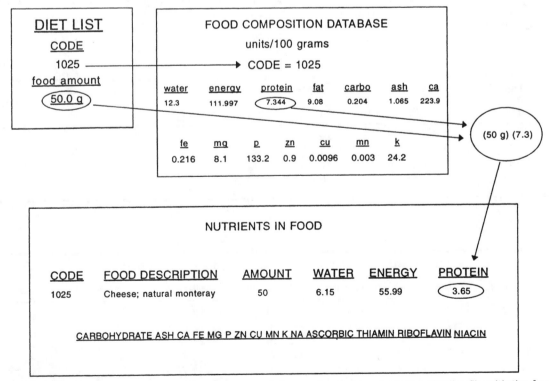

FIGURE 11-2.   The diet calculation program matches code numbers from the diet list file with the food composition file.

TABLE 11-4

Nutrient Content of Foods for Lunch: Menu Day 7

Meal	Food Item	Amount (g)	Energy (kcal)	Protein (g)	Fat (g)	Carbohydrate	Code
L	Bread, pita	50	142.00	4.55	1.50	27.00	3542.1
L	Turkey breast, rst slice	60	94.20	17.94	1.93	0.00	5186.0
L	Cheese, jack, sliced	30	112.00	7.34	9.08	0.204	1025.0
L	Cake, chocolate	94	337.50	4.23	14.60	52.10	526.4
L	Milk, low-fat	170	86.65	5.92	3.26	8.45	1080.0

TABLE 11-5

Nutrient Content of Menu Day 7

Variable	Amount
Food Amount (g)	1711.00
Water from Food (g)	1259.00
Energy (kcal)	2098.90
Protein (g)	77.50
Total Fat (g)	78.26
Carbohydrate (g)	283.71
Protein (% Energy)	14.77
Fat (% Energy)[1]	33.56
Carbohydrate (% Energy)	54.07
Saturated Fat (% Energy)	14.20
Total Monounsaturated Fat (% Energy)	10.10
Total Polyunsaturated Fat (% Energy)	10.90
P:S Ratio	0.4
Calcium (mg)	717.70
Calcium (% RDA)	59.75

[1]The sum of saturated, monounsaturated and polyunsaturated fat usually is less than the total fat content (ie, about 90%). Total fat values include not only saturated, monounsaturated, and polyunsaturated fatty acids but also mono- and diglycerides, phospholipids, and short chain and branched chain fatty acids.

TABLE 11-6

Macronutrient Distribution of a 2,200-kcal Diet by Meal

Meal	Energy (kcal)	Protein (g)	Fat (g)	Carbohydrate (g)
Breakfast	517	10.99	22.86	76.11
Lunch	721	13.73	41.35	47.12
Dinner	645	18.68	40.08	42.05
PM snack	298	4.72	18.05	79.30

TABLE 11-7

Statistics Report: Mean and Standard Deviation of Selected Nutrients (7-day Menu)

Variable	Unit	Days (N)	Minimum	Maximum	Mean	Std Deviation
Food Amount	g	7	1,547	1,715	1,647	81
Water	g	7	1,120	1,259	1,196	68
Energy	kcal	7	2,067	2,099	2,098	1
Protein	g	7	70	78	75	4
Fat	g	7	58	89	76	13
Carbohydrate	g	7	257	320	290	26

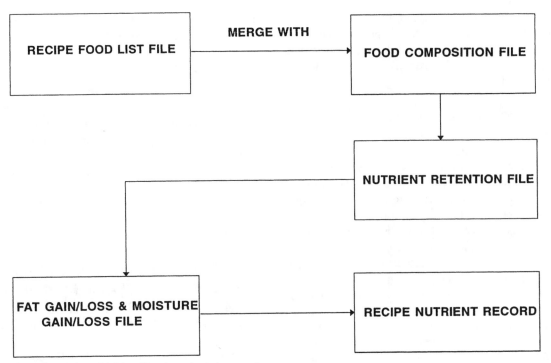

FIGURE 11-3.   Linking files to calculate a recipe.

puter can be used to report percentage of goal (that is, the fraction each calculated nutrient level is above or below its target). Sometimes, to achieve the target goal, the nutritionist may need to modify the menu by adding new foods, substituting foods, increasing amounts of foods, or eliminating foods from a menu. To do this on the computer, food intake amounts in the diet list file may need to be manually modified before another computer nutrient analysis is performed.

For some research studies, no matter how many times a diet is manipulated and recalculated, the target nutrient levels will never be achieved until a specialty item is used. For example, to feed a large amount of saturated fatty acids in a low-fat diet, a highly saturated margarine may need to be added to the menu. Most likely, this margarine will need to be specially prepared by a manufacturer for the study. Another example is a protocol that specifies study participants are to be fed three diets differing only in selenium content. Except for the selenium level of the diets, nutrient content and food quantities in all three diets must remain the same. To achieve these specifications, specially grown high-

selenium-content wheat and low-selenium-content wheat must be included in the diets. (Also see the discussion of modified and experimental foods in Chapter 12, "Producing Research Diets.")

Sometimes, in order to meet nutrient target levels, an investigator might use nutrient loss or retention information to create the control necessary for a research diet. Consider, for example, a study conducted to assess the effect of animal or plant protein sources on the vitamin B-6 requirement of young women (50, 51). Strictly controlled, conventional food, 3-day cycle diets with protein from animal or from plant sources were fed during four repletion periods. Both repletion diets were calculated to provide a 0.5 mg per day of vitamin B-6, and a multiple vitamin and mineral supplement devoid of vitamin B-6 was fed daily to the volunteers. The difficulty in designing this diet was that when protein intake levels were met, vitamin B-6 intake exceeded the target level. Through the use of nutrient retention information, special cooking procedures were devised to lower the vitamin B-6 content of the foods. All poultry, beans, and

TABLE 11-8

Missing Nutrient Values in Menu Day 7

Nutrient	Percent of Foods with Missing Value
Carbohydrate	0
Fat	0
Protein	0
Vitamin A (IU)	6
Vitamin A (RE)	24
Vitamin E	67

vegetables were boiled and drained three times before serving. Poultry was skinned and boiled prior to the three cooking treatments. Microbiological assay confirmed that the boiling procedure was effective in reducing the vitamin B-6 content in the foods tested.

Developing the Purchasing List

Once a diet is calculated and accepted for a research study, a purchasing list must be developed. It is critical that foods purchased for a research study are exact matches with the food items coded for the nutrient calculations. The simplest way to create this exact match list is to append and merge foods from all menus in the study into one file. The purchasing list in this file should identify each food used in a menu cycle, along with the food code, a full food composition description of the food, and the food amount to be served to one participant. A simple program can be written to help tabulate, by food code, the amount of each food needed on a weekly basis for the entire study. In addition, this tabulation program can be written to show the number of times each food is served during a menu cycle or the amount of food required at each calorie level. Furthermore, the purchasing list can be converted into an inventory list for use throughout the study or a work flow planner for the dietary staff.

Using Food Subsets to Develop Menus

From experience, the most efficient way to use a computer to design a research diet that will meet study specifications is to create two subsets of foods for each day's menu. One subset should consist of *core foods,* which are served on all diets and contain relatively small amounts of the nutrients under investigation. The other subset should contain *modifiable foods,* which are rich in the nutrients under study, and whose quantities and composition can be manipulated to accommodate most of the required variability in the experimental diets. The foods comprising these subsets, and the quantities needed, are determined through a series of iterations that bring the calculated diet successively closer and closer to the design targets.

Example: Following is background information for a test diet high in saturated fat. Consider a study requiring two double-blinded dietary treatments that differ in fat content. For a 2-week (14-day) menu cycle, the average energy distribution of both diets should be: 36% of calories from fat, 15% from protein, and 48% from carbohydrate. The average cholesterol content should be 400 mg/day. For the Saturated Fat Diet, the energy distribution (%kcal) of saturated (S), monounsaturated (M), and polyunsaturated (P) fatty acids should be: S 19%: M 11%: P 6%. For the Monounsaturated Fat Diet, the energy distribution from fatty acids is S 11%: M 19%: P 6%. Oleic acid (18:1) is the predominant monounsaturated fatty acid in the diet, and linoleic acid (18:2) is the predominant polyunsaturated fatty acid. The design target for the Saturated Fat Diet specifies that 3% of energy should be provided by stearic acid (18:0); there is no target value for the other saturated fatty acids.

Preliminary Activities

Menu designers should verify that the available food composition databases and software packages contain appropriate information for all potential study foods. The database should also include the composition of any foods prepared from special study recipes.

The designer chooses one energy level for calculating the sample diet; this typically is the most common calorie level, or the one that forms the best basis for adjusting the other energy levels. (The sample menus provided here are based on 3,000 kcal/day).

Separating the Foods for Each Menu into Core Food and Modifiable Food Subsets

The menu designer first identifies the foods that are candidates for use in each subset, then estimates likely portion sizes for each food.

In this example (see Table 11-9), the core foods contain relatively small amounts of fat, or their fat content cannot easily be adjusted through recipe changes. The modifiable foods subset contains foods such as baked goods, table spreads, and salad dressings, because these are excellent vehicles for presenting the special test fats (special margarines, oils, and shortenings) that are used to achieve the required fatty acid distribution.

The modifiable foods subset should provide most of the test nutrient needed to achieve the design target. In the example below, the modifiable foods subset is expected to provide about three fourths of total dietary fat, or approximately 90 g (810 kcal).

First Iteration: Quantities of Foods from Each Subset

The first iteration comprises the following steps:

1. Start with the core foods subset. Using the likely portion sizes as estimated above, calculate their nutrient content. (The core foods for the Saturated Fat Diet and their fat content are shown in Table 11-10.)
2. Repeat this process for the modifiable foods subset. (Fat-rich modifiable foods are shown in Table 11-11.) This first iteration yielded 83 g of fat, slightly below the target of 90 g.
3. Next, evaluate the results of the first iteration by adding the contributions from the two food subsets and compare the results with the target values.

In the example shown here (see Table 11-12), total fat was higher than desired (because the core foods subset contained slightly more total fat than originally expected), whereas saturated fat was lower than desired (because the modifiable foods subset contained less saturated fat than originally expected).

TABLE 11-9

Food Subsets for the Design of Fat-Modified Menus

Core Foods Subset	Modifiable Foods Subset[1]
Meats	Baked goods
Vegetables	Spreads
Grains	Salad dressings
Fruits	Snacks
Dairy products, low-fat	Dairy products, high fat
Eggs[1]	Eggs[2]

[1]In this example, the modifiable foods subset includes foods that have a high content of fat as well as foods whose fat composition or content is relatively easy to alter.
[2]Eggs (as whole eggs, yolks, and/or whites) can be used as needed in either subset to meet design specifications.

TABLE 11-10

Core Foods Subset for Saturated Fat Diet (3,000-kcal/day); Fat Content, First Iteration for Menu Day 3

Fat (g)	Portion (g)	Food Description[1]
0.061	103	Orange juice; added calcium, frozen concentrate, diluted 1:3
10.594	34	Sausage; pork, links or bulk, cooked
0.028	28	Jelly; other than guava
9.446	492	Milk; cow; pasteurized, fluid, 2% fat
9.513	90	Pork products; ham, cured, boneless, regular (approx. 11% fat)
0.550	50	Bread; rye, made with nonhydrogenated soybean oil
0.047	25	Lettuce; iceberg (includes crisp head types), raw
0.148	45	Tomatoes; red, ripe, raw, year-round average
5.355	150	Chicken; broilers or fryers, breast, meat only, cooked, roasted
4.052	20	Gravy, turkey; made with moderate oleic acid content mayonnaise (Test Fat)
0.250	250	Potatoes; baked, flesh and skin, without salt
0.066	60	Broccoli; frozen, spears, cooked, boiled, drained, without salt
0.104	55	Lettuce; iceberg (includes crisp head types), raw
0.148	45	Tomatoes; red, ripe, raw, year-round average
1.543	5	Eggs; chicken, yolk, raw, fresh
0.550	25	Bread, cracked wheat, made with nonhydrogenated soybean oil
4.723	246	Milk; cow, pasteurized, fluid, 2% fat
0.000	12	Sugar; beet or cane, granulated
0.597	166	Apples; raw, with skin
47.775	—	Total, all items

[1]Foods listed several times are served at different meals.

TABLE 11-11

Modifiable Foods Subset for Saturated Fat Diet (3,000-kcal/day); Fat Content, First Iteration for Menu Day 3

Fat (g)	Portion (g)	Food Description[1]
13.018	165	Blueberry muffins, made with coconut oil (Test Fat)
15.960	20	Margarine, high-saturated-fat (Test Fat)
9.448	14	Mustard spread, made with high-saturated-fat margarine (Test Fat)
20.557	75	Oatmeal cookies, made with high-saturated-fat margarine (Test Fat)
3.087	10	Eggs; chicken, yolk, raw
5.442	30	Chocolate mayonnaise cake, made with high-oleic-acid mayonnaise (Test Fat)
15.960	20	Margarine, high-saturated-fat (Test Fat)
83.472	—	Total, all items

[1]Foods listed several times are served at different meals.

TABLE 11-12

Core Foods + Modifiable Foods Subsets (Total Diet) for Saturated Fat Diet (3,000-kcal/day); Fat and Energy Content, First Iteration for Menu Day 3[1]

	Energy Distribution (% kcal)		Nutrient Content (g/3,000 kcal)	
	Target	Calculated	Target	Calculated
Calories	3,000	3,036	—	—
Fat, total	36	38.5	118	130
Fat, saturated	19	14.8	63	50
Fatty Acids				
Stearic	3	2.7	9	9
Oleic	11	13.1	36	44
Linoleic	6	6.9	19	23
Other[2]	16	13.6	54	46

[1]Values may not add to 100% because of rounding.
[2]Other fatty acids: exclusive of 18:0 (stearic), 18:1 (oleic), 18:2 (linoleic).

Subsequent Iterations: Adjust Items and Quantities of Subset Foods

Later iterations fine-tune the food amounts and measure calculated and target values for the diet:

1. Revise the type and amounts of foods in both subsets if the nutrient values of highest interest (in this case, total fat and saturated fat) do not meet target levels.
2. In later iterations, focus on the quantities and composition of the items in the Modifiable Foods Subset (see Table 11-13).
3. After each iteration, compare the calculated and target values for the entire diet (comprising both the core foods and modifiable foods subsets) to assess whether the goals have been reached.

In this example, several modifications were made to the foods comprising the subset: the high oleic acid mayonnaise chocolate cake was deleted; a portion of coconut oil was added; portion sizes of high-saturated-fat margarine were reduced; coconut oil-based salad dressing was added; and the quantity of egg yolk was reduced to adjust the cholesterol content. (Note: To construct a corresponding Monounsaturated Fat Diet, test fats rich in oleic acid would be used.) The results of these changes are shown in Table 11-14: after multiple iterations, the calculated composition of the entire sample menu, based on the contribution of all food subsets, is close to the target values. Note, for later discussion on chemical analysis of diets, the discrepancy between target and calculated values for total fat.

In actual practice, after the modifiable foods are ad-

TABLE 11-13

Modifiable Foods Subset for Saturated Fat Diet (3,000-kcal/day); Fat Content, Final Iteration for Menu Day 3

Fat (g)	Portion (g)	Food Description[1]
13.018	165	Blueberry muffins, made with coconut oil (Test Fat)
11.172	14	Margarine, high-saturated-fat (Test Fat)[2]
9.448	14	Mustard spread, made with high-saturated-fat margarine (Test Fat)
20.557	75	Oatmeal cookies, made with high-saturated-fat margarine (Test Fat)
1.543	5	Eggs; chicken, yolk, raw[2,3]
10.041	30	Salad dressing or dip, made with coconut oil (Test Fat)[2]
10.000	10	Coconut oil (Test Fat)[2]
11.97	15	Margarine, high-saturated-fat (Test Fat)[2]
87.749	—	Total, all items

[1]Foods listed several times are served at different meals.
[2]Amount changed or new food added. In this example, compare with food list in Table 11-11 and note: deletion of chocolate cake made with high-oleic-acid mayonnaise; addition of coconut oil test fat in several forms; decrease in portion size for high-saturated-fat margarine; and decrease in portion size of egg yolk (see footnote 3).
[3]Egg yolk decreased from 10 g to 5 g to effect a decrease in cholesterol content from 454 mg/day to 386 mg/day. (In this example, the design target for cholesterol is 400 mg/day.)

TABLE 11-14

Core Foods + Modifiable Foods Subsets (Total Diet) of Saturated Fat Diet (3,000-kcal/day) for Fat and Energy Content[1], Final Iteration for Menu Day 3[1]

	Energy Distribution (% kcal)		Nutrient Content (g/3,000 kcal)	
	Target	Calculated	Target	Calculated
Calories	3000	3019	—	—
Total Fat	36	39.9	118	134
Saturated Fat	19	18.2	63	61
Fatty Acids				
Stearic	3	2.7	9	9
Oleic	11	11.2	36	38
Linoleic	6	6.3	19	21
Other[2]	16	17.6	54	59

[1]Values may not add to 100% because of rounding.
[2]Other fatty acids: exclusive of 18:0 (stearic), 18:1 (oleic), 18:2 (linoleic).

justed the dietary levels of all relevant nutrients must be evaluated; further iterations may be necessary if any do not meet target values. The example shown in Tables 11-9 through 11-14 has been simplified for didactic purposes and focuses on dietary fat composition and content, but the protein and carbohydrate levels also are components of the overall dietary design and also must ultimately meet the requirements of the study design.

The complexity (ie, difficulty and cost) of the iterative calculation process varies with the dietary software packages and other computer support available. It often is advisable to first use simpler ways to estimate or otherwise "try out" contemplated changes in the core foods and modifiable foods subsets. One approach is to use a calculator. Also, if the user is familiar with linear programming, a linear equation can be written to calculate the amounts of food needed to meet target variable levels; this technique has the potential to reduce the needed number of computer iterations. (Also see the discussion of computer-assisted menu planning in Chapter 3, "Computer Applications in Controlled Diet Studies.")

Reviewing the Menu Cycle and Verifying Composition through Chemical Assay

The review process encompasses the following:

1. Summarize the calculated (estimated) nutrient content of the entire menu cycle, and calculate descriptive statistics such as mean, median, and range.
2. Verify nutrient content through direct chemical analysis.
3. Determine which menus fall within acceptable limits. Menus not meeting necessary design or production standards should be discarded or adjusted (reformulated or recalculated).
4. Calculate the menus for the other calorie levels that are needed to meet participants' energy requirements. Using menus that have been determined to be acceptable, scale

the portions as needed (ie, make proportional adjustments in the serving sizes for each food item).

The ultimate goal of this process is an entire cycle of menus whose average composition (determined by chemical assay) closely approximates the design target (see Table 11-15). It is not unusual to observe some variation between the calculated values and the assayed composition. Often this reflects the difference between the average values in the nutrient database used to calculate the diets compared with the composition of the specific foods used to construct the diets. (In Table 11-15, the assayed fat content is lower than the calculated fat content.) Using the foods subset approach provides a convenient means of creating such an appropriately designed cycle menu for each dietary treatment. Thus, on any given day of the study described in the example, all diets will have the same meats, vegetables, salads, and breads, but each treatment will provide baked goods, sauces, salad dressings, spreads, and dessert toppings with differing composition.

The painstaking process of estimation and refinement must be carried out separately for each study menu (this example only shows the iterations for Menu Day 3). Numerous (five or more) successive iterations may be necessary until the design targets are reached. So many factors can constrain the design of appealing diets that it is highly recommended that extra menus be designed; it is likely that several will not be usable. Not only must the calculations result in a satisfactory nutrient composition but the recipes and portion sizes must also be palatable as well as practical for delivering to the study participants.

Linear Programming Approaches

Research diets traditionally are formulated by first defining a list of foods to use in a diet and then calculating the nutrient composition of the proposed diet. As described earlier, if the

TABLE 11-15

Core Foods + Modifiable Foods Subsets (Total Diet) of Saturated Fat Diet (3,000-kcal/day), Average Composition of 14-day Menu Cycle[1]

	Energy Distribution (% kcal)			Nutrient Content (g/3,000 kcal)		
	Target	Calculated	Assayed	Target	Calculated	Assayed
Protein	15	15.1	15.2	112	113	114
Carbohydrate	48	46.0	48.7	352	345	365
Total Fat	36	39.9	36.1	118	134	120
Saturated Fat	19	18.2	17.2	63	61	57.5
Fatty Acids						
Stearic	3	2.7	2.7	9	9	9.1
Oleic	11	11.2	10.6	36	38	35.5
Linoleic	6	6.3	5.8	19	21	19.2
Other[2]	16	17.6	16.5	54	59	54.9

[1]Values may not add to 100% because of rounding.
[2]Other fatty acids: exclusive of 18:0 (stearic), 18:1 (oleic), 18:2 (linoleic).

total nutrient values exceed or fall below required values, food quantities are altered or exchanged and the diet recalculated. Calculations are repeated as often as necessary until a suitable diet meeting all nutrient levels is obtained. One way to simplify this tedious task is to allow the computer to calculate the research diet, a process called *linear programming*. (Also see the discussion of computer-assisted menu planning in Chapter 3, "Computer Applications in Controlled Diet Studies.")

Although linear programming techniques have been used successfully to calculate formula diets (51), using linear programming to formulate conventional food diets is a much more complicated task. In calculating a formula diet, the function of the linear program is to find estimates by fitting the linear equations with various iterations until all given conditions are satisfied. In formulating a conventional food diet, a linear program is first written to eliminate or select foods based on set nutrient criteria. Then, linear equations must be set for each target nutrient variable. A logical definition for frequency of use of foods and serving limits must also be set. A subset of foods must then be developed to be used in the linear equation to help adjust the nutrient requirements.

Once a diet is produced by linear programming, sample meals must be prepared and evaluated for portion size and palatability. For formula diets, it would be wise to generate several combinations of different ratios of chemical salts to produce several different formulas. From these formulas, the most palatable formula should be selected based on a taste test. (Also see Chapter 14, "Planning and Producing Formula Diets.")

CONCLUSION

This chapter has addressed various aspects of nutrient data and the use of computers to design research diets. Food da-

tabases provide data for an ever-increasing array of nutrients and for an ever-increasing number of food items. Nutritionists must have a full understanding of the degree of accuracy of these data, as well as the computer skills to form this basic information into carefully defined research diets. A skillful blend of science and art underlies the exercise of designing a simple yet tasteful research diet that creatively meets the scientific requirements of the protocol.

REFERENCES

1. National Research Council Food and Nutrition Board. *Recommended Dietary Allowances.* 10th ed. Washington, DC: National Academy of Sciences; 1989.
2. Yates AA, Schlicker SA, Suitor CW. Dietary reference intakes: the new basis for recommendations for calcium and related nutrients, B vitamins, and choline. *J Am Diet Assoc.* 1998;98:699–706.
3. *National Cholesterol Education Program Report of the Expert Panel on Population Strategies for Blood Cholesterol Reduction.* Bethesda, Md: US Department of Health and Human Services, NIH publication 90–3046; 1990.
4. Butrum RR, Clifford CK, Lanza E: National Cancer Institute dietary guidelines: rationale. *Am J Clin Nutr.* 1988;48:888–895.
5. Cleveland LE, Goldman JD, Borrud LG. *Data Tables: Results from USDA's 1994 Continuing Survey of Food Intakes by Individuals and 1994 Diet and Health Knowledge Survey.* Agricultural Research Service, US Department of Agriculture; 1996.
6. Woteki CE, Briefel RB, Kuczmarski R. Contributions of the National Center for Health Statistics. *Am J Clin Nutr.* 1988;97:320–328.
7. US Department of Health and Human Services. National Center for Health Statistics. NHANES III refer-

ence manuals and reports (CD-ROM). Hyattsville, Md: Centers for Disease Control and Prevention; 1996. Available from National Technical Information Service (NTIS), Springfield, Va. Acrobat.PDF format; includes access software: Adobe Systems, Inc. Acrobat Reader 2.1.

8. US Department of Health and Human Services. National Center for Health Statistics. *Third National Health and Nutrition Examination Survey, 1988–94,* Series 11 Number 1A, ASCII Version or Number 1A, SETS Version 1.22a. Hyattsville, Md: Centers for Disease Control and Prevention, July 1997. Available from the National Technical Information Service, Springfield, Va.

9. US Department of Agriculture. *Nutrient Database for Standard Reference,* Release 12 (SR-12). Riverdale, Md: Agricultural Research Service; 1998.

10. US Department of Agriculture. *Composition of Foods: Raw, Processed, Prepared. Agriculture Handbook No. 8.* Washington, DC: US Government Printing Office; 1976–1993.

11. Merrill AL, Watt BK. *Energy Value of Foods—Basis and Derivation.* Rev. US Department of Agriculture, Agriculture Handbook No. 74, 105 pp. Washington, DC: US Government Printing Office; 1973.

12. Perloff B. USDA's National Nutrient Data Bank. *Proceedings of the Fifteenth National Nutrient Databank Conference.* Blacksburg, Va: The CBORD Group, Inc; 1990:11–17.

13. Jones DB. *Factors for Converting Percentages of Nitrogen in Foods and Feeds into Percentages of Protein.* US Department of Agriculture, Cir. No. 83, Washington, DC; 1941.

14. *Improvement of Protein Nutriture.* Washington, DC: National Academy Press; 1974.

15. Li BW. Dietary fiber methodologies: status and controversial issues. *Proceedings of the Fifteenth National Nutrient Databank Conference.* Blacksburg, Va: The Cbord Group, Inc; 1990:19–29.

16. *Official Methods of Analysis,* 16th ed. Arlington, Va: AOAC International; 1995.

17. Dreher ML. *Handbook of Dietary Fiber: An Applied Approach.* New York, NY: Marcel Dekker, Inc; 1987.

18. Marlett JA. Content and composition of dietary fiber in 117 frequently consumed foods. *J Am Diet Assoc.* 1992;92:175–186.

19. Food Guide Pyramid: A Guide to Daily Food Choices. Washington, DC: US Department of Agriculture/US Department of Health and Human Services; 1992.

20. Colditz GA, Giovannucci E, Rimm EB, et al. Alcohol intake in relation to diet and obesity in women and men. *Am J Clin Nutr.* 1991;54:49–55.

21. Crouse JR, Grundy SM. Effects of alcohol on plasma lipoproteins and cholesterol and triglyceride metabolism in man. *J Lipid Res.* 1984;25:486–496.

22. Lieber CS. Perspectives: do alcohol calories count? *Am J Clin Nutr.* 1991;54:976–982.

23. Rumpler WV, Rhodes DG, Baer DJ, et al. Energy value of moderate alcohol consumption by humans. *Am J Clin Nutr.* 1996;64:108–114.

24. Brook M, Grimshaw JJ. Vitamin C concentrations of plasma and leukocytes as related to smoking habit, age, and sex of human. *Am J Clin Nutr.* 1968;21:1254–1258.

25. Kallner AB, Hartmann D, Horning DH. On other requirements of ascorbic acid in man: steady-state turnover and body pool in smokers. *Am J Clin Nutr.* 1981;34:1347–1355.

26. Heaney RP, Gallager JC, Johnston CC, et al. Calcium nutrition and bone health in the elderly. *Am J Clin Nutr.* 1982;36:986–1013.

27. Rose DP: Effects of oral contraceptives on nutrient utilization. In: Hathcock JN, Coon J, eds. *Nutrition and Drug Interrelations.* New York, NY: Academic Press; 1978.

28. Gershoff SN, Brusis OA, Nino HV, et al. Studies of the elderly in Boston. I. The effects of iron fortification on moderately anemic people. *Am J Clin Nutr.* 1977; 30:226–234.

29. O'Hanlon P, Khors MB. Dietary studies of older Americans. *Am J Clin Nutr.* 1978;31:1257–1269.

30. US Food and Drug Administration. *Food Standards: amendment of Standards of Identity for Enriched Grain Products to Require Addition of Folic Acid.* Washington, DC: Code of Federal Regulation, Title 21; 1996:136, 137.

31. Souci SW, Fachmann W, Kraut H. *Food Composition and Nutrition Tables 1986/87.* Stuttgart, Germany: Wissenschaftliche Verlagsgesellschaft; 1986.

32. Holland B, Welch AA, Unwin ID, et al. *McCance and Widdowson's The Composition of Foods.* United Kingdom; 1992.

33. Mangels AR, Holden JM, Beecher GR, et al. Carotenoid content of fruits and vegetables: an evaluation of analytic data. *J Am Diet Assoc.* 1993;93:284–296.

34. Holden JM, Gebhardt S, Davis CS, Lurie DG. A nationwide study of the selenium contents and variability in white bread. *J Food Comp Anal.* 1991;4:183–195.

35. Krebs-Smith SM, Guenther PM, Cook A, et al. *Foods Commonly Eaten in the United States: Quantities Consumed per Eating Occasion and in a Day, 1989–91.* NFS Report No 91–3. Riverdale, Md: US Department of Agriculture; 1998.

36. Judd JT, Clevidence BA, Muesing RA, et al. Dietary *trans* fatty acids and plasma lipids and lipoproteins of healthy adult men and women fed a controlled diet. *Am J Clin Nutr.* 1994;59:861–868.

37. Rand WM. Food composition data: problems and plans. *J Am Diet Assoc.* 1985;85:1081–1083.

38. Soergel D, Pennington JAT, McCann A, et al. A network model for improving access to food and nutrition data. *J Am Diet Assoc.* 1992;92:78–82.

39. Barr SL, Ramakrishnan R, Johnson C, et al. Reducing total dietary fat without reducing saturated fatty acids

does not significantly lower total plasma cholesterol concentrations in normal males. *Am J Clin Nutr.* 1992;55:675–681.

40. Carpentieri CR, Hannah J, Bente L, et al. Dietary compliance in an outpatient feeding study. *FASEB J.* 1994;8:A184.

41. Turner D. *Handbook of Diet Therapy.* Chicago, Ill: The University of Chicago Press; 1965:221.

42. Smith J, ed. *Nutrient Databank Directory.* 9th ed. Newark, Del: University of Delaware; 1993.

43. Shanklin D, Endres JM, Sawicki M. A comparative study of two nutrient data bases. *J Am Diet Assoc.* 1985;85:308–313.

44. Nieman DC, Nieman CN. A comparative study of two microcomputer nutrient data bases with the USDA Nutrient Data Base for Standard Reference. *J Am Diet Assoc.* 1987;87:930–931.

45. Eck LH, Klesges RC, Hanson CL, et al. A comparison of four commonly used nutrient database programs. *J Am Diet Assoc.* 1988;88:602–604.

46. Frank GC, Farris RP, Berenson GS. Comparison of dietary intake by 2 computerized analysis systems. *J Am Diet Assoc.* 1984;84:818–819.

47. O'Brien J. Problems in nutritional analysis. *Trends Food Sci Tech.* 1991;2:283–285.

48. Klensin JC. Information technology and food composition databases. *Trends Food Sci Tech.* 1991;2:279–282.

49. Matthews RH, Garrison YJ. Food yields summarized by different stages of preparation. *Agriculture Handbook No. 102.* Washington, DC: U.S. Department of Agriculture; 1975.

50. Kretsch MJ, Sauberlich HE, Newbrun E. Electroencephalographic changes and periodontal status during short-term vitamin B-6 depletion of young, nonpregnant women. *Am J Clin Nutr.* 1991;53:1266–1274.

51. Fong AKH. Food composition databanks: important considerations in designing metabolic research diets. *Proceedings of the 17th National Nutrient Databank Conference.* Baltimore, Md: The CBORD Group, Inc; 1992:90–104.

CHAPTER 12

PRODUCING RESEARCH DIETS

BEVERLY A. CLEVIDENCE, PhD; ARLINE D. SALBE, PhD, RD; KAREN TODD, MS, RD;
ALICE K. H. FONG, EdD, RD; LINDA J. BRINKLEY, RD; JANIS F. SWAIN, MS, RD; AND
CYNTHIA SEIDMAN, MS, RD

FOOD PROCUREMENT AND STORAGE

Procuring food is a fundamental aspect of producing research diets—one that is more complex and challenging than it might appear. A major priority in food procurement is to ensure constancy of the nutrients of interest throughout the course of the study. It is common to purchase food items from single lots, in quantities sufficient for the entire study. In some tightly controlled studies this includes all food items except those that are highly perishable (eg, milk or fresh fruit). In studies requiring less control, fewer food items—perhaps only test foods—are purchased and used with this degree of control.

    If a study is designed to feed all participants collectively (eg, 20 participants studied on an outpatient basis for 4 weeks), then a facility's ability to provide constancy of food items is typically limited by storage space. If the study is to be carried out in an intermittent or extended fashion (eg, 1 or 2 participants per month) constancy in food procurement is also limited by storage space, but it is further compounded by the need to guarantee food freshness and nutrient stability over time. Shelf-life, storage space, and freshness are critical considerations for most studies.

Purchasing According to Needs and Storage Capacity

Raw and Cooked Weight

When considering the quantity of food to be purchased, study designers must first be aware of whether the calculations for the nutrients of interest are based on the raw or cooked weight of the food items. When participants are studied individually, food may be prepared on a participant-by-participant basis. In this case, calculations may be based on raw weights, which simplifies the determination of quantity of food to be purchased. In larger facilities in which numerous participants are studied concurrently, however, foods may be cooked as a unit for multiple participants and then portioned prior to service. In addition, mixed dishes such as meat loaves, casseroles, soups, and sauces may be used if recipes are analyzed and scaled for the appropriate number of servings. If the cooked weight is known, then the appropriate calculations can be made to convert to raw weight after considering losses or gains during preparation and cooking.

Purchasing Sufficient Amounts of Food

In procuring food for research studies, it is prudent to err on the side of overpurchasing; running out of a food item can be a crisis for a well-controlled feeding study. Dietitians typically make a "best estimate" of the amount of each food item needed for a study and then ensure adequate quantities by adding a "safety" (or caution) factor. The best estimate is based on edible portions of foods as purchased; for example, an 8-oz (227-g) can of green beans may only contain 180 g edible weight of green beans. Lean cuts of beef may be further trimmed in the research kitchen to yield smaller portions.

The safety factor must be adequate to cover any differences between estimated and actual food requirements; safety factors are not a substitute for making best estimates that are as accurate as possible. Typically, estimated food requirements are increased by 25% to guarantee that sufficient quantities are purchased. This safety factor should account for the number of diets to be used for composites, food spoilage, food that might be unexpectedly wasted during preparation, and food that might be wasted because of meal delays. The size of this safety factor may vary depending on the particular food item. For example, a smaller safety factor would be needed for dry goods such as pasta, rice, and beans, which generally have a long shelf-life, and a longer safety factor would be needed for poultry.

The safety factor may also vary with the number of participants to be fed. In this situation, the principle of *economy of scale* must be considered: when planning for 10 participants, a safety factor of 25% may be sufficient, but when planning for 1 or 2 participants, a safety factor of 50% may be necessary. For example, a 25% safety factor applied to the amount of food consumed by 30 participants would easily provide sufficient food for triplicate composites of foods from each of two dietary treatments, whereas a 50% safety factor applied to the food consumed by 1 participant may be necessary if triplicate composites are to be made.

Storage Capacity and Shelf-Life

The capacity of the storage facility is of vital importance in considering the amount of food that can be purchased at one time. The purchasing agent must also consider the form in which these items are to be stored; eg, does the food need refrigeration or freezing; will it be kept in cans or as dry bulk items? Other considerations are these:

- Most meats will be portioned prior to freezer storage, whereas canned items typically do not need to be portioned until just prior to serving.
- Items such as breads and meats will require adequate freezer space.
- Canned items may be easiest to store because they require the least accommodation.
- Dry goods such as cookies, cereals, sugar, dry milk powder, rice, and pasta will need space that is reliably cool, dry, well-ventilated, and protected against insect invasion.
- Food items that come individually packaged in portion-controlled servings may stay fresher for a longer period than those packaged in family-sized or institutional por-

tions. However, items that come in portion-controlled servings may require reweighing prior to serving.

If storage capacity for all items is limited, then this factor may constrain the number of participants that can be studied at any one time. To minimize intraparticipant variability, it is essential that each participant eat exactly the same food over the course of his or her individual study. Although it is desirable for all participants in a research study to eat exactly the same food from a common lot regardless of when they are studied, this may not always be possible. Every effort, therefore, should be made to purchase the same brands of dairy products and staples and the same cuts of meat. If differing food lots are used for different participants throughout the course of a study, variance in nutrient intake among participants can be detected by assaying diet composites that have been collected over time.

The shelf-life of each food also must be considered when staff decide how much to purchase. Table 12-1 provides maximum storage times for foods typically stocked for research diets. In addition, many food items will have the "out-date" or last usable date stamped on the container, which provides additional information about expected storage times.

Dry goods and canned foods are subject to deterioration through the process of nonenzymatic browning. Nonenzymatic browning causes the formation of dark-colored pigments in foods as diverse as dry milk powder, canned fruit, fruit juice, corn syrup, and dehydrated meat. The Maillard condensation reaction between simple sugars and amino acids, reactions involving ascorbic acid, and caramelization reactions are examples of nonenzymatic browning. As a rule, browning is considered a distinct sign of deterioration in food and is an important factor limiting its shelf-life (1).

Maintaining Records of Food Sources

Detailed information about individual foods, including the manufacturer, exact food item, and lot number, should be included in participants' food records. Many food manufacturers can provide "cut sheets" detailing the nutrient composition of their food items. Cut sheets can be valuable sources of nutrient information, as well as excellent records of the exact food used. Even if nutrient composition is available from the manufacturer, however, it is usually recommended that essential items be chemically assayed for the main nutrients of interest. This information should then be a part of the permanent records of the research kitchen and added to the computer database.

Using the same food distributor over time can also help ensure consistency, especially for fresh meats, poultry, eggs, dairy products, vegetables, and fruits. The same distributor is more likely to be able to provide the same cultivar of broccoli from one study to the next, because it is possible to identify the grower from whom the broccoli was purchased in the past. In many institutional settings, however, pur-

TABLE 12-1

Recommended Storage Times

Food	Maximum Storage Time[1]
Canned Products	12 months
Dried Foods	
Cereals	6–9 months
Chips, cookies, crackers	12 months
Pasta, rice, beans	12 months
Powdered milk	3 months
Frozen Foods	
Bread	1–2 months
Butter, margarine	3–6 months
Fruits, vegetables	12 months
Beef, poultry	6–9 months
Ground meat, fish	1–3 months
Pork	3–6 months

Source: Adapted from West BB & Wood L. *Foodservice in Institutions.* 6th ed. New York: Macmillan; 1988.

[1]Storage times are based on foods stored in their original containers. If highly perishable products such as ground meat and fish are portioned prior to freezing, storage times should be decreased by half.

chasing from the same distributor is not always possible because of policies stipulating that food contracts be awarded to the lowest bidder. In that case, it may be helpful to meet with purchasing department personnel and storehouse managers to explain the unique needs of the research kitchen. Formal waivers from purchasing policies may be required.

Control of Food Variability Over Time

Although purchasing from single lots is common for research facilities, it is rare in general foodservice, so vendors may not appreciate the importance of providing foods from single lots. For single-lot purchases, it is imperative to clearly communicate to the vendor that a single-lot purchase is required. Upon delivery, single-lot purchases must be verified by checking each carton, package, and can. Lot numbers are imprinted on individual cans and packages and also indicated on the outside of the carton. Although it is best to purchase sufficient food of a single lot for an entire study, this may not be possible if storage space is limited. As a result, food items for all participants in an entire study may not be from the same lot. However, as mentioned earlier, it is essential that all the food of each type eaten by a given participant come from a single lot.

It is necessary to establish and maintain written specifications for each food item used in the research kitchen. Adherence to these written standards from one participant to the next will minimize variability among participants' diets. Written specifications for beef, for example, should indicate the grade, cut, percent fat, or trim standards. Specifications for chicken should indicate class, grade, cut, and weight. It is advisable to purchase chicken parts that are boneless and skinless to minimize processing in the research kitchen. Specifications for vegetables and fruits should indicate product, supplier or manufacturer, style, and can size. Specifications for packaged dry goods should indicate product, manufacturer, and weight as purchased.

Use of a single-source supplier is also desirable. For example, it is preferable to purchase ground beef from the same breed of animal raised by the same rancher. However, given today's US food distribution system, this is seldom possible; and, for many studies, it may also be unnecessary. If protein is the nutrient of interest, for example, ensuring that the cut, percent fat, and nitrogen analysis of the meat is the same from participant to participant (and verifying this by periodic composite assay) may be sufficient. If selenium is the nutrient of interest, however, the meat must come from animals raised by one rancher because the amount of selenium in beef is a reflection of the forage that the animals eat (2).

Seasonal food items can add variety and freshness to a repetitive meal plan. There may be considerable variability in the micronutrient composition of fresh foods (eg, the amount of vitamin C in fresh broccoli may vary with cultivar, soil conditions, time of harvest, transport time to distribution center, and amount of time prior to sale) (3). Thus, it is imperative in many studies that seasonal food items be purchased in quantities sufficient to last for an entire study. But food quality and nutrient stability may be of concern if too great a quantity of fresh food is purchased and expected to last over a long period of time. A useful example is that of broccoli used in a study of antioxidant vitamins: the amount of vitamin C in the broccoli would be expected to decrease as a function of storage time after purchase (3).

Procurement of sufficient broccoli for use during 1 week of a study may be acceptable, whereas purchasing sufficient fresh broccoli for use over 3 weeks would not be. As a result, weekly purchases would necessitate chemical assay of the vitamin C levels in each batch of broccoli and adjustment of quantities served on the basis of the analyzed values. If this process is too cumbersome, the investigator may find that a better alternative is to use a canned or frozen product that can be purchased in a single lot.

Fresh potatoes may be used for short-term, constant or metabolic diets if the potatoes are purchased in 50-lb or larger bags. The reason for this is that when potatoes are pulled from the ground, all the potatoes in a specific area of the field go into one 50- or 100-lb bag. Therefore, the composition of the potatoes from that bag should be comparable. However, sufficient storage space is vital if fresh, rather than instant, potatoes are used. For long studies, compositional changes that occur with storage must be considered.

PREPARATION TECHNIQUES FOR CONVENTIONAL FOOD DIETS

Whether conventional food or liquid formula diets are used, it is important to develop a procedure manual detailing food preparation techniques and recipes. The procedures are essential documents that represent the standards of operation of the research kitchen. Special procedures may be designed for individual studies, if necessary.

Weighing and Measuring

All research kitchens should have electronic analytical balances that are accurate to at least 0.1 g. If small amounts of substances such as vitamins and mineral supplements, stable isotopes, spices, herbs, and other similar items are to be weighed, then the balance must be accurate to 0.01 g. These balances must undergo weekly calibration checks, periodic inspection, and maintenance to confirm their accuracy. Typically, every food item should be weighed as accurately as possible prior to service, including liquids. Exceptions in some macronutrient studies may include foods such as broth, lettuce, celery, onion, and carrot sticks. Table 12-2 lists the weights of common serving sizes of various foods.

It is generally preferable to weigh rather than measure most food items because there may be considerable variability in the weight of fluid volumes. However, when micronutrient intakes are not of prime concern (eg, in a study comparing different dietary fats), a decision may be made to measure fluids in graduated cylinders. A graduated cylinder must first be placed on a level platform so that the graduations are at eye level. The bottom of the meniscus (the lowest point of the fluid level) is the point that should be read. Sometimes a small piece of white paper placed behind the cylinder can aid in detecting the meniscus.

Portion-controlled foods should not be considered accurately weighed unless frequent spot checks reveal that, in fact, a precise quantity is consistently delivered. The reported weight of portion-controlled foods—especially dry goods such as crackers and cookies, and condiments such as salt and pepper—is generally not sufficiently accurate for most research diet studies. For example, cereal boxes claiming to contain 21 g have been found to contain as much as 28 g of cereal; 4 cookies allegedly weighing 28 g weighed only 22 g; pepper packets weighed from 2 g to 4 g each. The degree of accuracy necessary for food weights will depend on the nutrient under consideration. For example, portion-controlled boxes containing ± 5 g of a fat-free, fortified breakfast cereal may be acceptable for a study controlling lipid intake, but this degree of accuracy would not be sufficient for a study of iron balance.

The water and fat content of foods can change during cooking, as can the content of some other nutrients. (Also see Chapter 11, "Designing Research Diets.") Thus, the kitchen staff must be careful to portion foods for participants in the same form (ie, raw or cooked) used to calculate the diets. For example, if the raw food was used to calculate nutrient content of a chicken breast, then this item must be portioned prior to food preparation.

Cooking Techniques

A major goal in food preparation for controlled feeding studies is to minimize variability among individual servings. Microwave cooking and oven roasting or baking in closed containers are methods that yield minimal losses and greatest reproducibility.

In large-scale studies, in which diets are planned for multiple participants at stepwise calorie levels, food may be purchased fresh or frozen, prepared, and then weighed out according to desired calorie level. In this setting, care must be taken to minimize losses during cooking and to ensure accuracy during portioning. Standardizing cooking times and temperatures will help to control batch-to-batch variability.

In small-scale studies, diets may be individually planned for each participant, with control exercised for calories as well as macro- and micronutrients. Food is often weighed first, frozen, thawed, and then prepared. Many facilities seek to avoid transferring food from one container to another after it has been weighed, and from the cooking vessel to the serving plate after the food has been cooked. A variety of dishes and containers, available from restaurant wholesalers, are suitable for food storage as well as cooking and serving. Many glass and ceramic products, for example, are freezer-, oven-, and microwave-safe. In addition, these containers make an attractive place setting.

Meat, Poultry, and Fish

Ground beef of a specified cut and percent fat content is a simple product to weigh in advance and store in a freezer.

TABLE 12-2

Approximate Weights of Common Serving Sizes of Various Foods[1]

Food	Serving Size	Weight[2]
Meat		
Chicken, breast, raw, ½ breast	1 piece	118 g
Chicken, breast, roasted, ½ breast	1 piece	86 g
Chicken, thigh, raw	1 piece	69 g
Chicken, thigh, roasted	1 piece	52 g
Chicken, drumstick, raw	1 piece	62 g
Chicken, drumstick, roasted	1 piece	52 g
Beef, chuck, pot-roasted, lean	1 slice	85 g
Beef, round steak, lean	1 slice	85 g
Beef, ground, 17% fat	1 patty	113 g
Frankfurter, beef and pork	1 link	57 g
Fruit		
Apple, raw with peel, 2.75″ diameter	1 whole	138 g
Apple, raw with peel, 3.25″ diameter	1 whole	212 g
Applesauce	½ cup	122 g
Pear, raw, Bartlett, medium	1 whole	166 g
Pear, raw, Bosc, small	1 whole	139 g
Pear, canned	1 half	79 g
Orange, California navel, peeled	1 whole	140 g
Orange, Valencia, peeled	1 whole	121 g
Peach, canned	1 half	98 g
Pineapple, canned	1 slice	47 g
Vegetables		
Green beans, canned	½ cup	68 g
Peas, canned	½ cup	85 g
Corn, canned	½ cup	82 g
Carrots, canned	½ cup	73 g
Spinach, canned	½ cup	107 g
Potatoes, mashed	½ cup	105 g
Potato, with skin, baked	1 whole	156 g
Potato, peeled, boiled	1 whole	135 g
Rice and Pasta		
Rice, white, cooked	½ cup	103 g
Rice, brown, cooked	½ cup	98 g
Rice, white or brown, uncooked	½ cup	93 g
Spaghetti, cooked firm	½ cup	70 g
Spaghetti, cooked tender	½ cup	70 g
Baked Goods		
Bread, white or whole wheat	1 slice	28 g
Saltine crackers	4 crackers	12 g
Hamburger bun	1 whole	43 g
Hot dog bun	1 whole	43 g
English muffin	1 whole	57 g
Bagel, 3.5″ diameter	1 whole	71 g
Blueberry muffin	1 whole	57 g
Cookies, chocolate chip	4 cookies	40 g
Cookies, sandwich type	4 cookies	40 g
Pound cake	1 slice, ½″ thick	28 g

continued

TABLE 12-2

Continued

Food	Serving Size	Weight[2]
Beverages		
Milk, whole	1 cup	244 g
Milk, skim	1 cup	245 g
Apple juice	1 cup	248 g
Orange juice	1 cup	249 g
Cranberry juice cocktail	1 cup	253 g
Spreads and Condiments		
Butter and margarine	1 tsp	5 g
	1 pat	5 g
	1 tbsp	14 g
Jam and preserves	1 packet	14 g
Peanut butter	1 tbsp	16 g
Sugar, white	1 packet	6 g
Coffee, instant dry powder	1½ tsp	2 g

[1]Adapted from *USDA Nutrient Database for Standard Reference Release 12,* Agricultural Research Service, Beltsville, Md (1998).
[2]Weights given are typical but approximate. For greatest accuracy, each item should be weighed prior to use.

Typical serving sizes range from 50 g to 120 g (Table 12-2). When meat is thawed prior to service, care should be taken to transfer all juices from the wrapper to the cooking dish. If the meat is to be grilled or fried, a portion of the participant's allotted butter for the day can be used to grease the grill or frying pan. Care should be taken that the fat does not splatter by cooking with low heat and/or covering the meat pan with a lid.

After the meat has been cooked to the desired doneness and removed to the dinner plate, a spatula should be used to remove all meat particles from the cooking surface. A small amount of deionized water—eg, 5 mL to 10 mL applied three times—can be used with a spatula to clean the cooking surface. This water (now "gravy") should then be poured over the meat. Meat cuts requiring individual preparation are seldom used in large-scale studies; instead, meats that can be cooked as one unit then portioned (eg, roasts and meat loaf) or that lend themselves to casserole preparations are typically preferred.

Chicken breasts from specific classes and grades (eg, fryers or roasters) should be purchased skinless and boneless to minimize waste and preparation time. The dietary staff should then trim all visible fat from, rinse, and dry the meat prior to weighing. Typical serving sizes range from 50 g to 120 g (Table 12-2). Chicken breasts can be prepared in the same manner as beef patties, using the same precautions. Condiments or sauces are often applied to the meat during the latter stage of cooking. If needed, chicken with sauce can be warmed in a microwave oven just prior to serving.

Fish fillets can be purchased flash-frozen in specified weights. These should be weighed into individual portions after thawing. They can be cooked directly in the microwave oven on the serving plate or grilled or fried following the same steps as for meats described earlier. Liquids remaining in the serving dish after the fish has been cooked should be consumed by the participant. Canned fish such as tuna should be drained in a colander for a specified time prior to weighing. Tuna packed in water without added salt should be used if sodium is the nutrient under investigation.

Vegetables and Fruits

Canned and frozen fruits and vegetables offer the most consistency in nutrient composition. They can be purchased in single lots in quantities sufficient for an entire study. For the best consistency, canned fruits should be packed in their own juices with no added sugar; vegetables should be canned in water with no added salt or sugar. Canned fruits and vegetables should be drained for a specified length of time and blotted dry prior to weighing. To preserve palatability, it is recommended that portioning of canned fruits and vegetables should take place no more than 1 day prior to serving. Typical serving sizes range from 60 g to 220 g (Table 12-2). Fruits should be weighed into serving dishes. Vegetables should be weighed into containers that can be used for microwave cooking and subsequent serving. Butter or margarine from the participant's allotment can be melted on the vegetables during microwave cooking. Salt or spices, if used, should be added by dietary personnel or the participant and thoroughly mixed into the vegetables prior to consumption.

Frozen fruits and vegetables are a good alternative to canned products because they too can be purchased in single lots to ensure nutrient consistency. However, frozen foods must be thawed and drained in a consistent manner prior to weighing in order to ensure an accurate weight. When sodium is the nutrient under investigation, frozen vegetables may contribute more than an acceptable level of sodium to the diet. In addition, there may be variability in the amount of sodium present, for example, in a given spear of frozen broccoli, depending on the number of cut surfaces exposed on that spear.

Fresh fruits and vegetables are acceptable for use in studies investigating macro- but not micronutrients. Micronutrient variability can be considerable in fresh fruits and vegetables, and it may be preferable to use canned or frozen products unless the investigator is willing to assay aliquots of each purchased batch of food prior to use. If fresh fruits and vegetables are used, the most accurate form of delivery entails weighing them in their trimmed, cored, and/or peeled state just prior to serving. However, for some studies it is sufficient to weigh fruits with peels or cores after applying a refuse factor (Table 12-3). If researchers are using potatoes and basing nutrient intake on the peeled weight, potatoes should be peeled prior to weighing and cooked in the microwave or boiled prior to serving.

Some participants object to the taste of reducing compounds such as ascorbic acid or lemon juice used to prevent oxidation of cut apples. Unlike most varieties of apples, which turn brown when cut, Cortland apples do not oxidize. This cultivar is grown in the northeastern United States and may be regionally limited in distribution. Cortland apples can be used fresh but also have good baking properties. The Golden Delicious variety does oxidize but much more slowly than most varieties. Golden Delicious apples are sweeter than Cortland apples and are available nationally.

Baked Goods

Baked goods are typically purchased in single lots and kept in frozen storage until needed. Desired quantities should be thawed and weighed prior to serving. For most research diet studies, bread may be toasted without significantly altering the nutrient composition of the food. However, losses may occur if the bread is crumbly and falls apart during toasting.

Dry Goods

Dry goods such as rice, pasta, instant potatoes, cereal, cookies, and snack food items should be purchased in single lots. Rice and pasta should be cooked in deionized water if minerals are under consideration in the study. Individual portions of preweighed dry material may be cooked in individual serving dishes. However, larger quantities may be cooked and portioned after cooking if care is taken to guarantee that the same recipe is always used (eg, 400 g dry macaroni to 12 L deionized water, cooked at a rolling boil for 10 minutes; weigh entire cooked product and divide by 8; weigh out 8 equal servings, each equivalent to 50 g dry macaroni). Mashed potatoes made from instant potatoes, deionized water, milk, and margarine should be weighed and mixed in the serving dish according to a predetermined recipe. Dry cereal should be weighed into the serving bowl. Cooked cereal should be weighed, dry mixed with deionized water, and cooked in the microwave oven in the serving bowl. Cookies and snack food items should be weighed prior to serving even if they are purchased in portion-controlled packages. Table 12-2 shows typical serving sizes for commonly used dry goods.

TABLE 12-3

Refuse Values for Selected Raw Fruits[1]

Fruit	Inedible Material	Percent[2]
Apples, with skin	Core and stem	8
Bananas	Skin	35
Blueberries	Stems and spoiled berries	2
Cherries, sour, red	Pits and stems	10
Grapes, American style	Total refuse	42
(slip skin)	Seeds	6
	Skin	34
	Stems	2
Grapes, European style		
(adherent skin)	Stems	4
Oranges, California		
Navels	Peel and navel	32
Valencias	Peel and seeds	25
Oranges, Florida	Peel and seeds	26
Pears, with skin	Core and stem	8
Plums, with skin	Pits	6
Strawberries	Caps and stems	6
Tangerines	Peel and seeds	28

[1] Adapted from *USDA Nutrient Database for Standard Reference Release 12,* Agricultural Research Service, Beltsville, Md (1998).
[2] Percent of total weight of the fruit, as purchased.

Condiments and Spices

Condiments and spreads such as butter, margarine, peanut butter, jams, jellies, mayonnaise, mustard, catsup, and salad dressings should be purchased in single lots and weighed prior to serving. Portion-controlled items should be re-weighed to maintain accuracy. There are a number of nu-trient-controlled condiments on the market, and because these items can add variety and palatability to a research menu, the nutrition coordinator is encouraged to investigate their availability.

Salt, sugar, and spices are also an important part of an appetizing diet. These items, each purchased from a single lot, can be used by the dietary staff and the participants to enhance the flavor of the diet. In most cases, one or more condiments can be preweighed for an entire day's service. Care should be taken that the condiment is not lost in transfer from the portion container to the food. In addition, investi-gators should be aware that spices and sauces can be hidden sources of nutrients. Paprika contains carotenoids; Worces-tershire sauce, which contains anchovies, provides small amounts of omega-3 fatty acids.

Beverages

Deionized water should be used in research diet studies if essential minerals are under investigation. For these tightly controlled studies, instant coffee and tea are reconstituted with a measured amount of boiled, deionized water. Brewed coffee is made in an electric coffeemaker using a weighed amount of coffee and deionized water. After the coffee is brewed for a timed period, individually weighed portions are served. Beverages such as canned soda may be used if pur-chased from the same lot. Portion-controlled milk, cream, and juices may be used, but many studies require that they be remeasured prior to being served. (See Chapter 15, "Meeting Requirements for Fluids.")

Mixed Dishes

Mixed dishes can provide much-needed variety during long menu cycles. However, unless the dish is prepared in-house, it is more difficult to minimize nutrient variability in mixed dishes. Some commercially prepared products such as frozen waffles, French toast, and pancakes may be acceptable breakfast alternatives if purchased in single lots for an entire study. For other mixed dishes, such as stews, casseroles, or soups, it may difficult to guarantee nutrient accuracy if the entire portion is not served. Homogeneous mixtures such as spaghetti sauce can often be used if the accompanying pasta and meat are weighed separately. Macaroni and cheese, chicken à la king, chicken salad, and similar dishes can also be prepared in "steps" with each ingredient weighed sepa-rately. However, this stepwise process will require additional time and staffing devoted to preparation.

An alternative to either conventional solid food diets or formula diets is the frozen diet (4). The frozen diet comprises standard meals that are created at defined calorie levels and then flash-frozen. These "TV-dinner" frozen meals can sim-plify food delivery, especially for short-term and outpatient studies. Special serving dishes such as partitioned aluminum foil or plastic containers that are microwave-safe should be used.

Although the planning and preparation needed to create these frozen diets is considerable, frozen meals may reduce the need for inpatient admissions. In addition to the prepa-ration, however, careful instructions and participant moni-toring in the outpatient setting are essential for a successful study.

TRACKING THE PRODUCTION PROCESS

Food Labels

When portioning the product for serving, the foodservice worker weighs the gram amounts indicated on the produc-tion sheet (see Chapter 13, "Delivering Research Diets," and Chapter 18, "Documentation, Record Keeping, and Recipes") for each participant at his or her designated cal-orie level. As the food is portioned and wrapped, a label bearing the code number for that food item is applied to each serving. If the study is masked, the label (Figure 12-1) on a participant's serving of food will show the generic descrip-tion and code (ie, spice cake, 420) rather than a full descrip-tion (spice cake with moderate *trans* margarine). The partic-ipant's calorie level (2,800), masked dietary treatment (blue), and menu number are also displayed.

Visually striking, clearly worded labels become particu-larly important when a facility is engaged in multiple con-current protocols. (Also see Chapter 20, "Staffing Needs for Research Diet Studies.")

Individual food labels can be computer generated—a great savings of time compared with making labels by hand—and color coded as appropriate. Alternatively, foods can be labeled with bar codes. This facilitates blinding par-ticipants to their assigned diets. Data encoded in the bar code is matched to information contained on the menu in the da-tabase. Thus, any error in treatment or calorie level and any missing or duplicated food item will be promptly spotted when the bar codes on a participant's tray are scanned. Bar codes can be generated directly from a database; for ex-ample, a database of daily menu items containing gram amounts served at each calorie level. Selected data file fields are incorporated into a label-generating facility of the pre-ferred database software, then printed onto adhesive labels. Office supply stores carry labels in a variety of sizes and colors that are suitable for computer printing on tractor feed or laser printers. (See Chapter 3, "Computer Applications in Controlled Diet Studies.")

Food Codes

Foods are frequently identified by code number as well as description. These codes usually are food database numbers or other codes assigned by the research kitchen staff. (Also

```
┌──────────────────────────────────────────────────┐
│                                                    │
│  SPICE CAKE 420              Menu 12               │
│  2,800                       kcal Friday           │
│  Blue                        Dinner                │
│  50 grams                                          │
│                                                    │
└──────────────────────────────────────────────────┘
```

FIGURE 12-1.   Label on food item served to a participant eating 2,800-kcal diet in a masked study.

see Chapter 13, "Delivering Research Diets.") Code numbers can serve as a convenient shortcut for the staff, lightening the work of writing or printing labels. The codes also can be an important part of the protocol, however, by preserving the masking of foods in a blinded study. For example, in a masked study comparing three test fats, the kitchen might prepare various baked goods as carriers of the test fats. The test margarines (no *trans* [ZERO], moderate *trans* [MOD], and high *trans* [HIGH] margarines) might be assigned the codes 10, 20, and 30, respectively. Spice cake, one of the vehicles for delivering these test fats, would be prepared with each type of margarine. Spice cake would be assigned the general code of 400, and the spice cakes made with the three test fats would be coded 410, 420, and 430, respectively. In the kitchen, both the code and full description (eg, 420, MOD spice cake) would be associated with the product.

During production and storage, foods are tagged with both codes and full descriptions. For example, a baker preparing spice cakes adds moderate *trans* margarine to the mixer, tags the mixer with the test fat code (ie, 20), and labels the baking pan with the appropriate code number and the full description of the product (ie, 420, spice cake w/MOD *trans* margarine). This prevents a possible mixup among cakes at the point of production. The code and description stay with the product as it is baked and during frozen storage. At temperatures normally used for baking and freezing foods, masking tape labels are stable and adhere well to aluminum baking pans. (The staff must take care to ensure that these production codes and labels are not seen by study participants.)

Chain of Custody

Proper use of production forms (see Chapter 18, "Documentation, Record Keeping, and Recipes"), codes, and labels will establish an effective "chain of custody" for all foods produced in the research kitchen. The chain of custody concept also is highly applicable to test materials used for research menus. This involves "logging in" test foods as they are received and used.

For example, in a research kitchen using three test fats, the amount and type of each fat is recorded in a log as it is received and the code number and full description are written on each container of fat. Direct access to the test materials can be limited to key personnel who serve as "gatekeepers," distributing the fats to foodservice workers

as they are needed. This control point ensures that the foodservice worker uses the correct test fat. It also allows for efficient record keeping, because the gatekeeper records the date and amount of test material used at the time it is passed into the custody of the foodservice worker. Any fat that is discarded (eg, a burned cake) is also noted in the log book. After the study, if questions arise about use of test materials, complete records will be available for review. (Chain of custody procedures are also used for quality control in handling and analysis of biological samples and food composites.)

SAFETY AND SANITATION

The safety and sanitation standards for research diets are the same standards that apply to all foodservice operations. Standards that have been established by such agencies as local and state health departments, the Joint Commission on Accreditation of Healthcare Organizations, and the Occupational Safety and Health Administration are the commonly used ones that should be followed in the research kitchen. These standards are extremely important in research diet preparation, particularly so because food for research diets is often handled many times prior to service and this may increase the risk of foodborne illness.

The Hazard Analysis Critical Control Point concept (HACCP), a system of continuous quality improvement in food safety, provides a model for integrating safety and sanitation measures into the preparation and production processes of research diets (5, 6). HACCP suggests identifying: (1) sensitive ingredients, (2) sensitive areas in food processing, and (3) sensitive points of personnel health and hygiene. Once these areas have been identified, critical control points are then categorized according to: (1) the potential for microbiological contamination, (2) sanitation requirements, (3) time-temperature constraints, and (4) employee hygiene.

Several examples, outlined here, demonstrate effective application of the HACCP model in the production of research diets. (Also see Chapter 21, "Performance Improvement for the Research Kitchen," for further discussion of the HACCP model.) The preparation of fresh boneless and skinless chicken breasts provides one such example. Chicken breasts are generally purchased fresh, trimmed, portioned into serving sizes, frozen for long periods of time, thawed, prepared, and finally served to the participant. Poultry is potentially hazardous because, as a protein source with a neutral pH, its risk of microbial growth is high. Poultry also is known to have a high rate of intrinsic salmonella contamination. Caution must therefore be taken that this meat is properly handled at every step in the process to avoid contamination and spoilage:

1. Employees should always wash their hands thoroughly prior to food handling.
2. Personnel should not have open cuts or sores on their hands and should not put their hands to their faces during the food production process.
3. Raw poultry should not be held in the temperature danger zone (7°C to 60°C, 45°F to 140°F) for more than 2 hours.
4. To avoid cross contamination, raw poultry should be cut on a sanitized cutting board. The board should not be used for ingredients other than raw meats. Cutting boards should be sanitized daily.
5. Poultry should be quickly washed, drained, dried, and packed into air-tight containers for freezing.
6. Freezer and refrigerator temperatures must be checked at least daily to guarantee that equipment integrity is maintained.
7. All frozen meats should be thawed in the refrigerator.
8. Poultry must be thoroughly cooked to a minimum of 74°C (165°F) for 15 seconds. A thermometer should be used to monitor quality assurance.

Exhibit 12–1 is an example of HACCP applied to this model. Following the principles of HACCP can help maintain food safety and sanitation standards in the food preparation process.

Another example of the HACCP concept is examining the way in which meals are prepared in large-scale foodservice systems. Frequently, meals are prepared in advance, with full cooking and food preparation taking place a day or two prior to service. Prepared meals are quickly chilled and held under refrigeration until they are reheated, often using a microwave oven, just prior to serving. A hazard analysis of this cook/chill process would identify potentially sensitive ingredients and critical time-temperature constraints in the system to minimize bacterial growth. The hazard analysis would include such points as:

- Foods must be cooked sufficiently and chilled quickly.
- Reheating must be thorough enough to destroy bacteria that may be present.
- Plastic disposable gloves should be worn when food handlers are preparing fresh foods such as salads or sandwiches that will not undergo heating prior to service.

Formulas that are prepared for research diets often do not have any heat treatment. A hazard analysis of this process must identify not only preparation control points but also safe sources of ingredients, especially for potentially sensitive protein components. When the formula is prepared in large batches, careful attention must be paid to the total time the mixture is held in the danger zone. The total holding time must include preparation time, freezing time, storage time, the time it takes to weigh the formula prior to service, and the time between service and participant consumption.

As with other potentially hazardous foods, formulas should be cooled according to published government guidelines (Food and Drug Administration, Food Code, US Public Health Service, US Department of Health and Human Services, Washington DC, 1997). Formulas that are heated must first be cooled within 2 hours from 60°C (140°F) to 21°C (70°F), and then further cooled within 4 hours from 21°C (70°F) down to 5°C (41°F) or lower. Formulas that are prepared at room temperature should be cooled from 21°C (70°F) to 5°C (41°F) or lower. Frozen formula should be thawed under refrigeration that maintains the mixture at tem-

EXHIBIT 12-1

The HACCP Checklist for Chicken Breast Preparation

Ingredient: Chicken Breast
Hazard Status: Potential for microbial contamination is *high*
Food Processing Requirements:

- Do not keep raw poultry in the danger zone (45°F to 140°F) for longer than 2 hours.
- Cutting board should be dedicated and marked "FOR POULTRY ONLY."
- Sanitize cutting board daily.
- Use airtight containers for packaging.
- Check freezer and refrigerator temperatures at least daily.
- Thaw frozen poultry in the refrigerator.
- Cook poultry to a minimum of 165°F—use a thermometer!

Personnel Requirements:

- Wash hands thoroughly prior to food handling.
- Check hands for open cuts or sores.
- Keep hands away from faces during the food production process.

peratures of 5°C (41°F) or less. (Also see Chapter 14, "Planning and Producing Formula Diets.")

Temperature-sensitive labels are available that can help to monitor time and temperature conditions. These labels use liquid crystal technology to identify products that have been exposed to adverse conditions and thus help to guarantee the safety of sensitive foods (sources include Monitor Mark Brand Product Exposure Indicators, 3M Packaging Systems Division, St Paul, Minn, also LifeLines Technology, Inc, Morris Plains, NJ).

Research diets prepared for outpatient studies present another potentially hazardous food safety situation. Possible problem areas include improper packaging and/or subsequent participant mishandling. Study participants should be instructed in proper food-handling techniques, food storage, and food preparation. Strict adherence to limiting the time that food remains in the danger zone to a 2-hour to 4-hour maximum is critical for food safety. Yet, depending on the amount and type of initial contamination, the growth medium, and the temperature, even a maximum of 2 hours in the danger zone cannot guarantee food safety. Willingness to follow safe food-handling procedures is a key characteristic of a compliant participant; screening materials, informed consent documents, and protocol instructions all must address the issue of food safety.

The ultimate responsibility and liability for safety and sanitation standards as they apply to research diets lies with the investigator in charge of the study. It is the chief dietitian's responsibility to ensure that food safety and sanitation standards are firmly established and documented in the facility. In addition, dietary staff must be formally trained and periodically retrained through in-service education sessions to ensure that the proper standards are maintained. The HACCP concept provides a model for monitoring food safety that is especially appropriate for the research kitchen.

USE OF MODIFIED FOODS AND EXPERIMENTAL FOODS

At times the diet design targets of the protocol cannot be achieved with the use of standard foodstuffs. For these cases, investigators may wish to consider using modified foods that differ from their traditional counterparts with respect to one or more nutrients or dietary compounds. These modified foods can be useful tools for changing levels of various nutrients in experimental diets. Some can be substituted for the traditional product with little or no devaluation of sensory properties. Others have altered cooking properties or palatability, reducing their acceptability.

The modified foods discussed in this section do not represent a comprehensive listing; rather, the intent is to give examples of experimental foodstuffs that have been used in controlled diet studies and to address issues relevant to feeding experimental foodstuffs to study participants. Additionally, the investigator will want to inquire about the safety of experimental foodstuffs for human consumption. At this writing, some of the foods mentioned here have not been approved for human consumption by the Food and Drug Administration, and some have been approved only for limited use.

Modified or experimental foods usually are far more expensive than standard items, often by more than a factor of 10. These costs must be considered when researchers plan the study's budget. In some cases costs of such foods may be prohibitive and a revised protocol is in order. At other times an experimental food product provides a key element of dietary control.

Plant Foods with Isotopic Labels or Altered Composition

The use of stable isotopes to label plant foods for human nutrition studies was recently reviewed by Grusak (7). Stable isotopes in general are considered inherently safer than radioactive isotopes, and their use is expanding to studies of nearly every category of nutrient, from macronutrients to vitamins, minerals, and water. Elements lending themselves to such studies include hydrogen, carbon, nitrogen, magnesium, calcium, iron, copper, and zinc. (Also see Chapter 16, "Compartmental Modeling and Balance Studies.")

Clinical investigators interested in using isotopically labeled plant products for controlled feeding studies should undertake product development through close collaboration with knowledgeable plant physiologists. For example, if labeled seeds are needed, it is best to select a cultivar (variety) whose seeds tend to mature at a fixed time rather than sequentially over an indeterminate time frame (7). In addition, depending on the nutrient and the means of administration, the tracer may preferentially concentrate in certain plant tissues (eg, stems, roots, leaves, or seeds). Stable isotopes can be incorporated into plant tissues as they grow ("intrinsic labeling") by culturing plants in labeled hydroponic medium, injecting isotopes into plant stems, or growing the plants in labeled gaseous atmosphere (a method used primarily for carbon-13 studies) (7). Although many varieties of plants lend themselves to labeling treatment, their growing habits or metabolic characteristics can affect how suitable they are for a particular protocol.

The stable isotope of carbon, ^{13}C, is naturally concentrated above background environmental levels (ie, in CO_2 from air) by certain plants, particularly corn and sugar cane. (Also see Chapter 14, "Planning and Producing Formula Diets.") ^{13}C can also be added to hydroponic cultures to produce isotopically labeled plant metabolites. Kale containing ^{13}C-labeled carotenoids have been grown in this way for studies of carotenoid absorption and metabolism (8).

Radioactive isotopes also are used to label foods when scientifically appropriate and are judged safe for subjects. For example, radiolabeled calcium chloride, incorporated into foods, has been fed to humans to assess relative absorbability of calcium from food sources (9). The tracer was added directly to milk (ie, *extrinsic* labeling) or incorporated into kale as it was grown hydroponically (ie, *intrinsic* labeling). Tissues of intrinsically labeled kale have a uniform distribution of the ^{65}Ca tracer.

Another way to test the effect of diets high or low in calcium is through supplementation of calcium in foods or use of low-calcium or calcium-substitute foods. Foods that have been supplemented with calcium include juices, dairy products, flours, and baked goods. In some food products, such as juices, participants can detect a difference in taste between the traditional and the calcium-supplemented product. Comparison diets that are low in calcium typically include few milk products; thus, soy milk (eg, Vita Soy®) can be useful as a low-calcium milk substitute.

Known geographical differences in the mineral content of local soils have been used to advantage in obtaining foods of specific composition. Wheat that is high in selenium has been grown in an area of South Dakota where the soil has a high selenium content. This high-selenium wheat and a low-selenium counterpart were incorporated into bread products and fed to men with low selenium status (10). The low- and high-selenium products were compared to each other and to other selenium supplements to assess the relative bioavailability of selenium. There was no difference in flavor or acceptability of the two wheat products in this study.

Wheat bran is a good source of dietary trace minerals, but it contains phytic acid that can form complexes with cations. Phytic acid has been implicated in reducing mineral bioavailability by binding several nutritionally important minerals including iron, zinc, calcium, and magnesium, thus making them unavailable for absorption. A modified product, dephytinized wheat bran from which phytic acid has been removed by promoting natural phytase activity, has been useful as an experimental food in evaluating the effect of phytic acid on apparent mineral absorption (11). The modified and traditional wheat brans were incorporated into muffins with no detectable differences in baking or sensory properties.

Foods Used to Reduce or Replace Dietary Fat

Many low-fat or fat-modified products are available commercially. Some products have reduced-fat content resulting from fat removal (eg, skimmed or low-fat rather than whole milk). In others, the fat is diluted, as when water replaces some of the fat in low-fat margarines, or air is incorporated into margarine and cream cheese to provide less fat for a given volume of product. In some products the type rather than the amount of fat is altered. In filled milk products, for example, vegetable oils are substituted for animal fats to retain properties of the original food (eg, milk that has the milk fat replaced with sunflower oil). However, filled milk products are not generally low in fat.

Producing fat-modified and low-fat cheeses has proven to be a technological challenge. The texture, body, and flavor of cheeses are largely dependent on the type and amount of fat as are their functional properties. Storage conditions can affect fat-modified foods as well as their traditional counterparts. For example, in contrast to full-fat mozzarella cheese, low-fat mozzarella is hard and less meltable (12). However, following refrigerated storage for 6 weeks, the texture and melting characteristics are more desirable. Frozen storage also affects sensory characteristics of cheeses.

Low-fat and skimmed milk, and cheeses made with these milks, have an obvious role in reducing the saturated fat content of diets. Conversely, traditional, full-fat products can be used as vehicles for delivering fat in diets designed to be higher in fat. Although participants are likely to object to the use of visible fats, such as butter, in higher-fat diets, they typically accept whole milk or cheese without complaint.

Protein-based fat substitutes include Simplesse® (Monsanto Corp, Chicago, Ill), Trail Blazer® (Kraft General Foods, Glenview, Ill), Lita® (Opta Food Ingredients, Louisville, Ken), and Dairy-Lo® (Pfizer Inc, Milwaukee, Wisc). Additionally, soy products including flour, grits, and protein concentrates are used in comminuted meat products (frankfurters, meat loaves) resulting in products with reduced proportions of animal fat. Meat analogs made of soy resemble meat in texture and flavor and have similar reduced-fat characteristics. Soy has a distinct taste but works well as a meat substitute in chili and other spicy foods. Recipes for use of protein-based meat substitutes are available (13).

Among the protein-based fat substitutes, Simplesse is one of the better known. This product, composed primarily of egg and milk proteins, has a fat-like texture that is due to the small size of its microparticles (0.1 to 3 micron spheres) (14). Protein particles of this size have a smooth mouth feel in contrast to larger particles, which feel gritty. The product is well suited for frozen desserts and salad dressings. Because the microparticles break down when heated, the product is not suitable for use in foods that must be cooked. Individuals who are allergic to egg or milk proteins may have reactions to Simplesse (15).

Carbohydrate-based fat substitutes include cellulose, gums, and the maltodextrins including Oatrim® (ConAgra, Omaha, Neb), Z-trim® (USDA, recent patent), Ricetrin® (Zumbro Inc, Faribault, Minn), and Paselli-SA2® (Avebe America Inc, Princeton, NJ). For example, Oatrim can be incorporated into products without affecting taste or texture. It is suitable for use in dairy products and salad dressings and can be used in baked goods because of its stability at high temperatures. The product is used as a meat extender because it enhances the water-holding capacity of products such as ground beef, promoting juiciness that is normally associated with fat content. The product is also a good source of soluble fiber.

Fat-based fat substitutes include Olestra® (Proctor and Gamble, Cincinnati, Ohio), Veri-Lo® (Pfizer Inc, Milwaukee, Wisc), and Dur-Lo® (Loders-Croklaan Inc, Glen Ellyn, Ill). The best known of these, Olestra, is a sucrose polyester; that is, a mixture of hexa-, hepta-, and octaesters formed from sucrose and long-chain fatty acids (16). Olestra provides no calories because it is not hydrolyzed by gastric lipases and is not absorbed. Olestra can be tailored to meet desired functional and sensory characteristics by varying the fatty acid composition, and, like conventional fats, can be used for cooking. The product is suitable for blinded studies because Olestra has the taste and consistency of fat. Study participants are unable to distinguish between Olestra and conventional dietary fat, and many participants can consume fairly high levels of Olestra without experiencing gastrointestinal side effects (17). However, sucrose polyesters appear to reduce absorption of dietary carotenoids (18).

The use of synthetic triglycerides—those created to contain specific fatty acids—is an option when the goal is to control the type of dietary fat. In contrast to natural fats, which contain an array of fatty acids, synthetic triglycerides can be tailored to provide a desired number and distribution of fatty acids. Synthetic fats have been useful in experimental diets designed to investigate the effects of specific fatty acids on blood lipids (19). However, it should be noted that in some synthetic fats, a large proportion of the triglyceride contains a saturated fatty acid in the middle position of the glycerol. (This is also true of natural fats that have been randomly reesterified—that is, the fatty acids removed from the glycerol and reesterified.) In nature that position on the glycerol molecule is, for the most part, reserved for polyunsaturated fatty acids. This difference in triglyceride configuration can influence lipid absorption and metabolism (20).

Foods Modified to Reduce Cholesterol Content

There are a number of ways to reduce the cholesterol content of eggs (21). Perhaps the most common methods involve removing the yolk and replacing it with either vegetable oils or nonoil ingredients. For most baked products, egg substitutes can successfully replace whole eggs. However, some recipes require egg yolk for their emulsifying properties (mayonnaise) or fat content (Hollandaise sauce). Egg substitutes that contain vegetable oils are not satisfactory replacements in recipes that require egg whites for foam-forming functions (angel food cake, meringues).

Because of their high cholesterol content and the localization of cholesterol in the yolk, eggs have been the major food targeted for cholesterol reduction. In addition, methods are under development for removal of cholesterol from butterfat (22, 23), so more cholesterol-modified foods may soon be available for experimental diets.

Experimental Foods Used to Increase Fiber Content of Diets

Dietary fibers are used in controlled feeding studies both as conventional foods and as experimental foodstuffs. As a rule, the insoluble fibers add bulk to the diet, enhancing fecal bulking and laxation, but they do not lower blood cholesterol levels as some soluble fibers do. Soluble fibers are widely studied; but, as experimental foodstuffs, they are frequently a challenge to successfully incorporate into recipes.

Gums in soluble fibers (for example, beta-glucan in oat fiber) can produce stiff gels in doughs and batters during the mixing process, making the product sticky and difficult to handle; the stickiness increases yet further with longer mixing times. Another problem associated with gums and gel formation is decreased volume in baked goods. For example, the volume of baked goods can be reduced by one-third to one-half when carboxymethyl cellulose, a particularly sticky gum, is incorporated into the recipe. On the other hand, volume is unchanged with other fibers, such as locust bean gum. To minimize gum development in food preparation, it is prudent to add the soluble fiber as the last ingredient in a recipe and to mix as little as possible after its addition. Leavening agents are commonly increased in recipes to counteract the decrease in volume associated with using gums.

Some fibers are better tolerated by study participants than others, and individuals vary in their ability to tolerate a given type and amount of fiber. Adverse reactions such as bloating, belching, and flatulence are common during the first week of a high-fiber diet, but these symptoms generally ameliorate during the second week as the activity of colonic bacteria that ferment polysaccharides changes in response to the higher-fiber diet (24).

Pilot Plant Production of Experimental Foods

Researchers often need to collaborate with colleagues in universities or in the food industry to produce experimental foods in forms that are needed for human feeding studies. Trade organizations (Exhibit 12–2) can provide information and assist in making contacts with food scientists who produce specialized products. Many universities, particularly land grant universities, have pilot plant facilities that may be suitable for producing specialized experimental foods. Professional societies for food scientists and some of the many trade and professional journals for food science and technology are listed in Exhibits 12–3 and 12–4, respectively.

Food Safety and Experimental Foods

The investigator must ensure that any experimental food fed to humans meets high standards of sanitation and safety. As with all foods, the experimental food must be processed in sanitary facilities using good manufacturing practices. The food must be safe from pathogens, hazardous chemicals, and other potentially harmful agents, and free of repulsive or offensive matter that is considered filth (25).

The investigator should be certain that the experimental food in question can legally be fed to humans. US regula-

EXHIBIT 12-2

Food-Related Trade Organizations

American Egg Board, Park Ridge, Ill. Promotes egg industry and demand for egg products. (847) 296–7043, http://www.aeb.org

American Frozen Food Institute (AFFI), McLean, Va. AFFI's Foundation for Frozen Food Research develops and coordinates scientific research in industry-wide, noncompetitive areas to increase understanding of the storing and thawing process of frozen food production. (703) 821–0770, http://www.affi.com

American Institute of Baking (ABA), Manhattan, Kan. Promotes education and research in the science and art of baking, bakery management, allied sciences, food processing sanitation, and safety for the benefit of all people. (785) 537–4750, http://www.aibonline.org

Food Marketing Institute (FMI), Washington, DC. Conducts programs in research, education, industry relations, and public affairs on behalf of its 1,500 members—food retailers and wholesalers and their customers in the United States and around the world. (202) 452–8444, http://www.fmi.org

Grocery Manufacturers of America (GMA), Washington, DC. GMA's member companies manufacture about 85% of supermarket goods. (202) 337–9400, http://www.gmabrands.com

Institute of Shortening and Edible Oils (ISEO), Washington, DC. Represents refiners of edible fats and oils. ISEO's 26 members represent approximately 90% to 95% of the edible fats processed domestically. (202) 783–7960, http://www.iseo.org

International Food Information Council (IFIC), Washington, DC. A nonprofit organization that communicates sound, science-based information on food safety and nutrition to health professionals, educators, government officials, journalists, and consumers. (202) 296–6540, http://www.ificinfo.health.org

National Cattlemen's Beef Association (NCBA), Chicago, Ill. Represents livestock marketers, growers, meat packers, food retailers, and food service firms. Conducts program of promotion, education, and information about beef, veal, pork, lamb, and associated meat products. (312) 670–9213, http://www.beef.org

National Fisheries Institute (NFI), Arlington, Va. The objective of NFI is to strengthen the US fish and seafood industry in its mission of supplying more and greater variety of high-quality fish and seafood products to the nation's consumers. (703) 524–8880, http://www.nfi.org

National Food Processors Association (NFPA), Washington, DC. Represents the scientific and technical interests of approximately 500 member companies that manufacture processed or packaged fruits and vegetables, meats, seafoods, juices, beverages, and specialty products. (202) 639–5900, http://www.nfpa-food.org

Refrigerated Foods Association (RFA), Atlanta, Ga. The RFA is an international association of manufacturers and suppliers of refrigerated foods. (770) 452–0660

Snack Food Association (SFA), Alexandria, Va. Represents manufacturers, distributors, and suppliers of snack foods. (703) 836–4500, http://www.sfa.org

United Fresh Fruits and Vegetables Association, Alexandria, Va. Provides a meeting place for members, customers, suppliers, and groups to exchange ideas and to associate; promotes the interests of its members; educates the public by promoting the benefits of increased consumption of fresh fruits and vegetables; and assists members and their employees in their professional development. (703) 836–3410

United Soybean Board (USB), Chesterfield, Mo. A team of approximately 60 farmer-members, working voluntarily in the areas of domestic marketing, production, new uses, and international marketing of soybeans. (800) 989–8721, http://www.unitedsoybean.com

---

tions regarding foods for human consumption are detailed in the Code of Federal Regulations (CFR) (25), which is revised at least once a year. To ensure that information is up to date, the latest issue of the CFR must be used in conjunction with subsequent amendments. The latest amendments can be traced through the "List of Code of Federal Regulations Sections Affected," which is issued monthly, and the "Cumulative List of Parts Affected," which appears in the Reader Aids section of the daily *Federal Register.* A summary of the principal laws and regulations that are enforced by the Food and Drug Administration (FDA) is available in nonlegal language (26).

The CFR describes conditions for safe use of food additives. A food additive is any substance that may be reasonably expected to become a component of food or affect the characteristics of food. US law requires that the safety

EXHIBIT 12-3

Professional Societies Concerned with Food Science and Experimental Foods

American Association of Cereal Chemists (AACC), St Paul, Minn. (612) 454–7250, http://www.scisoc.org/aacc

American Dairy Association, Rosemont, Ill. (847) 803–2000, http://www.dairyinfo.com

American Dietetic Association (ADA), Chicago, Ill. (800) 877–1600, http://www.eatright.org

American Meat Science Association, Kansas City, Mo. (816) 444–3500, http://www.meatscience.org

American Oil Chemists' Society (AOCS), Champaign, Ill. (217) 359–2344, http://www.aocs.org

AOAC International, Gaithersburg, Md. (703) 522–3032, http://www.aoas.org

American Society for Clinical Nutrition (ASCN), Bethesda, Md. (301) 530–7110, http://www.faseb.org/ascn

American Society for Nutritional Sciences (ASNS), Bethesda, Md. (301) 530–7050, http://www.nutrition.org

Institute of Food Technologists (IFT), Chicago, Ill. (312) 782–8424, http://www.ift.org

Poultry Science Association, Champaign, Ill. (217) 356–3182, http://www.psa.uiuc.edu

EXHIBIT 12-4

Trade and Professional Journals Concerned with Food Science and Experimental Foods

Cereal Chemistry
Cereal Foods World
Food Chemistry
Food and Nutrition Bulletin
Food Technology
International Journal of Food Science and Nutrition
International News on Fats, Oils, and Related Materials (INFORM)
Journal of Agricultural and Food Chemistry
Journal of The American Dietetic Association
Journal of the American Oil Chemists' Society
Journal of Applied Spectroscopy
Journal of the Association of Official Analytical Chemists International
Journal of Food Composition and Analysis
Journal of Food Science

of a food additive must be determined by the FDA before the additive may be used in food either indirectly (eg, as a result of processing or packaging) or directly. This law exempts from the definition of food additives those substances that are generally recognized as safe (GRAS) by qualified experts for the intended use in food.

Title 21, part 172 of the CFR contains a list of food additives permitted for direct addition to foods that are intended for human consumption. Title 21, part 182 of the CFR, identifies substances that are generally recognized as safe for human consumption. However, many unlisted substances may also be safe. If there is any question concerning the safety of an experimental food for human consumption, the investigator should seek an opinion from the FDA. Title 21, part 170 contains instructions for submitting a petition for affirmation of GRAS status, and Title 21, part 171 contains instructions for preparing a petition for approval of a food additive.

Some experimental foodstuffs may have characteristics that make them similar to pharmaceutical products. Investigators in these cases should inquire about whether it is necessary to develop a New Drug Application, which is handled by the FDA. Sufficient time in the study schedule must then be allotted for the approval process.

CONCLUSION

Many creative research diets have been designed using experimental foods. However, no matter how creative the study design, implementation is key to a successful research study. It is clear that accurately producing research diets requires considerable attention not only from the foodservice workers who "produce" meals but also from the principal investigator, the study coordinator, and from dietitians and lead cooks. Accurately and safely producing research diets requires unyielding attention to the details of food purchasing and storage, to weighing and cooking techniques, and dedication to uncompromised food safety and sanitation procedures.

REFERENCES

1. Berk Z, ed. *Braverman's Introduction to the Biochemistry of Foods.* Amsterdam, The Netherlands: Elsevier; 1976;149–67.

2. Kubota J, Allaway WH, Ganther HE, et al. Selenium in crops in the United States in relation to selenium responsive diseases of animals. *J Agric Food Chem.* 1967;15:448–453.

3. Vanderslice JT, Higgs DJ. Vitamin C content of foods: sample variability. *Am J Clin Nutr.* 1991;54:1323S-1327S.

4. St Jeor ST, Maddock RK, Jr, Tyler FH. Simplifying dietary procedures for research. *J Am Diet Assoc.* 1969; 55:357–360.

5. Bauman H. HACCP: concept development and application. *Food Technol.* 1990;44:156–158.

6. Bobeng BJ, David BD. HACCP model for quality control of entree production in hospital food service systems. *J Am Diet Assoc.* 1978;73:524–529.

7. Grusak MA. Intrinsic stable isotope labeling of plants for nutritional investigations in humans. *J Nutr Biochem.* 1997;8:164–171.

8. Fahey JW, Clevidence BA, Russell RM. Methods for assessing the biological effects of specific plant components. In: Food, Phytonutrients, and Health. Proceedings of a USDA Symposium. *Nutrition Reviews.* In press.

9. Heaney RP, Weaver CM. Calcium absorption from kale. *Am J Clin Nutr.* 1990;51:656–657.

10. Levander OA, Alfthan G, Arvilommi H, et al. Bioavailability of selenium to Finnish men as assessed by platelet glutathione peroxidase activity and other blood parameters. *Am J Clin Nutr.* 1983;37:887–897.

11. Morris ER, Ellis R, Steele P, et al. Mineral balance of adult men consuming whole or dephytinized wheat bran. *Nutr Res.* 1988;8:445–458.

12. Tunick MH, Mackey KL, Smith PW, et al. Effects of composition and storage on the texture of Mozzarella cheese. *Neth Milk Dairy J.* 1991;45:117–125.

13. ConAgra, Nine ConAgra Drive, PO Box 3100, Omaha NE 68103–0100.

14. Stargel W. Simplesse: all natural fat substitute. In: Stewart, MR, ed. *Proceedings of the Fifteenth National Nutrient Databank Conference.* Blacksburg, Va: The CBORD Group, Inc; 1990:165–168.

15. Sampson H. In vitro allergenicity/antigenicity testing of Simplesse in individuals with allergy to milk or egg proteins. *FASEB J.* 1989;3:A1254. Abstract.

16. Jones DY, Koonsvitsky BP, Ebert ML, et al. Vitamin K status of free-living subjects consuming Olestra. *Am J Clin Nutr.* 1991;53:943–946.

17. Glueck CJ, Hastings MM, Allen C, et al. Sucrose polyester and covert caloric dilution. *Am J Clin Nutr.* 1982;35:1352–1359.

18. Weststrate JA, van het Hof KH. Sucrose polyester and plasma carotenoid concentrations in healthy subjects. *Am J Clin Nutr.* 1995;62:591–597.

19. Bonanome A, Grundy SM. Effect of dietary stearic acid on plasma cholesterol and lipoprotein levels. *New Engl J Med.* 1988;318:1244–1248.

20. McGandy RB, Hegsted M, and Myers ML. Use of semisynthetic fats in determining effects of specific dietary fatty acids on serum lipids in man. *Am J Clin Nutr.* 1970;23:1288–1298.

21. Mast MG, Clouser CS. Processing options for improving the nutritional value of poultry meat and egg products. In: *Designing Foods. Animal Product Options in the Marketplace.* Washington, DC: National Academy Press; 1990:311–331.

22. Bradley RL. Removal of cholesterol from milk fat using supercritical carbon dioxide. *J Dairy Sci.* 1989; 72:2834–2840.

23. Micich TJ, Foglia TA, Holsinger VH. Polymer-supported saponins: an approach to cholesterol removal from butteroil. *J Agric Food Chem.* 1992;40:1321–1325.

24. Salyers AA. Polysaccharide utilization by human colonic bacteria. In: Furda I, Brine CJ, eds. *New Developments in Dietary Fiber, Physiological, Physicochemical, and Analytical Aspects.* New York, NY: Plenum Press; 1990:151–158.

25. *Code of Federal Regulations.* Title 21, parts 170–199. Office of the Federal Register, National Archives and Records Administration. Food and Drug Administration, Department of Health and Human Services, Washington, DC.

26. *Requirements of Laws and Regulations Enforced by the US Food and Drug Administration.* DHHS (FDA) publication 89–1115. Washington, DC: US Government Printing Office. Or online at http://www.access.gpo.gov/su_docs/

CHAPTER 13

DELIVERING RESEARCH DIETS

BEVERLY A. CLEVIDENCE, PHD; CARLA R. HEISER, MS, RD;
HELEN RASMUSSEN, MS, RD, FADA; RITA TSAY, MS, RD; JANIS F. SWAIN, MS, RD;
ALICE K. H. FONG, EDD, RD; SUSAN LEARNER BARR, MS, RD; KAREN TODD, MS, RD;
MARY JOAN OEXMANN, MS, RD; AND DAVID J. JENKINS, MD, PHD, DSC

Many investigators believe that the best way to ensure dietary control in research studies is to house the research participants and carefully control their food intake. This is an ever less feasible option because it is very expensive for the investigators and burdensome for the participants. However, research studies can be carried out quite successfully with free-living participants. For some studies, free-living participants are required to eat all (or most) meals at the feeding facility. In other studies, participants may eat all (or most) meals away from the facility.

Although some degree of control is lost when the dietary staff does not directly observe the participants' food consumption, careful attention to compliance can yield good results. An advantage of using free-living participants is that the recruitment pool can be broadened to include those bound by geography or physical limitations, the elderly, and members of religious communities.

This chapter addresses how to "deliver" research diets to study participants. (Techniques for managing the delivery of diets for multiple concurrent studies are discussed in Chapter 20, "Staffing Needs for Research Diet Studies.")

Topics include: methods for serving meals eaten at feeding facilities as well as for distributing food eaten away from the study site; practical ways to maintain masked study designs; eating techniques particular to controlled diet studies; and management approaches for problem situations that could affect compliance or nutrient intake. The discussion finishes with some "true tales" of mishaps.

FOODSERVICE AND DISTRIBUTION TECHNIQUES

On-Site Delivery

With the "prepared-tray" delivery system, trays are assembled by the kitchen staff and delivered to the dining room or to residents' rooms. This delivery method is popular in small facilities because it requires less space than the "cafeteria style" of service. The labor involved in tray assembly is not extensive if the number of study participants is small.

In many larger units, food is delivered in a cafeteria style. Participants collect designated foods, item by item, as they move down a cafeteria line. Food items are typically weighed, but in some circumstances ad libitum (ad lib) service may be appropriate. With this method, the labor involved in tray assembly is shifted from staff members to study participants.

For both methods, a quality control checklist should be used before the tray is released to the participant. (An example of a checklist is shown in Chapter 18, "Documentation, Record Keeping, and Recipes." Menus also can be used as checklists.) A foodservice supervisor or the research dietitian checks the trays to ensure that each food item is present at the appropriate calorie level and for the appropriate dietary treatment. After marking each item on the checklist against the food items on the tray, the person checking trays will easily spot missing or duplicated food items. When more than one person checks trays, it is advised that they initial the checklists to indicate responsibility for the accuracy of the corresponding tray; this allows mistakes to be traced. Empty trays should be returned to the cafeteria window and checked to be certain all foods and beverages have been completely consumed.

If there are any leftovers, the participants should be reminded of their obligation to eat all of each food item. If there are extenuating circumstances, and food or beverages are refused, the kitchen staff must weigh the returned items and enter the weight data into the computer by participant name or code number. Thus the participant's dietary record is amended by subtracting the weights of refused items from the total for that day. In rare circumstances, the food refusals may be chemically analyzed for adjusting nutrient intake records. It is important that the investigator be notified immediately when food is not consumed, especially if the volunteer is sick.

Occasionally, extra portions of food remain on the serving line after participants have eaten; this occurs when a subject drops out of the study or is absent, or when extra servings are inadvertently portioned. Although it can be tempting to keep these items. it is prudent to discard any leftover, portioned food at the end of the day. This control point prevents an unintended food item from being served on a subsequent day.

The following example demonstrates how one facility successfully combined the prepared tray and the modified cafeteria style of service to meet study needs (1–3). The goal of the study was to determine which foods, and the amount of each food, that participants would select when given several food items to choose among.

Example: The prepared-tray method of food delivery is used to deliver foods to participants for "skeleton meals" served at 8:00 AM, noon, and 5:00 PM in the dining room. Each participant receives a tray, marked with his or her name, containing certain food items. These items, which include milk, tossed salads, fruits, and condiments, are served to each participant at appropriate meals to supply needed nutrients and to increase palatability. On the breakfast tray, all participants are given a vitamin-mineral supplement to compensate for the unlikely possibility of nutritional deficiencies arising during the study.

In addition, participants select among six isocaloric food items offered in unlimited quantity at each meal. Food choices are placed on a large tray in the dining room to simulate a cafeteria style of foodservice. Each of the food items is preweighed into small containers, covered, and labeled for easy identification. Participants may eat as many portions of each food item as desired. The research kitchen staff brings more food items to the tray when any food choice is low. In this particular protocol, the same food items are served at each breakfast, lunch, and dinner throughout the study.

A microwave oven near the table is available to warm food. Noncaloric beverages such as black coffee, tea, decaffeinated coffee, and herbal tea are available. In this study of food selection, carbonated beverages are not allowed because they tend to induce a sensation of fullness that may prevent participants from eating all their food. Sugar-free lemonade is provided to each participant in a thermos between meals.

Participants are instructed to not share food, to report spillage, and to leave food choice containers, empty or with refusals, on their own tray. After each meal, the research kitchen staff collects the individual trays, counts and records the containers by checking the food identification number on the bottom of the containers (eg, B2 denotes a food coded 2 that is served at breakfast), and weighs any refusals. This information is entered into the daily meal record sheet, and the nutrient intake is calculated.

Off-Site Delivery

Food Safety Considerations

Food hygiene and safety are primary concerns when food is to be eaten away from the controlled environment of the study facility. It is the responsibility of the research dietitian to ensure that volunteers understand the importance of proper food handling and storage. During the screening interview, the dietitian should discuss issues of food safety, including safe temperatures for foods; special care of milk, meats, and other perishables; the amount of refrigerator and freezer space that will be needed at home to store food; and special cooking required. In some centers, issues of food storage and the facility's liability are addressed in the consent form document to ensure that participants understand the importance of proper food handling.

Containers for carrying foods home can vary depending on the length of time the subject travels before the food can be refrigerated and on the ease of transport. Paper or plastic shopping bags should have carrying handles and can be purchased in colors to differentiate among diets. This is advantageous for the participant and the foodservice worker retrieving the bags from the refrigerator. They should not be used, however, when the subject's travel time is more than an hour. For longer travel times and large storage needs, a food cooler used with reusable "blue ice" packs is the better alternative. Temperature-sensitive strips are available for monitoring food temperatures (MonitorMark®, 3M Packaging System Division, St Paul, Minn). A checklist (an example is shown in Chapter 18, "Documentation, Record Keeping, and Recipes") should be attached to show that all items are in the cooler and to identify when each item is to be eaten. The checklist includes instructions for food preparation and a phone number to call if problems arise. It is advisable to have a 24-hour hot line for participants to call regarding food problems. After hours and on weekends, the dietitian on duty can carry a beeper to ensure that calls are received.

Weekend Meals and Take-out Meals

Many protocols allow for take-out meals for all or some of the study. Any type of research diet can be prepared for take-out, but the more rigorous research diets are the most difficult for outpatient studies and require more work for the kitchen staff and the study participant. The usual strict quality control standards must be applied, and the food must be packaged in containers that will not leak or spill. The kitchen staff needs extra time to pack food for take-out. Participants have additional responsibility because they must heat meals and may be required to consume them at the specified times. Also, participants have the added temptation to consume unauthorized foods and beverages when away from the study facility.

Consumption of All Foods Away from the Feeding Facility

Delivering a Week's Food Supply

If subjects are particularly hard to recruit for a given study, this plan may be given as an option to individuals who are otherwise discouraged from participating. This delivery plan is practical for use in studies of homebound or frail individuals as well as participants who, because of geography or other daily commitments, are inconvenienced by the daily or twice-weekly visits to the feeding facility.

A drawback to this plan is the lack of frequent contact between participants and investigators or other staff members. (However, meetings with participants can be scheduled for purposes other than picking up food.) Another drawback is the effect on participant morale if some participants are perceived to have special privileges. It must be stressed that although this system of food delivery is appropriate for many studies of total diet composition (ie, macronutrient studies), it may not be appropriate for precise nutrient balance studies.

This plan is not so radical a departure from on-site feeding of free-living participants as it may seem. Feeding arrangements for free-living participants are structured in various ways, wherein volunteers may come in daily or Monday through Friday, consume one or more meals at the facility, and take home the remainder of the day's meals or snacks, as allowed. Additional data and sample collections (24-hour urine and stool specimens, daily weights and blood pressures) may make daily visits necessary. Other visit schedules may entail two or three trips to the research facility each week. Sometimes the entire week's food is packaged for home consumption and is disbursed to the participant at one weekly visit.

The monitoring of a volunteer's progress on a study is a crucial part of the success of any research study. However, daily visits sometimes focus on obtaining food at the expense of time for visiting with study personnel. If the volunteer designates one day for pickup of the week's food, other visits could be set aside for reviewing any compliance questions or for reviewing lab values. Because the purpose of such visits focuses on an exchange of information between the participant and the study's professional staff, this could be a more "caring" approach to a volunteer's participation.

The logistics of the food delivery system depend on the type of food offered. Typically, most food items (and particularly those food items needing the most precise measurements) are portioned at the feeding facility. The main dishes, foods that are difficult to portion, and foods that contain key nutrients for the study should be weighed precisely. Preweighed food items or entire meals can be sent home frozen, with instructions for cooking. Some items can be sent home in bulk. Directions for measuring these foods in household units can be provided, and volunteers can portion many items, including lettuce, milk, rice, and bread.

The alternative to daily visits to the test facility is beneficial in many ways. Food preparation is less dictated by a daily or a three times per week food pickup, and food preparation and staffing patterns can be more flexible. Volunteers can pick up food with one trip to the feeding facility and take the food directly home, thereby eliminating the possible inadequacy of refrigeration of food at the participant's job site, for example. Sending bulk food items reduces leakage and spillage that is common when items are individually portioned. Additionally, this lightens the workload associated with portioning foods; the kitchen staff can spend more time with the participants, thus adding an extra dimension to their jobs.

It is important to teach the participants appropriate techniques for measuring and preparing food items. These instructions are commonly included in an orientation workshop that is held during the first week of the study. It should also be mandatory for each volunteer to come to the facility every day of the first week of the research study to verify the appropriate energy level for weight stabilization as well as to review all food preparation techniques.

Courier Service

A courier service can be effectively used to deliver research diets to home-based participants. Dietary staff packages food items in three boxes for each study participant: (1) dry goods, (2) refrigerated goods (4°C) (bread, fruit, vegetables, dairy, etc), and (3) frozen goods (–20°C). All boxes are labeled with the participant's full name, address, and telephone number (conveniently printed on a sticker) together with a clearly visible courier delivery number. Boxes should also be labeled (eg, A, B, and C), and the courier should know the number of boxes to deliver to each participant. To avoid potential confusion, the number of boxes should be standard for all participants, if possible, regardless of caloric intake.

The courier should be instructed on the most convenient time for participants to receive delivery (nothing annoys participants more than being roused from bed to accept a delivery, and nothing frustrates the courier more than to be refused admission to an apartment because the occupant is not at home). A courier service once trained should be retained for further studies. The courier service can also be used for the retrieval of fecal and urine samples.

The courier system of food delivery has appeal in studies when special groups of participants are recruited; for example, patients with specific diseases or specific genetic characteristics. These individuals may be working full time and unable to visit a feeding facility on a daily basis. When the courier system is used, it is advisable that the participant always be in possession of an extra two days' supply of food to be kept for emergencies such as snow or floods that may prevent the courier from getting through.

Vending Machine Feeding Systems

Vending machines have been successfully used in studies of food intake regulation (1–3).

Example: Ten isocaloric food choices were made available to study participants through refrigerated vending machines. Food items were prepared, portioned, and wrapped with plastic wrap, then stocked into the individual slots of a vending machine. Items were restocked at least twice a day by the research kitchen staff so that items were consistently available to participants. Participants obtained any one of the food choices by entering their code number on the keypad attached to the machine. A microcomputer connected to the vending machine recorded the identity of the participant, the item of food removed, and the time that food was obtained.

Participants immediately consumed the whole portion upon its removal from the vending machine. If they could not finish the whole food portion at that time, they reported this to the staff. Participants had access to the vending machine 24 hours a day.

Considerations in Designing Vending Machine Feeding Systems
- Select food items tailored to the study population and the study hypothesis.
- Offer a variety of selections. Include at each meal food items that can be heated as well as those that can be eaten cold and provide microwave ovens and ice machines as needed.

- Assess the availability of the food items to be used. Manufacturers change their recipes and packaging sizes, so it is advisable to check the projected availability of the product.
- Consider each food choice with respect to the physical facility, operating system, staffing pattern, and storage space requirements. Making food items from original recipes is a good option if staffing for food preparation is adequate but storage space is limited. Otherwise, commercially prepared and packaged food items are recommended. (Note that composition of foods must be verified.)
- Select food items that can be weighed and portioned in advance and stored in a freezer or refrigerator. This saves time and avoids last-minute rushes that can cause errors.
- Devise recipes that can be produced in large quantity, then measure them into smaller portions.
- Identify packaging that is suitable for each food item (heat-sealable containers can be useful). Avoid using poor quality paper containers. They tend to absorb liquid or fat and can also affect the appearance of foods.
- Avoid foods that change in color or texture after being refrigerated. For foods that require warming, avoid items that develop an odd texture when heated in a microwave oven.
- Avoid food items with easily separated components; for example, a bagel and cream cheese. Participants may remove the cream cheese, thus altering the intended calorie level and nutrient content of the meal.

Unit Foods

Unit foods are food items such as muffins and cookies that mimic the nutrient content of a dietary treatment. Unit foods are typically used to adjust calories in a research study. For example, in a long-term feeding study examining the effect of a low-fat diet (25% fat, 15% protein, 60% carbohydrate) on serum lipoproteins, a muffin was designed to approximate this particular diet composition. When calories were needed, this muffin, portioned into 100-calorie units, was used. Examples of recipes for unit food items are given in Chapter 18, "Documentation, Record Keeping, and Recipes."

MASKING OR BLINDING DIETARY TREATMENTS

General Considerations

The technique of *masking* (sometimes called *blinding*) is frequently used in human research studies. The goal of masking is to prevent bias on the part of study participants or the data collector (the investigator measuring the clinical or cognitive parameter of interest). If the identity of the dietary treatment is withheld from both the participant and the data collector, the study is considered "double-blinded." A study is "single-blinded" when the identity of the treatment is withheld from either the participant or the data collector, but not both. In single-blinded studies, it is typically the participant rather than the data collector who is blinded, but occasionally the reverse is true. For example, study participants taking fish oil supplements may know whether they are receiving active treatment because of the supplements' smell and taste, but the treatment could be blinded to the data collector.

Masking is a valuable tool that adds credibility to diet studies, and it is a desirable study trait to employ when possible. Masking of participants prevents variation in compliance based on knowledge of the treatment. When participants provide data (eg, questionnaires evaluating emotional or cognitive parameters), masking prevents bias in responses. Masking of the data collector prevents bias in measurements.

Unfortunately, some experimental variables cannot readily be masked because of their taste (artificial sweeteners), smell (fish oils, thiamin), or texture (some dietary fibers). Others cannot be masked because of physiological effects; for example, the altered mental state produced by alcohol, the distinctive yellow color of urine after riboflavin ingestion, and some orange skin discoloration associated with long-term use of beta-carotene supplements.

Ethical issues to consider in masking subjects to treatments include the subject's "right to know" and safeguarding the well-being of the subject. Prior to committing to a research study, potential participants are typically informed of the study protocol, including dietary treatments, both verbally (at an information meeting) and in writing (as part of the informed consent document). At this time participants are also told whether the treatments are to be masked. Most participants accept this arrangement as fair, especially in conjunction with a crossover or Latin square design in which every participant cycles through every treatment.

Some investigators believe that the participant always has the right to know which treatment he or she is receiving and will tell the participant if asked. Others do not share this concern. If participants have been adequately informed about the diets and the masking procedures prior to the study, they rarely ask about the treatment codes. Dietitians and investigators need to share an understanding about when and how to break the code to participants. In addition, it is prudent, and in some studies essential, to establish procedures for monitoring treatment effects to ensure safety of the study participants. The criteria by which an individual investigator or a protocol oversight committee might "unmask" the study to ensure safety also should be developed before the study begins.

Practical Approaches

Masking is difficult in dietary fiber studies and in studies comparing the effects of different protein sources (eg, dairy vs red meat). In fiber studies, purified fibers or fiber supplements may be masked to participants by incorporating the fiber into standard foods such as breakfast cereals; the required technology usually necessitates help from industrial collaborators. Similarly, in highly flavored dishes such as chili or burgers, it is possible to use different protein sources (eg, vegetable proteins) in exchange for animal protein. Sometimes masking is not possible because the nature of the fiber or protein is to be assessed in terms of whole foods. In these cases, control foods should be chosen for similar macronutrient content and dietary function (eg, milk vs milk analogues) in the diet in order not to distort the meal pattern or alter the palatability or acceptability of the diet.

To mask dietary treatments in fat substitution studies, it is advisable to avoid food items with obvious changes in "mouth feel." For example, the flavor and mouth feel of butter as opposed to margarine or whole milk compared with skim milk are likely to be detected by participants, whereas these differences are less easily detected in baked products, particularly when the product is highly flavored (eg, through use of flavoring extracts).

Certain foods are particularly useful vehicles for adding fats or oils without compromising taste, texture, or masking. These include mashed potatoes; tuna salad; chicken salad; salad dressings; meatloaf; chili; spaghetti sauce; other mixed casseroles and rice dishes; and baked products such as muffins, quick breads, and cookies. (See also Chapter 18, "Documentation, Record Keeping, and Recipes.") Preparing portions in individual baking tins allows for participant-specific addition of ingredients. This strategy for individualization also works well in the case of preparation of individual pizzas, which can be baked with varying amounts of cheeses and pizza sauces prepared with differing amounts of oils or hard fats.

Coding diets by color, number, or letter is an effective way to mask dietary treatments. With this system, each dietary treatment is assigned a different code and references to specific diets are by code rather than by description of the dietary treatment. The topic of masking should be discussed with the foodservice workers. Like dietitians, they are not likely to be masked to dietary treatments, and they should be cautioned not to interpret codes for study participants.

In the following example, color coding is used in conjunction with the cafeteria style approach to foodservice. Note that although the calorie levels and gram amounts of each food item are displayed on the participants' menus in this example, participants are blinded to this information in many studies. (See the discussion of bar codes in Chapter 12, "Producing Research Diets.")

Example: As study participants enter the cafeteria line they pick up their menus from assigned slots in an accordion folder. This menu is used by the participants to identify food items to gather from the cafeteria line. The menu is printed on green or yellow paper with the color green corresponding to a diet high in monounsaturated fats and the color yellow to a diet high in saturated fats. Food items on the cafeteria line are also color coded, each bearing a green or yellow label. (See Chapter 12, "Producing Research Diets.") This label helps the participants to locate their food items on the serving line and facilitates the dietitian in checking their trays.

Exhibit 13-1 shows a "master menu" from which participants' menus are printed onto colored paper. As a precautionary measure, the word *green* is printed in the upper left corner of the menu. This ensures that the monounsaturated diets corresponding to "green" are not mistakenly copied onto the yellow paper. It should be noted that use of color codes is problematic if colors are similar or if any staff member or study participant is color blind.

Another caveat about masking treatments is that the description of food items should be limited on participants' menus. Exhibit 13-2 is a kitchen menu or production sheet (refer to Chapter 18, "Documentation, Record Keeping, and Recipes") used to portion food items by calorie levels. The detailed description of food items that appear on the kitchen menu is not present on the participants' menus. In contrast to the dietary staff, the participants only need to know which foods to gather; the fat content of the items is masked.

Thus, in this example, a salad dressing is listed as a single item on the participants' menu, whereas the two fat sources that are added directly to the salad dressing are detailed on the kitchen menu. On the participants' menu the two asterisks after "salad dressing" indicate that the code 31 dressing was modified by the addition of two ingredients. Notice also that the kitchen menu bears not only the color code and full description of menu items but, unlike the participants' menus, also bears the identification of the dietary treatment (monounsaturated).

In the study from which this example was drawn, the dietary treatments were masked to both the participants and the data collector. The primary investigator, the study coordinator, and the dietary staff were not masked; their knowledge of the treatments was necessary to ensure accurate delivery of test meals. Data were sent directly from the analytical laboratory (the data collector) to an independent statistician without passing through the primary investigator. The statistician, who had assigned the participant codes during the design of the study, received the data and conducted statistical analyses as designated in the study protocol. This system ensured that the resulting data could not be influenced by potentially biased parties (the data collector to whom treatments were masked and the primary investigator to whom treatments were not masked).

EATING TECHNIQUES

Thorough instructions detailing how study participants should consume their food are instrumental to the accuracy of tightly controlled feeding studies. Verbal instructions given by the dietitian or investigator enable the rationale and techniques to be explained to and discussed with the participant. This also affords staff the opportunity to assess participant comprehension and potential compliance. Written instructions should then be given to the participant to keep.

Most controlled feeding studies require participants to eat "all" of each food item given to them, but "all" can imply different degrees of thoroughness depending on the nutrients under investigation and the outcome variables to be assessed. The word can also mean different things to different participants.

The *scrape and wash technique* is used in metabolic balance studies in which a high degree of control is required, such as vitamin, mineral, and nitrogen balance studies. Although this eating technique breaks the rules for good table manners, it is employed to ensure that participants consume every morsel of food and liquid they are served. The following specific techniques are suggested:

- Participants should use a small, five-inch "icing spatula" (eg, Revere® or Corning®) to scrape up any particles of food remaining on the plate or dish, and eat the scrapings.
- Participants should save a piece of bread and use it to absorb any liquid remaining on the serving plate or dishes, and eat the bread.
- Participants should save a portion of allotted drinking water (distilled) and use it to rinse all beverage glasses, and drink it.
- Staff should use weighed salt, pepper, pectin, etc, very carefully so as not to lose a grain. If it is to be consumed in total, provide the participant with a cotton tipped swab to clean out the shaker at the last meal of the day or have it added to the food directly by the technician responsible for distributing the research diet. (When mineral intake is critical, the minerals, such as $NaCl$ or $KHCO_3$, may be mixed in a weighed amount of deionized water at a specific concentration and distributed on the meal tray.)

Some studies are well-controlled but require less stringent eating techniques. Examples follow:

- A protocol to study the effect of the type or amount of dietary fat may not require the scrape and wash technique because trace amounts of fat, rather than gram amounts, are left behind on the plate.
- If a participant left the crust of a meal's bread uneaten, he or she would be asked to eat it to comply with caloric intake requirements; however, a normal scattering of bread crumbs might be considered inconsequential.
- Small quantities of such foods as carrots or celery might be provided as "free items" in a lipid study because of their low caloric content and lack of fat; of course, this would not be appropriate in studies of fiber or carotenoids.
- Because the ideal quantity of lettuce for consuming a given amount of salad dressing is a matter of individual preference, participants might be given a generous serving of lettuce to ensure that all of the salad dressing is consumed. In many lipid studies, uneaten lettuce (without dressing) would not be challenged, because lettuce is not supplying critical nutrients, including calories. However, participants would be asked to eat all visible traces of salad dressing and margarine by picking up traces of these fat

EXHIBIT 13-1

Master Menu for a Participant Menu

This master menu is from a study using color coding to mask dietary treatments. The master menu is copied onto green paper and distributed to all participants eating the diet coded by the color green. As part of the masking procedure, this menu describes foods generically. The participants collect preweighed food items at their assigned calorie levels according to the food items designated on the menu. The calorie levels displayed on the menu typically include at least one level above and below the expected use (here, from 1,400 kcal to 4,400 kcal). The amount of each food item is shown in the body of the exhibit for incremental calorie levels. Amounts are in grams unless otherwise indicated. Amounts of milk are number of cartons plus number of grams.

Name | **DIET = 07 GREEN** | Date:

SECTION	CODE	FOOD DESCRIPTION	1,400	1,600	1,800	2,000	2,200	2,400	2,800	3,200	3,600	4,000	4,400	EXTRAS:
		BREAKFAST												EXTRAS:
1100	503	ORANGE JUICE	96	109	123	137	150	164	191	219	246	273	301	CUCUMBERS:
7	7064	SAUSAGE	16	18	20	23	25	27	32	36	41	45	50	CARROTS:
1100	242	BLUEBERRY MUFFIN	54	61	69	77	84	92	107	123	138	153	169	CELERY:
100	1149.1	JELLY, PKT	1 pkt	1 pkt	1 pkt	1 pkt	1 pkt	1 pkt	2 pkt	2 pkt	2 pkt	3 pkt	3 pkt	ONION PACKETS:
34		SPREAD	8.9	10.1	11.4	12.7	13.9	15.2	17.7	20.3	22.8	25.3	27.9	PICKLE RELISH:
1100	1079	MILK	1 + 0	1 + 26	1 + 59	1 + 92	1 + 125	1 + 158	2 + 0	2 + 53	2 + 118	2 + 184	3 + 0	KETCHUP:
		LUNCH												*Record extra amounts eaten
10	1013	HAM	42	48	54	60	66	72	84	96	108	120	132	
1100	104	RYE BREAD	23	27	30	33	37	40	47	53	60	67	73	
		MUSTARD, 2												
11	1125	LETTUCE	12	13	15	17	18	20	23	27	30	33	37	
11	1152	TOMATOES	21	24	27	30	33	36	42	48	54	60	66	
1100	542	OATMEAL BAR	35	40	45	50	55	60	70	80	90	100	110	
		DINNER												
5	5064	CHICKEN BREAST	70	80	90	100	110	120	140	160	180	200	220	
1100	629	CHICKEN GRAVY	9	11	12	13	15	16	19	21	24	27	29	
11	1167	BAKED POTATOES	117	133	150	167	183	200	233	267	300	333	367	
11	11095	BROCCOLI	28	32	36	40	44	48	56	64	72	80	88	
11	1125	LETTUCE	26	29	33	37	40	44	51	59	66	73	81	
11	1152	TOMATOES	21	24	27	30	33	36	42	48	54	60	66	
1	1125	EGG YOLK	2	3	3	3	4	4	5	5	6	7	7	
1100	31	SALAD DRESSING**	6.5	7.5	8.4	9.3	10.3	11.2	13.1	14.9	16.8	18.7	20.5	
1100	100	WHEAT BREAD	30	35	39	43	48	52	61	69	78	87	95	
1100	34	SPREAD	7.0	8.0	9.0	10.0	11.0	12.0	14.0	16.0	18.0	20.0	22.0	
1	1079	MILK	0 + 115	0 + 131	0 + 148	0 + 164	0 + 180	0 + 197	1 + 0	1 + 26	1 + 59	1 + 92	1 + 125	
300	2230	EXTRAS:												
9	9003	APPLE WITH SKIN	85	95	110	120	130	145	165	190	215	240	265	
100	2230	SUGAR, PKT	2	2	2	3	3	3	4	4	5	5	6	

EXHIBIT 13-2

Master Menu for a Kitchen Menu

This master menu is an example of a kitchen menu (or production sheet) that is used by the kitchen staff to portion individual food items for the calorie levels designated. The calorie levels displayed on the menu typically include at least one level above and below the expected use (here, from 1,400 kcal to 4,400 kcal). Note that in contrast to the participants' menu, where the goal is to mask dietary treatments, the kitchen menu displays the identification of the dietary treatment and the full description of food items (eg saturated margarine vs spread). The full description of the salad dressing is also displayed.

Date:

MONOUNSAT SECTION	CODE	DIET = 07 GREEN ENSUS FOOD DESCRIPTION	1,400	1,600	1,800	2,000	2,200	2,400	2,800	3,200	3,600	4,000	4,400	EXTRAS:
		BREAKFAST												
1100	503	ORANGE JUICE, W/CALCIUM	96	109	123	137	150	164	191	219	246	273	301	CUCUMBERS:
7	7064	SAUSAGE PORK LINK, CKD	16	18	20	23	25	27	32	36	41	45	50	CARROTS:
1100	242	BLUEBERRY MUFFIN. W/CANOLA OIL (CODE 42)	54	61	69	77	84	92	107	123	138	153	169	CELERY:
100	1149.1	JELLY. PKT	1 pkt	1 pkt	1 pkt	1 pkt	1 pkt	1 pkt	2 pkt	2 pkt	2 pkt	3 pkt	3 pkt	ONION PACKETS:
1100	34	MARGARINE, SATURATED	8.9	10.1	11.4	12.7	13.9	15.2	17.7	20.3	22.8	25.3	27.9	PICKLE RELISH:
1	1079	MILK, 2%	1 + 0	1 + 26	1 + 59	1 + 92	1 + 125	1 + 158	2 + 0	2 + 53	2 + 118	2 + 184	3 + 0	KETCHUP:
		LUNCH												
10	10135	HAM	42	48	54	60	66	72	84	96	108	120	132	
1100	104	RYE BREAD	23	27	30	33	37	40	47	53	60	67	73	
		MUSTARD, 2 PACKETS (OPTIONAL)												
11	11252	LETTUCE	12	13	15	17	18	20	23	27	30	33	37	
11	11529	TOMATOES	21	24	27	30	33	36	42	48	54	60	66	
1100	542	OATMEAL BAR COOKIES W/CANOLA OIL (CODE 42)	35	40	45	50	55	60	70	80	90	100	110	

		DINNER	70	80	90	100	110	120	140	160	180	200	220	
5	5064	CHICKEN BREAST	9	11	12	13	15	16	19	21	24	27	29	
1100	629	CHICKEN GRAVY + FAT. W/MOD OLEIC MAYO (CODE 29)												
11	11674	BAKED POTATOES WITH SKINS	117	133	150	167	183	200	233	267	300	333	367	
11	11095	BROCCOLI, SPEARS CKD	28	32	36	40	44	48	56	64	72	80	88	
11	11252	LETTUCE	26	29	33	37	40	44	51	59	66	73	81	
11	11529	TOMATOES	21	24	27	30	33	36	42	48	54	60	66	
1	1125	EGG YOLK	2	3	3	3	4	4	5	5	6	7	7	
1100	31	SALAD DRESSING, HIGH OLEIC POURABLE	6.5	7.5	8.4	9.3	10.3	11.2	13.1	14.9	16.8	18.7	20.5	
1100	29	MAYONNAISE, MOD OLEIC (ADD TO DRESSING)	4.7	5.3	6.0	6.7	7.3	8.0	9.3	10.7	12.0	13.3	14.7	ADD MAYO TO DRESSING
110041		COCONUT OIL (ADD TO DRESSING)	2.8	3.2	3.6	4.0	4.4	4.8	5.6	6.4	7.2	8.0	8.8	ADD OIL TO DRESSING
1100	100	CRACKED WHEAT BREAD	30	35	39	43	48	52	61	69	78	87	95	
1100	34	MARGARINE, SATURATED	7.0	8.0	9.0	10.0	11.0	12.0	14.0	16.0	18.0	20.0	22.0	
1	1079	MILK, 2%	0 + 115	0 + 131	0 + 148	0 + 164	0 + 180	0 + 197	1 + 0	1 + 26	1 + 59	1 + 92	1 + 125	
100	2230	EXTRAS:												
9	9003	APPLE WITH SKIN	85	95	110	120	130	145	165	190	215	240	265	
100	2230	SUGAR, PKT	2	2	2	3	3	3	4	4	5	5	6	

sources with bread. The use of distilled water would not be necessary nor would a water allotment be given.

- Coffee, tea, and diet beverages might be allowed free choice, within a given limit, as well as selected spices, including salt. Caution should be used that the spices allowed do not influence the outcome variables to be measured.

In studies of free-living participants, it is prudent to ensure that the foods that are vehicles for critical nutrients are wholly or primarily incorporated into those meals that are eaten at the facility. Most facilities discourage participants from taking out foods that are intended for consumption at the facility. When participants are allowed to take home foods ordinarily eaten at the facility, they may be required to record the items taken out (eg, by listing the items on the back of the menu). Participants should understand that this is not a simple issue of trust between the participant and the investigator but rather is one aspect by which the scientific community will assess the quality of the study.

Regardless of which eating technique is used in a study, it is important that the technique is applied consistently across all treatments, all dietary periods, and all volunteers. Participants' attention to the details of the eating technique can lapse during the course of the study. The research dietitian whose approach focuses on encouraging and reminding participants about eating techniques, rather than monitoring and scolding, is likely to have better cooperation.

COMMON PROBLEMS OF STUDY PARTICIPANTS EATING RESEARCH DIETS

Too Full, Too Hungry

Feeling either too full or too hungry is a frequent complaint of study participants, even though research diets usually are designed to maintain body weight. These symptoms are most likely to occur during the first days of the study—a time of adjustment both psychologically and physiologically. For some individuals, a study diet consisting of three meals a day may replace a habitual diet that was more calorically dense (fewer fruits and vegetables; more fats or candy). This change is likely to cause a too-full feeling. However, a premature decrease in the participant's energy intake may cause subsequent hunger and weight loss. On the other hand, if the distribution of calories among meals is markedly different from a participant's habitual diet, the participant may experience hunger between light and heavy meals.

A bloated or too-full feeling without weight gain can often be solved by allowing foods from heavier meals to be eaten at other times during the day. Similarly, the problem of hunger without weight loss is commonly solved by providing snacks between meals and by redistributing foods among meals. Adding foods with bulk may also help alle-

viate the feeling of hunger. The research dietitian should be vigilant to follow up on complaints of hunger. Not only is this unpleasant for the participant, but a hungry participant will be tempted to eat unauthorized foods. If a participant is losing weight and complains of hunger, the dietitian and study investigator should consider increasing the calorie level, even if the weight loss does not meet the criteria for a calorie increase. (See Chapter 17, "Energy Needs and Weight Maintenance in Controlled Diet Studies," for information on setting calorie levels.)

Depending on the diet composition and the study objective, these side effects may be inevitable. For example, some types of dietary fiber may cause discomfort from a too-full feeling, whereas a study designed to produce weight loss may cause hunger. During the planning phase of the protocol, criteria should be established for changing calorie levels, allowing food to be eaten between meal times, and acceptable use of medications for an upset stomach or constipation. During the orientation or screening interview, participants should be told that feelings of hunger or fullness may occur until diet adjustments have been made. This will ease anxiety of participants and reassure them that what they are experiencing is normal.

Food Refusal

Reasons that volunteers in a research study refuse to consume food are numerous. They include illness, food allergies, inadequate preparation of meals, poor meal quality, monotony, and dislike. In any event, incidents of food omission should be communicated to the investigator, and a decision should be made as to how to replace the food or whether to dismiss the participant from the study.

Food refusals should always be documented. The study records should be amended with an account of what food was not consumed, the weight of the refused food, and a recalculation of the day's intake. The participant's explanation for refusal is useful for documenting volunteer compliance, for assessing risk management issues in the case of food allergies or foodborne illnesses, and as a rationale for improving food quality or cooking procedures.

Displeasure with Calorie Changes

Weight gain and loss during nutrition research studies are variables that must be recognized either as needing to be controlled or of no consequence, depending on the objective of the study. Issues concerning body weight must be addressed with study participants during the recruitment phase. Unfortunately, many potential volunteers will think that a "diet study" is actually a "weight-loss study." If a study requires weight maintenance and a volunteer is expecting to lose weight while in the study, this can be distressing, particularly if the calorie level is increased because of weight loss. During the recruitment as well as the first few days of a study, the body weight range acceptable for each volunteer should be discussed privately with each participant. In studies in which weight is controlled by adding or deleting specific food items, choices should be offered to the participants so that they feel that they have a say in the matter. If a study is designed deliberately to provide excess calories, this should be clearly stated in the study protocol, the consent form, and verbally at the initial interview. Additionally, for participants who gain weight, provision should be made to offer optional dietary counseling to lose weight once the study is completed.

When a participant's calorie intake must be changed because of a change in body weight, it is advisable for the investigator or research dietitian to discuss the change with the participant in advance. Some participants will welcome the change because they felt the amount of food was too much or too little. However, it can be upsetting for a participant to unexpectedly find a change (particularly an increase) in his or her calorie level, especially if coupled with other life events that the participant cannot control. With an explanation of the anticipated change and a day's advance notice, most participants accept the change easily.

Calorie levels of diets can be masked to participants. (See the use of bar code labels for food items discussed in Chapter 12, "Producing Research Diets.") Blinding enables the investigator to alter a participant's energy intake without alienating the study participant. Although a participant may suspect that he or she is getting slightly more or less quantity of food items, the change may go unnoticed. Certainly the masked approach is more subtle than announcing the change. If calorie levels are to be masked, this, like other aspects of the diet, must be understood by participants before they commit to the study.

Take-out Meals

Requests for taking meals out—for work or weekends or beyond what the protocol permits—occur frequently. It is difficult to run a long-term study without allowing participants to occasionally take their food out on their request. If participants do not have this flexibility, there are likely to be problems in retention and future recruitment. Efforts should be made to accommodate the participants by packing some of their meals to take out. However, this step must be well-planned and managed; if not, control will be lost as an increasing number of meals are eaten away from the facility. If some participants are allowed to take meals out more often than others, this disparity will likely be noticed by participants and considered unfair.

When take-out is authorized, advanced notice should be given to the kitchen staff to allow for adequate time to pack meals; otherwise, transfer mistakes are likely to occur. Before permission is granted to the participant to take any meal out, certain assurances regarding the participant's eating techniques and habits should be obtained. Issues to be reviewed with the participant include compliance, food spillage, food safety, and appropriate reheating of food.

Emergency Meals

It is necessary to have contingency plans for keeping free-living participants on dietary treatments when it is not feasible for them to receive their meals in the usual way (eg, at a feeding facility or by courier). These events may include family emergencies, inclement weather (notably snow), lack of transportation, or errors of food omission. Providing one or two full days' meals for home storage can alleviate this potential break in a study protocol. Emergency meals are typically composed of foods that can be stored for a number of weeks without deterioration. Typically these include canned goods, frozen dinners, dry foods, and shelf-stable milk. In rare situations (death in the family, testing procedure conducted away from the facility), overnight air express may be the best means of providing study foods.

The research dietitian should ensure that each participant will have adequate storage space for frozen goods. Perishable items such as fresh fruits should not be included but may be listed on the emergency meal menu for optional use if they are available. If perishable foods are allowed, those approved foods should be listed along with the amounts to consume (in household measures). A research dietitian should contact participants to advise them of suitable substitutions.

Because emergency meals are tailored to the participant's dietary treatment, these meals must be distributed at the beginning of each treatment period. It is prudent to collect any unused emergency meals at the end of the dietary period. Otherwise, these meals may accumulate as participants switch over to different dietary treatments, and there is the potential for meals from different treatment phases to be confused with one another.

Studies Spanning Holidays

Studies are typically scheduled to avoid major holidays, particularly those associated with consumption of special foods and alcoholic beverages. When this is not possible, advance planning for these days is necessary. This may mean advance notice at the initial interview and again before the holiday that exceptions will not be made. Holidays are generally celebrated in dining facilities with appropriate decorations or party favors.

Commonly, some exceptions are made to the normal feeding procedure. For example, at Thanksgiving, participants may be allowed to eat specific foods at a traditional family dinner, whereas foods critical to the diet are provided from the feeding facility. In other situations, participants may be given a free meal on a holiday. Some investigators require that food records be maintained for any free-choice meal.

Holiday parties can be difficult for study participants, because celebrations are typically centered around food and, perhaps, alcohol. It is helpful if participants take approved snacks (those provided with their study diets) with them to parties. If a holiday such as New Year's Eve falls in the early days of a study period, one or two alcoholic drinks may not compromise the study results. However, as with any exception, it is important to give detailed instructions to the participant concerning what is and is not acceptable, and to record deviations from protocol in the participant's dietary record.

Illnesses

The study investigator must determine, on a case-by-case basis, whether a participant's illness during the study will compromise the study results. In some cases, a study physician or medical expert should be consulted before this determination is made. Sometimes participants are dismissed from studies because of unanticipated illnesses; more commonly, the illness (a cold or the flu) does not require the participant's dismissal. However, a contagious illness can compromise a study if it affects a large proportion of the participants. For this reason, some study investigators ask that participants take flu shots prior to the study. (The timing of the shots may be important.) Additionally, it is useful to provide a setting at the feeding facility where participants who have a contagious illness can eat away from other participants. Frequently, meals are sent home to participants during brief illnesses.

Participants should be cautioned not to force themselves to eat if they feel nauseated. If, because of illness, a research participant cannot consume all or part of a day's food, this must be noted in the participant's diet record. In some situations the illness may occur in a phase of the diet study where the investigator can "forgive" noncompliance that occurs because of illness, and the individual's participation may still be viable. Participants should discuss use of medication for an illness with the study investigator. All medications should be approved prior to use and documented in the study record as to type, dosage, and length of treatment.

Adverse Food Reactions

Adverse food reaction is the general term referring to both food intolerances (nonimmunologic reactions to foods) and food allergies (an abnormal immunologic reaction). Food intolerances are far more common in the general population than are food allergies, although many people believe that they are allergic to certain foods. Food intolerance reactions can be caused by enzyme deficiencies, toxins, infectious organisms, accidental contaminants, or pharmacologic substances. Strong intolerances also may be rooted in psychologically based aversions.

The symptoms for allergic and nonallergic reactions are not distinguishable. These reactions may be manifested as systemic (eg, headaches, irritability), gastrointestinal (eg, nausea, abdominal pain, vomiting, diarrhea, flatulence), res-

piratory (eg, rhinitis, asthma), or dermatologic symptoms (eg, hives, eczema) (4–6).

Food Allergies

Food allergies are more prevalent in children than in adults. Up to 4% of children younger than 6 years of age have food allergies (4), whereas 1% to 2% percent of adults do (5). Food allergies are more common in children with asthma and in atopic adults. Most allergic reactions are caused by relatively few foods: cow's milk, eggs, fish, shellfish, soybeans, tree nuts, and peanuts (4, 5). People who are sensitive to certain nonfood allergens are more likely to be reactive to certain foods. For example, those who are sensitive to ragweed pollen as an antigen commonly react to bananas and melons (watermelon, cantaloupe, honeydew), and those sensitive to birch pollen are more likely to react to apple, carrot, and hazelnut (4, 5).

Food Intolerances

Food intolerances are often caused by enzyme deficiencies and by sensitivity to agents used as preservatives, flavors, or color enhancers such as sulfites, nitrite and nitrate, monosodium glutamate, and tartrazine yellow (6). However the single most common food intolerance encountered in human feeding studies is lactose maldigestion or lactose intolerance. Dietitians planning studies conducted primarily among groups with a high prevalence of lactose maldigestion such as African Americans or Asians should consider menus that minimize the use of milk products. However, lactose maldigestion is frequently encountered in other populations, and all potential study participants should be queried about their tolerance for milk products.

For most people with lactose maldigestion, lactase is effective in relieving symptoms of gas, bloating, and diarrhea. Lactase is sold in tablet form (eg, Lactaid®, Lactaid Inc, Pleasantville, NJ, or Dairy Ease®, Sterling Winthrop Inc, New York, NY) to be taken with milk or other dairy products. Lactase is also sold in a liquid form designed to be added directly to milk. In feeding facilities this is less convenient, because for best results the lactase must act on milk lactose for 24 hours. Lactaid milk is now available in 1%, 2%, and 4% fat from the manufacturer in quarts and half-pints.

Individuals vary in the amount of milk and milk products that they can tolerate. Additionally, milk products such as yogurt with live cultures may not produce problems in participants who have lactose maldigestion. However, aversions to milk are not always related to adverse food reactions. Some participants are accustomed to drinking less milk than is typically served in diet studies; others simply dislike the taste or texture of milk. Depending on the goal of the study, it may be possible to substitute other foods for milk. (See the discussion of substitutions in Chapter 11, "Designing Research Diets.")

EXHIBIT 13-3

Sources of Information about Adverse Food Reactions

American Academy of Allergy, Asthma, and
Immunology
611 East Wells Street
Milwaukee, WI 53202
800-882-2762
http://www.aaaai.org

Asthma and Allergy Foundation of America
1125 15th Street NW, Suite 502
Washington, DC 20005
800-727-8462
http://www.aafa.org

The American Dietetic Association
216 West Jackson Blvd
Suite 800
Chicago, IL 60606-6995
800-877-1600 (for dietitians)
http://www.eatright.org

The Food Allergy Network
10400 Eaton Place, Suite 107
Fairfax, VA 22030
800-929-4040
http://www.foodallergy.org

American College of Allergy, Asthma, and Immunology
85 West Algonquin Road, Suite 550
Arlington Heights, IL 60005
800-842-7777
http://allergy.mcg.edu

National Eczema Association
1221 SW Yamhill, Suite 303
Portland, OR 97205
800-818-7546
http://www.eczema-assn.org

National Institutes of Health
Food allergy
Information Center
National Institute of Allergy and Infectious Disease
Building 31, Room 7A50
Bethesda, MD 20892-2520
301-496-5717
http://www.niaid.nih.gov

Lactose intolerance
National Digestive Diseases Information
Clearinghouse
2 Information Way
Bethesda, Md 20892-3570
301-496-3583
http://www.niddk.nih.gov

CONTROLLING EXTRANEOUS SOURCES OF NUTRIENTS AND OTHER CONFOUNDING SUBSTANCES

In addition to providing a well-planned diet for human feeding studies, the research dietitian and the study investigator must consider the influence of other sources of nutrients or nonnutritive substances that may affect the outcome of their study. This section addresses a number of those extraneous variables.

Vitamin and Mineral Supplements

Added nutrients, such as vitamin and mineral supplements, if not recognized or accounted for within a study protocol, can adversely affect interpretation of results from research studies. Volunteers are typically questioned at the initial screening regarding supplement use. Extra queries may be required concerning habitual use of "natural" or "alternative" products and supplemented sports drinks or other bev-

erages because participants may not view them as supplements. The principal investigator must determine whether any supplements will be allowed during the study and, additionally, must make it clear to the participant consuming the supplements when to discontinue them prior to participation. For some studies it is important that participants not take large doses of specific vitamins for a certain period of time prior to the admission date.

Supplements may need to be prescribed in conjunction with feeding studies, particularly when diets are designed to be low in certain nutrients. These preparations are generally tailor-made for the study specifications. If a commercial vitamin and mineral preparation is used for a research study, it is important to have it analyzed independently from its manufacturer. As part of a study protocol, a dietitian may be responsible for observing participants as they take supplements, thus adding an extra degree of control to the study.

Water and Seltzer Water

Controlling water source and quantity are important for mineral or electrolyte control/balance studies. Because the electrolyte content of tap water may be subject to variability, the use of deionized or distilled water is recommended. In such studies, a constant source and quantity of water should be used throughout the study. Intake and output records should be kept for any fluid balance study. For macronutrient studies, tap water, seltzer water, and spring water may be allowed ad lib. A number of flavored seltzers are now available, which can be used to add variety to diets, but these calorie-free beverages must be distinguished from sugar-containing sodas. A comprehensive discussion of water intake can be found in Chapter 15, "Meeting Requirements for Fluids."

Coffee, Tea, and Soft Drinks

Black coffee, tea, and diet soft drinks usually are considered to be noncaloric beverages and are thus allowed free choice, or within established guidelines, in many studies. The amount of each beverage should be kept consistent throughout the study, or a record of consumption should be kept. The methylxanthines contained in coffee, tea, cocoa, and some soft drinks include caffeine, theophylline, and theobromine. These are known to stimulate metabolic processes and affect the metabolism of free fatty acids, catecholamines, and creatinine. These beverages should be carefully monitored or avoided in metabolic research studies.

Instant coffee may be processed with gelatins and gums. Instant teas can include lemon flavor and sugar, saccharin, or aspartame. Considerations for the use of diet soft drinks relate to the sweetener contained in the product and its effects on the outcome variables to be measured. (See the discussion of artificial sweeteners.)

Alcohol

Alcoholic beverages are commonly not allowed in research diets because of their high energy content and their effects on various metabolic processes. This prohibition should be discussed with potential volunteers before they commit to a study. To the dietitian, the statement that "foods and beverages other than those provided by the study are not allowed" clearly means that alcohol is not to be consumed. However, some study participants may not understand this to include alcoholic beverages unless this is directly stated.

When consumption of alcoholic beverages is allowed, the type and amount of the beverage should be recorded. In studies that span a holiday that is associated with consumption of alcoholic beverages (eg, New Year's Eve), some investigators allow a limited number of alcoholic drinks, depending on the outcome variables to be assessed. The participant and investigator must have a mutual agreement regarding consumption of alcoholic beverages as part of religious rituals; frequency and amount of alcohol consumed at religious ceremonies should be determined and recorded.

Garnishes

Plate or tray garnishes for controlled diet studies must be planned in the context of the experimental diet. Many edible garnishes, such as parsley, watercress, and orange slices, contain levels of vitamins and minerals that are sufficient to destroy dietary control. When edible garnishes are used, the research dietitian must include them in the meal plan and the nutrient analysis and must ensure that participants eat the garnishes. Inedible garnishes such as paper flowers are generally a preferred option for adding color and interest while keeping a tight control on nutrient intake.

Chewing Gum

Gum is typically allowed but monitored. Regular chewing gum contributes trace amounts of carbohydrate. Sugarless gum is generally allowed ad lib because the content of calories and macronutrients is negligible. Gum can be useful for a participant on a liquid formula diet because it provides the chewing action the volunteer may miss and helps eliminate any aftertaste of formula diets. Labels should be read for type of sweetener and other additives to assess whether or not the additive will introduce an extraneous variable to the study. For instance, the sodium content of sugarless gum may affect electrolyte balance studies.

Hard Candy and Sugar

Hard candy typically has negligible nutritive value other than energy. In some situations hard candy can be used ad lib if its composition is not expected to affect electrolytes or nutrients under study.

Sugar allotments are typically included in controlled diets, but in determining the amount of the allotment investigators should consider participants' dental health. It is difficult to include an amount that pleases everyone; those who use sugar in coffee may want more than is allotted, whereas others may want less. Hard candy or jelly beans can be exchanged isocalorically for all or part of participants' daily sugar allotment, thus adding a small but welcome degree of control for the participants. (See the discussion of tradeoffs in Chapter 11, "Designing Research Diets.") Hard candy is also often used to clear objectionable aftertastes, such as those experienced after taking fish oil capsules.

Artificial Sweeteners

The artificial sweeteners typically permitted in research diets are saccharin and aspartame. However, because many people do not care for the taste of artificial sweeteners, participants should be informed at recruitment whether these sweeteners are to be used. The safety and relative sweetness of prominently used nutritive and nonnutritive sweeteners has been reviewed (7, 8). Saccharin is a nonnutritive synthetic sweetener that is 300 times sweeter than sucrose (7). It is heat stable and has a long shelf-life, but it has a slightly bitter aftertaste. Saccharin was used in most dietetic foods, liquid and solid form, prior to the approval of use of aspartame. Because it is a nonnutritive product and has little effect on the metabolism of most nutrients, saccharin-sweetened soft drinks, candy, and gum are allowed for most metabolic research studies.

Aspartame is a synthetic sweetener that is a dipeptide, providing 4 calories per gram. It is 200 times as sweet as sucrose and tastes similar to sucrose. Aspartame is used in most low-calorie dietetic foods now on the market because of its preferred taste. However, aspartame is unstable in liquid systems resulting in a decrease in sweetness with time. Aspartame is not usually used in baked goods because it breaks down at high temperatures. Because aspartame is a dipeptide it has some effects on amino acids and neurotransmitter metabolism. Therefore, a careful evaluation is necessary prior to permitting any aspartame-containing beverage, candy, or gum to be included in a metabolic research study involving amino acids or neurotransmitters.

Nonprescription Medications

Study volunteers are carefully screened for their use of prescription medications; however, they should also be screened for use of nonprescription medications. Because many nonprescription medications are casually used, participants should be made aware of the nutritional and/or biochemical impact of common medications, including antacids, laxatives, fibers, analgesics, and cough medicines. During the study period, the use of nonprescription medications should be discouraged, but if they need to be used, the brand name, composition, and incidence of usage should be reported.

Contraceptive Hormones and Hormone Replacement Therapy

Hormones can have a confounding effect on many outcome variables. Some studies accept women who are using hormones, whereas others do not. (See Chapter 8, "Women as Participants in Controlled Diet Studies.") In studies in which women using hormones are accepted, these volunteers are typically paired and then randomly assigned to the dietary treatments. The type and the amount of hormone used are routinely monitored. (See the daily record form discussed in Chapter 18, "Documentation, Record Keeping, and Recipes.")

For most studies it is important that the type and dosage of the hormones not change during the course of the study. A participant may have to be discharged from the study if a change is necessary.

Toothpaste and Dentifrices

The commercial dentifrices vary greatly in composition and ingredients, and their use can have an effect on metabolic research studies. For instance, toothpastes with baking soda formulas should be eliminated for sodium balance studies. Research volunteers should be instructed not to swallow any toothpaste. In some studies, for consistency, one brand of toothpaste is used by all participants throughout the entire study. Special dentifrices can be formulated for the study if no compatible commercial preparations can be found (Table 13-1). (Also see Chapter 12, "Producing Research Diets.")

Tobacco and Nicotine

Nicotine and curing compounds found in tobacco affect metabolic processes. Tobacco chewing and smoke inhalation habits should be carefully screened and monitored during controlled feeding studies. If studies accept volunteers who smoke, it is generally important that smoking status not change during the course of the study. Participants should be questioned about the use of nicotine gum and patches.

Other Sources

Food eaten during religious practices (communion wafers, sacramental bread, and wine) must also be approved and recorded in the participant's file. Licking prepasted stamps or stickers should be controlled or avoided for volunteers in trace mineral studies. Potential participants should be questioned in a nonjudgmental way at recruitment to determine whether they have pica, an appetite for nonfood items.

TABLE 13-1

Formulas for Dentifrice[1,2]

Ingredient	Amount
Sodium lauryl sulfate	30 g
Urea	80 g
Cinnamon water	1,000 ml
or	
Cinnamon oil	0.8 ml
Saccharin (soluble)	0.4 g
Methyl cellulose	20 g
Amaranth solution	1 ml
or	
Amaranth solution 1%	5 ml
Distilled water to volume	4,000 ml

[1] Adapted from Jones E. *A Dietetic Manual for Metabolic Kitchen Units.* Washington, DC: US Government Printing Office; 1969.
[2] To avoid mold growth, rinse container with ethanol.

CONCLUSION: TALES FROM THE REAL WORLD

Dinner with a group of research dietitians would lead to all sorts of stories about mistakes that were made and how problems were solved. What, for example, do you do when Bob has used Joe's salt shaker? This section relates some of those tales and tells how various mistakes or problems were handled. These are hints for avoiding the potholes of human nutrition research. (Fictitious names have been substituted for participants' actual names.)

Ellen Stevens and Fred Stevens were unrelated subjects in a free-living diet study. Fred, who was assigned to the green (no *trans* fatty acid) diet, accidentally picked up Ellen's weekend meals. Ellen, who was assigned to the blue (*trans* fatty acid) diet, discovered the mistake when she looked for her weekend cooler. Luckily, Fred was located before he ate the weekend food; otherwise, he would have been dropped from the study. Now the color coded cards that this facility uses on coolers bear first names in addition to last names and subject numbers. Additionally, concurrent use of blue and green color codes is being reconsidered because these colors are difficult for some individuals to distinguish, especially when they have a similar hue.

In portioning oranges for a study, the oranges were weighed with the peel attached and a refuse factor was used to determine the edible portion. The gram amounts displayed on the participants' food selection sheets indicated the weight of the orange with the peel for each calorie level and were therefore designated "orange with peel." Jane Fox was a participant committed to thoroughly complying with study protocol. She ate the orange and the peel for two menu cycles before the error in communication was discovered. No harm was done, and the participant enjoyed telling her tale.

A dinner tray was about to be delivered to an inpatient enrolled in a study that involved ascorbic acid depletion. The meal consisted of milk, chicken breast, rice, and canned corn, served on standard white hospital china. The cook, wanting to enliven the appearance of the meal and unaware of its high ascorbic acid content, added a sprig of parsley for color. Fortunately the tray was examined by a dietitian before service, and the parsley was removed. These research dietitians now recommend using paper garnishes.

When the staff plan menus for emergency meals or for take-out meals for weekends, special care must be given to provide foods that are relatively resilient to mishandling by participants. With food safety in mind, dietitians planning for an upcoming study intended to provide frozen dinners as part of the weekend take-out meals. Additionally, the participants were to be given a frozen dinner as part of their emergency meals. However, during recruitment of participants and query about storage space for frozen foods, it was found that several potential participants had inadequate freezers for storing frozen meals for even short periods of time. One couple who wanted to participate did not have a home freezer; they lived on a boat and used a simple ice chest as a refrigerator. Many participants engage in recreational activities on weekends that do not lend themselves to using frozen dinners. It is advised that dietitians discuss these problems and issues of food safety individually with participants.

Sometimes it is less labor intensive to send two employees to the grocery store, so that one may guard the shopping cart:

An employee picked up the 30 lb of specially ordered fish (Turbot) from the grocery store, but it was gone by the time she brought the van to the pick-up point. Another customer had made off with the next day's entree. Because this incident happened in a metropolitan area, it was possible to replace the Turbot. If it had not been recoverable, a readily available substitute would have been served and adjustments calculated for participants' diet records.

An employee was sent to a large grocery store to purchase 50 loaves of bread and a box of tea. After carefully counting the loaves, the employee left the grocery cart to search for tea on another aisle. The employee was perplexed to find only 46 loaves when they were counted at the feeding facility. The problem was traced to a cost-conscious shopper. According to the grocery clerk, a customer demanded a lower price for 4 loaves of bread in the "sale basket."

Perhaps every dietitian has a prize real-life story of "how the food item got away." Common ones include spilled or dropped items, or instances where the dog or the babysitter ate the food item. A favorite at one facility is from a participant who called to say that he would need to have his tuna replaced. He had left his lunch items on the window sill one November morning so that fellow employees would not take his food from a common refrigerator. A squirrel opened the Styrofoam container and ate the tuna, leaving behind peanuts, crackers, and other items more befitting a squirrel.

REFERENCES

1. Wurtman J, Lieberman H, Tsay R, et al. Calorie and nutrient intakes of elderly and young subjects measured under identical conditions. *J Gerontol.* 1988;43:B174–B180.
2. Wurtman J, Wurtman R, Reynold S, et al. Fenfluramine suppresses snack intake among carbohydrate cravers but not among non-carbohydrate cravers. *Int J Eat Disord.* 1987;6:687–699.
3. Tsay R, Cyr H. A novel method for measuring 24-hour patterns of food intake. *J Am Diet Assoc.* 1985;100. Abstract.
4. Sampson HA. Metcalfe DD. Food allergies. *JAMA.* 1992;268:2840–2844.

5. Sampson HA. Adverse reactions to foods. In Middleton E, Reed CE, Ellis EF, et al, eds. *Allergy: Principles and Practices.* 4th ed. St Louis, Mo: Mosby-Year Book, Inc. 1993;1661–1686.

6. Walder EC. Food allergy. *Am Fam Physician.* 1988;38: 207–212.

7. Position of The American Dietetic Association: use of nutritive and nonnutritive sweeteners. *J Am Diet Assoc.* 1993;93:816–821.

8. Kuntz LA. Achieving flavor parity with alternative sweeteners. *Food Product Design.* 1995;5:29–44. Northbrook, Ill: Weeks Publishing Company.

CHAPTER 14

PLANNING AND PRODUCING FORMULA DIETS

RITA TSAY, MS, RD; CYNTHIA SEIDMAN, MS, RD; HELEN RASMUSSEN, MS, RD, FADA; AND ABBY G. ERSHOW, ScD, RD

DECIDING TO USE A FORMULA DIET

Formula diets are well suited for use in strictly controlled studies. Of all the types of research diets, they provide the most accurate and constant intake of calories, macronutrients, vitamins, and minerals. These diets can comprise liquids (the most common option), solid foods, or both. Because formula diets are based on a limited number of ingredients, variability in nutrient content is minimal, and each ingredient can be analyzed for nutrient content to ensure that the composition of the diet is known with high accuracy. Formulas are convenient to use and can be adapted for many study designs. The dietary treatments are easily masked (or "blinded") and the recipes can be adapted to deliver numerous combinations of nutrients at markedly different dose levels.

Another advantage of formula diets is that they are economical. They maximize the number of participants and stud-

ies that can be accommodated with a minimum of work area and staff, because labor, kitchen space, and food-handling costs are low. In fact, once the recipe is calculated, the formula diet can be prepared in advance in bulk, frozen, and served as needed; some formulas can be stored at $-15°C$ for years without adversely affecting nutrient content (1). This means that storage space for the ingredients and the prepared formula is minimal. For example, a 40-L batch of liquid formula, which can be prepared in one hour by two foodservice workers, can supply 50,000 kcal. Costs associated with food composition analysis also are relatively low, because only a few component ingredients and the finished formula must be analyzed, as opposed to daily menus of different foods.

The main disadvantage of liquid formula diets is that most people prefer to eat solid foods, and the participants typically find that the regimen becomes increasingly monotonous over time. The lack of variety, lack of chewing, and the change in taste and texture from usual foods may contribute to participant dissatisfaction and lack of compliance. Formula diets also lack natural fiber, and tend to be low in starch and high in sugars. As a result, consumption of formula diets may change bowel habits, causing diarrhea, constipation, or other types of gastrointestinal discomfort such as flatulence, belching, nausea, and distention. These problems may resolve after a few days but often make it difficult to recruit and retain participants. Investigators considering use of formula diets must also decide whether these gastrointestinal side effects, or treatments for them, may ultimately influence study endpoints and thus confound interpretations of data. Concerns have been expressed that liquid-formula diets may differ from solid-food diets with respect to absorption and metabolism of nutrients (2, 3); more research is needed to clarify this poorly understood phenomenon.

Liquid formulas can be used to provide nutrients for protocols as short as 1 day (for example, postprandial fat load studies). The typical time span tolerated by participants is 3 to 6 months, but some participants have been maintained on liquid formula diets for several years (4).

WORKING WITH PARTICIPANTS

Screening

The success of a study starts with careful screening of potential participants. Highly motivated individuals are needed to undertake the rigors of formula diet protocols. For outpatient studies, motivation and support from family and friends should be evaluated and reinforced at the time of screening. It is helpful to have potential participants consume the entire volume of a single serving of a formula diet prior to committing to the study. This allows individuals to judge their tolerance of the formula and to evaluate their ability to adhere to the requirements of the study. If individuals are aware of the disadvantages of formula diets prior to the study, they are less likely to encounter problems later on.

A key step in the screening process is to review the formula ingredients with potential participants in order to eliminate individuals with allergies or intolerances to common ingredients, such as milk or egg protein.

Instructing the Participant

Water Intake

Participants on a liquid formula diet might be tempted to restrict their water intake, because they tend to have increased urinary output; they may wish to avoid carrying extra urine collection bottles. Nevertheless, participants should be advised to drink adequate amounts of water, particularly in hot weather, and to maintain adequate fluid balance when exercising. Calorie-free beverages may be allowed if the ingredients do not interfere with the study. It is best to provide water of known mineral composition (or deionized or distilled water) for studies where mineral intake is of interest. (See Sources of Nutrients; also see Chapter 15, "Meeting Requirements for Fluids.")

Free Foods

If they can be allowed, noncaloric items such as sugar-free chewing gum, bouillon, and herbal tea add variety and enhance participant compliance. Gum provides the chewing action that the participants may miss and also helps rid the mouth of aftertastes. Bouillon can be used as a source of sodium and can provide some warmth and saltiness to counter the monotony of the formula diet. Herbal teas offer yet more variety in flavor and may have a soothing and relaxing effect. The ingredients of any such teas must be reviewed to make sure they do not contain active ingredients that might interfere with study outcomes.

Eating Techniques

To ensure accurate intake of formula diets, participants are instructed on correct eating techniques. Participants should drink slowly without gulping to eliminate gagging and swallowing air, which may cause burping, nausea, and vomiting. Glasses or containers should be rinsed with water (distilled water for micronutrient studies), which also is drunk. Drinking the rinse ensures complete consumption of nutrients that otherwise might adhere to container surfaces. No visible formula residue should be left in the container.

Presenting the Diet

Volume and Number of Daily Meals

The volume of individual liquid formula meals depends on the tolerance of the study participants. As a general guideline, no more that 400 mL to 450 mL per serving is given to elderly participants and no more than 600 mL to 700 mL to young healthy adults. Individualized guidelines should be established for pediatric and other specialized populations.

Multiple isocaloric meals are recommended. The number depends on the total volume of the diet; the age and other characteristics of the study population; and the aims of the study. A regimen of four to five meals per day is acceptable to most participants. However, a schedule of three meals per day can be used if necessary by supplying part of the daily total calories as formulated solid food. (The use of solid food formulations is discussed later.)

Tray and Table Set-up

As with any meal, the appeal of formula diets can be enhanced through effective presentation. Colorful napkins or place mats, attractive glassware with unusual shapes, and appropriate garnishes (eg, paper flowers, twist of lemon rind if allowed) can add flair and make a positive impression on participants.

Compliance

As mentioned earlier, subjects prefer conventional food diets and this is a major factor affecting compliance with formula diets. Subjects consuming liquid formulas on an outpatient basis are more likely to have compliance problems, because they are routinely exposed to the temptations of more desirable foods. Even within the confines of a metabolic ward, participants have been known to drop out from a formula protocol when they smelled the aroma of food being prepared or served nearby for another study. Objective measures of compliance can be obtained by measuring urine osmolarity or by examining urine recovery of paraaminobenzoic acid added to the formula (5, 6). (Also see Chapter 24, "Biological Sample Collection and Biological Markers of Dietary Compliance.")

Designing Formula Diets

Planning the Production Mode

Liquid and Solid Forms

Liquid-formula diets are sometimes used in conjunction with specially formulated solid foods such as puddings (Exhibit 14-1), protein-free cookies (Exhibit 14-2), and unit muffins (see Chapter 18, "Documentation, Record Keeping, and Recipes"). These items offer a variety of textures, ease boredom, and allow for mastication of food while maintaining constant levels of nutrients. Solid foods are particularly useful in incorporating ingredients such as saturated fats, fiber, and certain complex carbohydrates, which are difficult to keep in homogeneous solutions.

Site-produced and Commercial Formulas

Formula diets usually are made in the research kitchen. The major advantages of on-site preparation of formulas are: (1) complete control of ingredients and (2) precise tailoring of the formula to the specifications of the study design. The needs of many studies, however, can be met by using commercial preparations. Among the numerous advantages of using commercial formulas, the first is financial: labor costs are minimal. Other advantages of using commercially prepared formulas include: rigorous sanitation standards at the manufacturing plant, manufacturer-solved issues of palatability and acceptability, and consistent texture and taste.

Storage requirements also may be simplified; already mixed dry powdered formulas that only need reconstitution with water or milk will require less storage space than their constituent dry basic ingredients. Liquid commercial formulas, of course, already contain the water component, a feature that adds both bulk and weight.

Purchased formulas can be considered if they provide a reliable nutrient composition in close accord with study goals. It is important in such cases to purchase single lots large enough for all study needs; to verify ingredient specifications with the manufacturer; to check that no recent processing changes in either content or handling have occurred; and to verify nutrient content by chemical analysis because it may vary somewhat from the labeling information. If the commercial formula is used as a base, rather than as a complete diet, pilot tests should be done to make sure that any added ingredients are fully compatible with the formulation. For example, a change in the type of fiber might alter the solubility of added mineral salts.

Meeting Nutrient Requirements and Study Goals

Macronutrients

There are two ways to tailor formula diets to meet macronutrient requirements: a single-formula method and an individualized-formula method.

Single-formula Method

When a constant nutrient composition is to be provided to all participants for the entire length of the study, one formula calculation can be used for all participants. Energy requirements are met by varying the amount of formula given. This method is commonly used to maintain energy homeostasis and to conduct baseline studies. The diet is first calculated to meet the protein goals of the diet protocol; protein is factored in first because many protein sources contain small amounts of fat (Table 14-1). The remainder of the calories is derived from carbohydrate and fat in amounts required to fulfill the study requirements.

Example:
- Liquid Formula B contains 15% protein, 40% fat, and 45% carbohydrate. Each 100 g of Formula B provides 4.7 g of protein, 5.6 g of fat, 14.1 g of carbohydrate, and 125 kcal (1.25 kcal/g). (See Exhibit 14-3.)
- Participant W, who requires 3,000 kcal daily, will receive 2,400 g of Formula B (3,000 kcal ÷ 1.25 kcal per g); Participant X, who needs 2,800 kcal a day, will receive 2,240 g of Formula B. (See Exhibit 14-3.)

Individualized-formula Method

When a specific level of a macronutrient is provided per kilogram of body weight, an individual formula calculation and recipe is needed for each participant. Other macronutrients are then distributed as a percent of the remaining calories.

Example:
- Liquid Formula C will be used for a dietary protocol requiring an isocaloric diet that provides 1.5 g protein per kilogram of body weight, 40% nonnitrogenous calories from fat, and 60% nonnitrogenous calories from carbohydrate. (See Exhibit 14-4.)
- Individually tailored recipe calculations are needed to make up Liquid Formula C for each participant. (See Exhibit 14-4.)

EXHIBIT 14-1

Solid Formulations: Puddings

BACKGROUND

- Puddings can be useful vehicles for providing complex carbohydrates or saturated fats that would not otherwise suspend in a liquid formula.
- Puddings should be used within three days of preparation. The mixtures do not freeze well and the texture is lost upon thawing.
- There are two ways to add saturated or hydrogenated fats to the pudding mix: (1) melt the fat and blend it into the pudding before the mix is brought to a boil; (2) finish cooking the pudding, remove it from the range, and blend in the solid fat; the fat will then be melted by the heat of the pudding.
- The Basic Pudding recipe is meant to provide a general approach to formulation. The ratio of starch, sugar, protein, and fat varies with each research diet protocol, so it may be necessary to experiment with the recipe to identify the best amount of liquid and the best order in which to add the ingredients.
- The protein-free puddings are useful for amino acid studies (such as described in Exhibit 14-5).

RECIPES

Basic Pudding

Ingredients	Quantities
Liquid (water or milk)	2,000 mL
Sugar	200 g–250 g
Protein source (optional)[1]	150 g–200 g
Starch	100 g–150 g
Fat	100 g–150 g
Flavoring extract	20 mL–30 mL

[1]The protein source can be egg (whole, whites, or yolks), milk powder, soy protein, etc.

Preparation Procedure

1. Mix liquid and half of the sugar to make a syrup. Bring to a boil, then lower the heat.
2. Beat eggs (or other moist protein source) until smooth. Add slowly to the hot sugar syrup, beating thoroughly after each addition. (It is helpful to first stir a small amount of the hot sugar syrup into the egg mixture. This will raise the temperature of the eggs and will prevent coagulation when they are added back into the syrup.)
3. Mix the remaining sugar (and any dry protein source) with the starch. Sift slowly into the liquid, mixing well.
4. Mix until smooth. Remove from heat.
5. Blend in fat and flavoring.
6. Pour appropriate quantity into serving dishes and cool.

Protein-free Wheat Starch Pudding (Lemon Flavor)

Ingredients	Quantities
Water	2,240 g
White sugar	1,054 g
Lemon juice	660 g
Wheat starch	312.4 g
Yellow food coloring	14 drops

Preparation Procedure

1. Combine all ingredients.
2. Cook over medium heat to a slow boil, stirring constantly.
3. Weigh out into serving dishes. Cool, cover, and refrigerate.
4. Yield: 27 servings, each weighing 152 g.

(*continued*)

EXHIBIT 14-1

Continued

Nutrient Content[1]	Amount
Protein	0.1 g
Fat	3.2 g
Carbohydrate	46.0 g
Energy	207 kcal

[1]For one 152-g serving.

Protein-free Cornstarch Pudding (Fruit Flavor)

Ingredients	Quantities
Water	2,240 g
Corn oil	240 g
White sugar	680 g
Cornstarch	140 g
Koolaid powder, unsweetened	24 g
Salt	14 g

Preparation Procedure

1. Weigh water and corn oil into separate bowls.
2. Weigh dry ingredients into large mixing bowl and transfer to a large (2-qt) saucepan.
3. Rinse the mixing bowl with some of the weighed water. Add to the saucepan, together with the rest of the water. Mix thoroughly and add the oil.
4. Cook over medium-high heat until thickened, stirring constantly.
5. Remove the mixture from the heat when it starts to bubble. Let it set for 5 minutes and stir again. (This step will help to keep the oil in suspension.)
6. Weigh out into serving dishes, stirring occasionally. Cool, cover, and refrigerate.
7. Yield: 19 servings, each weighing 160 g.

Nutrient Content[1]	Amount
Protein	0.1 g
Fat	12.2 g
Carbohydrate	40.1 g
Energy	266 kcal

[1]For one 160-g serving.

Vitamins and Minerals

The purified ingredients that are used to make formulas generally have a low vitamin and mineral content. The quantities of vitamins and minerals that are needed should first be calculated; the content of the formula can then be assayed directly or compared with predetermined nutritional standards, and the micronutrients supplied in the necessary quantities to make up any differences. There are two main ways to do this: (1) adding the vitamins and/or minerals directly to the formula or (2) giving the participant a pill or other form of supplement. Some pharmaceutical companies can produce customized vitamin and mineral preparations, such as a niacin-free vitamin. Research pharmacies at some facilities also may accommodate these special requests.

Micronutrients for formula diets should have high nutrient bioavailability. For example, calcium citrate might be chosen over calcium carbonate, which is not as well absorbed. It is also important to check the stability and solubility of any supplement. Some mineral salts may not dissolve readily; they may settle out if the formula is not consumed promptly after preparation. To avoid this problem, the formula should be stirred or shaken before serving; any residue adhering to stirring rods or spatulas should be consumed.

Fiber

Most formula diets are low in fiber; therefore, they have the potential to cause gastrointestinal discomfort. Fiber supple-

EXHIBIT 14-2

Solid and Liquid Formulations for an Egg-protein Diet: Protein-free Cookies and Liquid Formula A

BACKGROUND

- This diet uses egg protein as the main source of nitrogen.
- Part of the energy requirement is supplied by formulated solid food (protein-free cookies).
- The study protocol specifies the protein level as 1 g/kg body weight and the nonnitrogenous calorie ratio as 40% fat, 60% carbohydrate.
- The reference participant weighs 70 kg and has an estimated energy requirement of 3,150 kcal.
- The daily diet consists of three isocaloric meals, each containing protein-free cookies (2 cookies, uncooked total weight 90 g) and liquid formula A (599 g).

CALCULATIONS FOR DAILY DIET

Ingredient/Food	Weight (g)	Energy (kcal)	Protein (g)	Fat (g)	Carbohydrate (g)
Protein-free cookies (n = 6)	270[1]	1,195	1.1	60.8	164.7
Liquid Formula A[2]					
Egg white solids	72	273	60.0	0.0	3.2
Whole egg solids	20	118	10.0	8.2	0.8
Beet sugar	210	808	0.0	0.0	209.0
Orange sherbet[3]	195	273	2.1	3.9	59.3
Safflower oil	55	484	0.0	54.8	0.0
Koolaid® beverage, unsweetened (reconstituted)	1,245	0	0.0	0.0	0.0
Subtotal	1,797	1,956	72.1	66.9	272.3
Daily total (Cookies + Liquid Formula A)	2,067	3,151	73.2	127.7	437.0

[1]This refers to weight of unbaked (raw) cookie dough.
[2]The preparation procedure for Liquid Formula A is the same as for Liquid Formula C in Exhibit 14-4.
[3]Orange sherbet can be used to improve the flavor of liquid formulas. The small amount of protein in the sherbet usually will not affect study outcomes.

RECIPE

Protein-free Cookies

Ingredients	Quantities (g/batch)
Wheat starch	1,000
Beet sugar	300
Butter	454
Safflower oil	55
Baking powder	5.5
Salt	6
Water	80
Vanilla flavoring	10

Nutrient Content	Amount[1]
Energy	199.1 kcal
Protein	0.2 g
Fat	10.1 g
Carbohydrate	27.4 g

[1]Dough weight = 45 g raw, 41 g cooked.

Preparation Procedure

1. Mix sugar, butter, and oil together until smooth.
2. Add all dry ingredients and mix well.
3. Weigh raw dough for each cookie at 45 g.
4. Bake at 400°F for 15 minutes.
5. The cooked weight of each cookie averages 41 g.

TABLE 14-1

Selected Whey Protein Products

Product	Trade Name	Supplier	Nutritional Characteristics			
			Energy (kcal/100 g)	Protein (g/100 g)	Fat (g/100 g)	Carbohydrate (g/100 g)
Whey protein, concentrated	Pro Mod	Ross Laboratories Columbus, Ohio	424	75	9.1	10.2
Whey protein, caseinate	Propac	Sherwood Medical St Louis, Mo	400	76.8	8.0	5.2
Whey protein, ultra-filtered	Promix	Corpak, Inc Wheeling, Ill	400	75–78	6–8	8–10
Lactalbumin	Alatal 812	New Zealand Milk Products Petaluma, Calif	397	90.5	3.5	0.8

EXHIBIT 14-3

Single-formula Diet Using Liquid Formula B: Recipe and Preparation Procedures

BACKGROUND

- This diet provides all the participants with the same proportional distribution of energy from macronutrients: 15% protein, 40% fat, and 45% carbohydrate.
- Liquid formula B provides the entire daily diet.
- The quantity of formula is adjusted to meet the calorie requirements of individual participants.

CALCULATIONS FOR DAILY DIET

Subject	Energy Requirement (kcal/day)	Formula Portion[1,2] (g/day)	Macronutrient Distribution (% Energy)			Nutrient Intake (g/day)		
			Protein	Fat	Carbohydrate	Protein	Fat	Carbohydrate
Participant W	3,000	2,400	15	40	45	112.8	134.4	338.4
Participant X	2,800	2,240	15	40	45	105.3	125.4	315.8

[1]Formula Portion (g/day) = Energy Requirement (kcal/day) ÷ Energy density of formula (1.25 kcal/g).
[2]Energy density of Liquid Formula B: 1.25 kcal/g.

RECIPE

Liquid Formula B

Ingredients	Quantities[1]
Promix[2]	2.5
Corn oil	2.1
Polycose[3]	5.8
Water	29.6

[1]Weight in kg/batch.
[2]Promix (whey protein) (Corpac, Wheeling, Ill).
[3]Polycose (hydrolyzed cornstarch) (Ross, Columbus, Ohio).

Nutrient Content[1]	Amount
Energy	125 kcal
Protein	4.7 g
Fat	5.6 g
Carbohydrates	14.1 g

[1]Content per 100 g.

(continued)

EXHIBIT 14-3

Continued

Preparation Procedure (Batch Production)

1. Employee complies with hygiene measures (uses hairnet, washes hands, wears gloves).
2. Zero scale with bowls for dry ingredients and fat.
3. Weigh Polycose and Promix into one bowl.
4. Weigh corn oil into other bowl.
5. Remove these ingredients from scale and zero scale with a large bowl.
6. Weigh water into the large bowl.
7. Stir the dry ingredients with slotted spoon to blend Polycose and Promix. (Milk protein alone becomes lumpy when added to water.)
8. Pour water into the homogenizer; turn it on to obtain vortex in water.
9. Gradually blend dry ingredients into water.
10. Add corn oil. Turn off homogenizer. Rinse bowl three times with formula from the homogenizer to incorporate any residual oil into the formula.
11. Stir formula often with wire whip during mixing phase, after homogenization and before putting into quart-size storage containers.
12. Rapidly decant formula into quart containers (Conocups Tucker, Harrison, NJ), leaving a 2-in space on the top for expansion upon freezing. If producing more than one batch, refrigerate one batch while making the second.
13. To speed the cooling of formula to a safe temperature of 40°F or below, do not close the container. Place open containers on the coldest part of the freezer (where the circulating cold air originates) in order to enhance the cooling process.
14. When the formula temperature reaches 40°F (5°C), close the containers, clip them, and label with the number of the formula, the batch number, and the date made.
15. Freeze immediately.

---

ments can be added to a formula diet to promote more frequent bowel movements and to soften stools. Bulking agents should be carefully evaluated, however, for their potential effects on the gastrointestinal tract. This is especially critical for studies of nutrient absorption and mineral bioavailability.

Microcrystalline cellulose powder can be used as a source of fiber. Because of its thickening effect, it should be added to the formula at the time of service; it also can be offered as an additional supplement at meal time. Most participants find 20 g per day to be acceptable, administered either as a single 20-g dose or as two 10-g doses. *Alpha-cellulose* can also be given in amounts of 8 g to 10 g per day to increase stool bulk. *Methyl cellulose,* which is used less often, is more potent; it should not be used unless other sources have been evaluated and rejected. Typical doses of methyl cellulose are comparatively small (4 g per day).

Solute Load

Fluid and electrolyte homeostasis in living systems is maintained by the movement of water toward physiological compartments having higher concentrations of dissolved particles. Under free-living conditions with self-selected diets, healthy individuals will regulate their water balance through a variety of behavioral mechanisms that include the sensation of thirst, the drinking of water and other fluids, and the partially subconscious preference for salted or unsalted foods.

In a formula diet study, it is particularly important to evaluate and monitor the solute load because the protocol may constrain these mechanisms in several ways:

- The protocol may specify that all fluid be provided through the formula, rather than through *ad libitum* water consumption. This requirement deprives the participant of one of the most important physiological mechanisms for self-regulation of fluid balance.
- Formula diets often are made from highly purified ingredients, which may have a very low content of electrolytes in comparison with conventional foods.
- Unlike participants who are enrolled in many research protocols that use conventional foods, subjects who are enrolled in formula studies may not be permitted to add salt to their food, or they may consider it unappealing to add salt to a relatively sweet milkshake-like formula.

The solute content of a formula diet thus should be evaluated from several vantage points: first, the *enteric solute load,* which will influence gastrointestinal symptoms upon ingestion; second, the *renal solute load;* and finally, the *electrolyte content* of the entire diet.

The enteric solute load of a prepared formula is measured by its osmolality. *Osmolality* is a property of solutions that represents the number of dissolved particles per unit mass of solvent (ie, per kg water). One Osmol is defined as the number of dissolved particles required to depress the

EXHIBIT 14-4

Individualized Formula Diets Using Liquid Formula C, Recipe and Preparation Procedures

DIET DESIGNS FOR TWO REFERENCE PARTICIPANTS Y AND Z

BACKGROUND

- This formula diet uses egg protein as the main source of nitrogen.
- The study protocol defines the protein level as 1.5 g/kg body weight and the nonnitrogenous calorie ratio as 40% fat, 60% carbohydrate.

Subject	Body Weight (BW) (kg)	Energy Requirement (ER)[1] (kcal/day)	Macronutrient Requirements (g/day)			Energy Distribution (% kcal)		
			Protein	Fat	Carbohydrate	Protein	Fat	Carbohydrate
Participant Y	60	2,400	90	90.7	306	15	34	51
Participant Z	70	3,150	105	121	410	13	35	52

[1]Each participant's energy requirement is estimated using standard algorithms. (See Chapter 17, "Energy Needs and Weight Maintenance.").
[2]Protein requirement (g/day) = 1.5 g/kg BW × BW (kg).
[3]Fat requirement (g/day) = (40% of nonnitrogenous calories)* ÷ 9 kcal/g fat.
  *Nonnitrogenous calories (kcal/day) = ER (kcal/day) − (4 kcal/g protein × protein required (g/day)).
[4]Carbohydrate requirement (g/day) = (60% of nonnitrogenous calories) ÷ 4 kcal/g carbohydrate.

CALCULATIONS OF INDIVIDUALIZED FORMULA FOR PARTICIPANT Z

Ingredient/Food	Weight (g)	Energy (kcal)	Protein (g)	Fat (g)	Carbohydrate (g)
Egg white solids	105	398	87.5	0	4.7
Whole egg solids	30	176	15	12.4	1.2
Beet sugar	306	1,173	0	0	303.5
Safflower oil	102	900	0	101.8	0
Orange sherbet[1]	361	505	3.9	7.3	109.8
Koolaid beverage, unsweetened (reconstituted)	1,400	0	0	0	0
TOTAL	2,304	3,152	106.4	121.5	419.1

[1]Orange sherbet can be used to improve the flavor of liquid formulas. The small amount of protein in the sherbet will not affect study outcomes.
[2]The daily diet consists of four isocaloric meals, each containing 576 g of Liquid Formula C.

RECIPE

Liquid Formula C

Ingredients	Quantities (g/batch)[1]
Egg white solids	115.5
Whole egg solids	33
Beet sugar	336.6
Orange sherbet	397
Safflower oil	112
Unsweetened Koolaid® (reconstituted)	1,540

[1]Quantities are 110% by weight of each ingredient from the formula calculation in order to allow for losses such as those during transfer from blender to serving containers. Weight is in grams.

Preparation Procedure

1. Make a dry mix of the first three ingredients in a bowl.
2. Combine the remaining items in a blender with 1-gallon capacity. Mix for 3 minutes.
3. Add dry ingredients to the blender cup and mix for another 3 minutes.
4. Scrape down the lid, sides, and blades of the blender. Mix again for several minutes to ensure homogeneity of the formula.
5. Portion four servings of formula, each weighing 576 g, into four labeled serving containers. Cover containers with lids and refrigerate until serving time.

freezing point of one liter of water by 1.86°C (7). Osmolality (mOsmoles per kg water) is a *mass basis* expression of concentration, whereas *osmolarity* (mOsmoles per L solution) is a *volume basis* expression of concentration (6). Most dilute solutions have similar values for osmolality and osmolarity.

The macronutrient energy sources that suspend rather than dissolve in the formula (ie, lipids, complex carbohydrates, and proteins) have little effect on the solute load. Rather the most important contributors to the osmolality of the formula are the simple sugars, amino acids, and electrolyte salts (primarily sodium, chloride, and to a lesser extent magnesium, calcium, phosphate, and sulphate). The osmolality of formula diets can be estimated from algorithms that account for the formula recipe and the measured osmolality of each component ingredient (8, 9). Another approach, often used in the food industry, is to analyze a sample of the formula (and/or the component ingredients) in the laboratory with a vapor pressure or freezing point osmometer, making appropriate adjustments for viscosity, turbidity, and other types of interference from suspended solids (V Mustad, personal communication).

The osmolality of the formula diet should always fall within a certain range, or there will be major implications for safety and acceptability. (The constancy of the osmolality measurements over time can also serve as a quality control measure for formula diet production.) Formulas are considered *iso-osmolar* if they have a solute concentration similar to that of plasma and other physiological fluids (ie, approximately 275 mOsm/kg to 300 mOsm/kg).

Another simple and useful parameter for evaluating the concentration of the formula is the *energy density,* which reflects energy intake per unit of fluid or water. The usual daily total water allowance for mixed diets is approximately 1.5 mL/kcal (10). This value corresponds to an energy density of approximately 1.25 kcal/g formula (under the assumption that water comprises three-fourths of the weight of most formulas); additional fluids may be needed if this level is exceeded. The formulas used for enteral nutrition support, which resemble the formulas used for research diets, have a typical energy density of 0.5 kcal/mL to 2 kcal/mL and range in osmolality from a low of 120 mOsm/kg for polymeric mixtures (with intact protein, starch, and triglycerides) to a high of 650 for monomeric mixtures (with hydrolyzed starch, amino acids, and peptides) (11).

Dehydration and unpleasant gastrointestinal symptoms are the most serious consequences of imbalanced enteral solute loads. The ingestion of a hyperosmolar formula will draw water into the lumen of the gastrointestinal tract; this can cause nausea, rapid transit time, and diarrhea (11). Longer-term ingestion of such a formula may cause dehydration by forcing the kidneys to dilute the solutes in additional volumes of urine. Formulas that have a high content of salt, simple sugars, or amino acids often are hyperosmolar. To avoid this problem, the formula can be diluted or reformulated (for example, by using starch instead of sugar as a carbohydrate source); if the protocol allows, participants

should be encouraged to drink water or other noncaloric beverages. (See Chapter 15, "Meeting Requirements for Fluids.")

On the other hand, the research diet must provide electrolyte minerals (notably sodium, potassium, and chloride) in sufficient quantities to prevent deficiency (10), unless this is a planned aspect of the protocol. Long-term intake of a hypo-osmolar diet may result in excessive urine output, reduced plasma electrolytes, and other electrolyte imbalances (12). It may be necessary to supplement the diet with electrolyte salts in the form of pills or powder blends.

The renal solute load of the diet can be predicted from the electrolyte content and from nitrogen derived from all dietary sources, whether ingested as intact protein (such as casein) or as individual amino acids; carbohydrates do not enter into this calculation. It also is relatively simple to measure urinary osmolality as a way of checking renal solute load and risk of dehydration. Some researchers consider that a comparison between predicted and observed urinary osmolality can provide an objective measure of dietary compliance (6). (Also see Chapter 24, "Biological Sample Collection and Biological Markers of Dietary Compliance.")

Carbon-13 (^{13}C) Content

Stable isotopes are often used to trace the transformation and transport of biological compounds during the various steps of metabolic processing. (See Chapter 16, "Compartmental Modeling and Balance Studies.") Carbon is commonly chosen as the tracer element because of its preeminent role in the chemistry of organic molecules. About 99% of naturally occurring carbon comprises carbon-12 (^{12}C); other isotopes, including the stable isotope carbon-13 (^{13}C), are generally rare. Certain plants such as sugarcane and corn, however, tend to concentrate ^{13}C, and food products made from them are thus also enriched in ^{13}C. These include cane sugar, molasses, and all corn products (eg, cornstarch, corn syrup, and corn oil). Diets providing such foods can confound the results of studies using ^{13}C-labeled tracers because of alterations in the isotopic enrichment of metabolic products (such as expired CO_2 during fasting and feeding) (13). The research diet can be rendered ^{13}C-neutral by avoiding the use of any corn and sugarcane products.

Verifying Composition

Nutrient data for individual formula ingredients are readily available, and this facilitates calculating the formula prescription. However, for more accurate formulation of diets, laboratory analysis of selected ingredients should be performed prior to recipe calculation. For example, the fatty acid composition of some oils varies substantially, so in studies of fatty acids, it may be important to assess the profile of each fat and oil prior to use. Chemical verification after formulation is also recommended. (See Chapter 22, "Validating Diet Composition by Chemical Analysis.")

SOURCES OF NUTRIENTS

This section describes sources of *macronutrients* (water, protein, carbohydrates, and lipids). Sources of *micronutrients* are discussed in Meeting Nutrient Requirements and Study Goals. The food source for each nutrient is selected in accordance with the research question, the extent of control desired, and the physical and nutritional characteristics required. For example, the nutrient content of some food products varies with season (vitamin A in butter) or region (trace mineral content of wheat flour because of the wheat's growing area). Such foods will not provide consistency throughout the study and are not appropriate for certain protocols.

The supplier or manufacturer of each food product also must be carefully considered, because even purified sources of particular nutrients (such as protein) will often contain small amounts of other nutrients as well (such as fat); the levels of such "extraneous" nutrients will vary with the raw ingredients and processing method. Comprehensive listings are available that can simplify the task of choosing specialty food suppliers whose products meet the needs of the protocol (14).

Water

The decision to use tap or distilled water in liquid formula diets depends on study goals and outcome variables to be measured. Some investigators, particularly those who study minerals, use deionized water in formula and all other beverages. In other studies the source of the water is not particularly important, but investigators may prefer to keep it consistent with the source used in their prior studies to facilitate comparisons. (Also see Chapter 15, "Meeting Requirements for Fluids.")

Protein

Because of their high biological value and palatability, egg and milk are the most frequently used sources of protein in formula diets. Soy protein products and pure amino acids are less palatable and therefore are not as suitable for general-purpose formulas. Soy products and pure amino acids are more commonly chosen for protocols that evaluate their specialized properties or for situations in which egg or milk cannot be used.

Egg Protein

Egg white solids, which are usually used in the form of sprayed dried egg white, provide high-quality protein with a low mineral content. The amount of fat and carbohydrate in egg white solids is also small compared to other protein sources. Using egg white as the only source of protein, however, can have drawbacks: the formula tends to have an undesirable sulfur taste and a very foamy texture. To prevent the formation of lumps, the powder should be mixed first with other dry ingredients before water is added.

Whole egg solids supply a high-quality protein but also contain fats, cholesterol, vitamins, minerals, and trace amounts of carbohydrates. Unless strict control of lipids and vitamins is specified, a combination of egg white and whole egg solids is advised as the protein source for most formulas. Formulas that use whole egg as the sole protein source may have unacceptably high cholesterol content; reduction in the total cholesterol content can be achieved by replacing part of the whole egg with egg whites. Combining whole egg solids with egg white solids also can improve the taste and texture of the formula over those containing egg white alone (see Liquid Formulas A and C in Exhibits 14-2 and 14-4). The lecithin in the egg yolk serves as an emulsifier and promotes stability of the formula.

Egg white solids require no refrigeration and can be kept indefinitely at room temperature. Whole egg solids need no refrigeration for periods of up to 4 weeks if they are kept at room temperature (for example, on a cool dry shelf). If held for longer, storage below 50°F is recommended. Egg products suitable for formula diets may be obtained from Henningsen Foods Inc, White Plains, NY; Oskaloosa Food Products Corporation, Oskaloosa, Iowa; and Siegel Egg Products, Boston, Mass (14).

Milk Protein

Milk protein is available as processed caseins, whey proteins, and milk solids.

Caseins are the main proteins of milk. They are used principally as casein salts, of which sodium and calcium caseinates are the most common. In addition to providing a source of protein, caseinates function as emulsifiers and water binders (15). Because casein contains only trace amounts of water-soluble vitamins, it is preferable to egg solids in diets that are designed to be devoid of water-soluble vitamins. Caseinates contain fat and carbohydrate (lactose); amounts of these components must be evaluated in the context of specific studies. These proteins are hygroscopic and can absorb odors; temperatures below 25°C, relative humidities below 65%, and an odor-free environment are thus all essential to extend storage life. Casein products may be obtained from New Zealand Milk Products, Inc, Santa Rosa, Calif (14).

Whey proteins are obtained from skim milk after separation of casein during cheese production. Whey proteins have low water-binding capacities, permitting high protein concentrations without excessive viscosity (16). They also exhibit good emulsifying properties. The two main whey proteins are β-lactoglobulin and α-lactalbumin. Lactalbumins are water insoluble; therefore, they are difficult to use in liquid formulas. Lactalbumins are also hygroscopic and can absorb odors. Storage temperatures should be maintained below 25°C and relative humidities below 65%. Stocks should be used preferably within 6 months.

Some whey protein preparations contain substantial amounts of lactose; for certain protocols it may be necessary to obtain manufacturer's information about the lactose content and choose the supplier accordingly. Table 14-1 shows selected commercially prepared whey proteins and their energy values and macronutrient compositions.

Milk solids are produced by spray- or roller-drying processes, which remove the water fraction of whole milk. Dried milk offers convenience of transportation, utility, stability, and resistance to microbial growth. Another advantage is ease with which milk powder can be incorporated into many formulations. However, whole milk solids must be used with caution because the butterfat content makes the formula prone to develop rancid flavors during storage (16). Dried skim milk has excellent flavor, high nutritional value, and good functional properties such as water binding and emulsification. It is the most readily available form of nonfat milk solid and is easily obtained through retail grocery stores, wholesale food suppliers, and specialty suppliers such as Clofine Dairy and Food Products, Linwood, NJ (14).

Soy Protein

Soy protein contains nearly optimal proportions of all the essential amino acids for humans, including lysine and tryptophan, but has insufficient (limiting) amounts of cystine, methionine, and valine. Its digestibility is high, being equivalent to milk and superior to whole egg (17). The use of processed soy proteins in the formula diet has the additional benefit of being hypoallergenic for certain groups of individuals who are sensitive to milk or other proteins such as gluten.

Soy protein must be used cautiously, because it may contain biologically active constituents, such as estrogen-like compounds, which could confound the results of some studies. In addition, the high phytic acid content of many soy preparations renders them unsuitable for mineral absorption studies.

Isolated soy protein (ISP) can be used when a vegetable protein source is required in a formula diet. The isolate is prepared from soybean flour by extracting the protein and precipitating it to yield a product that is approximately 90% protein on a dry weight basis. It is virtually free of carbohydrate and fat. ISP is a bland, soluble powder with low viscosity and gelling properties. It is highly digestible, forms a stable suspension, and provides smooth mouth feel. Grains Processing Corporation (Muscatine, Iowa) and Protein Technologies International (St Louis, Mo) offer a wide range of ISP products (14).

Soy protein concentrate (SPC) is prepared by removing most of the water-soluble nonprotein constituents from defatted soy flakes. This yields a product that is approximately 75% protein on a dry weight basis. SPC is available from Protein Technologies, International (St Louis, Mo) (14).

Amino Acid Powders

Purified crystalline amino acids can be mixed in different ratios for studies of amino acid turnover or requirements. Crystalline amino acids are water-insoluble; therefore, they are not mixed directly into liquids. Instead, a liquid formula is used to provide nonprotein nutrients and calories, and amino acid mixtures are weighed and served as a solid item. (See Exhibit 14-5.) In order to mask their metallic and bitter taste, a similar amount (by weight) of beet sugar and a small amount of flavoring is typically added to each portion of the amino acid mixture. In some cases, tolerance and acceptance can be improved by making a gelled product, which is made by mixing the amino acid blend with water and a trace amount of carrageenan (Gelcarin SA 812, FMC Corporation, Rockland, Maine). Purified food-grade amino acids may be obtained from the Ajinomoto Company, Tokyo, Japan.

Carbohydrates

Carbohydrates typically provide the main source of calories in formula diets.

Simple Carbohydrates

Simple carbohydrates dissolve easily in liquid formulas. Dextrose and sucrose, in particular, are often used as a major source of calories and as a way of sweetening the formula. The type of simple carbohydrate selected depends on the degree of the sweetness desired; combinations of different sugars can be used to obtain the desired taste (Tables 14-2 and 14-3). The major sources are sucrose, glucose, dextrose, fructose, maltose, and lactose. Several of these (glucose, mannitol, lactose, sorbitol, and maltose) are chemically refined and are costly, so it is best to minimize their use. Sorbitol and mannitol are sugar alcohols that can have adverse gastrointestinal side effects because they are not completely absorbed. They usually are chosen as sweetening agents rather than as major sources of energy.

The relative sweetness of various sugars and syrups is sometimes expressed as a "dextrose equivalent" value. During the acid hydrolysis conversion of cornstarch to corn syrup, an array of simple sugars and small polysaccharides is formed (such as dextrin, dextrose, maltose, maltotriose, and maltotetrose). As the conversion proceeds, increasingly higher proportions of dextrose are formed. Stopping the process at various defined points yields a corn syrup having a particular dextrose content (ie, dextrose equivalent, or DE, value). Pure dextrose is assigned a DE value of 100. For corn syrup products, the DE value thus indicates the achieved degree of polysaccharide hydrolysis; a higher DE value indicates more complete hydrolysis, higher dextrose content, and greater sweetness (18).

Dextrose (D-glucose) is a dry corn sweetener that is made from cornstarch by the action of heat, acid, or enzymes, resulting in the complete hydrolysis of the cornstarch to its component D-glucose molecules. Purified, crystallized D-glucose is commonly available from chemical supply companies and specialty food suppliers as dextrose monohydrate (9% water by weight) or anhydrous dextrose (less than 0.5% water) (14).

Sucrose, a disaccharide composed of one molecule of glucose and one molecule of fructose, is extracted from sug-

EXHIBIT 14-5

Solid and Liquid Formulations for an Amino Acid Diet:
Amino Acid Blend, Protein-free Cookies, and Liquid Formula D

BACKGROUND

- This metabolic balance diet uses a specifically patterned amino acid blend as the main source of nitrogen.
- The study protocol defines the protein level as 1 g/kg body weight and the non-nitrogenous calorie ratio as 40% fat, 60% carbohydrate.
- The reference participant weighs 70 kg and has an estimated energy requirement of 3,150 kcal.

CALCULATIONS FOR DAILY DIET

Ingredient/Food	Weight (g)	Energy (kcal)	Protein (g)	Fat (g)	Carbohydrate (g)
Amino Acid Blend					
Amino acids	70.0	279.6	69.9	0.0	0.0
Beet sugar	80.0	308.0	0.0	0.0	79.6
Subtotal	150.0	587.6	69.9	0.0	79.6
Protein-free cookies (n = 6)[1]	270.0	1,194.8	1.1	60.8	164.7
Liquid formula D[2]					
Orange sherbet[3]	230.2	322.1	2.5	4.7	70.0
Safflower oil	64.8	575.7	0.0	64.8	0.0
Beet sugar	122.8	470.6	0.0	0.0	121.7
Koolaid®, unsweetened (reconstituted)	833.0	0.0	0.0	0.0	0.0
Subtotal	1,250.8	1,368.4	2.5	69.5	191.7
Daily total (Amino Acid Blend + Cookies + Liquid Formula D)[4]	1,670.8	3,150.8	73.5	130.3	436.0

[1]The recipe for protein-free cookies is shown in Exhibit 14–2.
[2]The preparation procedure for Liquid Formulas is shown in Exhibit 14–4.
[3]Orange sherbet can be used to improve the flavor of liquid formulas. The small amount of protein in the sherbet usually will not alter the outcome of the study.
[4]The daily diet consists of 3 isocaloric meals, each containing Amino Acid Blend (23.3 g amino acids and 26.7 g beet sugar), Protein-free cookies (2 cookies, uncooked total weight 90 g), Liquid Formula D (433.6 g).

arcane or sugar beets. The general composition and appearance of sucrose from these two plant sources are identical, but beet sugar contains less natural enrichment in ^{13}C and is therefore more appropriate for stable isotope studies. Sucrose is available in powdered, fine-grain, and coarse-grain forms, all of which have different dissolving properties. Brown sugars are less refined, retaining greater (dark) or lesser (light) amounts of molasses, which increases the water and mineral content and adds a distinct, strong flavor. Cane sugar is widely available from retail and wholesale grocers; pure beet sugar may be obtained from specialty suppliers (such as Western Sugar Company, Bayard, Nebr; Holly Sugar Corporation, Hereford, Tex; and Great Lakes Sugar Company, Fremont, Ohio) (14).

TABLE 14-2

Properties of Selected Carbohydrates[1]

Product	Solubility[2]	Sweetness[2]	Viscosity[2]	Dextrose Equivalents[3]
Starch	4	4	1	0
Maltodextrin	3	3	2	6–20
Corn syrup solids	2	2	3	20–58
Dextrose	1	1	4	100

[1]Adapted with permission from RS Igoe, *Dictionary of Food Ingredients,* 2nd ed (New York: Van Nostrand Reinhold; 1989), p 165.
[2]Range of values: 1 = greatest; 4 = least.
[3]For a discussion of dextrose equivalents, see Carbohydrates in this chapter.

TABLE 14-3

Relative Sweetness of Natural and Artificial Sweeteners[1]

Sweetener	Type	Sweetness Level (%)[2]
Saccharin	Artificial	300–400
Aspartame	Artificial	200
Fructose	Natural	150
Sucrose	Natural	100
Dextrose (glucose)	Natural	70
Sorbitol	Natural	55
Mannitol	Natural	50
Lactose	Natural	20

[1]Adapted with permission from RS Igoe, *Dictionary of Food Ingredients,* 2nd ed (New York: Van Nostrand Reinhold; 1989), p 181.
[2]Values are expressed in comparison with sucrose. Sucrose = 100%.

Complex Carbohydrates

At times the protocol requires use of a complex carbohydrate like cornstarch or wheat starch. For liquid formulas, this causes several types of problems. The first problem is that complex carbohydrates do not dissolve or suspend well in a cold liquid medium, so that a homogeneous mixture is hard to achieve. The second is that most liquid formulas made with complex carbohydrates have a thick, unpalatable texture because the uncooked starch granules swell but do not gelatinize. This problem can be alleviated by incorporating the cornstarch or wheat starch with other formula ingredients into cooked solid food forms, such as cookies and puddings.

Cornstarch is derived from the endosperm of corn and contains amylose and amylopectin starch molecules. Cornstarch is generally considered to be a good choice as a source of complex carbohydrate for a formula, provided its relatively high ^{13}C content does not pose a problem. (Also see the earlier discussion of ^{13}C.) Compared with other complex carbohydrate sources, cornstarch mixes more readily with water and other ingredients. Formulas made with cornstarch are not stable for freezing and thawing. Although cornstarch imparts a chalky taste to the formula, the taste can be masked with artificial flavorings. Highly purified cornstarch products are readily obtained from retail grocery stores as well as general and specialty wholesale suppliers (such as CPC International, Englewood Cliffs, NJ; Corn Products, Summit Argo, Ill; and American Maize Products, Decatur, Ill) (14).

Wheat starch produces lower viscosity and more tender gels than does cornstarch (15). Wheat starch imparts a pasty, chalky taste to formulas and thickens the formulas to an undesirable degree when not consumed immediately after preparation. Although not ideal for use in liquid formulas, wheat starch is preferred in solid baked formulations, such as cookies.

Maltodextrin is a spray-dried product. It is made from a purified, concentrated aqueous solution of nutritive saccharides obtained by hydrolysis of cornstarch. It usually has a DE of 20 or less. Maltodextrin is slightly sweet with no undesirable taste, and it disperses rapidly in cold water (Table 14-2). Specially processed maltodextrin (Amino Products, Philadelphia, Pa) can provide an effective avenue for emulsifying certain foods, nutrients, and ingredients. A wide range of maltodextrin products with differing DE values is available from Grain Processing Corp (Muscatine, Iowa). Several commercially available maltodextrin products are listed in Table 14-4.

Fats and Oils

Fats and oils play multiple functional roles in formula diets. They provide concentrated sources of calories and specific combinations of particular fatty acids, and are vehicles for flavoring agents and biologically active compounds such as antioxidants and fat-soluble vitamins. Oils are the most frequently used lipid sources in formula diets because they are liquid at room temperature and are readily incorporated into suspension (18). Because they usually have a more saturated fatty acid profile than oils, fats tend to be solid at room temperature. As a result, fats are not preferred as lipid sources for chilled liquid formula diets: their tendency to solidify at cool temperatures means that they will stick to the sides of preparation and serving containers, causing quantitative losses, and that they will leave an unpleasant coating in the mouth. For the same reasons, hydrogenated shortenings, which are commonly used in baked goods, are seldom used in liquid formulas.

There are many naturally occurring food fats and oils that can be chosen to obtain the desired combination of characteristics. Custom-made blends can also be produced by specialty manufacturers. (Information about the customized production of specialty fats and oils may be obtained from the Institute of Shortening and Edible Oils, Inc, 1750 New York Avenue, Washington, DC 20006.) The principal fatty acids of selected fats and oils are shown in Table 14-5. Several commercially available specialty oils are listed in Table 14-6.

Despite the technical problems already mentioned, some liquid formula protocols nevertheless require the use of saturated fats. The usual choices include butter, lard, and

TABLE 14-4

Selected Maltodextrin Products

Product	Trade Name	Supplier	Nutritional Characteristics	
			Energy (kcal/100 g)	Carbohydrate (g/100 g)
Maltodextrin	Sumacal	Sherwood Medical St Louis, Mo	380	100
	Moducal	Mead Johnson Evansville, Ind	380	100
	Maltodextrin 180	Grain Processing Corp Muscatine, Iowa	376	94
Cornstarch, hydrolyzed	Polycose	Ross Laboratories Columbus, Ohio	380	94
Corn syrup solids, deionized	Nutrisource Carbohydrates	Sandoz Minneapolis, Minn	320	100

margarine. Another alternative is anhydrous butterfat (also called *anhydrous milk fat* or *ghee*), which is the clarified fat portion of milk, cream, or butter. Anhydrous milk fat is produced from cream that has been spray-dried, then immediately centrifuged to remove traces of water (19). It is remarkably pure (ie, free of protein and carbohydrate) and can be kept for years at room temperature if stored and packaged appropriately. Anhydrous milk fat may be obtained from Clofine Dairy and Food Products, Linwood, NJ (14).

There are several ways of incorporating solid fats into formula diets. One way is to bring the fat into suspension by using an emulsifier such as lecithin (Lucas Meyer, Inc, Decatur, Ill). Another approach is to first melt the fat in a double boiler and then mix it manually into the formula using a food whip. The entire mixture is then homogenized under pressure (see the discussion under Equipment). The formula will remain stable at room temperature for many hours, but the emulsion is broken upon heating, freezing, and thawing; restoring the emulsion likely will require an additional blending process. Finally, as with the complex carbohydrates, using a solid food form such as a pudding or cookie can be an effective way of presenting a solid fat in a palatable preparation.

PRODUCING FORMULA DIETS

Choosing Suitable Ingredients

A starting point in the development of a formula diet is to identify available ingredients and to compile a reference list of potential formula components and their characteristics. Ideal ingredients (1) are easy to weigh, transfer, mix, and form into a homogeneous product; (2) have a well-defined nutrient composition that is constant among lots and shipments; and (3) come with manufacturer's product specifications that are detailed and accurate. Other characteristics of ingredients that should be considered include the shelf-life of the product, any special requirements for storage, and the likelihood of spoilage during storage or preparation. For example, deterioration of whole egg powder and whole milk powder has caused investigators to seek alternative sources of protein.

Some food ingredients are available in different forms for various uses; the investigator must identify the product that best suits the needs of the study. For example, egg white solids are available as nonfoaming and foaming types. Nonfoaming egg whites are preferable because foaming incorporates air during mixing, which can complicate measuring and handling. Casein is also available in various forms (eg, sodium caseinate and calcium caseinate).

Solutions, Suspensions, and Emulsifiers

Certain products in solid or powder form do not dissolve well in liquid (eg, amino acid powders or lard). The miscibility of the ingredients is crucial for production of a homogenized formula that provides an even distribution of nutrients. Ingredients that are not well dissolved will produce a gritty texture, and there is a great likelihood that the first portions decanted will differ in composition from the last.

Difficulties can occur in keeping certain ingredients in suspension. Starch and solid fats such as butter, margarine, and lard are difficult to incorporate into a liquid formula with an appealing taste and texture. The alternative is to combine the fat, the starch, and some of the sugar into formulated solid products like cookies or puddings. The remaining ingredients are served as a liquid formula that can maintain a stable suspension.

Some fat-containing food ingredients serve as emulsifiers in formula diets (eg, egg yolk solids, whole egg solids, and lecithin). When food ingredients do not provide adequate emulsification, an emulsifying agent such as polygly-

TABLE 14-5

Principal Fatty Acids of Selected Fats and Oils[1]

Oil or Fat[2]	Weight % of Each Fatty Acid													
	4:0	6:0	8:0	10:0	12:0	14:0	16:0	18:0	20:0	16:1	18:1	20:1	18:2	18:3
Soybean oil							11	4			24		54	7
Corn oil							11	2			28		58	1
Cottonseed oil						1	22	3		1	19		54	1
Palm oil						1	45	4			40		10	
Peanut oil[3]							11	2	1		48	2	32	
Olive oil							13	3	1	1	71		10	1
Low erucic acid rapeseed oil (canola)							4	2			62		22	10
Safflower oil							7	2			13		78	
Sunflower oil							7	5			19		68	1
Coconut oil		1	8	6	47	18	9	3			6		2	
Palm kernel oil			3	4	48	16	8	3			15		2	
Cocoa butter							26	34	1		34		3	
Butterfat[4]	4	2	1	3	3	11	27	12		2	29		2	1
Lard						2	26	14		3	44	1	10	
Beef tallow[5]						3	24	19		4	43		3	1
Menhaden oil[6]						9	19	4		13	16	2	2	1

[1]Table adapted with permission from: *Food Fats, and Oils.* 7th ed. Washington, DC: Institute of Shortening and Edible Oils; 1994. Fatty acid composition data determined by gas-liquid chromatography and provided by member companies of the Institute of Shortening and Edible Oils, Inc. Fatty acids (designated as number of carbon atoms:number of double bonds) occurring in trace amounts are excluded. Component fatty acids may not add to 100% because of rounding.

[2]Common names: C 4:0 = butyric; C 6:0 = caproic; C 8:0 = caprylic; C 10:0 = capric; C 12:0 = lauric; C 14:0 = myristic; C 16:0 = palmitic; C 18:0 = stearic; C 20:0 = arachidic; C 16:1 = palmitoleic; C 18:1 = oleic; C 20:1 = gadoleic; C 18:2 = linoleic; C 18:3 = linolenic.

[3]Peanut oil typically contains C 22:0 plus C 24:0 at 4%–5% of total fatty acids.

[4]Butter fat typically contains C 15:0 plus C 17:0 at about 3% of total fatty acids.

[5]Beef tallow typically contains C 15:0 plus C 17:0 at about 2% and C 14:1 plus C 17:1 at about 2% of total fatty acids.

[6]Data on menhaden oil from Bimbo AP. *J Am Oil Chem Soc.* 1987;64:706. Menhaden oil typically contains the omega-3 fatty acids C 20:5 (EPA) and C 22:6 (DHA) at about 13% and 8% of total fatty acids, respectively. In addition, the minor fatty acids C 22:1, C 18:4, C 20:4, and C 22:5 typically compose about 6% of total fatty acids.

TABLE 14-6

Selected Specialty Oils

Product	Source Oil	Trade Name	Supplier
Microparticulated lipid	Safflower oil	Microlipid	Sherwood Medical St Louis, Mo
Medium chain triglycerides	Fractionated coconut oil	MCT oil	Mead Johnson Evansville, Ind
	Fractionated coconut oil	Nutrisource Lipid-MCT	Sandoz Minneapolis, Minn
Long-chain triglycerides	Soybean oil	Nutrisource Lipid-LCT	Sandoz Minneapolis, Minn

cerol ester (Drew Chemical Corp, Boonton, NJ) or carrageenan (FMC, Inc, Philadelphia, PA) may be added to the formula to ensure a well-homogenized suspension (1).

Organoleptic Aspects

Mouth-feel and Taste-testing

The tactile oral sensation of a food is sometimes called its "mouth-feel." Liquid formula diets preferably should have a smooth texture that does not leave a sensation of "coating" in the mouth. Ingredients that may conflict with this goal are highly saturated fat sources, poorly soluble carbohydrates, fibers, and minerals.

Before settling on the final recipe for the product, the dietary staff and investigators or a panel of independent testers should consume a full serving of the product to assess its odor, texture, flavor, and its overall acceptability. The formula served at taste-testing should also be presented at the same temperature at which it will be served to the subjects. A final step in taste-testing is to present the formula to volunteers who have demographic and other characteristics similar to those of the anticipated study participants.

Flavor

Many participants prefer formulas that have a sweet, rather bland flavor, especially for a long-term study. Other participants may wish to have a choice of flavors to help relieve monotony. Variety in flavor can be provided by using flavor packs or extracts at the time of serving (Table 14-7). Slices of lemon can also be offered to cut the sweetness of a formula if the fruit does not interfere with the nutrients under study. Before any flavorings are added to a controlled formula diet, their chemical composition and any potential metabolic activity should be evaluated.

Flavor extracts, such as vanilla, lemon, almond, and orange, are available commercially. Local ice cream manufacturers can also provide a variety of flavorings. Flavor extracts may contain alcohol and may not be suitable for use in certain protocols.

Instant coffee powder (regular or decaffeinated) is another well-liked flavoring agent.

Vari-Flavor® Flavor Pacs (Ross Laboratories, Columbus, Ohio) provide five flavor options (cherry, lemon, orange, pecan, strawberry). Each 1-g packet contributes 4 kcal and trace amounts of minerals; contains dextrose, artificial flavor, and artificial color.

Koolaid® (Kraft General Foods, Inc, White Plains, NY) is a powdered soft drink mix. It contains citric acid, salt, calcium phosphate, and vitamin C. Koolaid powder is available in a variety of fruit flavors. There is a choice of naturally (sugar) sweetened, artificially sweetened, and unsweetened forms.

Vivonex flavor packs (Sandoz, Minneapolis, Minn) have five flavor options (cherry vanilla, raspberry, lemon-lime, orange-pineapple, and vanilla). Each packet contains 0.111 g (raspberry flavor) to 0.169 g (vanilla flavor) of aspartame, trace amounts of citric acid, dextrose, artificial colors, and flavors. Because aspartame contains phenylalanine, this product is not recommended for use in studies restricting phenylalanine. It is also not recommended for use in formulas that will receive heat treatment because aspartame decomposes at cooking temperatures. Aspartame decomposition can also occur in acidic mixtures that undergo prolonged storage.

Color

In formulas the appearance of the finished product should be consistent with standard expectations for colors that are associated with particular flavors or ingredients. For example, milk- and egg-based formulas are best developed to be off-white or in light tones of yellow or orange, which are typically associated with milk- and egg-based foods. Fruit flavors are sometimes associated with yellow, orange, red, and purple. Brown tones would be expected for coffee and chocolate flavors; green for mint flavor. Several of the flavoring blends listed in Table 14-7 also include compatible food colors.

Temperature

Formula feedings are typically served at 35°F to 40°F, or common refrigeration temperature. Not only are these temperatures in keeping with food safety standards, but the palatability of formulas is best in this range. Exceptions must be made for formulas that need to be warmed before serving because they contain certain ingredients such as lard and other saturated fats that may not remain in solution at this temperature. An alternative approach is to freeze the formula and serve it as a milkshake-like slush. As mentioned earlier, formulas that have been frozen and thawed may lose their homogeneous texture; the broken emulsions sometimes can be restored through vigorous shaking.

Recipes and Preparation Techniques

Once the formula ingredients have been determined, the recipes can be calculated and standardized preparation steps can be specified. The same ingredients are always used for any one formula, preferably all from the same lot, to attain consistency of nutrient composition throughout the protocol. The standardized format for recipes and preparation procedures should specify:

- Names and quantities of ingredients
- Expected yield; number of servings
- Nutrient composition for each serving
- Amount of water needed to achieve an appropriate concentration
- Type and amount of flavoring
- Weighing method
- Mixing procedures
- Types of storage and serving containers
- Type of serving utensils

TABLE 14-7

Extract Blends for Flavoring Formula Diets[1,2]

Flavor	Ingredient	Quantity[3]
Butternut	Banana extract	12 drops
	Coconut extract	12 drops
	Butter pecan extract	15 drops
	Brown food color	1 drop
Butternut spice	Banana extract	12 drops
	Coconut extract	12 drops
	Butter pecan extract	15 drops
	Cinnamon powder	2 shakes
	Brown food color	1 drop
Cinnamon nog	Cinnamon powder	1/16 Tsp
Cinnamon nut	Butter pecan	30 drops (¼ tsp)
	Coconut extract	12 drops
	Cinnamon powder	2 shakes
Cream de toffee	Rum toffee extract	12 drops
	Banana extract	6 drops
	Cinnamon powder	Pinch
	Brown food color	1 drop
Hawaiian basic	Banana extract	12 drops
	Coconut extract	9 drops
	Yellow food color	1 drop
Hawaiian comfort	Lemon extract	12 drops
	Coconut extract	6 drops
	Banana extract	6 drops
Hawaiian mint	Coconut extract	12 drops
	Peppermint extract	3 drops
	Banana extract	9 drops
	Yellow food color	1 drop
Mint julep	Wintergreen extract	12 drops
	Banana extract	12 drops
	Coconut extract	4 drops
	Green food color	1 drop
Montage	Black walnut extract	12 drops
	Rum toffee extract	6 drops
	Maple extract	9 drops
	Coconut extract	6 drops
	Peppermint extract	3 drops
Tutti frutti	Strawberry extract	15 drops
	Banana extract	9 drops
	Red food color	1 drop
Yellow winter	Wintergreen extract	9 drops
	Banana extract	12 drops
	Yellow food color	1 drop

[1] Recipes provided courtesy of Phyllis Stumbo, PhD, RD, University of Iowa GCRC, Iowa City, Iowa.
[2] Flavors can be added to each serving rather than to the entire day's formula.
[3] Quantity is suitable for flavoring one 180-ml serving of formula.

- Portion size and serving temperature
- Labeling and coding
- Handling and storage conditions
- Caveats and hints for avoiding problems

A minimum number of containers should be used during formula preparation in order to avoid omission errors, to limit loss of ingredients, and to minimize contamination. In mixing a liquid formula, the preparer should first add some water into the blender cup, then add the dry ingredients, blend the mixture for a few minutes, then add the remaining liquids. This process will prevent the dry ingredients from adhering to the surface of the blender cup. To allow for some waste and spillage in preparation, it is advisable to increase the weight of each ingredient (including water) by 5% to 10%. Gram weights rather than volume measures should be used to portion each serving.

To ensure a safe and palatable product, the formula should not be prepared more than 2 days in advance, unless it will be frozen. The prepared formula should be clearly labeled with the code or name of the formula and the date that it is mixed.

Quality control of formula diets may be achieved by sampling each batch or random sampling of different batches and assaying for key nutrients. A less expensive procedure is to document the weight of a predetermined volume of formula, monitor it on a weekly basis, and compare the results with the established standard. Testing the pH value of the formula is quick and simple and can also be used for quality control.

Equipment

Equipment selection for preparation of liquid formula diets depends on the composition of the formula and quantities required for the study. Large quantities of formula composed of protein, carbohydrate, fat, and water can be successfully mixed into a smooth and palatable consistency using a homogenizer. *Homogenizers* are processing equipment for the production of high-quality emulsions. They differ from blenders in the ability to break food particles into smaller molecules to obtain better suspension. The Standard Gaulin Model 15M single-stage Labscale Homogenizer (APV Gaulin Inc, Wilmington, Mass) is a high-energy, high-pressure machine that can yield up to 40 L per hour. The IKA Ultra-Turrax T65 (IKA Works Inc, Cincinnati, Ohio) achieves its dispersing effect through a high-speed, rotor-stator principle (rotations per minute) yielding approximately 20 L per batch. If a homogenizer is not available, smaller batches can be processed in a 1-gallon blender (Waring Products, New Hartford, Conn) if the fat is unsaturated and ingredients are easily solubilized.

Homogenization using high pressure and/or higher temperatures is beneficial, for example, when a study design cannot accommodate using emulsifiers to keep saturated fats in suspension. Companies that manufacture homogenizers typically provide technical support when problems arise.

For preparation of formulas in batches greater than 20 L, the following are required: a top-loading scale with large capacity (30 kg or otherwise larger than total batch weight) and a smaller electronic balance (capacity 6 kg) for weighing ingredients, a large vessel with a spigot at the base for ease in decanting, a wire whip for premixing, wax-coated paper containers with plastic clips for sealing before storage (Conocup; Tucker, Harrison, NJ), freezer-stable labels and markers, long-handled spatulas, and freezers capable of maintaining low temperatures ($-18°C$ or below) for long-term storage.

After defrosting, a formula can be aerated by mixing to a slurry in the half-gallon size Waring blender (model 36BL23) or the IKA Ultra-Turrax T65 (IKA Works, Inc, Cincinnati, Ohio).

Sanitation

Because the neutral pH and high protein content of formulas provide an excellent medium for the rapid growth of bacteria, the same rigorous standards and guidelines for food safety and sanitation must be followed for preparing formulas as for conventional foods (20). As with any other food, formula should not be held at "danger zone" temperatures of 5°C to 60°C (41°F to 140°F) for more than 4 hours during preparation, during short- or long-term cold storage, or during thawing. It thus is important to monitor the temperatures frequently while the prepared formula is cooling down or freezing.

Frozen formula also must be thawed in accord with safe food-handling practices, under refrigeration (20) with frequent shaking to maintain a uniformly cool mixture. In addition, all equipment used in preparing the formula must be kept meticulously clean. Care also must be taken to prevent contamination when staff repeatedly withdraws small quantities from bulk packages of dry ingredients (eg, boxes of powdered skim milk or dried egg white). Risk is highest when the container is opened and kept open and when the measuring utensil is inserted. Careful attention to storage conditions, holding temperatures and packaging, and advance portioning of dry ingredients into smaller clean containers can help to protect against this problem. It is prudent to carefully archive small samples of liquid formula in a freezer at $-20°C$ to $-80°C$. These samples may be an important resource in the event that a participant becomes ill and the safety of the formula must be checked.

Participants should be given written instructions concerning appropriate handling and storage of their formula. Those who must consume their formula off-site should be given a good-quality, nonbreakable Thermos®; the formula will stay cold for several additional hours if the empty Thermos is first chilled in the freezer before filling. A telephone number should be provided in case the participant has a problem that needs immediate attention.

CONCLUSION: RESEARCH APPLICATIONS OF FORMULA DIETS

In comparison with whole-food diets, formula diets are relatively easy to produce and deliver, and the composition can be controlled to a remarkable degree with modest cost. Provided that the nutrients of interest are available in purified or semipurified forms, formula diets can be considered when the complex background matrix of whole foods interferes with testing the hypothesis under investigation or when the composition of whole foods is too variable to deliver adequate dietary control. Formulas also are a means of evaluating food components (such as specific amino acids) that cannot easily be manipulated through whole foods. The tightly defined composition of formulas is useful for studies of nutrient balance and requirements, dose-effects of single nutrients, and between-nutrient interactions.

Formula diets usually are better suited to short-term applications because participants often find the monotony and limited sensory stimulation to be problematic (although some investigators have been successful in long-term feeding of formulas). Nevertheless, this time frame is highly compatible with many types of protocols, such as postprandial metabolism and absorption studies, nutrient load and tolerance tests, diagnostic test meals, and balance studies for nutrients with short equilibration time.

Considered from another perspective, there are research problems in which this lack of sensory variety may actually enhance the investigator's purposes. For example, some hypotheses are best tested under conditions that minimize variation in texture, taste, food volume, and visual perception of relative quantities and varieties of foods. Similarly, for many nutrients, the formula diet provides a convenient means of delivering a double-blinded intervention because changes in nutrient content are harder to perceive in the absence of associated food flavors.

The authors gratefully acknowledge the many helpful suggestions made by Janis Swain, MS, RD, and Carol Stollar, MEd, RD.

REFERENCES

1. Ahrens EH Jr. *Advances in Metabolic Disorders.* Vol 4. New York, NY: Academic Press; 1970.
2. Hegsted M. Dietary fatty acids, serum cholesterol, and coronary heart disease. In: Nelson GJ, ed. *Health Effects of Dietary Fatty Acids.* Champaign, Ill: American Oil Chemists' Society; 1991.
3. Clarke R, Frost C, Collins R, Appleby P, Peto R. Dietary lipids and blood cholesterol: quantitative meta-analysis of metabolic ward studies. *BMJ.* 1997;314(7074):112–117.
4. Liebel RL, Rosenbaum MD, Hirsch J. Changes in energy expenditure resulting from altered body weight. *N Engl J Med.* 1995;332:621–628.
5. Roberts SB, Morrow FD, Evans WJ, Shepard DC, Dallal GE, Meredith CN, Young VR. Use of p-aminobenzoic acid to monitor compliance with prescribed dietary regimens during metabolic balance studies in man. *Am J Clin Nutr.* 1990;51:485–488.
6. Roberts SB, Ferland G, Young VR, Morrow F, Heyman MB, Melanson KJ, Gullans SR, Dallal GE. Objective verification of dietary intake by measurement of urine osmolality. *Am J Clin Nutr.* 1991;54:774–782.
7. Randall HT. Water, electrolytes, and acid-base balance. In: Goodhart RS, Shils ME, eds. *Modern Nutrition in Health and Disease.* 5th ed. Philadelphia, Pa: Lea and Febiger; 1973:338.
8. Ferrett KA. Osmolality determinations of concentrated enteral nutrition formulas. *Nutr Support Serv.* 1982; 2(12):6–9.
9. Anderson K, Kennedy B. A model for the prediction of osmolalities of modular formulas. *JPEN.* 1986;10(6): 646–649.
10. Food and Nutrition Board, National Research Council. *Recommended Dietary Allowances.* 10th ed. Washington, DC: National Academy of Sciences; 1989.
11. Shike M. Enteral feeding. In: Shils ME, Olsen JA, Shike M, eds. *Modern Nutrition in Health and Disease.* 8th ed. Philadelphia, Pa: Lea and Febiger; 1993.
12. Oh MS. Water, electrolyte, and acid-base balance. In: Shils ME, Olsen JA, Shike M, eds. *Modern Nutrition in Health and Disease.* 8th ed. Philadelphia, Pa: Lea and Febiger; 1993.
13. Wolfe RR. *Radioactive and Stable Isotope Tracers in Biomedicine.* New York, NY: Wiley-Liss; 1992.
14. *Thomas Food Industry Register.* Vols 1, 2, and 3. New York, NY: Thomas Publishing Co; 1997.
15. Igoe RS. *Dictionary of Food Ingredients.* 2nd ed. New York, NY: Van Nostrand Reinhold; 1989.
16. Pomeranz Y. *Functional Properties of Food Components.* New York, NY: Academic Press; 1985.
17. Zapsalis C. *Food Chemistry and Nutritional Biochemistry.* New York, NY: Macmillan Publishing Co; 1986.
18. *Foods and Nutrition Encyclopedia.* 2nd ed. Boca Raton, Fla: CRC Press; 1994.
19. Mulder H, Walstra P. *The Milk Fat Globule.* Farnham Royal, Bucks, England: Commonwealth Agricultural Bureau; 1974.
20. Food and Drug Administration. *Food Code.* Washington, DC: US Public Health Service, US Department of Health and Human Services; 1997.

CHAPTER 15

MEETING REQUIREMENTS FOR FLUIDS

ABBY G. ERSHOW, ScD, RD

Water is the most essential of all nutrients. Investigators conducting a controlled diet study are obligated to ensure that participants have an adequate intake of water just as for all other nutrients except those under investigation.

Thirst is one of the most powerful of all physical drives, even more so than hunger, and is subjectively unpleasant. Because any continued experience of thirst will quickly derail the participant's adherence to the protocol, provisions must always be made to avoid this sensation. It is crucial that the participant not feel that water or fluids are being restricted except under special conditions of the protocol. Participants who are likely to be thirsty for any period of time should be given advance notice and suggestions for coping with the discomfort (for example, dissolving hard candy in the mouth). Conversely, if required intake is too high, participants may feel that they are "forcing fluids," with an accompanying sense of gastric fullness and the inconvenience of extra trips to the bathroom.

For many people, intake of beverages such as tea, coffee, soda, juice, or plain drinking water is a habitual behavior incorporated into the daily routine. This dietary pattern, which is distinct from thirst (1), has implications for well-controlled feeding studies, because participants may find it difficult to change this behavior to comply with the requirements of a feeding study. This can lead to problems with recruitment and adherence. It is preferable to allow the participants to control their own intake of beverages in general and water in particular.

ALLOWANCES AND SOURCES

Water Allowances

Water is required in the amount individuals need to allow normal physiological function without dehydration or over-heating. Recommendations for water intakes are, however, set not as requirements but as allowances, which include a generous safety margin. The Food and Nutrition Board, National Research Council (2), estimates the water requirement to be 1 mL (or gram) of water per kilocalorie of diet under ordinary circumstances, but recommends an allowance of 1.5 mL/kcal to cover most variations in need. Additional water beyond this level is needed when using certain types of medications or under conditions of heavy exercise, heavy sweating, hot weather, high protein intake, or high sodium intake. For example, a 200-mEq sodium diet (4,600 mg Na/day) might necessitate a water allowance of 40 mL/kg body weight.

Water requirements are also increased in illness associated with diarrhea, fever, vomiting, or polyuria. Lactation increases the need for water, as does pregnancy. Water intake must be carefully monitored for persons whose sensation of thirst may be blunted, such as elderly individuals or athletes exercising in hot weather (2). Some situations, such as use of antihistamine or decongestant medications, may lead to a sense of dryness in the mouth without much change in actual water requirements.

Typical Quantities and Sources of Water Intake

Intakes of total water from all dietary sources (solid foods and soups, plain drinking water, and other beverages) have been estimated for the US population using data from the 1977–1978 USDA Nationwide Food Consumption Survey (3, 4). Tables 15-1, 15-2, and 15-3 show these values expressed as total g/day, g/kg/day, and g/kcal/day (1 g water = 1 mL water). There is considerable variation among individuals, with a 3-fold to 4-fold range between the 5th and 95th percentiles of intake. Variations in intake partially re-

TABLE 15-1

Total Water Intake (g/day) by Age and Sex[1-3]

Sex	Age (yr)	Mean	SD[4]	Percentile Distribution				
				5	25	50	75	95
Males	<1[5]	1,152	324	642	922	1,127	1,344	1,731
	1–10[5]	1,594	517	848	1,235	1,531	1,895	2,538
	11–19	2,210	769	1,170	1,673	2,095	2,626	3,634
	20–64	2,515	916	1,310	1,889	2,374	2,976	4,244
	65+	2,407	778	1,329	1,886	2,305	2,832	3,799
Females	<1[5]	1,144	341	631	918	1,118	1,319	1,704
	1–10[5]	1,523	493	827	1,176	1,462	1,800	2,437
	11–19[6]	1,773	594	947	1,367	1,696	2,104	2,812
	20–64[6]	2,045	716	1,068	1,547	1,952	2,421	3,338
	65+	2,055	653	1,122	1,597	1,985	2,425	3,257
Pregnant women		2,076	743	1,085	1,553	1,928	2,444	3,475
Lactating women		2,242	658	1,185	1,833	2,164	2,658	3,353

[1]Total water intake from all sources (drinking water, beverages, and foods).
[2]1 g = 1 mL water.
[3]Adapted from Ershow AG, Cantor KP analysis (3) based on data from 1977-1978 USDA Nationwide Food Consumption Survey.
[4]SD = Standard deviation.
[5]Does not include breast-fed children.
[6]Does not include pregnant or lactating women.

TABLE 15-2

Total Water Intake (g/kg/day) by Age and Sex[1-3]

Sex	Age (yr)	Mean	SD[4]	Percentile Distribution				
				5	25	50	75	95
Males	<1[5]	153.0	52.9	86.1	114.9	146.2	178.8	247.7
	1–10[5]	76.4	32.8	34.5	53.3	70.2	93.5	137.2
	11–19	39.6	14.8	19.5	29.1	37.5	47.9	67.8
	20–64	32.3	12.4	16.2	23.7	30.2	38.7	55.3
	65+	32.9	11.3	17.2	25.3	31.6	39.0	53.5
Females	<1[5]	172.9	70.7	87.2	124.2	160.4	207.6	305.7
	1–10[5]	74.2	31.6	34.1	51.1	67.9	90.7	134.5
	11–19[6]	35.5	13.9	16.5	25.8	33.6	43.0	61.4
	20–64[6]	32.9	12.6	16.0	24.1	31.0	39.4	56.5
	65+	32.8	11.6	16.8	24.4	31.2	39.7	54.9
Pregnant women		32.1	11.8	16.4	22.8	30.5	40.4	53.5
Lactating women		37.0	11.6	19.6	28.4	35.1	45.0	59.2

[1]Total water intake from all sources (drinking water, beverages, and foods).
[2]1 g = 1 mL water.
[3]Adapted from Ershow AG, Cantor KP analysis (3) based on data from 1977-1978 USDA Nationwide Food Consumption Survey.
[4]SD = Standard deviation.
[5]Does not include breast-fed children.
[6]Does not include pregnant or lactating women.

flect physiological and environmental factors such as age, sex, season, region, body size, and pregnancy or lactation, but these account for only a relatively small fraction of the variance in water intake; other personal factors clearly play a large role as well. Day-to-day intakes of total water tend to be relatively constant for individuals (4).

In free-living US adults, the average total intake of water from *all* dietary sources is approximately 2 L per day for women and 2.5 L per day for men. This does *not* represent 2 L per day of drinking water; there is a widespread popular misconception that people need to drink 8 cups of water each day to meet their requirement. Most surveyed

TABLE 15-3

Total Water Intake (g/kcal/day) by Age and Sex[1-3]

Sex	Age (yr)	Mean	SD[4]	Percentile Distribution				
				5	25	50	75	95
Males	<1[5]	1.5	0.3	1.1	1.3	1.5	1.7	2.0
	1–10[5]	1.0	0.3	0.6	0.8	1.0	1.2	1.5
	11–19	1.0	0.3	0.6	0.8	0.9	1.1	1.5
	20–64	1.1	0.4	0.6	0.9	1.1	1.3	1.9
	65+	1.3	0.5	0.8	1.0	1.2	1.5	2.2
Females	<1[5]	1.6	0.6	1.0	1.3	1.5	1.7	2.1
	1–10[5]	1.0	0.3	0.6	0.8	1.0	1.1	1.5
	11–19[6]	1.1	0.4	0.6	0.8	1.0	1.2	1.8
	20–64[6]	1.4	0.9	0.7	1.0	1.3	1.7	2.6
	65+	1.5	0.6	0.8	1.1	1.4	1.8	2.6
Pregnant women		1.3	0.5	0.7	0.9	1.2	1.5	2.2
Lactating women		1.3	0.4	0.7	1.0	1.2	1.5	2.1

[1] Total water intake from all sources (drinking water, beverages, and foods).
[2] 1 g = 1 mL water.
[3] Adapted from Ershow AG, Cantor KP analysis (3) based on data from 1977–1978 USDA Nationwide Food Consumption Survey.
[4] SD = Standard deviation.
[5] Does not include breast-fed children.
[6] Does not include pregnant or lactating women.

participants clearly have an adequate intake of water; more than half the population consumed more than the 1 mL/kcal requirement estimated to be adequate under most circumstances. Plain drinking water, tea, coffee, and carbonated beverages provide the largest fraction of all dietary water (Table 15-4); approximately one-fourth derives from solid foods and soups.

Pregnant and lactating women do consume more total water than their nonpregnant, nonlactating peers, but the extra intake is relatively small (ie, a daily increment of less than 2 cups) (4). The average water content of pregnant and lactating women's diets is 1.3 mL/kcal to 1.4 mL/kcal, similar to that of nonpregnant, nonlactating women of similar age (4, 5). Thus, diets accounting for the increased energy needs of these conditions will generally provide adequate water as well.

Tapwater (consumed as plain water or used to prepare tea, coffee, and other foods and beverages) provides 55 ± 18% (mean ± SD) of total water intake in freely selected diets (3). This figure varies little with season, geographic location, or age. The tapwater intake of infants (younger than 1 year) will reflect the type of formula they drink; tapwater intake is low when ready-to-feed formula is used, whereas tapwater intake composes nearly all the water intake of babies drinking powdered formula. For adults 20 years to 64 years, the average tapwater intake is 1,366 g/day, supplied primarily by plain drinking water (674 g), coffee (395 g), tea (152 g), cooked grain products (45 g), and reconstituted citrus juices (27 g).

Water and Beverage Intakes and Allowances for Controlled Diet Studies

Two main aspects of water and beverage intake should be assessed for participants in a research diet study: (1) what the usual daily total water intake is, and (2) what the typical daily pattern of beverage intake is. Daily water intake should be assessed to ensure that the conditions of the study, which may entail complete provision of all beverages as well as food, meet the participant's requirements. The typical pattern of beverage intake should be assessed to help the study design fit better with the participant's established daily routines.

Assessing Intake

Total water intake can be assessed readily in the context of a standard 24-hour recall, with two special considerations. First, extra questions must be added to elicit information on water consumed. This entails asking about plain drinking water from tap, water fountain, or bottled water sources, and about extra ice added to foods or beverages. The 24-hour recall must include all foods and beverages, including plain water, tea, coffee, and unflavored carbonated waters.

Second, the database used for nutrient calculations must include information about the water (ie, moisture) content of the food. With this information, the total daily water intake can be calculated along with other nutrients of interest.

Typical patterns of beverage intake can also be assessed as part of the diet history (ie, food record or food frequency

TABLE 15-4

Dietary Sources of Total Water Intake by Age (Both Sexes)[1]

Age (yr)	Source[4]	g/day[2]								% of Total g/day	
					Percentile Distribution[3]						
		Mean	SD[5]	5	25	50	75	95		Mean	SD
1[6]	Food	250	198	0	72	236	381	633		21	16
	Drinking Water	197	186	0	0	240	240	480		16	14
	Other Beverages	701	235	333	558	693	839	1,085		63	19
	All Sources	1,148	332	631	920	1,120	1,339	1,727		100	—
1–10[6]	Food	409	175	175	283	384	506	727		27	10
	Drinking Water	505	354	0	240	480	720	1,200		30	16
	Other Beverages	645	247	283	483	630	784	1,083		43	14
	All Sources	1,559	507	838	1,210	1,497	1,843	2,507		100	—
11–19[7]	Food	515	230	204	349	487	638	933		27	10
	Drinking Water	664	483	0	320	560	880	1,600		31	17
	Other Beverages	809	382	289	566	756	984	1,490		42	15
	All Sources	1,989	719	1,025	1,489	1,874	2,369	3,336		100	—
20–64[7]	Food	545	239	223	375	509	678	992		26	10
	Drinking Water	674	555	0	320	560	960	1,760		28	17
	Other Beverages	1,024	539	358	668	925	1,267	2,001		46	17
	All Sources	2,243	839	1,133	1,665	2,109	2,663	3,793		100	—
65+	Food	575	243	238	406	542	711	1,028		27	10
	Drinking Water	776	554	0	400	720	1,040	1,920		33	17
	Other Beverages	849	381	310	604	807	1,032	1,523		40	15
	All Sources	2,199	1,196	1,700	2,109	2,616	3,482	4,370		100	—

[1]Adapted from Ershow AG, Cantor KP analysis (3) based on data from 1977–1978 USDA Nationwide Food Consumption Survey.
[2]1 g = 1 mL water.
[3]Percentile values for all sources are independent of values for individual sources (food, drinking water, and other beverages).
[4]Food category includes soups.
[5]SD = Standard deviation.
[6]Does not include breast-fed children.
[7]Does not include pregnant or lactating women.
0 = <0.5 g/day

questionnaire). Many people have well-established daily patterns of fluid intake, most notably for tea, coffee, soda, juice, and plain water. Some people take several discrete coffee breaks; others keep a bottle of water or soda at hand from which they sip throughout the day. A feeding study that interrupts these patterns will be more burdensome for the participant. If the study requires switching to noncaloric sodas or caffeine-free beverages, the participant may have difficulty adapting. A list of acceptable alternatives should be provided to guide the individual in choosing beverages. In addition, explaining the rationale for the study requirements will ease the transition for most people.

Alcoholic beverage intake generally is underreported, and extra probing may be necessary to obtain accurate information. It may be helpful to supplement a 24-hour recall or typical day's intake questionnaire with some food frequency questions directed at weekly patterns of intake, with special emphasis on weekend days and on different types of beverages, such as wine, beer, and distilled liquors. Some of this information should be obtained as part of screening pro-

cedures because heavy habitual consumers of alcohol often are unsuitable as participants in controlled diet studies.

Estimating Allowances

As mentioned earlier, a basic water allowance can be set at 1.5 g/kcal, which falls between the 75th and 90th percentile of intake for males and the 50th and 75th percentile of intake for females. A practical approach is to set the allowance at the 75th percentile of intake and quickly adjust up or down depending on whether the participant considers the level too high or too low. The 75th percentile for adult men is 3,000 g/day, 39 g/kg/day, or 1.3 g/kcal/day; for adult women it is 2,400 g/day, 40 g/kg/day, or 1.7 g/kcal/day) (Tables 15-1 through 15-3).

Basing intake on body weight can be convenient because this unit often is used for calculation of other nutrient intakes. This value can be adjusted after obtaining information about the participant's own typical daily intake of water, level of physical activity at work and leisure, tendency to perspire, and whether the work environment is hot. Season

TABLE 15-5

Dietary Sources of Total Water Intake by Pregnant and Lactating Women[1]

Age (yr)	Source[4]	Mean	SD[5]	Percentile Distribution[3] 5	25	50	75	95	Mean	SD
Pregnant	Food	483	214	191	323	455	612	867	25	11
	Drinking Water	695	525	0	320	640	960	1,760	32	19
	Other Beverages	897	497	274	546	820	1,130	1,818	44	17
	All Sources	2,076	743	1,085	1,553	1,928	2,444	3,475	100	—
Lactating	Food	558	268	254	382	499	678	1,175	25	9
	Drinking Water	677	492	0	240	560	1,040	1,600	29	18
	Other Beverages	1,008	512	307	719	913	1,215	1,885	46	18
	All Sources	2,243	658	1,185	1,833	2,164	2,658	3,353	100	—

Column groups: g/day[2] (Mean, SD[5], Percentile Distribution[3]: 5, 25, 50, 75, 95) and % of Total g/day (Mean, SD).

[1]Adapted from Ershow AG, Cantor KP analysis (3) based on data from 1977–1978 USDA Nationwide Food Consumption Survey.
[2]1 g = 1 mL water.
[3]Percentile values for all sources are independent of values for individual sources (food, drinking water, and other beverages).
[4]Food category includes soups.
[5]SD = standard deviation.
0 = <0.5 g/day

of the year has a surprisingly small overall effect on water intake, because adults generally replace hot drinks with cold with the change in seasons.

The diuretic effects of coffee, tea, and alcohol must be considered when planners estimate the water allowance for protocols that do not permit *ad libitum* (ad lib) intake. Total water intake may need to be higher if these beverages are used rather than plain water, uncaffeinated drinks, and alcohol-free drinks.

PROVIDING WATER AND BEVERAGES IN CONTROLLED DIET STUDIES

Drinking Water

Some studies allow the participant to consume plain water ad lib, and neither the source nor the quantities consumed are of interest. For other studies, source and quantities must be tightly controlled. Participants can be given bottled water of known composition in half-liter or liter bottles to carry with them throughout the day. For studies allowing water ad lib, it is important to provide more than is needed so that the participant will not run out. One liter of plain water per day is sufficient for 75% of adults; 2 L per day will accommodate all but the heaviest consumers (this quantity does not include the water provided through foods and other beverages). Remembering that water weighs 1 kg (2.2 lb) per liter, it is important not to burden the person with unnecessary amounts to carry.

Mineral balance studies must use water with defined mineral content for drinking, food preparation, and ice. Distilled or deionized water is frequently used for this purpose. Distilled water can be purchased in liter bottles or a distilled

water system can be installed in the research kitchen. Unfortunately, distilled or deionized waters taste flat and unappealing; having the water very cold can help participants accept the taste. Providing the water allowance as a flavored drink or with a small amount of lemon juice may be more appealing, but in this case all quantities must be consumed. Some commercial bottled waters may be sufficiently low in certain minerals that they can be used for such studies yet will taste better than distilled water. If bottled waters are used, however, they should be purchased in a single lot and the mineral content analyzed directly; compositional information from the label may not be accurate. Under these circumstances a considerable amount of storage space for water may be needed.

Other Beverages

The amounts and types of all beverages consumed in a research diet study must be defined as are all other foods. Some investigators allow ad lib consumption not only of plain water but also of unsweetened ("no-cal") carbonated drinks, tea, and coffee. These would not affect caloric balance but may affect mineral intake. If the participant is accustomed to adding sugar, milk, or cream to beverages it often is possible within the context of the study to add part of the milk or sugar allowance to the coffee or tea; the contribution of these additives must then be considered in the nutrient calculation of the diet.

Tea and coffee consumption frequently is limited during research studies because of the effects of caffeine, but they also contain other biologically active substances. For example, coffee is a rich source of niacin and potassium (6); tea contains substantial amounts of fluoride (7). Both contain tannin that may affect mineral absorption (8). Simply switching to decaffeinated versions may not eliminate these effects.

Carbonated beverages must be defined for the purposes of the study. Some types of "seltzer" are not plain carbonated water but rather are sweetened with sugar or corn syrup. The investigators also must decide whether to allow caffeinated sodas and artificially sweetened sodas as free or restricted items.

According to 1994 USDA survey data, alcoholic beverages typically provide 2% to 4% of daily energy for adult males and 1% to 2% for adult females (9). These figures likely are general underestimates and some individuals consume much more than these amounts. Alcoholic beverages often are not allowed within controlled diet protocols because of their complex and poorly characterized chemical composition, effects on behavior, and potential confounding of metabolic phenomena. However alcohol-free beers are available and may provide an acceptable substitute in some situations.

CONCLUSION: CONSIDERATIONS FOR PROTOCOL DESIGN

Water and fluid allowances, sources, and intakes should be evaluated carefully for different types of well-controlled dietary studies.

- In studies using liquid formula diets, the formula is likely to provide the largest source of water. Attempting to dilute the formula in the entire day's water allotment, however, will lead to an overly large volume of formula. Calculating the participant's individual water allowance will permit the dietitian to determine the osmolality of the entire diet; known volumes of drinking water can be provided to supplement the amount taken in through the formula. (Also see Chapter 14, "Planning and Producing Formula Diets.")

- Excretion studies or balance studies entailing 24-hour urine collections gain in precision from exact knowledge of water intake. Completeness of collection can be estimated better if the previous day's water intake is known. Appropriate instructions and data collection forms must be provided to the participants for recording all beverages, water, and foods consumed within a specified time period. (Also see Chapter 17, "Energy Needs and Weight Maintenance in Controlled Diet Studies.")

- Mineral balance studies must account for minerals present in water, just as in any other part of the diet. Controlled feeding studies of blood pressure may also have a similar design requirement. Water of known composition must be provided and used not just for ad lib consumption but also in the preparation of all foods, beverages, and ice. Depending on study requirements, this water can be tapwater, deionized water, or bottled water. In trace mineral studies, deionized water should be used for washing dishes. Regardless of the source, the water must be chemically analyzed for mineral content. For example, some softened waters have a high sodium content. The volume of all consumed water must also be a defined quantity, as with all other foodstuffs. Enough water must be provided so that the participant will not resort to undefined sources such as drinking fountains or sink taps.

- Some protocols require that the individual produce urine samples at timed intervals. For these studies, the water intake pattern must be manipulated so that large boluses of water or fluids are consumed at specific times of the day, with enough lag time to allow for absorption and renal clearance.

- Many protocols allow ad lib intake of tapwater but require that all other fluids and beverages be controlled. Tea, coffee, milk, juice, soups, and carbonated beverages are most likely to be regulated in this way.

- Well-accepted research diets are designed by considering typical patterns of intake for water and beverages, as well as for other foods. Portion sizes should resemble those frequently consumed by free-living individuals of similar body weight.

REFERENCES

1. Vokes T. Water homeostasis. *Ann Rev Nutr.* 1987;7:383–406.
2. Food and Nutrition Board, National Research Council. *Recommended Dietary Allowances.* 10th ed. Washington, DC: National Academy Press; 1989.
3. Ershow AG, Cantor KP. *Total Water and Tapwater Intake in the United States: Population-based Estimates of Quantities and Sources.* Bethesda, Md: Life Sciences Research Office, Federation of American Society for Experimental Biology; 1989.
4. Ershow AG, Brown LM, Cantor KP. Intake of tapwater and total water by pregnant and lactating women. *Am J Public Health.* 1991;81:328–334.
5. Stumbo PJ, Booth BM, Eichenberger JM, et al. Water intakes of lactating women. *Am J Clin Nutr.* 1985; 42:870–876.
6. US Department of Agriculture. *Nutrient Database for Standard Reference, Release 12 (SR-12).* Agricultural Research Service, Nutrient Data Laboratory, Beltsville Human Nutrition Research Center, Beltsville, Md (e-mail: http://www.nal.usda.gov/fnic/foodcomp).
7. Ma TS, Gwirtsman JJ. Determination of fluorine in tea. *Int J Environ Anal Chem.* 1972;2:133–138.
8. Mehansho H, Butler LG, Carlson DM. Dietary tannins and salivary proline-rich proteins. *Ann Rev Nutr.* 1987; 7:423–440.
9. Cleveland LE, Goldman JD, Borrud LG. *Data Tables: Results from USDA's 1994 Continuing Survey of Food Intakes by Individuals and 1994 Diet and Health Knowledge Survey.* Riverdale, Md: Food Surveys Research Group, Agricultural Research Service, US Department of Agriculture; 1996.

CHAPTER 16

COMPARTMENTAL MODELING, STABLE ISOTOPES, AND BALANCE STUDIES

DAVID J. BAER, PHD; ALICE K. H. FONG, EDD, RD; JANET A. NOVOTNY, PHD; AND MARY JOAN OEXMANN, MS, RD

COMPARTMENTAL APPROACHES TO NUTRITION RESEARCH

The systems studied in human nutrition research are complex collections of biochemical reactions, many of which share substrates, intermediates, and products. In contrast to animal studies, few tissues are available for analysis, thus limiting what can be studied directly in humans. Thus, a method is needed for inferring the dynamics of hard-to-observe physiological phenomena. Further, as information about metabolic processes is acquired, a system of "bookkeeping" is required to organize the data in a meaningful way. Compartmental modeling, which has become invaluable in biological investigations, provides such a bookkeeping system (1–3).

A *compartmental model* is a mathematically simulated description of a real-world system in terms of theoretical physiological spaces (such as plasma) and the transfers among them. Each component of the model corresponds to a component of the system being modeled. The relationships among the components of the model correspond to relationships among the components of the system of interest. For example, features of a doll correspond to features of a human. A doll possesses arms, legs, and a head in proportions similar to that of a human. However, not all features

of the human are present in the doll. Lungs, for example, are not important for the functioning of a doll and are therefore not included in the doll's construction. Similarly, a compartmental model includes features of the system that are important to the processes of interest but does not include features unrelated to the specific processes of interest. For example, a compartmental model of glucose metabolism will likely not include processes of protein synthesis.

The metabolic fate of nutrients can be studied by evaluating three components: input, intermediate processes, and output (see Figure 16-1). Measuring nutritional or dietary *input* requires food composition, quantities of food eaten, and compliance with the study diet to be well characterized. Typical measures of *intermediary metabolism* can include oxidation rates of nutrients, biochemical transformations, transport, and changes in nutrient stores. *Output* from the system is evaluated by measuring losses from the system, whether as nutrient mass or as energy.

For example, once a food is consumed, a proportion of the minerals in that food is absorbed and passes into the circulation while the nonabsorbed portion is eliminated in feces (see Figure 16-2) (4). Complete elimination of unabsorbed minerals may take 6 to 12 days. Some of the absorbed minerals will pass from the circulation into body tissues; some will be excreted in urine. Another path of excretory loss is from body tissues back into the gut via biliary or

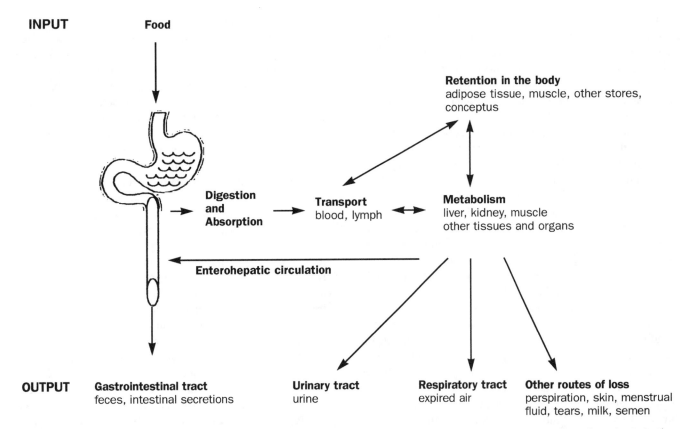

FIGURE 16-1. Physiologic pools in nutrient metabolism. This schematic figure summarizes the movement of nutrients in the body. Mass changes between input and output are the basis for calculating digestibility and nutrient balance.

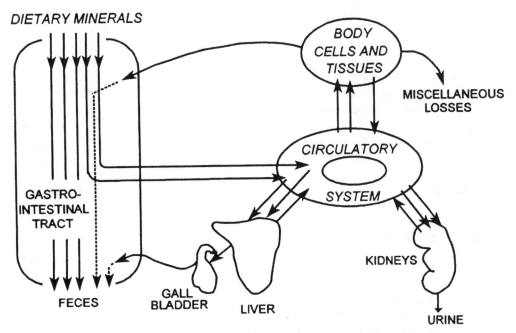

FIGURE 16-2. Absorption, distribution, and elimination of dietary minerals. Solid lines through the gastrointestinal tract represent unabsorbed minerals. Dotted lines represent endogenous minerals that are excreted into the gastrointestinal tract and eliminated with unabsorbed minerals.

Reprinted with permission from JR Turnlund, Bioavailability of dietary materials to humans: the stable isotope approach, *Crit Rev Food Sci Nutr,* 1991;30:387–396.

gastrointestinal (GI) secretions. Some of the endogenous minerals can be reabsorbed, but the majority pass into the feces. Once a mineral is absorbed into the body, it mixes with minerals from meals consumed recently and weeks, months, or years earlier. Thus, minerals excreted in feces, urine, and other routes are from a combination of recent and earlier intakes.

Whole-body nutrient economy is difficult to study in human subjects and generally requires the use of *balance study* methodology. The fundamental components of a balance study are the measurements of nutrient intake and nutrient output. This is a classic technique in human nutrition research. In fact, balance study methodology underlies several important lines of evidence for the determination of nutrient requirements (5–8): clinical or biochemical measures of nutrient status in relation to intake; biochemical measures of tissue saturation or of adequacy of molecular function in relation to intake; and knowledge of nutrient homeostasis and exchanges between body pools in relation to intake.

There also is a long tradition of using balance studies in animal nutrition research in order to link requirements for growth, maintenance, pregnancy, or lactation to the development of nutritionally adequate diets (9). Balance studies can be appreciated in a broader context by viewing them as a specialized form of compartmental modeling research, having the input and output compartments particularly well defined.

A recently developed methodology for enhancing compartmental studies uses *stable isotopes* (10). These naturally occurring, nonradioactive isotopes can be used to investigate the metabolism of energy, water, macronutrients, and micronutrients. Oral and intravenous doses of a nutrient can be tracked and distinguished from endogenous amounts of the nutrient already present in the body. Isotopic tracers thus permit additional information to be obtained on the metabolic fate of nutrients. When partnered with up-to-date analytical techniques and mathematical modeling methods, stable isotopes provide new research approaches for understanding nutrient transfer among different tissues and organs and *in vivo* metabolic processes.

This chapter discusses several types of compartmental modeling studies and the kinds of research questions such studies can answer. The focus of the information is on practical aspects to consider in study design and implementation.

CREATING A COMPARTMENTAL MODEL

Compartmental models consist of *pools* (compartments) of metabolites and *flows* (interactions) among pools. A pool is a kinetically distinct, homogeneous, well-mixed form of an analyte in the body. The compartments may or may not be associated with a physical space. For example, vitamin A in the liver is physiologically distinct (ie, found in a different physical location) from vitamin A in the plasma. In contrast, water in the extracellular space and water in the plasma are

physically distinct but not kinetically distinct (ie, having different half-lives) because the two body spaces exchange water freely. Moreover, two analytes may exist in the same physical space but be represented by distinct compartments in a model if their kinetic behavior differs. For example, vitamin A in the form of retinyl ester behaves differently than vitamin A bound to retinol-binding protein; therefore, these two would be represented as separate compartments even though they are both forms of vitamin A existing in the same physical space (the plasma).

The compartments interact by exchanging the analyte(s) of interest. The exchanges are represented by mathematical equations whose variables are the masses in the compartments and whose parameters describe the rate of exchange of material from the donor compartment to the recipient compartment. Material can flow into the system from the environment as oral ingestion or infusions, and material can leave the system irreversibly by urine or fecal loss, by metabolism, or by other means of loss. Flows between compartments may occur through simple partitioning of an analyte into different physical spaces or through processes of state conversions such as oxidation, binding, or delipidation.

An example of this concept is shown in Figure 16-3. In this two-compartment model of zinc kinetics, P (or p) represents the plasma pool; E (or e) represents the exchangeable pool (ie, the pool that exchanges between plasma and other tissues), Q (or q) represents isotope transported out of the system, and k is the rate constant representing the fraction of the pool that is replaced within a given time (t) (11). The fluxes between compartments can be described mathematically using differential equations. A good discussion of this topic is provided in Wolfe (5).

If the flows *into* the compartment balance the flows *out* of the compartment, the system is in steady state and there is no change in the pool size in any compartment. In states

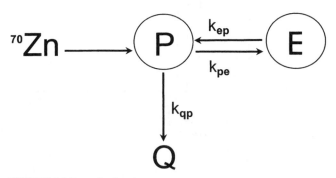

FIGURE 16-3.   A simple two-compartment model of zinc kinetics. The two compartments shown are plasma *(P)* and an exchangeable pool *(E)*. Isotope transported out of the model system is represented as *Q*. The rate constant, *K*, represents the fraction of the pool that is replaced within a given time.

Reprinted from W van Dokkum, et al, Study techniques, in FA Mellon, B Sandstrom, eds, *Stable Isotopes in Human Nutrition* (San Diego, Calif: Academic Press; 1996), by permission of the publisher, Academic Press.

of nutrient balance, the input mass (shown in Figure 16-3 as an intravenous dose of ^{70}Zn) will equal the output mass (shown in Figure 16-3 as Q).

The first step in creating a compartmental model is to create a schematic of the system of interest based on previous knowledge of the system. The schematic should include all measurable analyte pools and other pools that are important to the research question posed. Once the important pools are delineated, arrows are drawn among the pools to represent flows of material. The flows are then described by mathematical equations. Collaboration with an experienced mathematical modeler is essential to ensure that the correct equations are used and to avoid pitfalls in the assumptions used in deriving the model.

The mathematical equation that describes a particular flow from one compartment to another has a form that is determined by the characteristics of the exchange. Using this concept the measurement of size and rate of turnover of exchangeable body pools of an element can be derived. Thus far kinetic modeling has been used to examine many nutrients, including zinc (12), selenium (13), calcium (14), copper (15), vitamin A (16), and beta-carotene (17) metabolism. In some cases, such as in Figure 16-4, human whole-body copper metabolism, a model can be developed using kinetic modeling and balance study methodology. This figure shows a compartmental model of copper metabolism in adult men using enriched ^{65}Cu. The model predicted that enriched copper-65 masses were converted to total copper masses as in the following equations (14):

$$\text{Total copper-65} = \frac{\text{Predicted mass of enriched copper-65}}{\text{Copper-65 enrichment}}$$

$$\text{Total Cu} = \frac{\text{Total copper-65}}{0.3083 \text{ copper-65 in total Cu}}$$

Scott and Turnlund used ^{65}Cu in this study to develop a model of copper metabolism, the first in humans. The compartmental model was developed using CONSAM version 30.1 (18). The study was conducted in 5 young men who lived in a metabolic research unit for a 90-day period during which three different dietary levels of copper were fed. Copper-65 was administered orally 4 times and intravenously 3 times throughout the study. The model developed was simple, it used a simple recycling design, and it demonstrated that the amount of dietary copper consumed influences the flow of copper from one liver compartment to one plasma compartment and from that plasma compartment to the "other tissues" compartment. In this five-compartment (two plasma, two liver, and one "other tissues") model, tissue uptake of oral and intravenous copper differs, with the flow from plasma to a liver compartment varying with the route of administration. The circles represent compartments, the squares are delay elements, the triangle is the sum of the indicated compartments, and * is the site of the Cu tracer input. The authors hypothesized that plasma compartment 6 represents nonceruloplasmin-bound copper, whereas compartment 8 contains ceruloplasmin-bound copper. This model predicts that 65% of plasma copper is bound to cer-

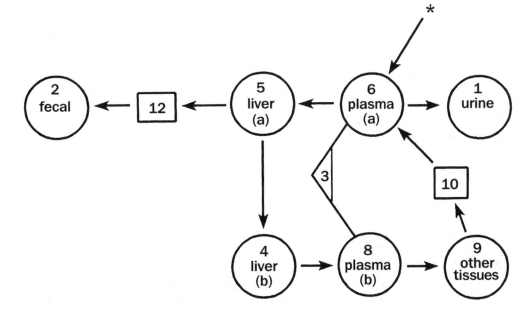

FIGURE 16-4.   Schematic representation of a compartmental model of copper metabolism in adult men. Circles represent compartments, squares are delay elements, the triangle is the sum of the indicated compartments, and the asterisk (*) is the site of input for the copper tracer.

Reprinted from *Journal of Nutritional Biochemistry,* vol 5, KC Scott and JR Turnlund, Compartmental model of copper metabolism in adult men, pp 342–350, 1994, with permission from Elsevier Science.

ulophasmin compared to 56% to 68% calculated from data. Similarly, the model predicted $4 \pm 1\%$ of total body copper would be present in plasma, very close to the 2% to 6% expected.

From this example, it is evident that the mathematics of compartmental modeling is complex and requires specially trained investigators. Jacquez (19) provides a good general introduction to compartmental modeling. Collins (20) reviews books, journals, and software packages focused on modeling. A complete and detailed description of the steps involved in the development of a compartmental model is described in Novotny et al (21). Software packages, such as Simulation, Analysis, and Modeling (SAAM) and CONSAM (the interactive conversational SAAM) (17) are now used not only to assist in data analysis but also to indicate parameters that must be incorporated into the basic experimental design of the study.

The power of computer mathematic simulation enables the modeler to develop a unified hypothesis of the functioning of the many complex processes that compose the system of interest. The model is then tested against experimental observation to be sure that the model mimics the system for every known situation.

Under ideal circumstances, once the model's behavior does not deviate from experimental observation in any case tested, the model can be used to investigate aspects of the system that otherwise would be experimentally inaccessible.

BALANCE STUDIES

It is assumed that a healthy adult who eats an adequate diet can thereby maintain equilibrium or balance for essential nutrients. This means that over a period of time, the amount of each of these substances that enters the body is equaled by the amount that leaves the body. By convention, when intake and output are equal, the subject is considered to be "in balance," a state in which nutrient or energy requirement have been met (no net change). When output exceeds input, the subject is in "negative balance," a state leading to depletion. When output is less than intake, the subject is in "positive balance," a state of nutrient accrual, growth, weight gain, anabolism, or repletion of stores. Equilibrium can be disturbed by changes in food intake, medications, physical activity, or disease, or by physiological states such as growth, pregnancy, and lactation.

For some nutrients, such as water, minerals, protein, fat, and energy, measuring nutrient or energy balance has provided an important means of understanding absorption and bioavailability. Balance studies of nutrients such as energy, nitrogen, and water also can provide clues to an individual's physiological state, such as growth. However, for other nutrients, a strictly defined concept of balance is less meaningful. For example, some of the vitamins (such as biotin, pantothenic acid, and vitamin K) (8) can be synthesized *in vivo* from intestinal bacteria, and diet only supplies part of total "input"; as a result, it is not possible to obtain precise quantitative data on the mass balance of these compounds.

Instead, in this case, balance studies may provide qualitative data about metabolism and requirements.

Specific time sequences of balance states can be established to address certain research questions. For example, nutrient requirements often are investigated using the following time sequence: negative balance is induced by feeding a diet known to provide inadequate levels of the nutrient under study; the diet then is altered until the point of balance (repletion or correction of deficiency) is established; and finally a state of positive balance is induced in which nutrient stores are established and intake exceeds requirement (22).

The balance technique is both time-consuming and labor-intensive. To measure balance precisely, one must determine the difference between the intake of nutrient and the amount excreted through urine, feces, and other routes, such as exhaled air, skin, hair, perspiration, menses, and other secretions. (In practice, measurement of total excretion is not always attempted because such collection conditions require complete research control that only a metabolic research unit can provide.) An additional complication is that nutrients undergo metabolic changes in the body, and the amount excreted as such may not equal the intake. Errors associated with the measurement of intake and output thus can cause a loss of precision and make it difficult to interpret the data.

Calculating Nutrient Balance and Availability

Nutrient balance (Formula 1) typically is calculated as the difference between the amount consumed and the amount excreted (23, 24):

(1) $$\text{Balance} = \text{Intake} - \text{Excreted}$$

Nutrient digestibility (Formula 2) also can be calculated from balance study data. In the simplest form, *true digestibility* is nutrient balance expressed as a fraction (or percent) of the amount consumed:

(2) $$\text{Digestibility} = \frac{\text{Intake} - (\text{Total excreted} - \text{Endogenous fecal excretion})}{\text{Intake}}$$

Because it is often difficult to separate the contribution of unabsorbed nutrients from the endogenous secretions and bacterial microflora of the gastrointestinal tract, a more common approach is to measure *apparent digestibility* and ignore the contributions of endogenous production.

Particularly in measuring the energy content of food or nutrients, further distinctions in apparent digestibility can be made if output from fecal and urinary sources is measured through bomb calorimetry. When only the energy output from feces is measured through bomb calorimetry, the data allow the calculation of the *digestible energy content* (Formula 3):

(3)   Digestible energy =

$$\frac{\text{Intake energy} - \text{Excreted energy (feces)}}{\text{Intake energy}}$$

When the energy content of both feces and urine is measured through bomb calorimetry, the *metabolizable energy content* (Formula 4) of the diet can be determined:

(4)   Metabolizable energy =

$$\frac{\text{Intake energy} - \text{Excreted energy (feces)} - \text{Excreted energy (urine)}}{\text{Intake energy}}$$

Net energy (Formula 5) is determined as the difference between metabolizable energy intake and heat increment (or the *thermic effect of food*):

(5)   Net energy = Metabolizable energy − Heat increment

The net energy is the energy available for productive purposes (growth, tissue repair, lactation, or pregnancy). Heat increment is the amount of energy released during digestive and metabolic processes associated with digestion and storage. The heat increment of a test meal can be measured by 6-hour calorimetry after ingestion of a test meal; however, this approach is limited to short-term measures.

Net energy (NE) (Formula 6) can also be determined as the ratio of the change (Δ) in retained energy (RE) at two (or more) levels of energy intake to the change in energy intake (IE).

(6) $$NE = \frac{\Delta RE}{\Delta IE}$$

Availability of a nutrient can be assessed by its digestibility (Formula 2), metabolizability (Formula 4), or net energy (Formula 5 or 6). These measures are most useful as direct comparisons between diets. Increasing digestibility is indicative of greater nutrient or energy availability. Although some foods may have the same digestibility, they may have different net energies as a consequence of nutrient interactions or of differences in the cost of digestion or metabolism. These formulas can be used to aid in the interpretation of differences that might be observed among diets containing various levels of fiber, energy, protein, fat, or carbohydrate.

Such formulas have been used in past investigations to determine protein and energy balance or requirements. In one study, through the usage of balance, digestibility, and metabolizable energy formulas, Calloway and Kretsch (25) examined protein and energy use. In the same study these investigators evaluated also whether absorption of protein and energy are different between poor rural Guatemalan inhabitants and healthy North Americans. Current and future investigative work in nutrition requirements or bioavailability evaluations will continue to rely on the usage of formulas, such as those provided above, to address many unresolved intake adequacy concerns.

Practical Considerations

Balance studies are carried out by keeping constant all possible influences that might disturb the balance and by varying or controlling only the one factor under investigation. It is essential that precise control and measurement of intake and output be made because small changes, rather than gross changes, are often expected. A slight error of overestimation of intake and a slight underestimation of excretion will cause a compounded error in the final balance calculation because "the two losses are additive, not self-canceling, as is generally supposed" (26).

Statistical issues for balance studies are not unique to this type of investigation. (See Chapter 2, "Statistical Aspects of Controlled Diet Studies.") In general, the experimental sequence of depletion, repletion, and balance states suggests using analysis techniques suited to designs in which the participant serves as his or her own control. This is particularly important because balance studies tend to enroll small numbers of participants and maximum statistical power must be gained from the design. Along with protecting against selection bias, randomized assignment of subjects to treatment sequences will allow adjustment for carryover effects. Repeated crossover treatments may also serve this purpose. If it is necessary to compare multiple dietary treatments, the protocol can be designed to combine the features of parallel-arm assignments with those of crossover designs to allow satisfactory comparison of treatment groups.

Adaptation to the Study Diet

Adaptation to a new diet is essential to allow for microbial changes in the gastrointestinal tract and to allow for enzymatic or secretory changes that may occur. Typically, subjects are allowed to adapt to a new diet for several days, but the length of the adaptation period often depends on the nutrient being altered. For many nutrients, an adaptation period of several weeks is required for metabolic changes to reach the new norm (27). An appropriate adaptation period is especially important when changes are made in the type or amount of dietary fiber. The symbiotic microbial population of the gastrointestinal tract, which ferments the fiber, must be provided enough time to adapt to the new diet.

When a change from a diet high in a substance to a diet low in the same substance takes place, there will be a transitional period before a new equilibrium is established. This adjustment period is best disregarded in evaluating the level of the new equilibrium, but important information can be gained from evaluating the rate of change and variability.

Sources of Error in Estimating Intake

The principal investigator and the research dietitian must be vigilant to see that errors are not introduced into balance studies. Some typical sources of error associated with nutrient intake and output are outlined here.

Controlling and Measuring Intake

A crucial factor in measuring nutrient balance is the accurate measurement of nutrient intake through accurate characterization of the ingested diet. Underestimating intake can produce a false negative balance, whereas overestimating intake can cause the incorrect conclusion of positive nutrient balance.

Maintaining a constant diet, and thus a consistent and predictable food and nutrient intake, is another important aspect of balance studies. Because changes in intake of some nutrients can alter rate of passage and hence absorption, care must be given to maintaining a constant level of intake prior to and during the balance period. It is best if the experimental and the control diets are closely matched for all nutrients except the nutrient to be investigated. When the diet consists of conventional foods, the greatest error in estimating nutrient intake is caused by day-to-day variations in the composition of the foods. This variation stems from the chemical variability of the food items as well as variation in weighing of food items. Use of formula diets or pureed/blended diets minimizes both types of errors. (Also see Chapter 14, "Planning and Producing Formula Diets.") If the amount of variation is expected to be high and unpredictable, it may be necessary to purchase food from specific production lots and also to collect food samples daily for chemical analysis. (Also see Chapter 22, "Validating Diet Composition by Chemical Analysis.")

For vitamin studies, unless nutrient retention values are available for the cooking method used, it is advisable to calculate the nutrient content of the diet using data for cooked forms of the food. Laboratory assay of the diet, as mentioned earlier, will yield yet more accurate data.

Food Preparation

Food preparation for balance studies must achieve the highest possible degree of precision because the state of nutrient balance is calculated by comparing the absolute nutrient intake with the absolute nutrient output (ie, loss). Thus it is critical that balance study diets deliver the specified *absolute* levels of nutrients, whereas for other study diets such precision may not be necessary or practical.

Basic techniques for balance diets are similar to those for other research diets. See Chapters 11 ("Designing Research Diets"), 12 ("Producing Research Diets"), and 13 ("Delivering Research Diets"). Additional precision is gained by using foods that have very consistent nutrient content, calculating the diet with database values for the foods in the forms that will be weighed out (ie, cooked or raw), and evaluating the potential for nutrient loss each time foods are transferred (ie, from storage containers to cookware to tableware to participant).

Extra precautions are required to prevent environmental contamination in trace mineral studies. Supplies and equipment (such as cookware, food storage containers, detergents, water for cooking and washing, and tableware, including disposable paper and plastic items) must be selected, and perhaps tested as well, to ensure that study minerals are not released into the food.

Plate Residues

Invisible "returns" will remain even after meticulous scraping with a spatula. Isaksson and Sjogren (28, 29) found daily mean losses for nitrogen to be 0.1 g, calcium to be 20 mg, sodium to be 2.7 mEq, and potassium to be 1.1 mEq. These losses can be much higher if the participant neglects to scrape and rinse the plates and glasses and drink the resulting rinse water. This error can be reduced by carefully explaining eating procedures to the participants before the start of the study and by establishing a system to check the participants' dishes for visible food particles after each meal. (Also see the discussion of eating techniques in Chapter 13, "Delivering Research Diets.")

Unauthorized Food Intake

Unauthorized food intake and omission of study foods are common problems during the initial days of a study as participants adjust to the study protocol. Hunger due to inaccurate calorie adjustments promotes consumption of unauthorized foods. Occasionally, deliberate or even malicious intake or omission of foods occurs—particularly when a participant's dissatisfaction with any part of the routine is not appreciated quickly enough by the staff. (Also see Chapter 13, "Delivering Research Diets.")

Sources of Error in Estimating Output

The two primary routes of loss for most nutrients are feces and urine. For some nutrients, there may be other appreciable routes of loss that need to be accounted for in order to obtain accurate balance measurements. For example, sodium loss associated with sweating can be significant, especially during short-term studies.

Fecal Collections

When feces represent a significant route of loss of the nutrient of interest (eg, macronutrients, some minerals), it is imperative to collect samples for analysis. Feces can be collected into plastic disposable freezer containers or into self-sealing plastic bags. Once collected, feces can be stored in Styrofoam coolers containing dry ice until they can be brought to the facility for additional processing, storage, pooling, and analysis. Temporary storage on wet ice is acceptable if the analyte of interest is relatively stable. Wet ice may not provide a cold enough holding temperature to minimize microbial fermentation, however, which can compromise the analysis of certain nutrients (eg, fiber, fatty acids). Thus, nutrient changes can occur after defecation and before proper sample storage.

The required length of time for collection depends on the menu cycle and the rate of food passage. If menus do not change from day-to-day, then the length of collection can be as short as 3 to 4 days, after an appropriate adaptation period. However, even when diet is relatively constant, there still might be physiologic variation in absorption and excretion. Therefore, when nutrient balance over an entire menu cycle is the research outcome of interest, it is preferable to collect all feces resulting from that menu cycle. Thus, if the menu cycle is 7 days long, then the subjects should consume all 7 days of meals, and the corresponding feces should be included in the fecal composite.

The length of time between bowel movements as well as the mineral or other nutrient content for each bowel movement varies. This variability causes fluctuation in the balance value of nutrients commonly excreted in feces (calcium, magnesium, phosphorus, and trace minerals). To obtain a reliable measure of fecal output, one can use an inert fecal marker such as polyethylene glycol (PEG) (30, 31). (Also see Chapter 24, "Biological Sample Collection and Markers of Dietary Compliance.")

Nontoxic dye markers can be used also to demarcate the beginning and end of the fecal collection period and to identify stool samples corresponding to specific days of the diet. Brilliant blue, carmine (red), or indigo carmine (blue) dyes are commonly used fecal markers. These markers can be given to the subjects in gelatin capsules. Small amounts of marker (approximately 200 mg) are sufficient for detection in the feces. Participants typically swallow the dye capsules at two time points, one marking the beginning of the test period and the second marking the end of the test period. Transit time (ie, from the time the food with the marker is eaten to the time the corresponding stool is produced) varies among individuals with a usual range of 1 to 4 days. All stool samples are collected from the time the dye marker first appears until the appearance of the second marker. The duration of collection varies among studies; for calcium balance, a 72-hour collection has been recommended (30).

Although these markers are used to help visually detect when collection should begin, they are often not the most reliable indicators to use. Color-blind subjects find the markers difficult to see. Also, depending on the foods consumed by a subject, the colors of the markers may blend with the excreted waste.

The failure to collect all feces during a study is extremely difficult to prove. Inadequate fecal collections can cause errors in balance determinations for elements in which the net absorption is small compared to the intake.

Urine Collections

Urine can contain appreciable amounts of urea, some minerals, and vitamins. Thus, total urine collections are necessary for balance measurements of many nutrients. However, for free-living studies in which complete collections are not possible, timed sample urine collections may be useful. Sometimes timed or random urine samples are necessary to check whether energy or total food intake is sufficient. In such a case, the urine is checked for ketone bodies. In the case of doubly labeled water methodology, post-dose urine samples are collected at set times on the day of dosing and

for 14 days afterward. In metabolic studies where complete collections are possible, urine would be collected for 24 hours daily.

In these studies, there is considerable individual variation in urine output, and there can be significant intraindividual variation as well. In normal healthy individuals, daily urine volume can range from 1,000 ml to 3,000 ml or more, depending on daily fluid intake. It is important to provide enough collection containers. For example, a subject making 24-hour urine collections returned completely full 1-gallon containers of urine daily. Upon questioning, it was learned that he was disposing of additional urine. The subject, who was employed in a service job requiring many hours in transit, habitually consumed unusually large volumes of fluid as he drove to his multiple job sites.

Once collected, samples can be stored on ice in coolers or on dry ice. For nitrogen balance studies, it might be necessary to acidify (usually with hydrochloric acid) urine after collection to minimize loss of ammonia generated from urea. Ammonia loss will result in a false positive balance of nitrogen and energy balance.

Errors caused by inadequate collection of urine are difficult to demonstrate. One solution to ensure completeness of urine collection is to feed para-amino-benzoic acid (PABA) and use this marker as a urine completeness validity check. (See Chapter 24, "Biological Sample Collection and Markers of Dietary Compliance.") Measures of compliance with urinary collection also can be based on a metabolic constant. Creatinine, for example, is excreted in proportion to muscle mass. However, a 5% to 10% day-to-day variation in urinary creatinine excretion is common (some of this variation may be caused by diet, such as the level of meat intake), and this reduces the precision of creatinine determination as an index of completeness of urinary collection.

Another technique to check for consumption compliance is through the urinary osmolality test. The osmolar load of urine is based on compounds, such as nitrogen, sodium, and potassium, derived from foods. A lower than predicted value for urinary osmolality suggests the subject did not eat all of the food provided; a higher value suggests the subject ate unauthorized foods. The disadvantage of this method is low precision and that it requires performing more than 6 days of 24-hour urine collection. (See Chaper 24, "Laboratory Quality Control in Dietary Trials.")

Other Sources of Nutrient Loss

As illustrated in Figure 16–1, there are many other potential routes of nutrient loss in addition to feces and urine. These include blood (phlebotomy, menses, injury), sweat, tears, saliva, hair, skin and dermis, and pulmonary exhalations. In most cases, these losses are negligible and difficult to measure.

Take, for example, the small but cumulative losses of nitrogen from various routes. If in determining nitrogen balance, the dermal and miscellaneous losses are disregarded, the total error in balance is about 0.5 g nitrogen per day for sedentary men in a comfortable environment. Nutrient losses in sweat and desquamated cells of hair, skin, and nails can be determined to account for the dermal losses. Calloway, Odell, and Margen (32) found that an average value of this error is 149 ± 51 mg of nitrogen per day for sedentary men. Nitrogen losses in tooth brushing, toilet tissues, plate wastes, and exhaled ammonia were found to amount to about 115 mg per day. The loss of nutrients from blood varies widely from study to study depending on the amount of blood drawn during the study, but Calloway, Odell, and Margen found a loss of 32 mg N/100 ml of blood. In addition, these investigators found other sources of nitrogen loss to include saliva (0.9 mg N/g), semen (27 mg N/ejaculate), and menstrual fluid (900 mg N/period).

Typical Applications of Balance Methodology

Zinc, Copper, and Iron Balance in Elderly Males

Turnlund et al (33) conducted a study of zinc, iron, and copper balance in elderly men to evaluate the adequacy of dietary recommendations for these elements for the elderly. The researchers attempted to eliminate a number of sources of error thought to contribute to unreliable and inconsistent results of balance studies by including long adaptation periods on constant mineral intake and balance periods of 21 days. The mineral balance study was part of a larger study on the protein, energy, and mineral requirements of elderly men.

The study comprised two 6-week metabolic periods. The only difference in the two metabolic periods was the protein intake: 9 g to 19 g of nitrogen per day in period 1 dependent on habitual protein intake, and 70 mg nitrogen/kg body weight in period 2. Two 3-week balance studies for

zinc, copper, and iron were carried out in 6 elderly males who were confined to a metabolic unit for a total of 12 weeks with constant dietary mineral intake. The diet used in the study was adequate in all nutrients and consisted of formula drinks, peaches, low-protein rusks with margarine, tea, coffee, and vitamin supplements. The nutrients of interest were made into solutions that were added to the formula drinks.

The subjects were observed during meals and care was taken to ensure complete consumption of all food offered. The subjects rinsed all dishes with deionized water and rinse water was consumed. Twenty-four-hour urine collections were collected in polyethylene bottles, and feces were collected for 3-day periods in polyethylene containers. Feces were homogenized in a colloid mill and acidified with 1% high-purity hydrochloric acid (HCL). Urine was acidified also with 1% high-purity HCL. Sweat and integumenatry collections were made for two 3-day periods. Subjects bathed and rinsed with deionized water containing 25% polyoxyethlene-23-lauryl ether before collections and wore cotton suits of long underwear that were covered with disposable, plastic-coated coveralls to avoid contamination of the underwear. The clothing was pretreated by soaking in 0.1 N HCL for 3 days; after wear, clothes were removed and soaked again in 0.1 N HCL that had been tested for zinc, copper, and iron levels. The bathwater and laundry soaking solutions were combined and aliquots taken for analysis. Blood was drawn during screening of subjects and at the end of the 6th and 12th weeks of the study.

In this study, mean zinc and copper balance for the 6 males was close to 0:0.1 mg/day for zinc and 0.06 mg/day for copper. (See Tables 16-1 through 16-4: zinc balance and serum zinc table, copper balance, serum copper, and ceruloplasmin table, and iron balance and blood parameters.) Iron balance appeared to be negative (mean of –0.44 mg/day) despite improved blood iron parameters for the majority of the subjects. Determinations of zinc, copper, and iron

TABLE 16-1

Intake and Excretion of Zinc, Copper, and Iron in Elderly Men

	Dietary Intake (mg/day)[1]	Fecal Excretion (mg/day)	Urinary Excretion (mg/day)
Zinc			
Metabolic period 1	15.4 ± 0.3	14.1 ± 0.4	0.7 ± 0.1
Metabolic period 2	15.5 ± 0.3	14.6 ± 0.5	0.8 ± 0.1
Copper			
Metabolic period 1	3.24 ± 0.14	3.18 ± 0.14	<0.015
Metabolic period 2	3.28 ± 0.11	3.22 ± 0.06	<0.015
Iron			
Metabolic period 1	10.0	9.87 ± 0.29	<0.1
Metabolic period 2	10.0	10.4 ± 0.16	<0.1

[1]Values represent mean ± SEM. (There was no SEM reported for iron intake.)
Source: Turnlund J, Costa F, and Margen S. Zinc, copper, and iron balance in elderly men. *Am J Clin Nutr.* 1981;34:2641–2647. © *Am J Clin Nutr,* American Society for Clinical Nutrition.

TABLE 16-2

Zinc Balance and Serum Zinc Concentration in Elderly Men

	Subject						
	1	3	5	6	7	8	Mean
Balance (mg/day)							
Metabolic period 1	−0.5	+1.8	+0.7	+0.3			
Metabolic period 2	−0.8	+1.1	−1.1	+1.3	−1.0	+1.0	0.1 ± 0.5
Serum Zn (µg/ml)							
Prestudy	0.7	0.9	1.0	0.6	0.7	0.8	
End study	0.9	1.0	1.2	1.1	0.9	0.9	
Change	+0.2	+0.1	+0.2	+0.5	+0.2	+0.1	0.2 ± 0.1[1]

[1]Mean ± SE of change.
Source: Turnlund J, Costa F, and Margen S. Zinc, copper, and iron balance in elderly men. *Am J Clin Nutr.* 1981;34:2641–2647. © *Am J Clin Nutr,* American Society for Clinical Nutrition.

TABLE 16-3

Copper Balance, Serum Copper, and Ceruloplasmin Concentration in Elderly Men

	Subject						
	1	3	5	6	7	8	Mean
Balance (mg/day)							
Metabolic period 1	−0.27	+0.08	+0.15	+0.07			
Metabolic period 2	−0.02	+0.16	−0.17	+0.22	+0.12	+0.04	0.06 ± 0.06
Serum Cu (µg/ml)							
Prestudy	1.3	1.2	1.0	1.0	0.4	1.0	
End study	1.7	1.1	0.8	0.9	0.9	1.0	
Change	+0.4	−0.1	−0.2	−0.1	+0.5	0	0.1 ± 0.1[1]
Ceruloplasmin (mg/dl)							
Prestudy	41	37	28	32	32	34	
End study	43	26	23	30	24	35	
Change	+2	−9	−5	−2	−8	+1	−3.5 ± 1.9[1]

[1]Mean change ± SE of change.
Source: Turnlund J, Costa F, and Margen S. Zinc, copper, and iron balance in elderly men. *Am J Clin Nutr.* 1981;34:2641–2647. © *Am J Clin Nutr,* American Society for Clinical Nutrition.

losses from sweat and the integument were not considered as reliable because for some subjects the bath and laundry water had a higher mineral content *before* washing and laundering occurred (ie, the "blank" samples) than did the water samples collected *afterward*.

The authors concluded that these losses were relatively small in most subjects and did not contribute significantly to trace mineral losses. They also concluded that daily intakes of 15 mg zinc and 3 mg copper were approximately sufficient to maintain balance in the studied sample of elderly men. Iron intake of 10 mg/day resulted in an average negative balance, although 5 of 6 subjects had improved markers of iron status during the study. This finding highlights the complexities of interpreting balance data for in-

dividuals, in contrast with balance data for the entire experimental group.

Nitrogen Balance Studies

Protein status is determined by conducting nitrogen balance studies. Proteins are nitrogenous compounds, and nitrogen serves as a surrogate for protein. Each 100 g of protein contains 16 g of nitrogen. Thus, food protein can be mathematically converted to nitrogen (N = Protein × 0.16); food, urine, or fecal nitrogen can be mathematically converted to protein (Protein = N × 6.25).

Urinary nitrogen (primarily from urea) typically represents about 90% of the dietary protein intake. Nitrogen bal-

TABLE 16-4

Iron Balance and Blood Parameters in Elderly Men

	Subject						
	1	3	5	6	7	8	Mean ± SEM
Balance (mg/day)							
Metabolic period 1	−1.04	+0.20	−0.08	+0.08			
Metabolic period 2	−0.59	−0.13	−0.80	−0.13	−0.01	−0.95	−0.44 ± 0.16
(Serum Fe (µg/ml)							
Prestudy	0.5		0.9	1.3	1.3	0.6	
End study	0.6	1.6	2.0	1.4	1.4	1.7	
Change	+0.1		+1.1	+0.1	+0.1	+1.1	+0.5 ± 0.2[1]
Hb (g/dl)							
Prestudy	12.6	13.9	14.1	13.4	15.1	11.6	
End study	12.5	16.3	16.3	14.1	15.9	12.8	
Change	−0.1	+2.4	+2.2	+1.3	+0.8	+1.2	+1.3 ± 0.4[1]
Hematocrit (%)							
Prestudy	38.8	41.2	41.4	39.9	43.6	34.8	
End study	37.7	47.1	46.9	41.5	47.2	39.8	
Change	−1.1	+5.9	+5.5	+1.6	+3.6	+5.0	+3.4 ± 111[1]
Total iron-binding capacity (µg/dl)							
Prestudy	333		273	240	225	393	
End study	264	285	255	230	225	288	
Change	−69		−18	−10	0	−105	−40 ± 20[1]
Saturation (%)							
Prestudy	15		34	59	57	16	
End study	23	54	78	56	63	60	
Change	+8		+44	−3	+6	+44	+20 ± 10[1]
Serum transferrin (mg/dl)							
Prestudy	265	290	223	240	200	366	
End study	295	320	255	230	255	335	
Change	+30	+30	+32	−10	+55	−31	+18 ± 13[1]
Total serum protein (g/dl)							
Prestudy	7.0	7.1	7.2	7.4	8.1	7.8	
End study	7.3	7.7	7.9	7.6	8.5	7.3	
Change	+0.3	+0.6	+0.7	+0.2	+0.4	−0.5	+0.3 ± 0.2[1]

[1]Change ± SE of change.
Source: Turnlund J, Costa F, and Margen S. Zinc, copper, and iron balance in elderly men. *Am J Clin Nutr.* 1981;34:2641–2647. © *Am J Clin Nutr,* American Society for Clinical Nutrition.

ance can thus be approximated by analyzing 24-hour urine collections for nitrogen and comparing to the nitrogen content of the diets consumed. As with minerals, the remaining nitrogen is excreted in the stool and sweat. In some nitrogen balance studies, the protein and nonprotein nitrogen pool present in the blood should also be considered; phlebotomy procedures will alter the size of this pool. Collected blood can be weighed after it is drawn into a syringe and the nitrogen loss estimated and subtracted from the intake (32).

Fecal nitrogen losses can sometimes be large dependent on the diet being consumed. However, large losses do not necessarily mean negative balance status. Past investigations have reported that rural Guatemalans with low D-xylose absorption values have large fecal losses of nitrogen, fat, and total energy. However, in spite of large fecal nitrogen loss, subjects could be in nitrogen equilibrium. Calloway and Kretsch (25) fed healthy men a fiber-free formula diet providing egg protein (0.57 g/kg) and a rural Guatemalan diet providing 0.875 g protein per kg body weight. The Guatemalan diet consisted of black beans, corn tortillas that were lime-treated, white rice, sweet wheat rolls, white cheese, dried whole egg, butterfat, chicken consommé, frozen sum-

TABLE 16-5

Stable Isotopes Commonly Used in Nutrition Research[1]

Element	Stable Isotope (Mass Number)	Protons (atomic Number)	Neutrons	Natural Abundance (%)
Hydrogen	1	1	0	99.98
	2	1	1	0.02
Carbon	12	6	6	98.89
	13	6	7	1.11
Nitrogen	14	7	7	99.63
	15	7	8	0.37
Oxygen	16	8	8	99.76
	17	8	9	0.04
	18	8	10	0.20
Sulfur	32	16	16	95.00
	33	16	17	0.76
	34	16	18	4.20
Iron	54	26	28	5.82
	56	26	30	91.66
	57	26	31	2.19
	58	26	32	0.33
Zinc	64	30	34	48.86
	66	30	36	27.81
	67	30	37	4.11
	68	30	38	18.57
	70	30	40	0.62
Selenium	74	34	40	0.87
	76	34	42	9.02
	77	34	43	7.58
	78	34	44	23.52
	80	34	46	49.82
	82	34	48	9.19

From Wolfe RR. *Radioactive and Stable Isotope Tracers in Biomedicine.* New York, NY: Wiley-Liss; 1992. Copyright © 1992 John Wiley & Sons. Adapted with permission of Wiley-Liss, Inc, a subsidiary of John Wiley & Sons, Inc.

[1]An example of a commonly used radioactive isotope in nutrition research is ^{3}H (tritium). The three isotopes of this nuclide are unstable and undergo spontaneous changes that result in the generation of radioactive energy.

mer squash, canned pumpkin, frozen banana, lemon juice, sugar, and coffee powder. For comparison, an egg formula diet was fed at the higher protein level with and without oat bran. Complete 24-hour urine and fecal collections were carried out throughout the study. Urine and fecal samples were analyzed for nitrogen and energy contents. Diets were separately analyzed for all nutrients under study. Metabolic balances were computed from analyzed dietary intakes and the average urinary and fecal excretion. Routine hematological parameters were measured. Nitrogen lost was estimated for each blood sample taken.

Study results showed that by the addition of oat bran, fecal excretion of dry matter and energy doubled and digestibility of energy and protein was reduced by up to 4%. Fecal dry matter, nitrogen, and energy excretions in the Guatemalan diet were nearly four times as high as with the for-

mula diet. These investigators found that protein digestibility of the Guatemalan diet was 78% and total digestible energy was 92%. At 0.875 g of protein per kg, the intake level maintained nitrogen balance in spite of large fecal losses of nitrogen and energy.

STABLE ISOTOPE STUDIES

The stable isotopes used in nutrition research are naturally occurring elements that are found in relatively low concentrations in the environment (see Table 16-5). For example, most of the oxygen in the environment (99.76% natural abundance) contains 8 protons and 8 neutrons (oxygen 16, ^{16}O). The commonly used stable isotope, ^{18}O, contains 8 protons and 10 neutrons and has a natural abundance of

0.204%. Because the mass of these two isotopes is different, the enrichment of ^{18}O can be measured with a mass spectrometer. Stable isotope research relies on enriching the background concentration of a naturally occurring atom and measuring changes in enrichment.

Stable isotopes are fundamentally different from radioactive isotopes. The nucleus of a radioactive isotope is unstable and spontaneously emits particles and electromagnetic radiation. Unlike the nucleus of a radioactive isotope, the nucleus of a stable isotope does not change or decay with time. A neutron in the nucleus of radioactive isotopes breaks down by releasing particles and energy, and in this process the radioactive isotope is converted to another element. For example, a uranium-238 nucleus releases a stream of helium-4 nuclei, and the remaining fragment is a thorium-234 nucleus. The energy carried in the released particles can be damaging to body components, such as DNA, and therefore radioactive isotopes are rarely used in human studies.

Modeling Nutrient Metabolism with Stable Isotopes

Use of stable isotopes in research endeavors is costly because the synthesis of compounds labeled at a specific location is a technically complicated process. Compartmental modeling has provided an effective means of analyzing data from stable isotope studies and maximizing the amount of information these expensive experiments can yield.

Once the preliminary equations have been derived, as described earlier in this chapter, the model's initial conditions are determined. The initial conditions are estimates of the state of the system at the beginning of the experiment. Initial conditions include values for pool sizes and estimates of transfer coefficients (rate coefficients between compartments). The initial pool sizes for the stable isotope are usually set to zero because the isotopes used are in low abundance and thus negligible in the subject when the study begins, and the initial pool sizes for the system at steady state are entered based on previously published literature values.

The initial conditions combined with the estimates of transfer coefficients provide the means for calculating flows of material through the system for each time interval. The stable isotope dose or infusion is mathematically entered into the system; then the equations are solved systematically in proper order to yield the mass of isotope moving to and from each compartment in each time interval. The calculations are reiterated in sequence to produce a model time course of the stable isotope mass in the various compartments. The model-predicted masses of the stable isotope are compared to those measured experimentally. Differences between model prediction and experimental measurement are used to modify the model parameters and structure to improve the model prediction. Once the model prediction is close to the experimental measurements, a least-squares fitting routine is performed to minimize the difference between the model prediction and the experimental measurement.

The results of the model include rates of flows among compartments, sizes of storage pools of the analyte in the body, other steady-state pool sizes of the analyte, daily irreversible utilization (from which we can learn nutrient requirement), levels of absorption of a nutrient from the GI tract, and other information about nutrient metabolism. The model therefore provides access to information that was previously inaccessible.

Logistical Aspects of Stable Isotope Studies

Stable isotope experiments and their accompanying compartmental models should be planned simultaneously so that the model requirements can guide the experimental design. An initial plan of the modeling strategy can help determine sampling sites, sampling frequencies, means for optimizing the observed response of the labeled nutrient, and so on. In human studies, sampling sites are chosen to be relatively noninvasive. Collections commonly include urine, feces, and plasma. These need only be collected if the nutrient is expected to appear in each of these types of samples. Fat and muscle biopsies can also be collected, if necessary, but with limited frequency. Viable cells can be collected from the oral (buccal) epithelium or from feces. The specific sites sampled in a given study are based on the expected appearance of the labeled nutrient in those locations.

Sampling frequency must be increased during times when the mass of labeled nutrient is changing rapidly in the sampled pools. For example, several hours after ingestion of a labeled nutrient, there may be a rapid rise of that nutrient in the plasma. Samples must be collected sufficiently often to clearly define the rise and fall of the nutrient level in the plasma. At later time points, when the level of labeled nutrient is changing less rapidly, the sampling frequency can be reduced.

The dose of the isotope to be used in a study depends on the natural abundance of the enriched and reference isotopes. It is also dependent on the content of the element expected in samples to be analyzed, the length of time detectable enrichment is required, and the precision of the analysis technique used to determine the isotope ratios. When extrinsic labeling with stable isotopes is used to measure absorption, it is important that the label be administered in a manner that creates optimal conditions for isotopic exchange.

The stable isotope-labeled nutrient can be delivered to the subject in several ways (11). The isotope-labeled nutrient can be enclosed in a small gelatin capsule for ingestion (21), mixed into a food or drink (34), or injected into a vein (either as a bolus or at a constant rate over several minutes or hours) (35). When the test nutrient is mixed with a food, it is important that no residue remain in the food container; the container must be rinsed with water, which is then consumed by the subject or wiped clean with bread that is subsequently eaten. Some studies serve the stable isotopes in formula or blended foods. Others use solid foods but in homogeneous forms. The isotope solution is usually added during preparation of the test foods or dripped onto the meal components and mixed carefully with them.

Labeling is usually conducted several hours before serving the food in order to allow sufficient time for equilibrium to occur. Another method is to administer the isotopes in a larger volume of solution together with the test meal. This technique, however, might not be the best design when studying gastrointestinal uptake, because solutions are often more efficiently absorbed than are solid foods.

Sometimes the dose is provided through *intrinsically labeled* food, rather than using an oral dose (*extrinsic labeling* method). Plants are labeled intrinsically by incorporating the isotope into the growing plant; animal products are labeled by injection or via the feed provided to the animal. Examples of intrinsically labeled foods include peas labeled with iron-57, spinach with iron-57, goat's milk with zinc-67, and chicken meat and eggs with iron-57 and zinc-67. Some groups have reported differences in absorption between intrinsic and extrinsic tags (36, 37). The reasons for the discrepancy are unknown. Nevertheless, most recent studies in humans have revealed good agreement between intrinsically and extrinsically added tracers of Zn, Ca, Mg, and Cu (38–40). (See Chapter 12, "Producing Research Diets," for additional discussion of isotopically labeled foods.)

The naturally occurring stable isotope of carbon, carbon-13, is naturally concentrated by a certain plants, notably sugarcane and corn (5). Food products derived from these plants also are rich in carbon-13. Researchers using this isotope for metabolic studies may wish to avoid confounding by providing a diet devoid of these foods. (Also see Chapter 14, "Planning and Producing Formula Diets," for a discussion of this issue.)

The investigator has considerable flexibility in selecting which isotope to enrich. The number of choices is limited only by the number of isotopes the element has. Usually the rare isotopes are used for enrichment, but very rare isotopes are not always preferred because of analytical difficulties. For minimal analytical error, the level of isotope signal should be equal to twice (or more) the level of background variance. Van Dokkum et al (11) provide detailed information about the selection and preparation of isotopes such as calcium, iron, and molybdenum.

Safety Issues

Because the composition of the nucleus of a stable isotope does not change or decay, there is no harm from radioactivity. Some commonly used stable isotopes may have biological effects; however, effects are not observed until these isotopes have been administered at high doses. For example, deuterium oxide (water with deuterium replacing hydrogen) is harmless in small amounts but may cause dizziness or changes in growth rate when consumed in large doses (41). When used in humans as *in vivo* tracers, stable isotopes do not present identifiable risks. Further, the isotope itself does not require special means of disposal.

However, when studies use stable isotopes in a research protocol, it may be advantageous to avoid using the term *isotope* for describing the research methods to subjects. Some subjects may interpret this term analogous to radiation, and it may evoke ungrounded fear. The terminology that has been successfully used in describing the use of hydrogen-2 (deuterium) and oxygen-18 to subjects is:

Heavy water weighs slightly more than the water you normally drink, but it contains exactly the same elements and number of atoms as all other water (two atoms of the element hydrogen and one atom of the element oxygen). But in heavy water, some of the hydrogen and oxygen atoms weigh more than in the water that you normally drink. Heavy water occurs naturally, so you consume a small amount of it in all of the water you drink. By giving you a cup of water with a higher level of heavy water than you normally drink, we can use very sensitive instruments to measure the amount eliminated in your urine. (Adapted from an IRB-approved protocol used by the Diet and Human Performance Laboratory, USDA Beltsville Human Nutrition Research Center, Beltsville, Md.)

Typical Applications of Stable-isotope Methodology

Using Doubly Labeled Water to Measure Energy Expenditure

One example of the important application of stable isotopes in nutrition is the measurement of energy expenditure of free-living subjects using the doubly labeled water method (42). The doubly labeled water method was developed to study energy expenditure in laboratory rodents during the 1950s (43, 44). Its application for use in humans gained popularity beginning in the 1970s. With the advent of better and less expensive analyses, this method has become an important tool for energy metabolism research.

The method is based on measuring the turnover of ^2H (deuterium) and ^{18}O. Both isotopes are administered in the form of water. The ^{18}O is eliminated in equal amounts as both water and carbon dioxide (the enzyme carbonic anhydrase keeps the ^{18}O in equilibrium between CO_2 and H_2O). The deuterium is eliminated as water. Thus, the difference in the rates of elimination is the rate of carbon dioxide production. Based on estimates of or measured food or respiratory quotient (CO_2 production ÷ O_2 consumption), the rate of oxygen consumption can be calculated. Energy expenditure is calculated using standard equations based on the rate of carbon dioxide production and oxygen consumption.

Typically, a sample of blood or urine is collected to measure background isotopic enrichment and the dose is administered. Samples of urine (spot samples usually collected once daily) are collected for 14 days (approximately two half-lives for the isotopes) and the isotopic enrichment of deuterium and ^{18}O are determined in these samples. This method requires little intervention, and it is easy for subjects to complete the collections.

Using Stable Isotopes to Enhance Balance Studies

Compartmental modeling with stable isotopes can be a useful adjunct to balance studies. The selenium metabolism studies of Patterson et al provide a good example of how these techniques can be combined (45). In this case, an oral dose of selenium-74 was given to the study participants. Fecal and urine samples were collected and analyzed for selenium-74. Plasma samples were also collected and analyzed for the stable isotope. The data collected from the balance portion of the study were combined with the data from the plasma samples, and a model of selenium metabolism was developed. The model was able to predict the rates of movement of selenium through body pools, levels of storage at steady state, and rates of elimination of selenium from the body.

Stable isotope tracers and compartmental modeling have been used to enhance studies of whole-body copper metabolism in humans. In a series of labeled copper studies including young men, elderly men, young women, and pregnant women conducted at the Western Human Nutrition Research Center, Turnlund et al were able to show that copper absorption is influenced markedly by the amount of dietary copper (15, 31, 46–50). These studies showed that the absolute amount of copper absorbed increases as the amount in the diet increases; when intake is low, however, compensation occurs and absorption is much more efficient, with a higher percentage being absorbed. This result suggests that the amount of dietary copper is the primary factor influencing absorption. In addition, these studies showed that endogenous copper excretion is markedly affected by dietary copper intake and fecal copper losses reflect dietary copper.

Thus, copper turnover is high when intake is high. But in contrast, the studies found that urinary copper changes little or not at all with increased dietary copper. This means that when copper intake is high, more is excreted through feces but not urine. Whereas urinary copper does not change with high intakes of copper, it does drop significantly with a low-copper diet. Finally, through the use of isotopes these studies found that several indexes of copper status also change with changes in copper intake. Plasma copper, ceruloplasmin concentration and activity, and urinary copper declined significantly with a low copper intake of 0.38 mg per day.

Vitamin A and beta-carotene metabolism in humans has also been studied using kinetic models based on the use of stable isotopes (51). Burri and Park hypothesized that preformed vitamin A from meat and milk sources might be metabolized differently than vitamin A derived from beta-carotene. A total of 14 healthy adult women, living in a metabolic unit, participated in these studies. Subjects were given one of two treatments: a bolus dose of deuterated retinyl acetate in a capsule containing corn oil and d-4-retinyl acetate, or a bolus dose of d-8-beta-carotene in a capsule containing corn oil. Timed blood samples were collected up to 57 days depending on the isotope measured. Serum levels of deuterated stable isotopes of retinol (d-4-retinol) and beta-carotene (d-8-beta-carotene) were measured using a high-precision technique of isotope-ratio mass spectrometry. Compartmental models of vitamin A and beta-carotene metabolism in women fed known concentrations of vitamins and carotenoids were developed.

Dietary changes of beta-carotene intake did not influence the turnover rate of retinol in the four-compartment model developed. However, steady-state masses and residence times of retinol changes occurred in several compartments. In the working compartmental model for beta-carotene, the kinetics of d-4-retinol formed from beta-carotene is more complicated than the preformed d-4-retinol. In addition, investigators suggested that d-8-beta-carotene readily converts into d-4-retinol with high interindividual variability.

CONCLUSION

Compartmental models, in conjunction with stable isotope methodology, can be expected to continue to provide an expanding variety of data about nutrient metabolism in humans. Their major advantage as tracers in modeling studies is that they do not decay. Thus, samples can be stored indefinitely, as long as the nutrient of interest does not deteriorate in the biological sample. Stable isotopes of several elements also can be administered simultaneously to develop multicompartmental models of intermediary metabolism and nutrient interactions. Isotopes provide a unique methodologic advantage in that specific foods can be given appropriate intrinsic labels, while entire meals can be tagged with other extrinsic labels, and the two types of labeling doses do not interfere with one another.

Traditional balance study methodologies, in combination with the newer techniques of compartmental kinetic modeling and stable isotope applications, have the potential to advance our understanding of energy balance, vitamin kinetics and metabolism, vitamin and mineral interactions, and interactions between micronutrients and macronutrients. Stable isotopes are completely safe, so they open up the opportunity to conduct experiments in people of diverse ages and physiological conditions. Refinement of these approaches for research on infants, children, adolescents, the elderly, and pregnant or lactating women thus may be a means of obtaining the long-sought data needed to establish nutrient requirements for these population groups.

REFERENCES

1. Green MH, Green JB. The application of compartmental analysis to research in nutrition. *Ann Rev Nutr.* 1990;10:41–61.
2. Collins JC. Resources for getting started in modeling. *J Nutr.* 1992;122:695–700.
3. Green MH. Introduction to modeling. *J Nutr.* 1992;122:690–694.
4. Turnlund JR. Bioavailability of dietary minerals to humans: the stable isotope approach. *Crit Rev Food Sci Nutr.* 1991;30(3):387–396.

5. Hegsted DM. Balance studies. *J Nutr.* 1975;106:307–311.

6. Duncan D. Some aspects of interpretation of mineral balances. *Proc Nutr Soc.* 1967;26:102–106.

7. Isaksson B, Sjogren B. A critical evaluation of mineral and nitrogen balances in man. *Proc Nutr Soc.* 1967;26:106–116.

8. Food and Nutrition Board, National Research Council. *Recommended Dietary Allowances.* 10th ed. Washington, DC: National Academy Press; 1989.

9. Maynard LA, Loosli JK, Hintz HF, Warner RG. *Animal Nutrition.* 7th ed. New York, NY: McGraw Hill Book Company; 1979.

10. Wolfe RR. *Radioactive and Stable Isotope Tracers in Biomedicine.* New York, NY: Wiley-Liss; 1992.

11. van Dokkum W, Fairweather-Tait SJ, Hurrell R, Sandström B. Study techniques. In: Mellon FA, Sandström B, eds. *Stable Isotopes in Human Nutrition.* San Diego, Calif: Academic Press; 1996.

12. Lowe NM, Green A, Rhodes JM, Lombard M, Jalan R, Jackson MJ. Studies of human zinc kinetics using the stable isotope ^{70}Zn. *Clin Sci.* 1993;84:113–117.

13. Martin RF, Janghorbani M, Young VR. Kinetics of a single administration of ^{74}Se-selenite by oral and intravenous routes in adult humans. *J Parenteral Enteral Nutr.* 1988;12:351–355.

14. Abrams SA, Esteban NV, Vieira NE, Sidbury JB, Specker BL, Yergey AL. Developmental changes in calcium kinetics in children assessed using stable isotopes. *J Bone Min Res.* 1992;7:287–293.

15. Scott KC, Turnlund JR. Compartmental model of copper metabolism in adult men. *J Nutr Biochem.* 1994;5:342–350.

16. Green MH, Green JB. Quantitative and conceptual contributions of mathematical modeling to current views on vitamin A metabolism, biochemistry, and nutrition. *Adv Food Nutr Res.* 1996;40(3):3–24.

17. Novotny JA, Dueker SR, Zech LA. Compartmental analysis of dynamics of beta-carotene metabolism in an adult volunteer. *J Lipid Res.* 1995;36(8):1825–1838.

18. Berman M, Beltz WF, Greif PC, Chabay GR, Boston RC. *CONSAM User's Guide.* Washington, DC: US Government Printing Office; 1983. PHS publication 1983–421–132, 3279.

19. Jacquez J. *Compartmental Analysis in Biology and Medicine.* Ann Arbor, Mich: University of Michigan Press; 1988.

20. Collins J. Resources for getting started in modeling. *J Nutr.* 1992;122:695–700.

21. Novotny JA, Zech LA, Furr HC, Dueker SR, Clifford AJ. Mathematical modeling in nutrition: constructing a physiologic compartmental model of the dynamics of beta-carotene metabolism. *Adv Food Nutr Res.* 1996; 40:25–54.

22. Sauberlich HE, Dowdy RP, Skala JH. *Laboratory Tests for the Assessment of Nutritional Status.* Boca Raton, Fla; CRC Press; 1974.

23. National Research Council. *Nutrition Energetics of Domestic Animals and Glossary of Energy Terms.* Washington, DC: National Academy of Sciences; 1981.

24. Blaxter K. *Energy Metabolism in Animals and Man.* Cambridge University Press, Cambridge, UK: Cambridge University Press; 1989.

25. Calloway DH, Kretsch MJ. Protein and energy utilization in men given a rural Guatemalan diet and egg formulas with and without added oat bran. *Am J Clin Nutr.* 1978;31:1118–1126.

26. Wallace W. Nitrogen content of the body and its relation to retention and loss of nitrogen. *Fed Proc.* 1959;18:1125–1130.

27. Schneider BH, Flatt WP. *The Evaluation of Feeds Through Digestibility Experiments.* Athens, Ga: University of Georgia Press; 1975.

28. Isaksson B, Sjogren B. A critical evaluation of the mineral and nitrogen balances in man. *Proc Nutr Soc.* 1967;26:106–116.

29. Isaksson B, Sjogren B. On the concept of "constant diet" in metabolic balance studies. *Nutr Dieta.* 1965;7:175.

30. Pak C, Stewart A, Raskin P, et al. A simple and reliable method for calcium balance using combined period and continuous fecal markers. *Metabolism.* 1980;29:793–796.

31. Turnlund J, Keyes W, Anderson H, et al. Copper absorption and retention in young men at three levels of dietary copper by use of stable isotope ^{65}Cu. *Am J Clin Nutr.* 1989;49:870–878.

32. Calloway D, Odell A, Margen S. Sweat and miscellaneous nitrogen losses in human balance studies. *J Nutr.* 1971;101:775–786.

33. Turnlund J, Costa F, Margen S. Zinc, copper, and iron balance in elderly men. *Am J Clin Nutr.* 1981;34:2641–2647.

34. You CS, Parker RS, Goodman KJ, Swanson JE, Corso RN. Evidence of cis-trans isomerization of 9-cis-beta-carotene during absorption in humans. *Am J Clin Nutr.* 1996;64:177–183.

35. Storch KJ, Wagner DA, Burke JF, Young VR. Quantitative study in vivo of methionine cycle in humans using [methyl-^{2}H$_3$] and [1-^{13}C]-methionine. *Am J Physiol.* 1988;255:E322-E331.

36. Janghorbani M, Istfan NW, Pagounes, JO, Steinke FH, Young VR. Absorption of dietary zinc in man: comparison of intrinsic an extrinsic labels using a triple isotope method. *Am J Clin Nutr.* 1982;36:537–545.

37. Fairweather-Tait SJ, Fox TE, Wharf SG, Eagles J, Crews HM, Massey R. Apparent zinc absorption by rats from foods labeled intrinsically and extrinsically with ^{67}Zn. *Br J Nutr.* 1991;66:65–71.

38. Egan CB, Smith FG, Houk RS, Serfass RE. Zinc absorption in women: comparison of intrinsic and extrinsic stable-isotope labels. *Am J Clin Nutr.* 1991;53:547–553.

39. Liu YA, Neal P, Ernst J, Weaver C, Rickard K, Smith DL, Lemons J. Absorption of calcium and magnesium

from fortified human milk by very low birth weight infants. *Pediatr Res.* 1989;25:496–502.

40. Weaver CM, Heaney RO, Martin BR, Fitzsimmons ML. Extrinsic vs intrinsic labeling of the calcium in whole wheat flour. *Am J Clin Nutr.* 1992;55:451–454.

41. Windholz M, ed. *Merck Index.* 10th ed. Rahway, NJ: Merck and Co; 1983:424–425.

42. Schoeller DA, Ravussin E, Schutz Y, Acheson KJ, Baertschi P, Jequier E. Energy expenditure by doubly labeled water: validation in humans and proposed calculation. *Am J Physiol.* 1986;250:R823-R830.

43. Lifson N, Gordon GB, McClintock R. Measurement of total carbon dioxide production by means of $D_2^{18}O$. *J Appl Physiol.* 1955;7:704–710.

44. Lifson N, McClintock R. Theory and use of the turnover rates of body water for measuring energy and material balance. *J Theor Biol.* 1966;12:46–74.

45. Patterson BH, Levander OA, Helzisouer K, McAdam PA, Lewis SA, Taylor PR, Veillon C, Zech LA. Human selenite metabolism: a kinetic model. *Am J Physiol.* 1989;257:R556-R567.

46. Turnlund JR, Michel MC, Keyes WR, Schutz Y, Margen S. Copper absorption in elderly men determined by using stable ^{65}Cu. *Am J Clin Nutr.* 1982;3:587–591.

47. Turnlund JR, Keyes WR, Peiffer GL, Scott KC. Copper absorption, excretion, and retention by young men consuming low dietary copper determined by using the stable isotope ^{65}Cu. *Am J Clin Nutr.* 1998;67:1219–1225.

48. Turnlund JR, Scott KC, Peiffer GL, Jang AM, Keyes WR, Keen CL, Sakanashi TM. Copper status of young men consuming a low-copper diet. *Am J Clin Nutr.* 1997;65:72–78.

49. Turnlund JR, Keen CL, Smith RG. Copper status and urinary and salivary copper in young men at three levels of dietary copper. *Am J Clin Nutr.* 1990;51:658–664.

50. Turnlund JR. Human whole-body copper metabolism. *Am J Clin Nutr.* 1998;67(suppl):960S–964S.

51. Burri BJ, Park JK. Compartmental models of vitamin A and β-carotene metabolism in women. In: Clifford AJ, Muller HG, eds. *Mathematical Modeling in Experimental Nutrition. Adv Exp Med Biol.* 1994;455:225–238.

CHAPTER 17

ENERGY NEEDS AND WEIGHT MAINTENANCE IN CONTROLLED FEEDING STUDIES

SACHIKO T. ST JEOR, PHD, RD, AND PHYLLIS J. STUMBO, PHD, RD

Abbreviations

AF	Activity factor
BEE	Basal energy expenditure
BMI	Body mass index
BMR	Basal metabolic rate
EE	Energy expenditure
FFM	Fat-free mass
LBM	Lean body mass
PA	Physical activity
REE	Resting energy expenditure
RMR	Resting metabolic rate
TEE	Total energy expenditure
TEF	Thermic effect of food
WHO	World Health Organization

Weight maintenance is of paramount importance in a controlled diet study, unless weight change is part of the experimental design. Because significant changes in body weight may be accompanied by changes in metabolism and/or nutritional status that alter study outcomes, care should be taken to preserve energy equilibrium throughout the study. Stability of body weight and body composition within a finite range requires energy intake and expenditure to be carefully controlled. In addition, participants must be clearly and frequently informed that the study design requires constant weight so they do not perceive the study as an opportunity to lose weight.

Typically diets are developed to be "isocaloric" and caloric levels are adjusted when a weight gain or loss is observed over a 4-day period (1). There is debate, however, regarding what constitutes significant weight change and whether adjustments in the overall caloric level might directly affect important factors such as body composition and/or metabolism of macronutrients, mainly fat (2, 3). This chapter discusses energy prescriptions for controlled diets; evaluation of weight changes; adjusting energy intake; and recommendations for maintenance of energy balance. (Also see Chapter 16, "Compartmental Modeling, Stable Isotopes, and Balance Studies," for a discussion of laboratory-based techniques for assessing energy balance, such as doubly labeled water and calorimetry. Energy requirements for children are discussed in Chapter 9, "Children as Participants in Feeding Studies.")

ENERGY PRESCRIPTIONS

The concept common to metabolic studies that "the diet must be adequate in all nutrients except those under investigation" is especially true for energy. Fortunately, because energy is eventually reflected in body weight changes, adequacy of energy intake is more easily monitored than most nutrients. However, efforts should accurately predict energy needs initially so that adjustments in energy intake will not be necessary once the controlled diet study has begun.

There is no well-established protocol for determining when weight changes become large enough to require adjustment in calories. The literature also is not specific regarding exactly how methods are implemented. For example, a recent article reported only that "the energy intake was adjusted so that each subject maintained his weight constant throughout the study" (4). In a survey of persons attending a series of research methodology workshops sponsored by the American Dietetic Association (ADA) and the National Heart, Lung, and Blood Institute (NHLBI) in 1991 ("Workshop Survey"), respondents suggested a variety of approaches as summarized in this chapter. Most respondents employ predictive equations and/or food diaries along with activity factors to estimate energy needs. (See *J Am Diet Assoc,* 1992;92:156–157 for a brief summary of this workshop.)

Energy Balance Equations

Dietary intake = Total energy expenditure (TEE)

Usual dietary intake is frequently estimated by 24-hour recalls, food records, and/or food frequencies (5). Assessment of usual dietary intake can provide important information regarding food preferences, dietary patterns, and usual levels of nutrients consumed. This information can be used in the formulation of menus to increase adherence to diets that may be monotonous because of restricted food choices and frequent repetition of standard menus. Food records (generally 7 days in length) have been used to establish an individual's usual pattern of energy intake because weekly patterns in energy intake as well as other nutrients have been shown to recur (6, 7). However, food records are generally not suitable for estimating the specific caloric need for individuals because the precision of the estimate is low and because energy requirements may change under study conditions. For example, the participant's usual level of physical activity may decrease during the study. Thus, the level of energy intake for each participant is based on estimates of total energy expenditure as described next.

Total energy expenditure (TEE) measured per 24 hours consists primarily of 65% to 70% resting energy expenditure (REE), which is approximately 10% above the basal metabolic rate (BMR) or basal energy expenditure (BEE); plus 20% to 30% physical activity (PA); plus 10% to 15% thermic effect of food (TEF) (8, 9):

$$TEE = REE \ (BEE + 10\%) + PA + TEF$$

$$REE = 1.1 \times (BEE)$$

Predictive Equations

The basal metabolic rate (BMR) represents energy use during the inactive, stress-free, fasting state. It is measured in a thermally neutral environment, upon awakening and before eating in the morning, in subjects who are at or near energy intake for weight maintenance. Because it is difficult to meet all of these conditions, the resulting measured energy expenditure is usually referred to as the resting metabolic rate (RMR). Metabolic rates can be calculated directly from respiration chamber measurements of either heat exchange or oxygen and carbon dioxide exchange. However, less cumbersome methods are preferable; the most convenient of these use predictive equations that take advantage of readily obtained information such as age, gender, and body size.

The method most widely used to calculate basal energy needs employs the predictive equation for BEE developed by Harris and Benedict in 1919 in a population of 136 males (64 ± 10.3 kg, 27 ± 9 years) and 103 females (56.5 + 11.5 kg, 31 ± 14 years) (10).

Harris-Benedict Equations for Basal Energy Expenditure (BEE):

Females: = 655 + 9.46 weight (kg)
            + 1.86 height (cm) − 4.68 age (yr)

Males: = 66.47 + 13.75 weight (kg)
           + 5 height (cm) − 6.76 age (yr)

Although the Harris-Benedict equation is still used for estimating energy requirements, it reportedly overestimates REE by approximately 5% to 15% in recently studied populations (11–16). Efforts have been made to develop predictive equations that update these original Harris-Benedict equations for current populations of typical body size, composition, and levels of physical activity, while applying improved technology and equipment (indirect calorimetry). Consistently, lean body mass (LBM) has been the best predictor of REE and simplified equations have evolved predicting REE from LBM alone. However, LBM or fat-free mass (FFM) are not routinely or easily measured, which limits their use for estimating REE. Recent observations also indicate that the relative metabolic activity of the various components of FFM (ie, skeletal muscle vs organs) is not constant throughout the life span and that age-adjusted FFM should be incorporated into equations for more accurate prediction of REE (17).

The Mifflin-St Jeor equations were more recently developed on a population of 498 healthy participants, including females (n = 247) and males (n = 251) aged 19 to 78 years (45 ± 14 years), and provide a useful alternative method for calculating REE (16). The sample also included normal weight (n = 264) and obese (n = 234) individuals. Thus weight, age, and sex-specific differences were better addressed (16). Furthermore, the equations have been simplified and the inclusion of weight, height, and age account for approximately 71% of the observed variability in REE. However, the limitations of predictive equations for REE must be considered, and indirect calorimetry is recommended when it is available and affordable.

Mifflin-St Jeor Equations for
Resting Energy Expenditure (REE):

Females: REE = 10 weight (kg) + 6.25 height (cm)
                − 5 age (yr) − 161

Males: REE = 10 weight (kg) + 6.25 height (cm)
               − 5 age (yr) + 5

REE values for a wide range of age, height, and weight groups have been calculated using the Mifflin-St Jeor equations and are shown in Table 17-1. REE estimates obtained from this table, multiplied by a factor for activity levels, can be used to approximate TEE. Thermogenesis is not included as a separate factor in the approximation of TEE because values for REE are approximately 10% higher than values for BMR.

TABLE 17-1

Predicted Resting Energy Expenditure (REE) (kcal/24 hr) by Age and Weight[1]

Weight (lb)	Age		
	18–29 Yr	30–59 Yr	60+ Yr
Women[2,3]			
100–109.9	1,228	1,032	1,016
110–119.9	1,274	1,078	1,062
120–129.9	1,319	1,123	1,107
130–139.9	1,365	1,168	1,153
140–149.9	1,410	1,214	1,198
150–159.9	1,455	1,259	1,243
160–169.9	1,501	1,305	1,289
170–179.9	1,546	1,350	1,334
180–189.9	1,592	1,396	1,380
190–199.9	1,637	1,441	1,425
200–209.9	1,683	1,487	1,471
210–219.9	1,728	1,532	1,516
220–229.9	1,774	1,578	1,562
230–239.9	1,819	1,623	1,607
240–249.9	1,865	1,668	1,653
250–259.9	1,910	1,714	1,698
Men[4,5]			
120–129.9	1,565	1,459	1,352
130–139.9	1,610	1,505	1,398
140–149.9	1,655	1,550	1,443
150–159.9	1,701	1,596	1,498
160–169.9	1,746	1,641	1,534
170–179.9	1,792	1,686	1,580
180–189.9	1,837	1,732	1,625
190–199.9	1,883	1,778	1,671
200–209.9	1,928	1,823	1,716
210–219.9	1,974	1,869	1,762
220–229.9	2,019	1,914	1,807
230–239.9	2,064	1,959	1,852
240–249.9	2,110	2,005	1,898
250–259.9	2,155	2,050	1,943
260–269.9	2,201	2,096	2,034
270–279.9	2,246	2,141	2,080
280–289.9	2,292	2,187	2,125
290–299.9	2,337	2,232	
300–309.9	2,383	2,278	2,171
310–319.9	2,428	2,323	2,216
320–329.9	2,474	2,369	2,262
330–339.9	2,519	2,414	2,307
340–349.9	2,564	2,459	2,352
350–359.9	2,610	2,505	2,398

[1]These values were generated using equations published in: Mifflin MD, St Jeor ST, Hill LA, et al (16).

[2]Women: Predicted REE (kcal/24 hr) = (10 × weight [kg]) + (6.25 × height [cm]) − (5 × age [yr]) − 161.

[3]Mean height values for age ranges listed here are: 65.5″ (18–29 yr); 64.5″ (30–59 yr); and 64″ (60+ yr). Mean height varies slightly in each weight range. Adjustments should be made for those taller or shorter than indicated. Values for mean height derived from data published in: St Jeor ST, ed. *Obesity Assessment: Tools, Methods, Interpretations; A Reference Case; The Reno Diet-Heart Study.* New York, NY: Chapman and Hall; 1997:629.

[4]Men: REE (kcal/24 hr) = (10 × weight [kg]) + (6.25 × height [cm]) − (5 × age [yr]) + 5.

[5]Mean height values for age ranges listed here are: 70.5″ (18–29 yr); 70.5″ (30–59 yr); and 69″ (60+ yr). Mean height varies slightly in each weight range. Adjustments should be made for those taller or shorter than indicated. Values for mean height derived from data published in: St Jeor ST, ed. *Obesity Assessment: Tools, Methods, Interpretations; A Reference Case; The Reno Diet-Heart Study.* New York, NY: Chapman and Hall; 1997:629.

Equations for predicting REE on the basis of body mass index (BMI; weight (kg) $\div$ height^2[m^2]) have also been developed using the same study population (18).

Females: REE = (BMI $\times$ 28.15)
$\quad\quad\quad$ − (Age $\times$ 6.44) + 905

Males: REE = (BMI $\times$ 28.15)
$\quad\quad\quad$ − (Age $\times$ 6.44) + 1,290

The predictive value for these BMI-based equations is favorable ($r^2 = 0.62$); they correctly classify 87% of individuals to within 300 kcal of their measured REE. Interpretation of the regression coefficients indicates an increase of + 28 kcal per unit of BMI, a decrease of − 6.44 kcal per year of age, and an increase of + 385 kcal for males compared with females (18). REE values for a range of BMI and age groups are shown in Table 17-2.

Physical Activity (PA) and Activity Factors (AF)

Most methods for estimating total caloric need involve either increasing REE by a factor reflecting an individual's overall activity level or by assigning energy values for specific activities. For most individuals, REE is about two-thirds of total energy need, with physical activity accounting for about one-third of need. The World Health Organization (WHO) factorial method recommends dividing an individual's day into periods of sleep, light, moderate, or heavy activity and applying separate factors to BMR for number of hours spent at each activity level.

In practice, the method for allotting additional calories for activity depends on the availability of accurate information about time spent in various activities. Our survey mentioned earlier indicated that equations for predicting BEE or REE plus one overall activity factor (AF) to predict TEE or 24-hour energy expenditure were most frequently used.

The AF applied to the BEE or REE ranged from 1.3 to 1.7; some researchers also make additional adjustments in AF to account for age effects. The level of activity is generally assessed using interviews, questionnaires, and/or objective measures such as activity monitors or other tools for assessing leisure time activities. In controlled diet studies, the "usual" activity level is frequently characterized or prescribed and subjects are classified as having light, moderate, or heavy activity. Thus, the lower factor of 1.3 $\times$ REE is frequently used to reflect sedentary or light activity and is recommended for establishing the baseline TEE. Severity and duration of moderate and heavy activity can then be evaluated and expressed as additional energy expended (kcal/kg/hr) and added to the baseline TEE (l9, 20).

The commonly used WHO method for predicting energy expenditure utilizes 1.6 − 1.7 $\times$ REE for moderate activity, 1.5 − 1.6 $\times$ REE for light activity, and 1.3 $\times$ REE

for a minimum level, which is defined as 10 hours a day at rest and 14 hours of light activity (such as sitting, standing, driving, typing, lab work, sewing, and cooking).

Doubly labeled water shows promise for improving predictions of energy requirements. It uses an indirect calorimetric method that measures CO_2 production by determining the difference in elimination rates of H-2 (deuterium) and O 18 from labeled body water (21, 22). (Also see Chapter 16, "Compartmental Modeling, Stable Isotopes, and Balance Studies.") Although the doubly labeled water method has received favorable attention, particularly for the assessment of free-living participants, its practical application is limited by the high cost and complex procedure involved. Reassuringly, the validity of prediction equations was reaffirmed by a recent evaluation of the WHO method in confined and free-living subjects with BMR and TEE by continuous respirometry, 4-day records of intake and activities, body weight, and urine collections (23). Agreement between measured and predicted 24-hour EE was reported within ± 2% for group results and ± 10% for individuals and was improved by an additional ± 5% when the equations used measured rather than predicted BMR. No differences were found in the 24-hour EE quotients between males and females and overall maintenance requirements were below the 1.5 $\times$ BMR generally recommended. Thus, the mean value of 1.27 $\times$ BEE for subjects in whom no physical exercise was prescribed provided an acceptable estimate of TEE in the 13 subjects (7 male and 6 females). On the other hand, the cost of physical activity has been negatively correlated with body weight and with percent body fat (24) and is most strongly associated with lean body mass (25); the increase in EE in the obese can be reflected by an overall increase in BMR (26). The obese may not be less active than normal weight subjects (27) and the same (or a slightly higher) AF $\times$ REE has been recommended.

Thermic Effect of Food (TEF)

The thermic effect of food is approximately 10% of TEE and varies with the type of food component (carbohydrate, protein, or fat) eaten. Attention has focused on the role of macronutrient composition of the diet in energy requirements (28), differential substrate oxidation (3), and the role of fat intake in obesity (29). Of particular importance is the possibility that body weight can be lost by reducing dietary fat without restricting food intake (30), and that dietary fat may play an independent role in obesity beyond dietary energy intake and balance (31, 32). The high caloric density, lower thermogenic effect, and higher metabolic efficiency of fat compared to protein and carbohydrate are thought by some to facilitate energy storage as adipose tissue (29). Others, however, do not believe that the percentage of energy from fat has any significant influence on energy requirements to maintain weight (28, 32). Clearly, more research is needed in this area; but if a defined, eucaloric diet is used, with the macronutrients remaining stable as a

TABLE 17-2

Predicted Resting Energy Expenditure (REE) (kcal/24 hr) by Age and Body Mass Index (BMI)[1]

BMI[2] (kg/m²)	Age					
	18–29 Yr	30–39 Yr	40–49 Yr	50–59 Yr	60–69 Yr	70+ Yr
Women[3]						
18	1,260	1,190	1,125	1,061	996	932
19	1,289	1,218	1,153	1,089	1,024	960
20	1,317	1,246	1,181	1,117	1,053	988
21	1,345	1,274	1,210	1,145	1,081	1,016
22	1,373	1,302	1,238	1,173	1,109	1,045
23	1,401	1,330	1,266	1,201	1,137	1,073
24	1,429	1,358	1,294	1,230	1,165	1,101
25	1,457	1,387	1,322	1,258	1,193	1,129
26	1,486	1,415	1,350	1,286	1,222	1,157
27	1,514	1,443	1,378	1,314	1,250	1,185
28	1,542	1,471	1,407	1,342	1,278	1,213
29	1,570	1,499	1,435	1,370	1,306	1,242
30	1,598	1,527	1,463	1,399	1,334	1,270
31	1,626	1,555	1,491	1,427	1,362	1,298
32	1,654	1,584	1,519	1,455	1,390	1,326
33	1,683	1,612	1,547	1,483	1,419	1,354
34	1,711	1,640	1,576	1,511	1,447	1,382
35	1,739	1,668	1,604	1,539	1,475	1,410
36	1,767	1,696	1,632	1,567	1,503	1,439
Men[4]						
18	1,645	1,575	1,510	1,446	1,381	1,317
19	1,674	1,603	1,538	1,474	1,409	1,345
20	1,702	1,631	1,566	1,502	1,438	1,373
21	1,730	1,659	1,595	1,530	1,466	1,401
22	1,758	1,687	1,623	1,558	1,494	1,430
23	1,786	1,715	1,651	1,586	1,522	1,458
24	1,814	1,743	1,679	1,615	1,550	1,486
25	1,842	1,772	1,707	1,643	1,578	1,514
26	1,871	1,800	1,735	1,671	1,607	1,542
27	1,899	1,828	1,763	1,699	1,635	1,570
28	1,927	1,856	1,792	1,727	1,663	1,598
29	1,955	1,884	1,820	1,755	1,691	1,627
30	1,983	1,912	1,848	1,784	1,719	1,655
31	2,011	1,940	1,876	1,812	1,747	1,683
32	2,039	1,969	1,904	1,840	1,775	1,711
33	2,068	1,997	1,932	1,868	1,804	1,739
34	2,096	2,025	1,961	1,896	1,832	1,767
35	2,124	2,053	1,989	1,924	1,860	1,795
36	2,152	2,081	2,017	1,952	1,888	1,824

[1]These values were generated using equations published in: Harrington ME, St Jeor ST, Silverstein LJ. Predicting Resting Energy Expenditure from Body Mass Index: Practical Applications and Limitations. Proceedings of the Annual Conference of the North American Association for the Study of Obesity, Cancun, Mexico; 1997. *J Obesity Res.* 1997;5:175,A066(suppl).

[2]Body mass index (BMI) = weight (kg) ÷ height² (m²).

[3]Women: Predicted REE (kcal/24 hr) = (BMI $\times$ 28.15) − (Age $\times$ 6.44) + 905.

[4]Men: Predicted REE (kcal/24 hr) = (BMI $\times$ 28.15) − (Age $\times$ 6.44) + 1,290.

percent of calories throughout the study period, no adjustments are currently recommended to compensate for different substrate mixtures.

EVALUATION OF WEIGHT CHANGES

The definition of what constitutes a *significant* weight change and how to determine the *energy equivalent* of a unit of body weight is approximate at best. Researchers vary in how frequently they monitor weights of subjects consuming constant diets with some evaluating weight daily, whereas others check weight biweekly or weekly. In the NHLBI-ADA workshop survey mentioned earlier, either initial body weight or a weight range constituted the baseline weight. Respondents considered weight change to be significant when it was ± 2% or 5 lb overall, when weekly variations were 3 lb, or when there was a change of 2 lb in 3 days. When weight changes exceed the critical level, recommendations were to "raise (or lower) to the next calorie level." Although these values are expressed in a variety of ways, they revolve around 1 kg per week as the "critical" weight change, with an absolute limit of 2.25-kg weight change overall before calorie adjustments are made. The "next calorie level" was ± 250 kcal/day to 300 kcal/day reflecting an approximate energy equivalent or net balance of ± 0.45 kg/wk.

Investigators must carefully assess fluid balance. Weight changes can be easily influenced by hydration (1 L of water weighs 1 kg), so changes in diet formulation, fluid retention, bowel irregularity, minor increases in activity, and hormonal fluctuations with the menstrual cycle can cause fluctuations in body weight. Daily fluctuations in weight should be evaluated before investigators increase or decrease calories. A history of weight ranges (including highest and lowest adult body weights), weight fluctuations, usual and desired weights, and dieting history should be documented and can provide valuable insight into weight management and facilitate timely intervention.

Small weight changes should be viewed with caution because interventions of even 250 kcal can cause abnormal and unwanted changes over the course of the study. It is useful to graph or track weights (daily, weekly, monthly) because small changes can be additive and reach significance if they are not monitored over time (33). It is important to consider that day-to-day fluctuations of 0.5 kg have been commonly observed in normal subjects for a variety of reasons, but a change of 1.0 kg has been quite rare. Body weight is apparently less stable in obese subjects (34).

DIETARY TECHNIQUES FOR MANAGEMENT OF WEIGHT MAINTENANCE

The method most frequently reported in the workshop survey described earlier to correct for weight gain or loss

was to introduce a "unit food" that conforms to the overall macronutrient specifications of the diet and is used to provide additional energy when needed. Unit foods are generally in the form of cookies, muffins, puddings, or other palatable and easily administered supplements to the diet and are provided in "units" of 100 kcal to 300 kcal.

An alternative method is to increase the entire diet to provide an increase in all nutrients. In this case, the gram weights of all foods are increased by the factor required to achieve the desired calorie level.

The unit food system is advantageous because menus prepared ahead require minimal change. However, several sequential increases may produce a diet with excessive quantities of the supplemented food item.

CONCLUSION: RECOMMENDATIONS FOR MAINTENANCE OF ENERGY BALANCE

In summary, recommendations for maintenance of energy balance in metabolic studies are:

- Use a predictive equation for energy balance supplemented with a diet and activity record to assess typical food pattern and activity level. (The Mifflin-St Jeor equation is recommended starting with a baseline activity factor (AF) of 1.3 for light activity. The same AF can be used for men and women, obese and normal weight individuals.)
- Monitor weight changes over time with graphing techniques (see Figures 17-1 and 17-2). Consider usual weight fluctuations and history of highest and lowest adult body weight, weight ranges, and desired body weight. If weight fluctuates more than 1 kg per week, the energy level of the diet should be adjusted. Caloric adjustments should occur in as small as 100-kcal increments.
- Dietary management requires patience, close monitoring, and cooperation with the participant. Dietary increases may be absolute (by unit foods to provide kcal supplements) or proportional (increase of all foods) to meet the goals of the study.

Behavioral, psychological, and environmental as well as physiological and medical factors need to be considered because they influence the delicate energy balance equation and differ from individual to individual.

REFERENCES

1. Reimer A, Tillotson J, Loughney MD, et al. *Clinical Center Diet Manual, 1963.* Washington, DC: Superintendent of Documents, US Government Printing Office, PHS publication 989:17.
2. Jeejeebhoy KN, Detsky AS, Baker JP. Assessment of nutritional status. *JPEN.* 1990;14:193S–196S.

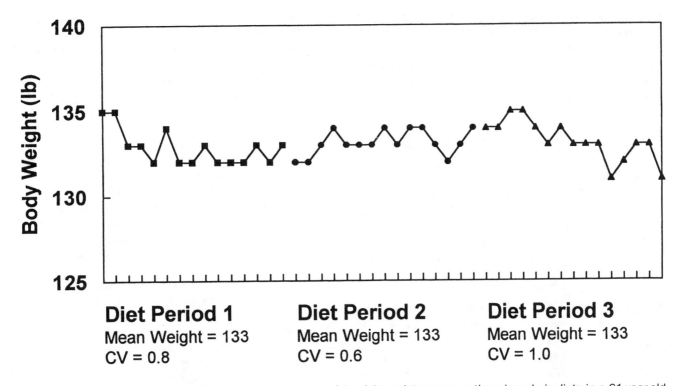

FIGURE 17-1.   This controlled feeding study shows successful weight maintenance on three isocaloric diets in a 61-year-old female. Weight was measured twice weekly. Coefficient of variation (CV) = (SD ÷ Mean) × 100. All diet periods lasted 8 weeks. Break between diet periods 1 and 2 was 6 weeks. Break between diet periods 2 and 3 was 4 weeks.

Source: Courtesy of SS Jonnalagadda and PM Kris-Etherton, Nutrition Department, Pennsylvania State University, University Park, Pa.

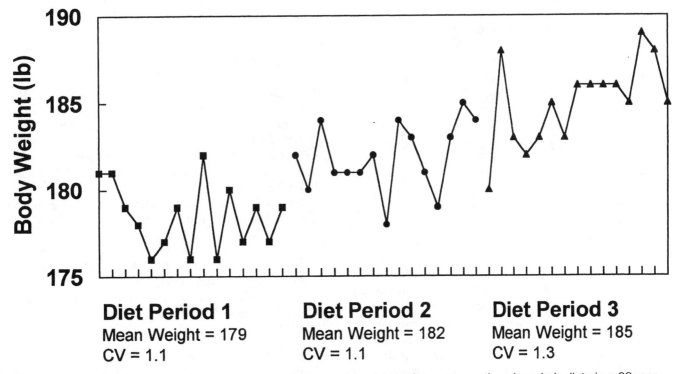

FIGURE 17-2.   This controlled feeding study shows unsuccessful weight maintenance on three isocaloric diets in a 28-year-old male. Weight was measured twice weekly. Coefficient of variation (CV) = (SD ÷ Mean) × 100. All diet periods lasted 8 weeks. Break between diet periods 1 and 2 was 6 weeks. Break between diet periods 2 and 3 was 4 weeks.

Source: Courtesy of SS Jonnalagadda and PM Kris-Etherton, Nutrition Department, Pennsylvania State University, University Park, Pa.

3. Hill JO, Peters JC, Reed GW, et al. Nutrient balance in humans: effects of diet composition. *Am J Clin Nutr.* 1991;54:10–17.

4. Denke M, Grundy S. Effects of fats high in stearic acid on lipid and lipoprotein concentrations in men. *Am J Clin Nutr.* 1991;54:1036–1040.

5. Willett W, ed. *Nutritional Epidemiology.* New York, NY: Oxford University Press; 1990:396.

6. Tarasuk V, Beaton GH. The nature and individuality of within-subject variation in energy intake. *Am J Clin Nutr.* 1991;54:464–470.

7. St Jeor ST, Guthrie HA, Jones MB. Variability in nutrient intake in a 28-day period. *J Am Diet Assoc.* 1983;83:155–162.

8. Ravussin E, Burnand B, Schutz Y, et al. Twenty-four hour energy expenditure and resting metabolic rate in obese, moderately obese, and control subjects. *Am J Clin Nutr.* 1982;35:566–573.

9. Jequier E, Schutz Y. Long-term measurements of energy expenditure in humans using a respiration chamber. *Am J Clin Nutr.* 1983;38:989–998.

10. Harris JA, Benedict FG. *A Biometric Study of Basal Metabolism in Man.* Washington, DC: Carnegie Institution of Washington (Carnegie Institute of Washington publication 279); 1919.

11. Daly JM, Heymsfield SB, Head CA, et al. Human energy requirements: overestimation by widely used prediction equation. *Am J Clin Nutr.* 1985;42:1170–1174.

12. Cunningham JJ. A reanalysis of the factors influencing basal metabolic rate in normal adults. *Am J Clin Nutr.* 1980;33:2372–2374.

13. Cunningham JJ. Body composition and resting metabolic rate: the myth of feminine metabolism. *Am J Clin Nutr.* 1982;36:721–726.

14. Owen OE, Kavle E, Owen RS. A reappraisal of caloric requirements in healthy women. *Am J Clin Nutr.* 1986;44:1–19.

15. Owen OE, Holup JL, D'Alessio DA. A reappraisal of the caloric requirements of men. *Am J Clin Nutr.* 1987;46:875–85.

16. Mifflin MD, St Jeor ST, Hill LA, et al. A new predictive equation for resting energy expenditure in healthy individuals. *Am J Clin Nutr.* 1990;51:241–247.

17. Weinsier RL, Schutz Y, Bracco D. Reexamination of the relationship of resting metabolic rate to fat-free mass and to the metabolically active components of fat-free mass in humans. *Am J Clin Nutr.* 1992;55:790–4.

18. Harrington ME, St Jeor ST, Silverstein LJ. Predicting Resting Energy Expenditure from Body Mass Index: Practical Applications and Limitations. Annual Conference Proceedings, North American Association for the Study of Obesity. Abstract. Cancun, Mexico, 1997. *J Obesity Res.* 1997;5:175, A066, suppl.

19. WHO (World Health Organization). *Energy and Protein Requirements. Geneva: Report of a Joint FAO/WHO/UNU Expert Consultation.* Technical Report Series 724; 1985.

20. Food and Nutrition Board, National Research Council. *Recommended Dietary Allowances.* 10th ed. Washington, DC: National Academy Press; 1989:24–38.

21. Schoeller DA. Measurement of energy expenditure in free-living humans by using doubly labeled water. *J Nutr.* 1988;118:1278–1289.

22. Livingstone MBE, Prentice AM, Coward WA, et al. Simultaneous measurement of free-living energy expenditure by the doubly labeled water method and heart-rate monitoring. *Am J Clin Nutr.* 1990;52:59–65.

23. Warwick PM, Edmundson HM, Thomson ES. Prediction of energy expenditure: simplified FAO/WHO/UNU factorial method vs continuous respirometry and habitual energy intake. *Am J Clin Nutr.* 1988;48:1188–1196.

24. Ferraro R, Boyce VL, Swinburn B, et al. Energy cost of physical activity on a metabolic ward in relationship to obesity. *Am J Clin Nutr.* 1991;53:1368–1371.

25. Astrup A, Thorbek G, Lind J, et al. Prediction of 24-hr energy expenditure and its components from physical characteristics and body composition in normal-weight humans. *Am J Clin Nutr.* 1990;52:777–783.

26. Welle S, Forbes GB, Statt M, et al. Energy expenditure under free-living conditions in normal-weight and overweight women. *Am J Clin Nutr.* 1992;55:14–21.

27. Tyron, WW. Activity as a function of body weight. *Am J Clin Nutr.* 1987;46:451–455.

28. Leibel RL, Hirsch J, Appel BE, et al. Energy intake required to maintain body weight is not affected by wide variation in diet composition. *Am J Clin Nutr.* 1992;55:350–355.

29. Sheppard L, Kristal AR, Kushi LH. Weight loss in women participating in a randomized trial of low-fat diets. *Am J Clin Nutr.* 1991;54:821–828.

30. Kendall A, Levitsky DA, Strupp BJ, et al. Weight loss on a low-fat diet: consequence of the imprecision of the control of food intake in humans. *Am J Clin Nutr.* 1991;53:1124–1129.

31. Tucker LA, Kano MJ. Dietary fat and body fat: a multivariate study of 205 adult females. *Am J Clin Nutr.* 1992;56:616–622.

32. Romieu I, Willett WC, Stampfer MJ, et al. Energy intake and other determinants of relative weight. *Am J Clin Nutr.* 1988;47:406–412.

33. Obarzanek E, Lesem MD, Goldstein DS, et al. Reduced resting metabolic rate in patients with bulimia nervosa. *Arch Gen Psychiatry.* 1991;48:456–462.

34. Garrow JS. *Energy Balance and Obesity in Man.* London, England: North-Holland Publishing Company; 1974:184.

This work was supported in part by Grant No. HL34589, National Heart, Lung, and Blood Institute, National Institutes of Health.

PART 4

THE RESEARCH KITCHEN

Chapter 18

Documentation, Record Keeping, and Recipes

Beverly A. Clevidence, PhD; Arline D. Salbe, PhD, RD; Karen Todd, MS, RD; Alice K. H. Fong, EdD, RD; Linda J. Brinkley, RD; Janis F. Swain, MS, RD; and Cynthia Seidman, MS, RD

The Need for Documentation

Extensive records accrue during the course of each human feeding study. These records, which specify the many details of the study, should be compiled to form a permanent file that is organized in a unique manner suitable to each research center. Because the permanent study file must contain documentation that could answer post-publication inquiry into study methods and procedures, it is essential to keep all records until the data have been published and sufficient time has passed for colleagues to challenge the results. Investigators and dietitians thus should make every effort to leave records that can be clearly interpreted in their absence. Personnel may be employed at several facilities over the course of their careers, but study records remain at the facility of origin to be used by others. In practical application, permanent files are typically kept as historical documentation long after the study has been published. Data for addressing new research questions can often be taken from archived permanent study files if pertinent detailed records have been maintained.

The forms in this chapter have been used by research dietitians to develop and implement diet studies. They are intended to serve as starting points for the development of specialized forms tailored to the unique needs of each research center. (Also see Chapter 3, "Computer Applications in Controlled Diet Studies," for a discussion of computer-generated forms.)

The Permanent Study File

A permanent study file (or notebook) should be prepared for each study and maintained in the dietary offices. The file should be readily available to the principal investigator and the study coordinator, but access may be limited to most others if it contains confidential information about individual subjects. The following are examples of the types of information included in such files:

- **Study protocol:** The protocol should be provided by the principal investigator. Any modifications or updates should be documented.
- **Diet summary:** The summary describes the general characteristics and purpose of the diet, the methods used to adjust energy intake, supplements used, test meal procedures, and other pertinent information.
- **Nutrient summary:** This section includes a summary of the calculated nutrient content of the diet, preferably with a comparison to the Recommended Dietary Allowances (RDA). The calculated nutrient content is based on the reference calorie level of the diet unless otherwise specified by the principal investigator. Nutrient summaries for the daily intakes and for the entire menu cycle for each

dietary treatment are also included. The name and version of the database used to calculate nutrient content of menus should be identified.

- **Menus:** A detailed master menu is included that shows at least one energy level, and preferably all the levels, used for the entire menu cycle. A record of foods and brand names purchased for the study, quantity specifications of food used (to facilitate future studies), and any changes made in the diets during the study should also be included. A summary evaluation of the diets (along with recommendations for possible changes that would improve management, palatability, etc) is useful in planning future studies.

- **Diet composites for chemical analysis:** This section should describe all diet composites, the corresponding menus, and the dates the composites were prepared, with reference to location of more complete listings. The procedure for making the composites and information on analyzed and calculated nutrient content should be included. If validation phase composites were assayed, the study file should include the analytical results, the menu, and details of modifications made for the actual study meals.

- **Interview forms and procedures:** The dietary interview forms for each participant and all dietary instructions provided to the participants should be placed in the file.

- **Body weight records:** The method used to determine participant energy needs should be described. Weight and energy intake graphs or computer printouts for individual participants should be included. (See also Chapter 17, "Energy Needs and Weight Maintenance in Controlled Feeding Studies.") The protocol for weighing the participants, including the type and brand of scale used, state of dress, etc, should be described. If dietary energy changes were made to maintain constant body weight, the criteria for doing so should be listed.

- **Prestudy food record and study intake records:** The location of food intake records and participant daily intake summaries should be referenced. The specific version of the nutrient database should be documented.

- **Emergency meals:** Copies of menus for "emergency meals" used for weather or other emergencies as well as food records associated with participants' emergency travel (eg, a death in the family) should be described.

- **Recipes:** All recipes used in the study should be included.

- **Suppliers:** The names and addresses of suppliers of any special food products (eg, casein, gluten flour) should be listed.

FORMS FOR PLANNING, PRODUCING, AND DELIVERING RESEARCH DIETS

Properly designed forms can be enormously helpful in managing the logistical sequence of research diet studies. A form for planning diet studies is shown in Exhibit 18-1; with it, the investigator and dietitian can document agreed-upon features of the study protocol.

Forms are used to plan workloads and ensure accurate completion of kitchen tasks:

- Exhibits 18-2 and 18-3 are examples of work schedules for four foodservice workers: two who work an early shift, two who work a late shift.

- Exhibit 18-4 is a checklist to be initialed by the foodservice workers who complete daily housekeeping tasks.

- Exhibit 18-5 is an example of a production sheet that is provided at each workstation. For each participant, food items are weighed or portioned as indicated. In many studies foods are weighed in proportion to participants' calorie levels. The "kitchen menu" shown in Chapter 13, "Delivering Research Diets," is another example of a production sheet that displays gram amounts of foods by calorie level.

- Exhibit 18-6 is a form used in conjunction with a quality control program to avoid errors created by use of a wrong recipe ingredient or improper label. Prior to weighing ingredients for a recipe, the foodservice worker has a coworker check and initial that the proper ingredients are used. Labeling steps are similarly double-checked. This allows mistakes to be traced so that errors are corrected and employees can be retrained if necessary.

Many types of quality control forms are also needed to ensure correct delivery of meals to participants:

- Exhibit 18-7 is an example of a menu given to study participants. At some facilities such menus are pinned to a common bulletin board to announce the day's meals. At the facility supplying this form, it is also used as a tray check. In a metabolic ward setting, the study participant, together with the foodservice worker who delivers the meal tray, checks each item on the tray against the listed food items to ensure complete delivery of foods.

- Exhibit 18-8 is a form used in the quality assurance/quality control process to avoid errors of omission or duplication of food items served to study participants. The form serves as a check that the tray or take-out container is complete. In the facility supplying this form, several foodservice workers assemble the trays, checking off the items as they are added to the tray.

- Exhibit 18-9 is an example of a form that is given to participants with their take-out meals. The form serves several purposes: (1) It is a checklist for take-out meals. Dietary employees check the appropriate slot on the form as the corresponding food item is put into the take-out container. (2) This form identifies which foods the participants are to eat at each meal. (3) At the bottom of the form, pertinent information for participants is provided. In this case instructions for reheating meals are included. Food safety messages or emergency telephone numbers might also be included.

Finally, a daily record form like the one shown in Exhibit 18-10 is used to document participants' deviations from

EXHIBIT 18-1

Diet Formulation Questionnaire

The purpose of this questionnaire is to ensure that:

- The diet is nutritionally adequate.
- No extraneous constituents interfere with the outcome of the study.
- The diet design fulfills the purpose of the study.

I. OVERVIEW OF PROTOCOL

A. Nutrient(s) under investigation (include target levels or requirements):

_____

_____

_____

B. Subjects:

	Number	Age Range	Weight (% ideal)	Other Characteristics
Males				
Females				

C. Design of the Study:

Number of feeding periods: _____

Length of feeding periods: _____

Length of depletion phase: _____

Length of repletion phase: _____

Prestudy periods? _____ No _____ Yes (specify) _____

Follow-up studies? _____ No _____ Yes (specify) _____

D. Type of Diet (check):

_____ Formula diet

_____ Conventional foods (whole)

_____ Conventional foods (pureed)

_____ Combination of formula and conventional foods

E. Comments:

_____

_____

II. NUTRIENT SPECIFICATIONS

	Amount	or	Other Information

A. Energy

  1. Intake goal

    a. kcal/day

    b. kcal/kg/day

  2. Basis for requirement (check)

    _____ BMR $\times$ 1.5

    _____ BEE $\times$ 1.5

    _____ Additional allowance for vigorous activity

    _____ kcal/kg body weight

    _____ Prestudy food records

B. Protein

  1. Intake goal

    a. g N/kg body weight

    b. % kcal

  2. Source(s) (check)

    a. Formula diet

      _____ Egg albumin

      _____ Na/Ca casein

      _____ Soy protein

      _____ Amino acids

(continued)

EXHIBIT 18-1

Continued

	Amount	or	Other Information

b. Conventional food diet
_____ Animal
_____ Plant
_____ Textured protein
_____ Low-protein products

C. Carbohydrate
1. Intake goal
   a. g/day _____
   b. % kcal _____
2. Distribution
   a. % complex _____
   b. % simple _____
3. Source
   a. Complex _____
   b. Simple _____

D. Fat
1. Intake goal
   a. g/day _____
   b. % kcal _____
2. Fatty acid specifications
   a. P:S ratio _____
   b. ___% polys, ___% monos, ___% sats _____
3. Type of fat to use (check)
   _____ Corn oil
   _____ Coconut oil
   _____ Cottonseed oil
   _____ Olive oil
   _____ Peanut oil
   _____ Safflower oil
   _____ Vegetable shortening
   _____ Other

E. Fiber
1. Intake goal
   a. g/day _____
2. Source
   _____ Alpha cellulose
   _____ Methyl cellulose
   _____ Raffinose
   _____ Bran
   _____ Pectin
   _____ Other

F. Vitamins (daily intake goal)
1. Daily intake goal
   A _____
   B-1 (thiamin) _____
   B-2 (riboflavin) _____
   B-3 (niacin) _____
   B-6 _____
   B-12 _____
   Folate _____
   C _____
   D _____
   E _____
   Other _____
2. Any specific chemical forms required?

(continued)

EXHIBIT 18-1

Continued

	Amount	or	Other Information

G. Minerals and Electrolytes
1. Daily intake goal
   Calcium _____ _____
   Phosphorus _____ _____
   Magnesium _____ _____
   Iron _____ _____
   Zinc _____ _____
   Sodium _____ _____
   Potassium _____ _____
   Chloride _____ _____
   Iodine _____ _____
   Selenium _____ _____
   Other _____ _____
2. Any specific chemical salts required?
   _____
   _____
   _____

H. Supplements
1. Reason for use:
   _____
   _____
2. Needed components and amounts:
   _____
   _____
3. Type(s) and source(s):
   _____
   _____

III. MEAL, MENU, AND PROTOCOL SPECIFICATIONS

A. Meal Schedule
1. No. of meals per day _____ _____
2. No. of hr between each meal _____ _____
3. No. of snacks per day _____ _____
4. Preferred hours for snacks and meals
   _____
   _____
   _____
   _____

B. Water Allowance
1. Minimum intake goal (ml/day) _____ _____
2. Source (check)
   _____ Tap
   _____ Bottled
   _____ Distilled
3. Measurements of intake (check)
   _____ No (ad lib)
   _____ Yes (specify): _____

C. Beverage Allowance
1. Total caffeinated beverages
   (c/day) _____
2. Coffee
   a. Amount (c/day) _____
   b. Type (check)
      _____ Decaffeinated
      _____ Brewed
      _____ Filtered
      _____ Instant
3. Tea
   a. Amount (c/day) _____

(continued)

EXHIBIT 18-1

Continued

	Amount	or	Other Information

b. Type (check)

_____ Decaffeinated

_____ Regular

_____ Instant

_____ Bottled

4. Soft drinks   _____

a. Amount (12-oz
   cans/day)   _____

b. Type (check)

_____ Regular

_____ Sugar-free

c. Flavor (check)

_____ Cola

_____ Seltzer

_____ Orange

_____ Lemon

_____ Root beer

_____ Other

D. Other Allowances and Restrictions

1. Indicate whether allowed (check)

_____ Non-nutritive sweeteners

_____ Chewing gum, regular

_____ Chewing gum, sugar-free

_____ Flavorings

_____ Candy

_____ Fruit juice

_____ Canned fruit

_____ Bread

_____ Other

2. Any specific items that would interfere with the study?

E. Biomarkers

1. Type (check)

_____ PABA

_____ PEG

_____ Fecal markers

2. Other comments

F. Load Tests

1. Purpose

2. Type

3. Frequency

4. Dose

5. Intake adjustments needed

G. Comments

EXHIBIT 18-2

Duty Schedule for Two Employees Assigned to First Shift

HOURS: 6 AM to 2:40 PM

6:00	Check temperatures of refrigerators and freezers.
6:05	Unlock all cabinets, refrigerators, and freezers.
7:00	Prepare outpatients' breakfast. Start weighing for lunch. Clean dining room tables.
7:30	Serve breakfast to outpatients.
7:45	BREAKFAST BREAK for first employee (Person A).
8:00	Collect breakfast trays from dining room. Weigh leftover foods and record in book. Clean dining room tables. General duties.[1]
8:30	Start breakfast preparation for inpatients.
9:00	Deliver trays to patients' rooms. BREAKFAST BREAK for second employee (Person B). Take dirty dishes to main kitchen.
9:30	Collect breakfast trays. Continue lunch preparation. Pack dinner take-outs and snacks for outpatients. General duties.
11:00	COFFEE BREAK.
11:15	General duties.
11:45	Set up trays for outpatients. Clean dining room tables.
12:00	Serve lunch.
12:15	Set up trays for inpatients.
12:30	Serve lunch. Collect trays from dining room. Clean dining room tables.
12:35	LUNCH BREAK. Take dirty dishes to main kitchen.
1:05	Collect trays from patients' rooms. Weigh ingredients for custard. Prepare dressing for next day. Transfer frozen entrees to refrigerator for next day. General duties.
2:40	END OF SHIFT.

[1]General duties: Wash, dry, and put away dishes. Refill distilled water. Record items that need to be ordered. Weigh coffee, margarine, sugar, etc. Trim and wrap meats. Do advance preparation as needed. Help others as needed. Record freezer, refrigerator temperatures. Perform other assigned duties.

study protocol. The form is filled in each morning by study participants. Use of medications and other deviations are noted in a computer log of "daily comments" that is maintained by the study coordinator. A scientist who obtains unusual laboratory results on a given date may, for example, ask the study coordinator whether medications were taken that week; this question can be readily answered by checking the notes on the daily record form.

RECIPES FOR RESEARCH DIETS

The general format for research diet recipes should be standardized for each research kitchen. Recipe elements should include:

- Menu name for the finished product.
- Database food code number for each ingredient.

EXHIBIT 18-3

Duty Schedule for Two Employees Assigned to Second Shift

HOURS: 10:20 AM to 7:00 PM.

10:20	Weigh liquids for lunch and dinner. Help Person A if preparation for the day is not finished. General duties.[1]
12:00	LUNCH BREAK.
12:30	Help Person A collect trays from patients' rooms. Weigh for next day.
1:00	Pick up supplies from downstairs. Put away supplies. Continue weighing for next day. Help Person A prepare dressing. General duties.
2:00	COFFEE BREAK.
2:15	Bake custard in main kitchen. Arrange the trays in refrigerator for next day's meals. General duties.
4:00	DINNER BREAK for third employee (Person C).
4:30	Set up trays for inpatients.
5:00	Serve inpatients' dinner.
5:30	Set up trays for outpatients. Clean dining room tables.
6:00	Serve outpatients' dinner. DINNER BREAK for fourth employee (Person D).
6:30	Collect trays from dining room. Clean dining room tables. General duties.
7:00	END OF SHIFT.

[1]General duties: Wash, dry, and put away dishes. Refill distilled water. Record items that need to be ordered. Weigh coffee, margarine, sugar, etc. Trim and wrap meats. Do advance preparation as needed. Help others as needed. Record freezer, refrigerator temperatures. Perform other assigned duties.

- Full description of each ingredient.
- Weight (in metric units) or volume of each ingredient.
- Specific directions for preparations, cooking, packaging, and storage.
- Oven or stove temperatures.
- Specific utensils and equipment needed.
- Yield.
- Nutrient content by database calculation.
- Nutrient content by chemical assay (if available).

For the sample recipes provided in this chapter, nutrient content calculations were performed using USDA databases, print version *Agricultural Handbook 456* or electronic version SR-11 *(Nutrient Database for Standard Reference)*, Agricultural Research Service, US Department of Agriculture, Riverdale, MD 20737, or Nutritionist III (First Databank, The Hearst Corporation, San Bruno, CA 94066).

The recipes appearing in this section were generously shared by research dietitians from across the country. Although the recipes have been checked for accuracy, users are encouraged to test them in their own facilities and to confirm nutrient calculations using their own databases.

Many of the recipes are for baked products because of their common use as vehicles for delivering dietary fats. Most are also appropriate for general research diets. Other recipes are for main dishes, low-sodium recipes, a low-protein recipe for fruit topping, and unit foods. Unit foods are baked goods that have the macronutrient composition of the overall research diet. They are used to increase calorie intake without altering the nutrient composition of the diet.

Quality checks for recipes that are used at the University of Iowa GCRC are listed here. (Information provided courtesy of Phyllis Stumbo, PhD, RD, and Cathy Chenard, MS, RD, University of Iowa Medical School, Iowa City, IA.) These "checks" are included in recipe directions to help spot any recipe preparation errors that may occur. The recipes in this section that include checks are Greg's Herb Butter, Greg's Low-sodium Vinegar and Oil Salad Dressing, and Shuli's Low-protein Fruit Topping.

EXHIBIT 18-4

Checklist for End of Shift

Persons B and C:	Init.	Init.	Init.	Init.	Init.	Init.	Init.
Stock paper cups, disposable containers, etc, in cabinet							
Replace all kitchen towels							
Rinse out dishwasher basket							
Replenish condiments in dining room							
Clean and sanitize: (1) can opener							
(2) range and oven							
(3) scales							
(4) dining room tables, chairs, carts							
(5) sinks							
(6) microwave							
(7) cabinets: outside/inside							
Person A:	Init.	Init.	Init.	Init.	Init.	Init.	Init.
Throw out leftover foods: baked potato, roast beef, etc							
Throw out old produce							
Clean toasters							
Throw out outdated dairy products, egg, milk, whip cream, yogurt							
Clean and sanitize: (1) warmer							
(2) counters							
(3) range and oven							
(4) dining room tables, chairs, microwave							
(5) chopping boards							
Produce sink: clean/sanitize; let water and garbage disposal run for 5 minutes							
Replenish condiments in dining room							

- After ingredients are combined but before cooking or baking, the actual weight of ingredients in the bowl or pan is compared with the "theoretical" weight (sum of ingredient weights). If they are very different, the recipe is discarded and prepared again. (See Shuli's Low-protein Fruit Topping.)
- After the recipe is prepared and all servings are weighed, the weight of leftover food is compared to the "theoretical" waste. (Theoretical waste = Recipe total weight − [Serving weight × Number of servings].) The actual waste is usually less than the theoretical waste because of spills and food adhering to utensils and containers. However, a large discrepancy may indicate that servings were weighed incorrectly or an incorrect number of servings was weighed. (See Shuli's Low-Protein Fruit Topping and Greg's Herb Butter.)
- When servings are prepared individually rather than in bulk, the finished product is reweighed and compared to

EXHIBIT 18-5

Production Sheet

Name: _____ Protocol: _____

Breakfast

Cranberry juice	240 g
$MgSO_4 \cdot 7H_2O$	1 g
Corn flakes	20 g
Scrambled eggs:	
Eggbeaters	19 g
Egg whites	122 g
Salt-free margarine	7 g
Salt-free bread, toast	52 g
Salt-free margarine	10 g
Jelly	1 pkg
Brewed coffee	1 cup
Mocha Mix	58 g
Distilled water	530 g
Sugar	1 pkg
Pepper	1 pkg

Lunch

Sandwich:	
Salt-free bread	48 g
Salt-free margarine	7 g
Tuna salad	77 g
Lettuce	1 leaf
Tomato	1 slice
Applesauce	150 g
Pear nectar	130 g
Salt-free vanilla cookies	27 g
Distilled water	530 g

Dinner

Beef casserole	166 g
Salt-free margarine	6 g
Salt-free bread	15 g
Salt-free margarine	5 g
Peas	69 g
Pears	132 g
Brewed coffee	1 cup
Mocha Mix	11 g
Sugar	1 pkg
Distilled water	530 g
Pepper	1 pkg

the theoretical serving weight. (See Greg's Low-sodium Salad Dressing.)

- When a recipe requires cooking or baking (as with spaghetti noodles, spaghetti sauce, and cakes), the product weight is recorded before and after cooking, and then the actual cooked weight/raw weight ratio is compared with the value assumed in calculating the recipe's nutrient composition. If the two yields differ greatly, the serving weight is adjusted to reflect this. For example, it is difficult to boil spaghetti sauce to an identical weight each time it is prepared. When calculating the nutrient composition of spaghetti sauce, one may have assumed that the total cooked weight would be 1,000 g; but when it is prepared, the actual cooked weight might be 1,125 g. To account for the additional water in this batch of spaghetti sauce, one would adjust the serving weight by a factor of 1.125 (ie, 1,125 ÷ 1,000). Instead of serving 100 g of spaghetti sauce as originally planned, 112.5 g (ie, 100 × 1.125) would be served.

EXHIBIT 18-6

Quality Control Form for Verifying Accuracy of Recipe Ingredients and Food Labels

Recipe	Weighed by: Init/Date	Ingred. Checked by: Init/Date	Frozen Batter Labeled by: Init/Date (2 People)	Cooked by: Init/Date	Cooked Product Labeled by: Init/Date (2 People)
Crisco Cookies	DA 1/1/99	HM-1/1/99	FL-1/1/99 GS-1/1/99	DA-1/2/99	HM-1/2/99 BH-1/2/99

EXHIBIT 18-7

Menu

Name: _____ Protocol: _____

Breakfast

Cranberry juice
Corn flakes
Mocha Mix
Scrambled eggs
Salt-free toast
Margarine
Jelly
Brewed coffee
Sugar
Distilled water
Pepper

Lunch

Tuna sandwich on salt-free bread
Applesauce
Pear nectar
Salt-free vanilla cookies
Potato chips
Distilled water

Dinner

Beef casserole
Salt-free bread with salt-free margarine
Peas
Canned pear
Brewed coffee
Mocha Mix
Sugar
Distilled water

8 PM Snack

Saltine crackers with salt-free margarine
Salt-free vanilla cookies

EXHIBIT 18-8

Tray Check Form or Checklist[1]

SUBJECT: PROTOCOL:

Breakfast	1/1	1/2	1/3	1/4	1/5	1/6	1/7	1/8	1/9	1/10
Cranberry juice										
Corn flakes										
Mocha Mix										
Scrambled eggs										
Salt-free toast										
Salt-free margarine										
Jelly										
Brewed coffee										
Sugar										
Distilled water										
Pepper (1 pkt)										
Lunch										
Tuna sandwich										
Potato chips										
Applesauce										
Pear nectar										
Salt-free vanilla cookies										
Distilled water										
Dinner										
Casserole										
Salt-free bread/margarine										
Peas										
Canned pear										
Brewed coffee										
Sugar										
Mocha Mix										
Distilled water										
8 PM Snack										
Saltines/margarine										
Salt-free vanilla cookies										
Distilled water for next day										

[1]Tray checklists often display the amounts served. This aids in finding discrepancies (eg, 3 cookies vs 2, 150 g rice vs 100 g).

EXHIBIT 18-9

Checklists and Instructions for Take-out Meals

Fat20A	
Lunch:	
Turkey sandwich	
Chicken noodle soup	
Salad	
Dressing	
Apple juice	
Peaches	
Angel Food cake	
Dinner:	
Meatloaf/gravy	
Rice	
Broccoli	
Cranberry Juice	
Apple slices	
Salad	
Dressing	
Milk	
Snacks:	
Lemonade	
Graham crackers	
Applesauce	

Fat20B	
Lunch:	
Roast beef sandwich	
Canned pear	
Kit-Kat	
Hard cooked egg	
Grape juice	
Orange juice	
Milk	
Dinner:	
Chicken a la King	
Rice	
Zucchini	
Salad	
Dressing	
Canned pineapple	
Cranberry juice	
Snacks:	
Pound cake	
Canned peaches	
Milk	

Fat20C	
Lunch:	
Lentil casserole	
Rice	
Salad	
Dressing	
Parmesan cheese	
Graham crackers	
Hard cooked egg	
Corn	
Mandarin orange	
Peach nectar	
Dinner:	
Spaghetti	
Parmesan cheese	
Peas	
French bread	
Butter	
Milk	
Orange juice	
Snacks:	
Whole wheat bread	
Jelly	
Banana	
Apple juice	

USE OF DUOTHERM DISPOSABLES

1. Do not use ovenware on stove top, under broiler, in toaster oven, during oven preheat cycle, or with oven temperatures above 450°F.
2. For safety, always use potholders to remove plate after heating.
3. To heat plate:

Microwave

1. Pop lid to allow steam to escape.
2. Microwave on medium power until hot.

Conventional Oven

1. Remove lid.
2. Cover with foil.
3. Bake at 350°F for 20 minutes or until hot (add time for frozen dinners).

These plates do not need to be returned but can be reused.

EXHIBIT 18-10

Daily Record Form

NAME _____ SUBJECT NUMBER _____ DATE _____

Please provide the following information covering the past 24 hours.

HEALTH

Have you been sick or had medical treatment? Yes _____ No _____

If so, describe: _____

Have you taken any medication? Yes _____ No _____

Record the total amount taken (for the day) of the following:

Aspirin _____ Tylenol _____ Advil _____ Antacids _____

Other over-the-counter medicines: Name _____ Amount _____

Prescription medications: Name _____ Amount _____

DIET

Record anything you ate or drank that was not provided by the study:

_____

_____

Record the amounts of the following that you drank:

Diet Sodas _____ Regular Coffee _____ Decaf Coffee _____

Regular Tea _____ Decaf Tea _____

EXERCISE

Did you engage in any vigorous physical exercise? Yes _____ No _____

What type? _____ For how long? _____

FOR SMOKERS ONLY

Record the amount that you smoked:

Cigarettes _____ Cigars _____ Pipe _____

FOR WOMEN ONLY

Did you take hormones for birth control or hormone replacement therapy?

Yes _____ No _____

If so, what (name)? _____

Dosage _____

Recipe 1: Unit Cookie, Oatmeal

Courtesy of Irving Center for Clinical Research, Columbia University; Wahida Karmally, MS, RD, CDE, and Maliha Siddiqui, MS.

Comment: Recommended for studies of macronutrients. Unit foods are used to increase calorie levels while maintaining nutrient composition of the diet. This recipe produces an energy distribution of protein, 15%; carbohydrate, 55%; and fat, 30%.

Food Code	Ingredients	Weight (g)
561	Sugar, granulated	100.0
122	Olive oil	32.0
1889	Coconut oil (melt before weighing)	14.0
1871	Oatmeal, regular, raw	208.0
531	Nut, walnut, Persian/English, ground	20.0
66	Milk, nonfat, instant, dried	90.0
811	Cinnamon, ground	8.0
681	Baking powder	2.4
97	Egg, white	138.0
2041	Vanilla	12.0
	Total raw weight	624.40

Directions:

1. Preheat oven to 350°F.
2. Cream together sugar and oils.
3. Add dry oatmeal, ground nuts, and nonfat dried milk (do not reconstitute), cinnamon, and baking powder. Mix well.
4. Add egg white and vanilla. Mix well.
5. Weigh cookie dough to a raw weight of 31 g per cookie.
6. Bake on ungreased cookie sheet for 10 minutes. Be careful not to overbake.
7. Cool completely before freezing/storage.

   Yields 18 cookies, 31 g raw weight each.

Nutrient Analysis (by Nutritionist III). Nutrient analysis is based on raw weight.

Nutrients	Units	per 100 g
Food energy	kcal	346
Protein	g	13.3
Fat	g	11.5
Carbohydrate	g	48.4
Saturated fat	g	3.3
Polyunsaturated fat	g	2.6
Monounsaturated fat	g	5.1
Cholesterol	g	2.5
Calcium	mg	222
Phosphorus	mg	324
Potassium	mg	417
Sodium	mg	160

Recipe 2: Unit Muffin, Banana

Courtesy of Irving Center for Clinical Research, Columbia University; Wahida Karmally, MS, RD, CDE, and Maliha Siddiqui, MS.

Comment: Recommended for studies of macronutrients. Unit foods are used to increase calorie levels while maintaining nutrient composition of the diet. This recipe produces an energy distribution of protein, 15%; carbohydrate, 55%; and fat, 30%.

Food Code	Ingredients	Weight (g)
502	Wheat flour, all-purpose, enriched	35.0
561	Sugar, granulated	110.0
1611	Baking soda	2.0
822	Salt	2.0
811	Cinnamon, ground	8.0
814	Nutmeg, ground	2.0
531	Nut, walnut, Persian/English, ground	22.6
235	Banana, raw, pureed	140.0
122	Olive oil	30.0
1889	Coconut oil (melt before weighing)	14.0
2041	Vanilla	12.0
97	Egg, white	440.0
1871	Oatmeal, regular, raw	140.0
	Total raw weight	957.6

Directions:

1. Preheat oven to 375°F.
2. Combine flour, sugar, baking soda, salt, spices, ground nuts, pureed banana, oils, and vanilla.
3. In a separate bowl, beat egg whites with an electric beater until fluffy.
4. Stir oatmeal into flour mixture; fold in egg whites.
5. Weigh muffin mixture (46 g) into paper cups. Tare balance between each weighing.
6. Place muffin cups in tins and bake for 20 to 25 minutes until done.
7. Remove from tins. Cool completely before freezing/storage.

   Yields 20 muffins, 46 g raw weight each.

Nutrient Analysis: (by Nutritionist III). Nutrient analysis is based on raw weight.

Nutrients	Units	per 100 g
Food energy	kcal	208
Protein	g	8.1
Fat	g	7.1
Carbohydrate	g	29.2
Saturated fat	g	2.1
Polyunsaturated fat	g	1.6
Monounsaturated fat	g	3.1
Cholesterol	mg	0
Calcium	mg	25.1
Phosphorus	mg	90
Potassium	mg	196
Sodium	mg	215

Recipe 3: Unit Muffin, Applesauce

Courtesy of Irving Center for Clinical Research, Columbia University; Wahida Karmally, MS, RD, CDE, and Maliha Siddiqui, MS.

Comment: Recommended for studies of macronutrients. Unit foods are used to increase calorie levels while maintaining nutrient composition of the diet. This recipe produces an energy distribution of protein, 15%; carbohydrate, 55%; and fat, 30%.

Food Code	Ingredients	Weight (g)
502	Wheat flour, all-purpose, enriched	34.0
1611	Baking soda	2.0
822	Salt	2.0
811	Cinnamon, ground	8.0
814	Nutmeg, ground	2.0
561	Sugar, granular	110.0
1871	Oatmeal, regular, raw	140.0
531	Nut, walnut, Persian/English, ground	22.4
97	Egg, white	440.0
122	Olive oil	30.0
1889	Coconut oil (melt before weighing)	14.0
227	Applesauce, unsweetened	300.0
2041	Vanilla	12.0
	Total raw weight	1,116.4

Directions:

1. Preheat oven to 375°F.
2. Combine flour, baking soda, salt, spices, sugar, oatmeal, and ground nuts.
3. Beat whites and add to fats, applesauce, and vanilla. Stir until mixture is barely moist.
4. Add raw weight portion of batter (55 g) one at a time to paper cups, taring balance between additions.
5. Place cups in muffin tin and bake for 20 to 25 minutes or until done.
6. Cool thoroughly before wrapping for freezer/storage. Yields 19 or 20 muffins, 55 g raw weight each.

Nutrient Analysis: (by Nutritionist III). Nutrient analysis is based on raw weight.

Nutrients	Units	per 100 g
Food energy	kcal	178
Protein	g	6.9
Fat	g	6.1
Carbohydrate	g	25.0
Saturated fat	g	1.8
Polyunsaturated fat	g	1.4
Monounsaturated fat	g	2.6
Cholesterol	mg	0
Calcium	mg	21
Phosphorus	mg	76
Potassium	mg	138
Sodium	mg	184

Recipe 4: Shuli's Low-protein Fruit Topping

Courtesy of University of Iowa GCRC; Cathy Chenard, MS, RD, LD; and Phyllis Stumbo, PhD, RD, LD.

Comment: Recipe adapted from "Easy Crumb Topping" in Schuett VE, *Low Protein Cookery for Phenylketonuria*, 3rd ed (Madison, Wis: The University of Wisconsin Press; 1997). © 1997. Adapted by permission of the University of Wisconsin Press. This recipe is recommended for low-protein diets.

Food Code	Ingredients	Weight (g)
___[1]	Rusk, low protein, crushed fine	50
19334	Sugar, brown	30
02010	Cinnamon, ground	0.5
02021	Ginger, ground	0.5
02025	Nutmeg, ground	0.5
01001	Butter	40
	Total raw weight of ingredients	121.5
	Total weight, prepared recipe	119.0

[1]Manufacturer's data, Aproten Low Protein Rusks: Dietary Specialties, Inc (Rochester, NY).

Directions:

1. Weigh rusk crumbs, brown sugar, and spices into bowl. Stir.
2. Record weight of a ___ qt microwave-safe bowl: ___ g.
3. Weigh butter into bowl. Cover with plastic wrap. Microwave on high power until butter softens.
4. Add rusk crumbs/sugar/spice mixture to softened butter. Stir until well mixed.
5. Weigh bowl and topping. Calculate actual recipe weight as percent of theoretical recipe weight (should be about 100%):

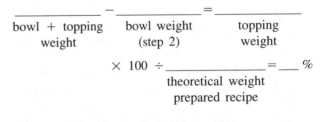

6. Weigh into plastic bags or small container: ___ g × ___ servings. Label and date.
7. Record waste: ___ g (theoretical waste about ___ g). Discard.

    Yields approximately 3 servings, 36 g each.

Note: Recipe may be frozen. Margarine or unsalted butter may be substituted for butter.

Suggested portion size: 24–48 g topping for 80 g canned fruit.

Nutrient Analysis: (by USDA Nutrient Database for Standard Reference except as noted).

Nutrients	Units	per 100 g	per 24-g serving
Food energy	kcal	517	124
Protein	g	0.8	0.2
Fat	g	31.3	7.5
Carbohydrate	g	61.1	14.7
Saturated fat	g	19.4	4.7
Monounsaturated fat	g	9.0	2.2
Polyunsaturated fat	g	1.2	0.3
Cholesterol	mg	83	20
Calcium	mg	45	11
Phosphorus	mg	36	9
Sodium	mg	300	72
Potassium	mg	130	31

Recipe 5: Greg's Herb Butter

Courtesy of University of Iowa GCRC; Cathy Chenard, MS, RD, LD, Phyllis Stumbo, PhD, RD, LD.
Comment: Recommended for general use.

Food Code	Ingredients	Weight (g)
04136	Butter	200
02032	Pepper, white	2
02029	Parsley, dried	0.5
02020	Garlic powder	2
	Total raw weight	204.5

Directions:

1. Weigh butter into mixing bowl; cover with plastic wrap. Leave at room temperature for about 15 minutes to soften.
2. Weigh white pepper, dried parsley, and garlic powder into butter.
3. Stir until thoroughly blended or use hand mixer.
4. Weigh 5 g herb butter into plastic containers, or weigh herb butter onto preweighed slices of bread or rusk. Wrap in plastic wrap. If necessary, cut slice in half and fold buttered sides to the center so butter does not stick to plastic wrap. Prepare ___ servings.
5. Affix label and freeze.
6. Record waste: garlic butter ___ g (theoretical waste about ___ g).
   Yields 40 servings, 5 g each.

Notes: Herb toast is best when warmed in oven or microwave. Recipe can be frozen. Margarine or unsalted butter may be substituted for butter. Suggested portion: 5 g to 10 g.

Nutrient Analysis: (by USDA Nutrient Database for Standard Reference).

Nutrients	Units	per 100 g	per 5-g serving
Food energy	kcal	705	35
Protein	g	1.1	0.1
Fat	g	79.3	4.0
Carbohydrate	g	1.0	0.1
Saturated fat	g	49.4	2.5
Monounsaturated fat	g	22.9	1.1
Polyunsaturated fat	g	2.9	0.1
Cholesterol	mg	214	11
Calcium	mg	28	1
Phosphorus	mg	27	1
Sodium	mg	809	40
Potassium	mg	45	2

Recipe 6: Greg's Low-sodium Vinegar and Oil Salad Dressing

Courtesy of University of Iowa GCRC; Cathy Chenard, MS, RD, LD, Phyllis Stumbo, PhD, RD, LD.
Comment: Recommended for low-sodium diets.

Food Code	Ingredients	Weight (g)
04518	Corn oil	12.0
02407	Distilled vinegar	8.0
19335	Sugar, granulated	1.0
09153	Lemon juice	0.5
	Herb mixture #1 (see below)	0.1
	Herb mixture #2 (see below)	0.4
	Total raw weight	22.0

Herb Mixture #1

02029	Parsley, dried	1.0
02023	Marjoram, dried	1.0

Herb Mixture #2

02020	Garlic powder	2.0
02026	Onion powder	3.0

Directions, Herb Mixture 1 and 2:

1. Weigh ingredients into container; stir to mix well.
2. Cover, label, and date. Store in cupboard until needed.

Directions, Salad Dressing:

1. Tare scale with 1-oz plastic medicine cup.
2. Weigh ingredients into cup. Mix. Affix plastic lid.
3. Prepare ___ servings total at 22 g each.
4. Label and date each container.
5. Refrigerate. Shake before serving.
   Yields 1 serving.

Quality Control Check (before labeling):

1. Tare scale with an empty 1-oz medicine cup and lid.
2. Weigh each salad dressing container and compare the actual weight to the theoretical weight of the serving of salad dressing.
3. If actual and theoretical weights differ by more than 1 g, discard dressing and prepare a new serving.

Nutrient Analysis: (by USDA Nutrient Database for Standard Reference).

Nutrients	Units	per 100 g	per 22-g serving
Food energy	kcal	512	113
Protein	g	0.3	0.1
Fat	g	54.6	12.0
Carbohydrate	g	8.2	1.8
Saturated fat	g	6.9	1.5
Monounsaturated fat	g	13.2	2.9
Polyunsaturated fat	g	32.0	7.0
Cholesterol	mg	0	0
Calcium	mg	12	3
Phosphorus	mg	8	2
Sodium	mg	3	1
Potassium	mg	38	8

Recipe 7: Low-sodium Sugar Cookies

Courtesy of Brigham and Women's Hospital GCRC; Janis Swain, RD.
Comment: Recommended for use in low-sodium diets.

Food Code	Ingredients	Weight (g)
92300[1]	Sugar, granulated	100.0
04131	Margarine, salt-free, unspecified oil	230.0
20081	Wheat flour, white, all-purpose, enriched	270.0
	Total raw weight	600.0

[1]Code is from USDA *Agricultural Handbook 456.*

Directions:

1. Preheat oven to 350°F.
2. Cream margarine and sugar. Add the flour and mix well.
3. Roll dough into bread loaf shape in foil and refrigerate overnight.
4. Weigh dough in 20-g portions. Bake 350°F for approximately 20 minutes.
5. Cool, then wrap individually in foil and freeze.
   Yields approximately 29 cookies, 20 g raw weight each.

Nutrient Analysis: (by USDA Nutrient Database for Standard Reference except as noted).
   Note: nutrient analysis is based on uncooked weight.

Nutrients	Units	per 100 g	per 20-g serving
Food energy	kcal	502	100
Protein	g	4.8	1.0
Fat	g	31.2	6.2
Carbohydrate	g	51.1	10.2
Calcium	mg	13	3
Magnesium	mg	10	2
Potassium	mg	58	12
Sodium	mg	2	0.4

Recipe 8: Sugar Cookies

Courtesy of Stanford University Medical Center GCRC; Patricia Schaaf, MS, RD.
Comment: Recommended for diets to modify carbohydrate, protein, fat, and cholesterol.

Food Code	Ingredients	Weight (g)
20081	Wheat flour, white, all-purpose, enriched	313.0
71300	Baking powder	6.0
89630	Salt	5.0
02010	Cinnamon, ground	2.0
92300	Sugar	258.0
04559	Shortening, soybean (hydrogenated) and palm oils	106.0
01123	Egg, whole, fresh	50.0
01124	Egg, whites, fresh	50.0
02052[1]	Vanilla, imitation without alcohol	4.5
	Total raw weight	794.5

[1]Most of the alcohol in flavoring extracts evaporates during baking and thus does not contribute calories. For this reason, the code for vanilla without alcohol is often used to calculate nutrient content of a recipe even when flavoring extracts with alcohol are used.

Directions:

1. Preheat oven to 375°F.
2. Mix together flour, baking powder, salt, and cinnamon in mixing bowl.
3. In separate mixing bowl, beat together sugar and shortening. Gradually add whole egg, egg whites, and vanilla. Beat until well blended.
4. Stir in dry ingredients.
5. Refrigerate approximately 1 hour or until well chilled.
6. Drop raw, weighed portions of dough onto lightly greased baking sheet. (Weight of dough used depends on the individual's diet.) Flatten dough lightly with a fork dipped into water.

7. Bake cookies 8 minutes or just until slightly brown. After 4 minutes rotate baking sheet so cookies brown evenly.
8. Cool completely on rack before freezing/storage.
   Yields 15 cookies, 50 g raw weight each.

Nutrient Analysis: (by USDA Nutrient Database for Standard Reference except as noted).

Note: Nutrients in recipe based on raw weight.

Nutrients	Units	per 100 g
Food energy	kcal	402
Protein	g	5.5
Fat	g	14.4
Carbohydrate	g	63.1
Saturated fat	g	4.3
Polyunsaturated fat	g	2.1
Monounsaturated fat	g	7.1
Cholesterol	mg	26.8
Calcium	mg	88
Phosphorus	mg	73
Potassium	mg	173
Sodium	mg	348

Recipe 9: Banana Bread

Courtesy of Stanford University Medical Center GCRC; Patricia Schaaf, MS, RD.

Comment: Recommended for diets to modify carbohydrate, protein, fat, and cholesterol.

Food Code	Ingredients	Weight (g)
04065	Margarine, corn oil	90.0
92300[1]	Sugar, granulated	160.0
01123	Eggs, whole, fresh	100.0
09040	Banana	245.0
20081	Wheat flour, white, all-purpose, enriched	250.0
71300[1]	Baking powder	12.5
	Total raw weight	857.5
	Total cooked weight	753.0

[1]Code is from USDA *Agricultural Handbook 456.*

Directions:

1. Preheat oven to 350°F.
2. Cream together margarine, sugar, and eggs. Mash bananas; add to creamed mixture.
3. Sift together flour and baking powder. Add to creamed banana mixture; beat until smooth.
4. Lightly spray an 8½ × 4½ inch Teflon loaf pan with vegetable oil. Pour batter into prepared pan. Bake 40 minutes.
5. Cool slightly before removing from pan.
6. Cool completely on rack before freezing/storage.
   Yields 15 slices, 50 g each.

Nutrient Analysis: (by USDA Nutrient Database for Standard Reference except as noted).

Note: Nutrient analysis is based on cooked weight (753.0 g) rather than uncooked weight (857.5 g). When actual weights differ from theoretical weights, the weight of the portion to be served is adjusted to reflect the actual weight of the product as described at the beginning of this chapter section; or nutrient analysis is modified based on actual weight.

Nutrients	Units	per 100 g
Food energy	kcal	340
Protein	g	5.5
Fat	g	11.4
Carbohydrate	g	54.9
Saturated fat	g	2.2
Polyunsaturated fat	g	3.2
Monounsaturated fat	g	5.2
Cholesterol	mg	56.4
Calcium	mg	122
Phosphorus	mg	95
Potassium	mg	189
Sodium	mg	297

Recipe 10: Pound Cake

Courtesy of Stanford University Medical Center GCRC; Patricia Schaaf, MS, RD.

Comment: Recommended for diets to modify carbohydrate, protein, fat, and cholesterol.

Food Code	Ingredients	Weight (g)
01001	Butter	223.1
92300[1]	Sugar, granulated	425.0
01123	Eggs, whole, fresh	250.0
20081	Wheat flour, white, all-purpose, enriched	270.0
89630[1]	Salt	1.4
71300[1]	Baking powder	1.0
02022	Mace, ground	0.5
02025	Nutmeg, ground	1.1
02052	Vanilla, imitation without alcohol	5.5
——[2]	Brandy	16.5
	Total raw weight	1,194.1
	Total cooked weight	1,086.0

[1]Code is from USDA *Agricultural Handbook 456.*
[2]In-house value used; flavoring extracts may be substituted and code for vanilla used.

Directions:

1. Preheat oven to 325°F.
2. Cream together butter and sugar until light and fluffy. Add eggs in 4-portion increments and beat well after each addition.
3. In separate bowl, blend together flour, salt, baking powder, mace, and nutmeg. Add to batter mixture; mix well.

4. Add vanilla and brandy; blend thoroughly.
5. Lightly spray 9-inch Teflon loaf pan with vegetable spray. Pour batter into loaf pan.
6. Bake 45 minutes; then cover cake lightly with foil and bake 25 minutes more or until a toothpick inserted into the center of the cake comes out clean. Do not overbake.
7. Cool slightly before removing from pan.
8. Cool completely before freezing/storage.
   Yields 14 slices, 75 g cooked weight each.

Nutrient Analysis: (by USDA Nutrient Database for Standard Reference except as noted).
Note: Nutrient analysis is based on cooked weight (1,086 g) rather than uncooked weight (1,194.1 g). When actual weights differ from theoretical weights, the weight of the portion to be served is adjusted to reflect the actual weight of the product as described earlier in this chapter; or nutrient analysis is modified based on actual weight.

Nutrients	Units	per 100 g
Food energy	kcal	429
Protein	g	5.6
Fat	g	19.3
Carbohydrate	g	58.5
Saturated fat	g	11.2
Polyunsaturated fat	g	1.0
Monounsaturated fat	g	5.7
Cholesterol	mg	142.8
Calcium	mg	26
Phosphorus	mg	74
Potassium	mg	62
Sodium	mg	259

Recipe 11: Sponge Cake

Courtesy of Stanford University Medical Center GCRC; Patricia Schaaf, MS, RD.
Comment: Recommended for diets to modify carbohydrate, protein, fat, and cholesterol.

Food Code	Ingredients	Weight (g)
01124	Egg white, fresh	180.0
92300[1]	Sugar, granulated	200.0
09216	Lemon/Orange peel, grated	2.0
01125	Egg yolk, fresh	90.0
14429	Boiling water	60.0
02052	Vanilla, imitation without alcohol	5.0
——[2]	Flour, cake	96.0
71300[1]	Baking powder	5.0
89630[1]	Salt	1.5
	Total raw weight	639.5
	Total cooked weight	525.6

[1]Code is from USDA *Agricultural Handbook 456.*
[2]In-house data.

Directions:

1. Preheat oven to 350°F.
2. Beat egg whites until stiff but not dry. Set aside.
3. Mix sugar and fruit peel together.
4. Beat egg yolks until very light. Add sugar/fruit peel mixture gradually.
5. Beat in boiling water. When mixture cools, add vanilla.
6. Sift together cake flour, baking powder, and salt. Add flour mixture to yolk mixture and stir until blended.
7. Fold in beaten egg whites.
8. Pour batter into clean 10-inch tube pan. Bake in lower third of oven for 45 minutes.
9. When cake is done, remove from oven and immediately reverse pan. Allow cake to cool upside down for 1½ hr or until cake drops from pan.
10. Cool completely on rack before freezing/storage.
    Yields 10 slices, 50 g cooked weight each.

Nutrient Analysis: (by USDA Nutrient Database for Standard Reference except as noted).
Note: Nutrient analysis is based on cooked weight (525.6 g) rather than uncooked weight (639.5 g). When actual weights differ from theoretical weights, the weight of the portion to be served is adjusted to reflect the actual weight of the product as described earlier in this chapter; or nutrient analysis is modified based on actual weight.

Nutrients	Units	per 100 g
Food energy	kcal	295
Protein	g	7.8
Fat	g	5.4
Carbohydrate	g	53.7
Saturated fat	g	1.6
Polyunsaturated fat	g	0.7
Monounsaturated fat	g	2.0
Cholesterol	mg	219.3
Calcium	mg	89
Phosphorus	mg	118
Potassium	mg	88
Sodium	mg	270

Recipe 12: Ginger Thins

Courtesy of Stanford University Medical Center GCRC;
Patricia Schaaf, MS, RD.

Comment: Recommended for diets to modify carbohydrate,
protein, fat, and cholesterol.

Food Code	Ingredients	Weight (g)
04065	Margarine, corn oil	100.0
92290[1]	Sugar, brown	156.0
01125	Egg yolk, fresh	45.0
83390[1]	Molasses, light	60.0
20081	Wheat flour, white, all-purpose, enriched	265.0
18372	Baking soda	2.5
02011	Cloves, ground	1.0
02010	Cinnamon, ground	1.0
02021	Ginger, ground	1.0
	Total raw weight	631.5
	Total cooked weight	584.0

[1]Code is from USDA *Agricultural Handbook 456.*

Directions:

1. Preheat oven to 350°F.
2. Cream together margarine, brown sugar, egg yolk, and molasses.
3. Mix together in separate bowl, flour, baking soda, cloves, cinnamon, and ginger. Add to creamed mixture.
4. Refrigerate dough for approximately ½ hr for easy handling.
5. Shape dough into approximately 1-in balls and place on lightly greased cookie sheet. Press balls down with a fork. Be sure "cookie form" is uniform and attractive.
6. Bake for approximately 8 minutes.
7. Cool on cookie sheet.
   Yields 18 cookies, 30 g cooked weight each.

Nutrient Analysis: (by USDA Nutrient Database for Standard Reference except as noted).

Note: Nutrient analysis is based on cooked (584.0 g) rather than uncooked (631.5 g) weight. When actual weights differ from theoretical weights, the weight of the portion to be served is adjusted to reflect the actual weight of the product as described at the beginning of this chapter section; or nutrient analysis is modified based on actual weight.

Nutrients	Units	per 100 g
Food energy	kcal	443
Protein	g	6.2
Fat	g	16.7
Carbohydrate	g	67.7
Saturated fat	g	3.2
Polyunsaturated fat	g	4.6
Monounsaturated fat	g	7.6
Cholesterol	mg	98.7
Calcium	mg	78
Phosphorus	mg	103
Potassium	mg	269
Sodium	mg	178

Recipe 13: Oatmeal Cookies

Courtesy of Stanford University Medical Center GCRC;
Patricia Schaaf, MS, RD.

Comment: Recommended for diets to modify carbohydrate,
protein, fat, and cholesterol.

Food Code	Ingredients	Weight (g)
92290[1]	Sugar, brown	145.0
92300[1]	Sugar, granular	200.0
04065	Margarine, corn oil	227.0
01125	Egg, yolk, fresh (about 8)	137.0
02052	Vanilla, imitation without alcohol	10.2
20081	Wheat flour, white, all-purpose, enriched	250.0
71300[1]	Baking powder	3.0
08120	Oatmeal, regular, dry	180.0
	Total wet weight	1,152.2
	Total cooked weight	1,064.0

[1]Code is from USDA *Agricultural Handbook 456.*

Directions:

1. Preheat oven to 350°F.
2. Cream together sugars and margarine.
3. Add egg yolks and vanilla.
4. Sift together flour and baking powder; add to the mixture. Mix well.
5. Add dry oatmeal and stir until blended.
6. Bake on ungreased cookie sheet for 10 minutes. Be careful not to overbake.
7. Cool completely on rack before freezing/storage.
   Yields 20 cookies, 50 g cooked weight each.

Nutrient Analysis: (by USDA Nutrient Database for Standard Reference except as noted).

Note: Nutrient analysis is based on cooked weight (1,064 g) rather than uncooked weight (1,152.2 g). When actual weights differ from theoretical weights, the weight of the portion to be served is adjusted to reflect the actual weight of the product as described earlier in this chapter; or nutrient analysis is modified based on actual weight.

Nutrients	Units	per 100 g
Food energy	kcal	473
Protein	g	7.5
Fat	g	22.4
Carbohydrate	g	61.6
Saturated fat	g	4.4
Polyunsaturated fat	g	6.2
Monounsaturated fat	g	10.1
Cholesterol	mg	164.7
Calcium	mg	66
Phosphorus	mg	180
Potassium	mg	153
Sodium	mg	240

Recipe 14: Basic Muffin Loaf

Courtesy of Stanford University Medical Center GCRC; Patricia Schaaf, MS, RD.

Comment: Recommended for diets to modify carbohydrate, protein, fat, and cholesterol.

Food Code	Ingredients	Weight (g)
20081	Wheat flour, white, all-purpose, enriched	438.0
89630[1]	Salt	3.4
92300[1]	Sugar, granulated	48.0
02010	Cinnamon, ground	3.7
71300[1]	Baking powder	11.0
01086	Milk, skim with nonfat solids added, fluid	367.6
92290[1]	Sugar, brown	55.0
04518	Corn oil	54.4
01123	Eggs, whole, raw	100.0
	Total raw weight	1,081.1
	Total cooked weight	944.0

[1]Code is from USDA *Agricultural Handbook 456*.

Directions:

1. Preheat oven to 375°F.
2. Mix flour, salt, granulated sugar, cinnamon, and baking powder.
3. Heat milk (warm). Add brown sugar, oil, and beaten eggs.
4. Add milk mixture to the flour mixture and stir until barely moistened. Do not over mix.
5. Pour batter into a Teflon loaf pan (8½ × 4½).
6. Bake 40 minutes or until done.
   Yields 18 slices, 50 g cooked weight each.

Nutrient Analysis: (by USDA Nutrient Database for Standard Reference except as noted).

Note: Nutrient analysis is based on cooked weight (944.0 g) rather than uncooked weight (1,081.1 g). When actual weights differ from theoretical weights, the weight of the portion to be served is adjusted to reflect the actual weight of the product as described at the beginning of this chapter section; or nutrient analysis is modified based on actual weight.

Nutrients	Units	per 100 g
Food energy	kcal	294
Protein	g	7.5
Fat	g	7.4
Carbohydrate	g	48.8
Saturated fat	g	1.2
Polyunsaturated fat	g	3.7
Monounsaturated fat	g	1.9
Cholesterol	g	45.8
Calcium	mg	146
Phosphorus	mg	129
Potassium	mg	153
Sodium	mg	293

Recipe 15: Lemon Cookies

Courtesy of Stanford University Medical Center GCRC; Patricia Schaaf, MS, RD.

Comment: Recommended for diets to modify carbohydrate, protein, fat, and cholesterol.

Food Code	Ingredients	Weight (g)
01001	Butter	50
04065	Margarine, corn oil	250
04518	Corn oil	150
92300[1]	Sugar	300
01123	Eggs, whole, fresh	75
01124	Egg whites, fresh	25
——[2]	Lemon extract	10
——[2]	Food color, yellow	3–4 drops
20081	Wheat flour, white, all-purpose, enriched	600
	Total raw weight	1,460.0

[1]Code is from USDA *Agricultural Handbook 456*.
[2]Values not available from USDA Nutrient Database for Standard Reference. In most cases the code for vanilla (02052) can be substituted for lemon extract. Because the amount of food color is small and the ingredient is not nutrient rich, this ingredient may be eliminated during the calculation, or a code for water can be substituted.

Directions:

1. Preheat oven to 350°F.
2. Cream together butter, margarine, and corn oil.
3. Add to above creamed mixture: sugar, whole eggs, egg whites, lemon extract, and yellow food color. Cream well.
4. Add flour and mix well.

5. Drop raw weight portion of dough (weight depending on individual's diet) onto an ungreased baking sheet. Press down with a fork; shape attractively.
6. Bake for 10 to 13 minutes.
7. Cool slightly before removing from baking sheet.
8. Cool completely on rack before freezing/storage.
   Yields 45 cookies, 30 g raw weight each.

Nutrient Analysis: (by USDA Nutrient Database for Standard Reference except as noted).
Note: Nutrients in recipe based on raw weight.

Nutrients	Units	per 100 g
Food energy	kcal	478
Protein	g	5.3
Fat	g	27.8
Carbohydrate	g	52.2
Saturated fat	g	5.7
Polyunsaturated fat	g	10.5
Monounsaturated fat	g	10.2
Cholesterol	mg	29.3
Calcium	mg	32
Phosphorus	mg	62
Potassium	mg	131
Sodium	mg	206

Recipe 16: Chocolate Drop Cookies

Courtesy of Stanford University Medical Center GCRC; Patricia Schaaf, MS, RD.
Comment: Recommended for diets to modify carbohydrate, protein, fat, and cholesterol.

Food Code	Ingredients	Weight (g)
01001	Butter	50.0
04065	Margarine, corn oil	115.0
04518	Corn oil	60.0
92300[1]	Sugar	300.0
01123	Eggs, whole, fresh	100.0
02052	Vanilla, imitation without alcohol	10.0
20081	Wheat flour, white, all-purpose, enriched	320.0
19165	Cocoa powder	60.0
18372	Baking soda	5.0
02010	Cinnamon, ground	3.0
89630	Salt	3.0
	Total raw weight	1,026.0

[1]Code is from USDA *Agricultural Handbook 456.*

Directions:

1. Preheat oven to 350°F.
2. Cream together butter, margarine, oil, and sugar. Stir in eggs and vanilla. Beat until light and fluffy.
3. In a separate bowl, mix flour, cocoa, baking soda, cinnamon, and salt. Stir into creamed mixture; blend thoroughly.
4. Drop batter in weighed portions (depending on the individual's diet) onto an ungreased baking sheet.

5. Bake for approximately 10 minutes.
6. Cool slightly before removing from baking sheet.
7. Cool completely on rack before freezing/storage.
   Yields 30 cookies, 30 g raw weight each.

Nutrient Analysis: (by USDA Nutrient Database for Standard Reference except as noted).
Note: Nutrients in recipe based on raw weight.

Nutrients	Units	per 100 g
Food energy	kcal	450
Protein	g	5.4
Fat	g	23.4
Carbohydrate	g	55.0
Saturated fat	g	5.1
Polyunsaturated fat	g	6.5
Monounsaturated fat	g	7.3
Cholesterol	mg	52.1
Calcium	mg	51
Phosphorus	mg	104
Potassium	mg	242
Sodium	mg	282

Recipe 17: East Indian Cauliflower

Courtesy of Stanford University Medical Center GCRC; Patricia Schaaf, MS, RD.
Comment: Recommended for carbohydrate and lipids studies.

Food Code	Ingredients	Weight (g)
04518	Corn oil	15.0
02024	Mustard seeds, black	3.5
02014	Cumin seeds	1.3
———[1]	Asafoetida (Hing)	0.6
02043	Turmeric powder	1.0
11329	Green chili peppers, hot	7.0
89630	Salt	3.0
11135	Cauliflower, fresh	185.0
11529	Tomato, fresh, chopped	135.0
	Total raw weight	351.4[2]

[1]In-house data; not available from USDA *Nutrient Database for Standard Reference.*
[2]Added water (30 g, step 4 of directions) dissipates as steam and is therefore not included in the total raw weight.

Directions:

1. Heat vegetable oil in pan.
2. Add black mustard seeds and cumin seeds and heat until seeds pop.
3. Add asafoetida (Hing), turmeric, freshly chopped green chili peppers, and salt. Stir. Heat well.
4. Stir in fresh pared cauliflower florets and 30 g water.
5. Steam until cauliflower is just tender (do not overcook).
6. Add chopped tomato.
7. Stir gently to combine.
   Yields 4 servings, 85 g each.

Nutrient Analysis: (by USDA Nutrient Database for Standard Reference except as noted).
Note: Nutrients in recipe based on raw weight. Added water (30 g) is assumed to dissipate as steam.

Nutrients	Units	per 100 g
Food energy	kcal	66
Protein	g	1.7
Fat	g	4.9
Carbohydrate	g	5.2
Saturated fat	g	0.6
Polyunsaturated fat	g	2.7
Monounsaturated fat	g	1.3
Cholesterol	mg	0
Calcium	mg	27
Phosphorus	mg	45
Potassium	mg	297
Sodium	mg	366

Recipe 18: Low-salt Salisbury Steak

Courtesy of University of North Carolina GCRC; Marjorie G. Busby, MPH, RD, LDN.
Comment: Recommended for low-salt diets and general research diets.

Food Code	Ingredients	Weight (g)
4938	Ground beef, lean (see below)	75.0
633	Onion, chopped fine	3.4
37	Tomato catsup, low sodium	10.0
818	Pepper, black	0.005
	Total raw weight	88.405

Directions:

1. To match this code, beef is ground to specifications at the feeding facility. (Top round of beef is trimmed to remove most visible fat, then ground.)
2. Mix all ingredients well; make into a patty. Handle as little as possible.
3. Spray skillet with vegetable spray; "fry" until done. Yields 1 serving.

Nutrient Analysis: (by Nutritionist III).
Note: Nutrient analysis is based on uncooked weight.

Nutrients	Units	per 100 g	per 88.4 g serving
Food energy	kcal	123	109
Protein	g	19	17
Fat	g	3.6	3.2
Carbohydrate	g	1.8	1.6
Potassium	mg	372	329
Sodium	mg	112	99

Recipe 19: Low-salt Beef Gravy

Courtesy of University of North Carolina GCRC; Marjorie G. Busby, MPH, RD, LDN.
Comment: Recommended for low-salt and low-fat research diets.

Food Code	Ingredients	Weight (g)
5048	Broth, instant, low-sodium	15.0
1821	Water, boiling	550
503	Wheat flour, all-purpose, enriched	50.0
818	Pepper, black	0.005
	Total raw weight	615.0

Directions:

1. Dissolve beef broth in boiling water.
2. Stir sifted flour into about ⅓ cup of beef broth; blend thoroughly.
3. Add remainder of broth; blend in blender. Add pepper.
4. Place mixture in glass container; microwave 4 to 4½ minutes or until mixture boils, stirring several times.
5. Stir until smooth; weigh 30-g portions into medicine cups; label, date and freeze.
6. To use, place frozen "cube" in microwave for 1½ minutes.
   Yields approximately 20 servings, 30 g each.

Nutrient Analysis: (by Nutritionist III).
Note: Nutrient analysis is based on uncooked weight.

Nutrients	Units	per 100 g	per 30-g serving
Food energy	kcal	37	11
Protein	g	1.0	0.3
Fat	g	0.3	0.1
Carbohydrate	g	7.4	2.2
Sodium	mg	9	3
Potassium	mg	9	3

Recipe 20: Baked Chicken Breast

Courtesy of University of North Carolina GCRC; Marjorie G. Busby, MPH, RD, LDN.
Comment: Recommended for general research diets.

Food Code	Ingredients	Weight (g)
4946	Chicken breast, deboned and skinned	90
822	Salt	0.25
818	Pepper	0.005
817	Parsley	0.05
816	Paprika	0.25
	Total raw weight	90.55

Directions:

1. Thaw chicken; flatten.
2. Place chicken on plastic wrap.
3. Sprinkle seasonings over chicken; wrap chicken loosely.
4. Place chicken in microwavable dish; cut 2 small slits in plastic wrap.
5. Microwave for 3 minutes, turn and microwave for 2 minutes more; serve.
   Yields 1 serving.

Nutrient Analysis: (by Nutritionist III).

Note: Nutrient analysis is based on uncooked weight.

Nutrients	Units	per 100 g	per 90-g serving
Food energy	kcal	194	175
Protein	g	29.4	26.5
Fat	g	8	7
Carbohydrate	g	0.2	0.2
Sodium	mg	177	159
Potassium	mg	252	227

Recipe 21: Lemon Baked Chicken

Courtesy of University of North Carolina GCRC; Marjorie G. Busby, MPH, RD, LDN.

Comment: Recommended for general research diets.

Food Code	Ingredients	Weight (g)
4946	Chicken breast, deboned and skinned	90
263	Lemon juice	15
822	Salt	0.25
818	Pepper	0.005
817	Parsley	0.05
813	Garlic powder	0.25
	Total raw weight	105.55

Directions:

1. Thaw chicken, flatten.
2. Place chicken on plastic wrap.
3. Sprinkle lemon juice and seasonings over chicken; wrap chicken loosely.
4. Place chicken in microwavable dish; cut 2 small slits in plastic wrap.
5. Microwave for 3 minutes, turn and microwave for 2 minutes more; serve.
   Yields 1 serving.

Nutrient Analysis: (by Nutritionist III).

Note: Nutrient analysis is based on uncooked weight.

Nutrients	Units	per 100 g	per 105-g serving
Food energy	kcal	170	178
Protein	g	25.2	26.5
Fat	g	6.6	6.9
Carbohydrate	g	1.1	1.2
Sodium	mg	154	162
Potassium	mg	228	239

Recipe 22: Macaroni and Cheese

Courtesy of University of North Carolina GCRC; Marjorie G. Busby, MPH, RD, LDN.

Comment: Recommended for general research diets.

Food Code	Ingredients	Weight (g)
2872[1]	Macaroni noodles, cooked	42.0
115	Margarine, hard, pat	7.0
503	Wheat flour, all-purpose, enriched	5.0
50	Milk, whole	120.0
3	Cheddar cheese, grated	45.0
350	Bread crumbs, whole wheat	8.0
818	Black pepper	0.005
	Total raw weight	285.0

[1]The food code used for nutrient analysis is for raw macaroni; 42 g of dry macaroni noodles (see directions) is expected to yield a cooked weight of approximately 100 g.

Directions:

1. Bring 2 cups of distilled water to a boil on high heat. Add 42 g of dry macaroni noodles to water. Cook on medium high heat for 15 minutes. Drain noodles in a colander for 10 minutes.
2. Make white sauce: In microwave, melt margarine on power level 30 in Pyrex measuring cup until melted; stir in flour with wire whip; microwave on high power for one minute.
3. Microwave milk on power level 70 until warm; add milk to margarine-flour mixture; microwave on 70 until thick; stir with wire whip every 45 seconds.
4. Add grated cheese and stir until cheese is melted.
5. Spray casseroles with vegetable spray; put drained macaroni in casserole; add sauce; top with bread crumbs. Add pepper.
6. Bake at 375°F until browned, about 10 to 15 minutes; serve or cover with aluminum foil and freeze.
7. To reheat, bake frozen at 375°F for 30 minutes.
   Yields 1 serving.

Nutrient Analysis: (by Nutritionist III).

Note: Nutrient analysis is based on uncooked weight.

Nutrients	Units	per 100 g	per 285-g serving
Food energy	kcal	161	458
Protein	g	7.1	20.1
Fat	g	9.1	25.8
Carbohydrate	g	13.0	37.0
Saturated fat	g	4.7	13.3
Polyunsaturated fat	g	0.8	2.4
Monounsaturated fat	g	2.8	7.9
Cholesterol	mg	22.6	64.4
Calcium	mg	173	493
Phosphorus	mg	144	410
Potassium	mg	108	308
Sodium	mg	158	450

CHAPTER 19

FACILITIES AND EQUIPMENT FOR THE RESEARCH KITCHEN

CARLA R. HEISER, MS, RD; MARLENE M. WINDHAUSER, PhD, RD, FADA; AND
BEENA LOHARIKAR, MS, RD

THE PLANNING PROCESS

Whether planners are building, remodeling, or contracting kitchen space for research food preparation, thoughtful planning and execution will result in cost savings and improved time management. This chapter highlights considerations for facility design that can be applied to projects as small as redesigning the layout of a cooking area for an existing kitchen or as large as new construction or complete renovation of an existing facility. Most of the information generally applies to small or large research kitchens, but special considerations are noted for those designed for large-volume food preparation.

Planning is integral to the development of a well organized, cost-effective kitchen plan. First, careful consideration of the scope and complexity of facility requirements enables appropriate selection of the planning team (1). Research managers and lead nutrition staff should be included in this panel to help identify common logistical problems and to discuss budgetary issues (2).

A planning team might also include the following individuals:

- Member of board of directors for the research institution (general resource allocation and compatibility with current and future projects).
- Architect (layout and design issues).
- Cook or food technician (site-specific experience).
- Restaurant consultant (time, space, motion, and service issues).
- Subcontractor or general contractor (logistics, planning, and inspection codes).

- Manufacturer representatives or equipment dealers (access to the parent companies' resources, input regarding price and features).
- Engineer (expertise in physical plant systems, ie, heating, air conditioning, and electrical).
- Health department official (addresses health regulations and installation specifications) (1, 2).

If it is not possible to recruit a health inspector for the planning team, an architect, contractor, or consultant could act as a liaison to the local health office. In the university setting the capital resources manager may work with health agency staff who can ensure health codes are met throughout the design phase. When architects, consultants, or contractors are not needed, as is the case for small projects, it remains important to address health regulations and installation specifications. All major or minor structural, electrical, and plumbing alterations must pass building and fire codes.

Planning the research kitchen begins by considering space and function (Exhibits 19-1 and 19-2). The next step is to forecast production and menu requirements. An analysis of space and equipment needs can then be further elaborated. Realistic costs can be forecast based on the identified criteria. Effective remodeling also requires revisions of pre-existing design drawbacks. Former "mistakes" are often transposed or, worse yet, additional ones can be included in the new design. Considering the pros and cons of current kitchen designs results in a more efficient, cost-contained plan.

Future expansion also should be considered during the planning stage, when designing for change is possible. Inexpensive remodeling can then be easily done as needs

EXHIBIT 19-1

Worksheet for Calculating Capacity and Space Requirements[1]

CAPACITY REQUIREMENTS[2]

Number of participants		_____
Meals and snacks/participant/day		× _____
Meals and snacks served/day	Total =	_____

SPACE REQUIREMENTS[3]

Storage area
    Nonperishable food[4] (0.33 sq ft to 0.5 sq ft/meal)   _____
    Perishable food[5]
    Refrigerator (0.5 sq ft to 1.0 sq ft/meal)   + _____
    Freezer (0.75 sq ft to 1.5 sq ft/meal)   + _____

Nonfood: (0.09 sq ft/meal)[6]   + _____

All storage (1.0 sq ft to 3.0 sq ft/meal)   Total =   _____

Preparation area (1.1 sq ft to 1.5 sq ft/meal)[7]   + _____

Serving area[8] (0.57 sq ft/meal)   + _____

Dishwashing and sanitation areas[9] (0.58 sq ft/meal)   + _____

Dining area (12 sq ft to 14 sq ft/participant/seating)   + _____

All areas   Total =   _____

[1] Adapted from Pannell D (6).
[2] Capacity represents seating and serving needs.
[3] Actual storage requirements for large research kitchens (facilities feeding 25 to 100 participants) are underestimated by these figures.
[4] Nonperishable food is stored dry and at room temperature.
[5] Depending on type of meal service, refrigerator/freezer space allotments may be reversed (ie, balance space for food served on day of preparation vs advanced prep area and frozen items). Space estimates are for walk-in units.
[6] Estimates for nonfood storage may be increased for carry-out containers and disposables.
[7] Estimates for preparation area include refrigeration and may be increased for multiple ovens and other large equipment.
[8] The figures for estimating serving and dishwashing areas may be increased to meet the needs of large feeding programs. Less space is required when dishwashing and meal service are done in shifts.
[9] Verify requirements set by state sanitation codes.

change. Flexible planning is exemplified by modular designs that use movable equipment, tabletops, and service components to facilitate rearrangement. Equipment contracts also can include provisions for future upgrades.

SPACE AND EQUIPMENT

Kitchen Layout

A primary focus of kitchen design is work flow, that is, the actual steps between food procurement, preparation, and cleanup. Simply mapping flow of materials and traffic patterns points out inherent flaws with existing kitchen setups. For example, arranging the sink, range, and cold storage in a triangle configuration facilitates work flow among stations; direct paths between these functional kitchen areas avoid wasted steps. This design solution minimizes backtracking and crossover of kitchen staff (3).

In facility designs each area must be considered according to its specific function (4). Layouts can then accommodate preparation, cooking, storage, and cleanup tasks. Stations require a work table, cutting surface, and adequate storage space. In addition, the placement of a sink and garbage disposal amid areas is useful to enhance work flow. Floor space is needed for tray carts, waste containers, and other movable equipment. A work pattern among production areas must be established that accommodates staff movement and effective use of equipment.

EXHIBIT 19-2

Space Requirements and Considerations for a Cafeteria-style Tray Service Area[1]

Lane space	30 in
Tray slide	12 in
Serving counter width	2 ft to 3 ft
Work space	4 ft
Back counterspace	2½ ft
Holding equipment (cold and hot food)	Depends on number of meals served per day
	Depends on equipment specifications
Self-service areas	Depends on number of meals served per day
	Requires tray and utensil areas
	Requires dessert, salad, and condiment areas

Adapted from Pannell D (6).

Generally, 3 ft to 6 ft of aisle space is required between island or work counters and wall cabinets because open cabinet or equipment doors increase width requirements (3, 5). Consultants can verify state code specifications for aisle width. Additional factors that may be considered in aisle layout are to:

- Avoid arranging aisles along bare walls: space is minimized and work areas are only accessible from one side.
- Consider using equipment with sliding doors: work space is maximized because doors do not open into aisles.
- Design aisles at right angles: total aisle space is otherwise decreased.
- Locate aisles away from high-volume work areas: work flow and productivity are maximized and risk of accidents is lowered.

Plans should first focus on the hot-food preparation area; then development of subsequent workstations can proceed (3). Because the cooking station frequently becomes multifunctional, this area requires adequate storage and counterspace for food preparation and equipment. Placing ovens in close groups provides a more efficient arrangement for ventilation, utility hook-up, maintenance, and sanitation. Oven capacity and storage space should be sufficient for a variety of cookware and utensils.

Similarly, work areas can be arranged with productivity in mind. Adequate storage and work space are desirable in all work centers. Certain pieces of equipment are necessary in each work area (Exhibit 19-3), so the specific layout will be affected by equipment installation and utility hook-up. These requirements need to be considered to determine the best physical arrangement (5). For large facilities, a quantity food production area with ovens and other large equipment may be shared while several work areas are used independently.

Four different configurations are commonly used to arrange work areas: the straight and parallel lines or the L and U shapes (see Figure 19-1). There are advantages and disadvantages to each arrangement; however, the straight line

is considered the best with regard to time and space efficiency. Similarly, the L shape uses a limited space while providing a convenient work surface. This arrangement may be used to create a workstation that is separate from the traffic aisle. For example, L shapes are useful in sanitation areas. On the other hand, the U-shape layout offers a large surface area, but it adds more steps walking in and out of the workstation. Lastly, parallel or back-to-back tables are convenient and used frequently in kitchen plans. These arrangements maximize available space and provide ample work surfaces by affording two-sided access.

For larger facilities to accommodate simultaneous feeding studies, two or more L- or U-shaped work areas, or "bays," are desirable. Each bay area may be similar in design or specialized for the food preparation function. Duplicate equipment may be needed for each area.

An island, strategically placed, enhances the efficiency of a work area. Islands that are 4½ ft × 8 ft are functional, whereas narrow islands do not provide sufficient work space for a research kitchen. Islands can be placed among cooking, refrigeration, and sanitation areas to facilitate food preparation and work flow. Islands should be electrically wired to accommodate equipment requirements.

Counterspace is an additional priority in designing floor plans. Research kitchens differ from other kitchens in that they require more counterspace for portioning food items. To prepare meals for 5 to 10 participants, 6 ft to 9 ft of continuous counterspace is recommended in the food preparation center and 3 ft to 6 ft in the cooking area. The amount of counterspace needed increases when staff prepare meals for more participants. Adequate counterspace allows for food processing, preparation, and weighing portions. Additional counterspace may be required if meals are packaged for take-out to accommodate bags, boxes, or coolers.

Because counters may double as hot-food holding and serving areas, countertops next to cooking areas should be heat resistant. In addition, a generous number of electrical outlets should be installed along the wall behind the equipment or backsplash. Horizontal strips can be used to accom-

EXHIBIT 19-3

Equipment Considerations

MAJOR EQUIPMENT

Cooking Area

Comment: Cooking and baking requirements will dictate the type and amount of oven equipment purchased. Residential versions are sufficient for many small facilities.

Suggested Items

Range (2 to 4 burners)
Conventional oven
Convection oven (single-cavity units (18 in $\times$ 20 in $\times$ 23 in) or double-cavity units (36 in $\times$ 40 in $\times$ 46 in))
Deck oven
Hood and air filter
Vegetable steamer
Steam kettle

Cold Preparation Area

Comment: Commercial reach-in refrigerators and freezers are manufactured in one-, two-, or three-compartment sections. Purchase options include full-size or half doors and adjustable shelving or tray slides. Walk-in versions can also be considered for larger studies or facilities. Space requirements and installation costs require further investigation. Another option is to contract walk-in space from a main kitchen.

Additional freezer space may be required for studies that require frozen storage with infrequent food pickup; refrigerated space may be required to hold take-out meals. A $-70°F$ freezer is necessary for storing food composites. Walk-in space from the hospital or main kitchen may be negotiated for short-term programs. Movable stainless steel cages that can be secured are efficient for using space and resources well.

Guidelines for Determining Capacities

Number of Participants	Reach-in Refrigerator	Reach-in Freezer	Walk-in Refrigerator	Walk-in Freezer
< 25	1-46.5 cu ft	1-46.5 cu ft	N/A	N/A
25-50	2-46.5 cu ft	3-46.5 cu ft	88 sq ft	N/A
50-100	4-46.5 cu ft	2-46.5 cu ft	100 sq ft	120 sq ft

Sanitation Area

Suggested Items

Deionizer
Dishwasher
Garbage disposal
Sinks
Ice machine
Water distiller

Minor Equipment

Suggested Items

Blender, industrial
Top-loading balances
Mobile tray, silverware, and dish storage carts
Microwave ovens
Appliances—coffee maker, mixer, food processor, and toaster
Stoneware and sturdy service ware
Slicers
Carts and tray racks

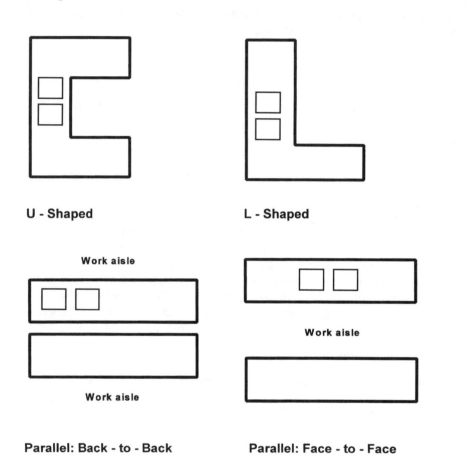

Straight - Line

U - Shaped

L - Shaped

Work aisle

Work aisle

Work aisle

Work aisle

Parallel: Back - to - Back

Parallel: Face - to - Face

□□ **indicates location of sinks**

FIGURE 19-1.   Common arrangements for work centers.

modate multiple appliance hook-ups. This type of outlet placement eliminates the need for extension cords or connections in the floor, decreases the potential for clutter and accidents, and facilitates sanitation (1). An electrician should review floor plans to make sure sufficient power is provided, particularly for high-voltage equipment, but even small appliances require substantial energy.

Counters should be 3 ft high, a comfortable work level for most adults. Cooking areas may include a lower counterspace for baking purposes or for housing large appliances. This lower section in a baking area facilitates kneading and rolling dough and helps prevent lower back injuries. It can be placed between the preparation area and the cooktop or in the middle of the preparation area (3). Marble surfaces are commonly recommended for baking purposes to facilitate product preparation, cleanup, and sanitation.

Ventilation and Climate Control

Ventilation and climate control must be adequate to minimize heat generated from major appliances. Air and water cooling systems are common requirements. Economic and environmental issues underscore the need to implement a heat recovery system that recycles heat lost by refrigeration, air conditioning, and ice making, and from heat pump systems. Recovered energy is used for partial heating of dishwashing water. This system should reduce the substantial costs of heating water (1). In addition, the kitchen staff can work more efficiently when the ambient temperature is comfortable.

Work Surfaces

Easy-to-clean wall and floor surfaces are recommended. Ceramic or glazed tiles are appropriate wall surfaces; quarry or unglazed ceramic tiles are appropriate for floors because they are grease resistant, durable, low maintenance, and less slippery than other floor coverings when wet (4). Quarry and unglazed ceramic tiles are most useful in high-volume research kitchens or in areas with heavy traffic (3). In the small-scale research kitchen, it may not be necessary to use high-durability floors because there may not be as much traffic or equipment movement as is evident in a commercial or hospital kitchen. Resilient floor materials may be considered as appropriate alternatives in this case. Although these coverings require routine maintenance, initial cost savings over quarry or ceramic tiles are considerable.

Specifications for food, nonfood, and splash contact surfaces have been defined by the National Sanitation Foundation (NSF, 3475 Plymouth Rd, Ann Arbor, MI 48105; phone: (313) 769-8010; toll free: (800) NSF-MARK; fax: (313) 769-0109; Web address: http://www.nsf.org). Food contact surfaces must be smooth, nontoxic, corrosion resistant, stable, and nonabsorbent. They cannot impart color, odor, or taste, and they cannot modify foods in any way. Splash surfaces and surfaces that do not contact food need to be made of smooth, corrosion-resistant materials that do not crack or chip (5). Also, splash surfaces need to be easy to remove (1).

Stainless steel meets the criteria for food contact surfaces. It is a commonly used and widely accepted surface in commercial kitchens and has become an industry standard because of its versatility and durability (2). It can be purchased as is or custom fabricated. Because stainless steel is heat-, stain-, and chip-proof, it requires little maintenance and repairs are infrequent. Stainless steel, which is approximately four times the cost of the plastic laminate surfaces, can be expensive. However, the benefits of stainless steel clearly outweigh the expense.

Artificial stone surfaces such as Fountainhead,® Gibraltar,® and Corian® satisfy NSF standards, but they are somewhat porous. This characteristic decreases their application in commercial kitchens. These synthetic surfaces have many desirable characteristics; they are heat, stain, and scratch resistant and easy to repair. Like stainless steel, they are manufactured to order. Therefore, artificial stone splashboards and countertops can be made without seams and with raised or rolled edges to avoid spills and maximize sanitation. The cost of synthetic surfaces is high—slightly more expensive than stainless steel. A combination of these two surfaces can meet health and sanitation codes and serve the research kitchen well.

Sanitation Area

Sinks with two to four compartments are required to meet sanitation codes for washing large utensils and pots. In smaller facilities, two-compartment sinks may be sufficient when pots are washed off-site. Accommodations also must be made for soiled and clean utensils, waste removal, and recycling. The sanitation area should provide sinks, dishwasher, and cabinets for storage of dishes, utensils, glassware, and cleaning supplies (1). Garbage disposals may or may not be permitted depending on state or local sanitation codes. Other equipment that may be placed in this area includes a hand-washing sink, water deionizer, and ice machine.

Dishwasher capacity will determine the necessary type of model. Commercial models are undercounter, semiautomatic rack types, or automatic rack conveyors. Adequate clearance space is required for loading and unloading dishwashers. Because an open undercounter dishwasher door should not obstruct aisle space or work flow, the dishwasher should not be installed on an angle, especially when it is placed next to the sink area (3). A second consideration for dishwasher installation is water temperature. Often a booster is required to attain temperatures high enough for washing and sanitizing.

Counterspace in the sanitation area should be at least 3 ft to 6 ft long. These specifications include the dishwasher surface area. Countertops should be apportioned on either side of the sink area to separate soiled from clean utensils (3).

Well-equipped and organized workstations also allow for a better use of staff time. Frequently used utensils, appliances, and cookware must be stored between knee and shoulder heights, close to where they are needed. Nonfood items and cleaning supplies are stored separately. Bulky items such as carts and coolers for take-out meals can be stored adjacent to the kitchen. Storage criteria are also dictated by health department codes.

Selecting and Storing Equipment

Well-equipped, logically organized workstations allow for better use of staff time. Kitchen equipment (Exhibit 19-3) should be selected according to necessity, the condition of present equipment, and the possibility of reducing energy and operating costs. The costs of upgrading from home-quality to institutional-quality equipment are often justified by improved durability, capacity, and energy efficiency as well as superior health and safety standards. This is especially true for high-volume research kitchens.

For a small-scale research kitchen, equipment purchases may include range tops and ovens, food processors, and smaller-capacity refrigeration units. Purchases of institutional dishwashers, coffee makers, mixers, toasters, and larger refrigeration units should be considered. Many facilities use a combination of institutional and household equipment in an effort to meet requirements for capacity yet contain costs.

Wall-mounted equipment and equipment racks enhance sanitation by eliminating equipment legs or stands. Mobile

TABLE 19-1

Considerations for Dry Storage[1]

Criteria	Recommended Specifications
Temperature	50°F–70°F
Ventilation	Air turnover, 6 times per hour
Lighting	No direct sunlight; less intense lighting
Environment	Humidity 50%–60%
	Minimize extraneous heat
Shelving	Rust-proof, off the floor and away from the ceiling, ie, steel wire shelves (per state and local specifications)

[1]Adapted from Pannell D (6).

equipment is helpful when components are used in more than one work area. On the other hand, removing the wheels from seldom-moved equipment can foster better sanitation and maintenance, because less dust and dirt can accumulate beneath and among the pieces of equipment (3).

The NSF also defines sanitation and safety standards for commercial equipment construction. Therefore, the NSF seal of approval has become an industry standard. Comprehensive information about commercial equipment is also provided from manufacturers. By identifying the many types of available kitchen equipment, consultants can provide useful advice before purchase decisions are made.

Examples of good space savers are movable under-counter shelving; deep, pull-out drawers for base cabinets; "tray" cabinets with vertical dividers for storing awkward items including lids and cutting boards; drawer dividers to organize utensils; lazy susans and swing-out shelves for corner cabinets; undersink compartments; and undercounter cart storage. For less frequently used appliances, overhead storage may be permissible if compatible with safety codes (3).

Regular temperature monitoring and back-up alarm systems should be part of the cold storage plan whether on-site or off-site. Power failures are common and must be protected against. Considerable cold storage space is also needed for research diet studies. Adequate refrigerator space is required for raw food items as well as prepared meals. Frozen storage space needs to accommodate food lots and prepared entrees or baked products because many research kitchens use cook/chill procedures. For large facilities, walk-in refrigerators and freezers are a must! For example, long-term storage of bulk frozen meat, purchased from a single lot, might be arranged with a local butcher or frozen storage warehouse or rental refrigerator trailer. Mobile locked cages can be especially useful for shared storage spaces.

Food Storage

Storage space requirements for controlled diet studies are remarkably high. Because specified ingredients with known nutrient composition are a strict requirement of research diets, research food inventories must be maintained sepa-

rately from the regular foodservice supplies (see Table 19-1). For example, in long-term micronutrient balance studies, adequate space must be allotted for batch lots of canned fruits and vegetables. Therefore, dry storage space requirements may be considerable. The length of the research study and the number of participants also determine the amount of storage space required; longer, larger studies need far more room. Special arrangements can be set up for additional dry storage.

A threefold increase in storage capacity can be achieved with proper planning and well-designed shelving. Mobile, locked, stainless steel cages are excellent for storage of some items because they effectively maintain and secure separate inventories. Storage space may need to be partitioned when several studies with large inventories are ongoing. Dry storage areas that accommodate pallets of food might be necessary. Many investigators find they must arrange additional off-site food storage.

Staff Office Areas

Ideally, staff offices are located near the research kitchen to enhance work flow, quality assurance monitoring, and communication among nutrition and kitchen staff as well as locales for participant and family counseling. Outpatient facilities or conference rooms can be used as needed for large group meetings or clinic visits.

Ample office space is needed to maintain participant records, study files, and educational materials. Participants' records and other confidential information must be stored in securable file cabinets. Office layouts should foster individual and small group interactions among participants and clinicians. Space is also required for obtaining anthropometric measurements and for computer work.

Dining, Serving, and Reception Areas

Estimates for dining room space are based on the number of participants, meal census, the type of meal service, and the arrangement of tables. Twelve to 14 sq ft is usually necessary per participant (5). Therefore, 350 sq ft is required to accommodate 25 participants. Additional space may be needed for guests who accompany study participants. More participants can be accommodated by having multiple seatings for any given meal. Considerable space savings result by employing a continuous meal service and using rectangular rather than round tables. A space allowance of 8 to 10 sq ft per participant is then possible. Serving space can be conserved through off-site delivery of research diets. Space requirements for meal assembly will increase, however, when packaging bulk "to go" meals and plating advance preparation items. Exhibit 19-2 outlines requirements and considerations for a cafeteria-style service area.

Dining, serving, and reception areas should be checked 'carefully to ensure that unpleasant odors from the kitchen garbage disposals and laboratories do not intrude. It may be necessary to revise ventilation systems to avoid these problems. Similarly, temperature control is important; it is preferable to enable staff to adjust the temperature if participants find it too hot or cold in the dining room.

The trend toward larger diet studies and outpatient feeding trials means that expanded food distribution facilities and space for staff interaction with research participants must be considered. A well-furnished, comfortable lounge area is ideal for studies that require extended clinic visits. Additional provisions include a television, VCR, telephone, and typewriter or computer. Similarly, a children's area for special activities can be planned as part of studies that include families with children.

HUMAN FACTORS

Atmosphere

Another consideration of facility planning is the development of a pleasant work environment and dining atmosphere, which fosters employees' careful menu preparation and participants' compliance with diets. Factors include:

- Environment: lighting, noise, ventilation, temperature.
- Physical layout: floor plans and traffic patterns.
- Interior design and décor.
- Table settings and furniture.
- Dining areas: shape and size of rooms.
- Sanitation (4).

The menu type and meal delivery system are major factors to consider in designing a research kitchen. These two factors and the expectations of staff and participants provide useful insight into proper facility design. For example, when a participant pool consists of men and women who will receive partial meals-to-go as well as enjoy on-site dining, areas designated for food pickup, table dining, and tray disposal are required. Meal pickup may be cafeteria style or window service. Participants appreciate dining in an area that is quiet, well-lit, and tastefully decorated with comfortable tables and chairs.

Lighting and Color

Effective lighting helps to mitigate design problems, accent desirable areas, and improve the overall environment. The best system for lighting a research kitchen and dining facility incorporates direct and indirect lighting. Fixtures or spotlights are examples of direct light. Indirect light from daylight, estimated by the total glass area of windows and skylights, should also be considered in planning additional lighting requirements.

Studies show that environment plays a key role in enhancing worker productivity, morale, sanitation, and performance. Decreased strain and fatigue, accidents, training time, employee turnover, and absenteeism are additional benefits of a well-lit work environment. Professional lighting designers can be consulted to provide insight on the best approaches for illuminating kitchen and dining areas.

Light requirements are dictated by the size of work areas and the contrast and reflection of work backgrounds. Visual acuity is affected by the type and intensity of light sources and placement of fixtures. Fluorescent bulbs are economical and commonly used to light large work areas. Soft white and pink bulbs (2:1) are often used in kitchens to improve the appearance of food material and skin tones. Table 19-2 lists specific lighting requirements for kitchen and dining areas.

Light intensity and glare vary with appliance finishes and countertops. For example, stainless steel may potentiate high-intensity lighting. The reflection of direct lighting on stainless surfaces should be minimized because glare leads to fatigue and eye strain. Proper fixture placement minimizes glare, shadows, and poor contrasts. Less glare is apparent when fluorescent fixtures are arranged parallel to the line of vision. Similar results are realized when bright lights are set overhead at an angle less than 60° from the center of visual acuity. Glare can also be reduced by using several low-intensity light sources or by using grid covers that divert light rays.

Walls should reflect 50% to 60% of available light if equipment is dark and 50% to 70% if stainless steel or light colored equipment is used. Floors should be moderately light and reflect 25% of light; kitchen ceilings should reflect 85% to 95% of light (4). Soft yellow or cream and peach colors are recommended for kitchen walls to complement natural food and skin tones; ceilings should be painted off-white.

Noise

The environment for kitchen and dining areas should be designed to minimize noise. It is important to establish a balanced acoustic level. Noise in dining rooms can be controlled by drapes, carpeting, table pads, and acoustic ceiling tiles.

Similarly, kitchen clamor is tempered by locating loud equipment away from main work areas and dining facilities. Undercoating tables with liquid asphalt or using plastic mesh mats beneath tables and using acoustic tiles, veneers, or panels on upper walls or ceilings also reduces kitchen noise (5).

TABLE 19-2

Lighting Requirements in Different Kitchen Areas[1]

Kitchen Areas	Average Light Levels (Foot Candles)
Storage (to discern package labels)	20
Storage (to discern case labels)	15
Work areas (to discern large print)	25
Work areas (to discern detailed print)	40
Sanitation areas	85
Offices	125
Service areas	75

Adapted from Avery AC (5).

Security

It is a sad reality that theft and vandalism occur frequently in research kitchens. Valuable small equipment (such as analytical balances, scales, computers, knives, and blenders), and expensive supplies (such as meat and spices) are particular targets. Whenever possible, small items must be secured with locking cables, drawers, and cabinets; refrigerators, freezers, and walk-in dry or cold storage should also be lockable. Distribution of keys and security codes must be appropriately conservative. Most experienced investigators have had to contend with at least one incident that has resulted in loss of time, money, data, and trust. Not just unknown intruders but also participants and staff have been implicated on some of these occasions.

Data and specimen security also is of high priority. Some research kitchens are located close to patient examination areas and laboratories. Secure areas for participants' personal belongings and coats may be needed. Confidential paperwork must be kept in locked file cabinets and otherwise protected from prying eyes. Computer file data must be protected appropriately. Freezers with stored biological samples must be locked and must have backup emergency alarm and phone-tree systems in the event of power failures, vandalism, or other damage that can affect the research.

The cost of losing the samples or data from a well-controlled feeding study is nearly incalculable if one considers both the high budget requirements and the enormous human effort that has been expended on the part of staff and participants.

CONCLUSION: ALTERNATIVES TO NEW CONSTRUCTION OR REMODELING

If there is insufficient space in which to prepare food in an existing kitchen, work priorities can be adjusted. For example, most cooking and baking can be done during off-peak meal service times, and satellite kitchens can be used for preparation and arrangement of foods in research menus. Bulk meal delivery on an outpatient basis may also be considered depending on study criteria.

Another approach to new construction or remodeling is to contract space from a foodservice unit (such as a hospital kitchen, university dormitory, cafeteria, or sorority or fraternity facility). Large feeding studies may be effectively managed in this way. In this situation, trained staff and dedicated equipment are necessary. Food purchasing, plans, and accommodations for work and storage space arrangements must be highly developed. Written contracts that clearly define terms and conditions are required prior to initiating diet studies as part of an existing foodservice operation.

Whenever space, personnel, or funds are limited, the nutrition research staff will need to be especially creative and flexible. Diet studies that stretch the limits of routine research meal preparation can be accommodated with careful planning.

The authors gratefully acknowledge the helpful contributions of Karen Todd, MS, RD.

REFERENCES

1. Birchfield JC. *Design and Layout of Food Service Facilities.* New York, NY: Van Nostrand Reinhold; 1988.
2. Lawrence E. *The Complete Restauranteur—A Practical Guide to the Craft and Business of Restaurant Ownership.* New York, NY: Penguin Books USA, Inc; 1992.
3. North American Association of Food Equipment Manufacturers (NAFEM). *An Introduction to the Foodservice Industry.* 2nd ed. Chicago, Ill: NAFEM; 1990. (http://www.nafem.org)
4. Kazarian EA. *Food Service Facilities Planning.* 3rd ed. New York, NY: John Wiley; 1989.
5. Avery AC. *A Modern Guide to Food Service Equipment.* New York, NY: Van Nostrand Reinhold; 1985.
6. Pannell D. *School Food Service Management.* 4th ed. New York, NY: Van Nostrand Reinhold; 1990.

CHAPTER 20

STAFFING NEEDS FOR RESEARCH DIET STUDIES

DARLENE FONTANA, MS, RD; COLLEEN MATTHYS, RD; PATRICIA ENGEL, MS, RD; BEVERLY A. CLEVIDENCE, PHD; KAREN TODD, MS, RD; AND ABBY G. ERSHOW, ScD, RD

STUDY DESIGN AND INTENSITY OF EFFORT

The work of the nutrition research kitchen is time-consuming and labor-intensive, and requires a high degree of precision and meticulous attention to detail. The nutrition research team thus needs to be highly motivated and well trained to ensure that protocols are executed correctly. The size of the team and the number of staff with particular skills are best determined by evaluating the study's "design elements"—that is, the operational features that distinguish one protocol from another. Because the activities required for research diet studies are so different from those of typical institutional foodservice, the time and personnel estimates in this chapter are based on the authors' own experience.

The following aspects of study design ("design elements") should be assessed when planners consider each study's staffing requirements:

- **Is the study conducted on an inpatient (resident) or outpatient (nonresident) basis?** Inpatient studies generally require staff coverage for 2 or 3 shifts, 7 days per week. Outpatient studies, however, can be surprisingly labor intensive because considerable effort is needed to coordinate participants' schedules, package the foods for take-out, accommodate food pickup times, monitor quality assurance procedures, and address compliance issues. On the other hand, outpatient studies tend to enroll larger numbers of participants and may realize economies of scale, particularly in procurement of food and other supplies.
- **Which nutrients are to be controlled?** The amount of time to design the diet increases when more nutrients are designated for control. In addition, certain nutrients are more difficult to manipulate, which means that the re-

search kitchen will be engaged in more complex production techniques.
- **Are nutrition screening or dietary intake assessments part of the protocol?** Compared to height and weight, the more complex anthropometric measurements such as skinfold thickness or lean body mass take more time. If dietary intake data are to be collected, the frequency and method should be determined. Any need for counseling or intervention also will directly alter the demand for professional staff time.
- **What data collection instruments will be used?** Some studies require the research dietitian to design specific instruments. This can be time-consuming as the instrument is developed, tested, and refined.
- **What is the "size" of the study?** To estimate each study's staff requirements, it is necessary to determine the total length of the study, the number of diet periods, and the total number of participants enrolled at any time. Some studies may have high staffing needs for short periods of time; others have low staffing needs for longer periods of time. Protocols that require simultaneous multiple diets will be more labor intensive.
- **How complex is the diet protocol?** The precision of the study diet determines the staff time required. Consideration should be given to: the diet protocol specified (ie, metabolic balance, constant, controlled nutrient, weighed, estimated, or liquid formula); the length and number of diet study periods; the menu design (ie, 1-day fixed menu, cycle menu, or self-selected menu); recipe development and standardization; quality assurance procedures; and the number of diet composites required for nutrient analysis.

Information about the study's design elements and other features of the research plan, derived from answers to these questions, can be used to rank protocols by intensity of effort. (See Tables 20-1, 20-2, and 20-3.) Time and labor es-

TABLE 20-1

Design Elements Classification Guide for Outpatient (Nonresident) Studies[1]

Design Element	Low Effort	Medium Effort	High Effort
Number of subjects	<10	10–30	>30
Length of study	Days to weeks	Weeks—4 months	>4 months
Diet complexity	Standard house or therapeutic diets with routine cafeteria or tray service	One nutrient altered or restricted	Multiple nutrients altered or restricted
	One dietary treatment produced and served	Two concurrent dietary treatments produced and served	Three or more concurrent dietary treatments produced and served
	Foods not weighed	Limited number of test foods weighed	All food items weighed to meet caloric needs of individual subjects
	No need to produce specialized test foods	One specialized food produced to deliver test nutrients	Multiple specialized foods produced to deliver test nutrients
	No meals eaten off-site	Some meals packed for off-site consumption	Many meals packed for off-site consumption
Menu cycle length	1 day	2–7 days	>7 days
Diet composites	Limited number of high-priority foods are composited	One day's menu from each treatment is composited in duplicate for analysis before the study begins	Individual days' menus and/or complete menu cycles for each treatment are composited before the study and throughout each diet period
Number of dietary staff	<5	5–10	>10
Nutrient intake questionnaires (Qx)	Single Qx with long-turnaround data analysis	Multiple Qx with medium-turnaround data analysis, or single Qx with short-turnaround data analysis	Multiple Qx with short-turnaround data analysis
Method for assessing energy requirements	Predictive equations (eg, Harris-Benedict)	Calorimetry by doubly-labeled water method	Multiple food records analyzed by computer
Body composition measurements	Single assessment	Single assessment	Multiple assessments
	Anthropometric measurements (eg, height, weight, skinfold thickness)	Laboratory measurements (eg, bioelectrical impedance, hydrostatic weighing, DEXA)[2]	Anthropometric and laboratory measurements
Biological samples	1–2 blood samples	Multiple blood samples	Multiple collections of blood, urine, feces, etc
		24-hr urine collections	Any invasive procedure

[1]This classification guide was developed by Beverly Clevidence, PhD, at the Beltsville Human Nutrition Research Center, US Department of Agriculture, Beltsville, Md.
[2]DEXA, dual-energy X-ray absorptiometry.

TABLE 20-2

Protocol Intensity Ranking Guide[1]

Protocol Features	Low Intensity	Medium Intensity	High Intensity
Diet design	Special diet for simple, one-component study; not individualized	Special diet for individual subjects	Any protocol with "medium" ranking and additional component
Setting	Inpatient or outpatient	Inpatient or outpatient	Inpatient or outpatient
Meal production	Regular meals or snacks only	Special diets with one restriction	Special diets with multiple restrictions
	Standard therapeutic meals (eg, low-fat, diabetic)		Weighed diets with computer analysis
Anthropometric measurements	One-time bioelectrical impedance tests or skinfold thickness measurements	Sequential bioelectrical impedance or skinfold thickness measurements	Combined body composition measurements (eg, hydrostatic weighing, skinfold thickness)
		Hydrostatic weighing with residual volume measurement	
		Calorimetry	
Nutrient data services	Single nutrient intake questionnaire with simple data analysis	Multiple nutrient intake questionnaires with simple data analysis	Multiple nutrient intake questionnaires with complex data analysis
	Subject-kept food diaries	Calorie counts with analysis by food exchange groups	Calorie counts with computer analysis
	Long turnaround time for data analysis	Medium turnaround time for data analysis	Short turnaround time for data analysis
Other		Activities include analysis and reporting of data	Activities include study and protocol design, writing grant applications, hiring and supervising staff, writing data publications
			Dietitian(s) must be certified for data collection and testing

[1]This ranking guide was adapted from a model originally developed by the late Donna Nickel, MS, RD, at the behest of the Dietitians' Administrative Committee (Karen Todd, MS, RD, chairperson), General Clinical Research Center Program, National Center for Research Resources, Bethesda, Md.

TABLE 20-3

Examples of Intensity-Ranked Protocols[1]

Protocol Features	Low-Intensity Protocol: "Serotonergic Mediation of Dimethyl Tryptamine Effects in Humans"	High-Intensity Protocol: "Trial of Ca^{2+} Supplementation in Pregnancy for the Prevention of Preeclampsia and Preterm Birth"
Number of subjects	24	900
Setting	Inpatient (IP)	Outpatient (OP)
Subject days or visits	4 IP days/ subject (2 IP days/ visit x 2 visits/subject)	4 OP visits/ subject
Meal production	Regular meals (some vegetarian) One meal per subject	No meals provided
Nutrient data services	None	Nutrition research manager hires/supervises 0.5 FTE dietitian(s) for study. Dietitian(s) certified annually to obtain two 24-hour recalls per subject.
Clinical services	None	Referral to hospital obstetrics/gynecology department if necessary

[1]These examples were adapted from a set originally developed by the late Donna Nickel, MS, RD, at the behest of the Dietitian's Administrative Committee (Karen Todd, MS, RD, chairperson), General Clinical Research Center Program, National Center for Research Resources, Bethesda, Md.

timates can then be adjusted up or down accordingly. Ranking studies in this manner is especially useful when staff are synchronizing the effort for multiple simultaneous protocols. (The guidelines provided throughout this chapter are generally geared toward medium-intensity protocols.)

THE PERSONNEL ORGANIZATION OF CONTROLLED DIET STUDIES

The organizational structure of the nutrition research unit should ensure that the core functions of a controlled feeding protocol can be achieved. These functions include: scientific management; institutional management and financial support; ethical, scientific, and financial oversight; recruitment and management of participants; preparation and delivery of the dietary intervention; laboratory analysis; and data management and analysis.

There are many ways of assigning the responsibilities needed to achieve these functions (see Exhibit 20-1). Similarly, a wide variety of institutions, with widely varying internal organizational structures, can provide appropriate settings. Among these are private research foundations, university laboratories, and industry laboratories. The organizational structure needed to conduct a single study, such as one that may be supported by a single research grant, is relatively simple (see Figure 20-1).

If multiple concurrent studies are undertaken, more delegation of responsibility is needed, with a more hierarchical approach and, perhaps, more narrowly defined position descriptions and job titles (see Figure 20-2). The National In-

stitutes of Health General Clinical Research Centers (GCRCs) have a unique organizational structure that is mandated by the funding agency (see Figure 20-3).

Under ideal circumstances, the professional nutrition staff and the principal investigators for specific studies will develop strong collegial relationships that are personally rewarding and scientifically productive, with respectful acknowledgment of areas of responsibility and expertise. In most settings, doctoral-level principal investigators have overall responsibility for the study, playing the key role of initiating the research program and obtaining funds. The principal investigator develops the study's main scientific hypotheses, lays out the basics of the research plan, oversees data analysis and interpretation, and arranges for review of human subjects protection. (The oversight roles of the principal investigators and medical officers are addressed in Chapter 5, "Ethical Considerations in Dietary Studies.") The principal investigator and the nutrition research manager together must ensure that the study's hypotheses are reflected in the dietary design and that the research kitchen and the biochemical laboratory have a smoothly coordinated working relationship.

Nutrition Personnel

By considering the particular skills and responsibilities of the personnel who are employed in the nutrition research kitchen, it generally is possible to make a distinction between the managerial and the staff categories. The principal functions, responsibilities, and guidelines for several dif-

EXHIBIT 20-1

Responsibilities of Study Personnel[1]

Research Coordinator/Study Coordinator
Manages clinical feeding study. Works closely with principal investigator and biostatistician to develop research and recruitment strategies and to establish study schedule. Manages data flow between laboratory and biostatistician. Works directly with research dietitian, subject coordinator, and biomedical coordinator to elicit compliance with study goals and objectives. May be responsible for ordering and purchasing supplies.

Subject Coordinator
Works closely with study participants during recruitment and screening. Promotes retention and compliance throughout the study. Acts as a liaison among study participants and research management staff. (These responsibilities can also be assigned to the research coordinator when appropriate.)

Biomedical Coordinator
Coordinates and schedules biological sample collection. Manages laboratory personnel and data collection and analysis.

Medical Technician
Draws blood samples and collects other biological samples from study participants. Must be appropriately qualified according to rules of sponsoring institution.

Biochemical Laboratory Technician
Performs chemical and other assays on biological samples according to study protocol.

Biostatistician
Works closely with principal investigator to develop optimal study design to achieve research objectives and to determine the most powerful data analysis approach. Conducts statistical analysis of study data.

Data Management Assistant
Assists biostatistician with data management activities (coding, data input, programming, data analysis).

Research Dietitian/Administrative Dietitian/Senior Research Dietetic Technician
Develops study diet according to research objectives. Works directly with food production technicians to monitor quality of food products. Trains and manages food production technicians and food service assistants. May share responsibilities for purchasing food and supplies.

Food Production Technician/Dietetic Technician/Nutrition Technician/Nutrition Research Manager
Prepares and portions special foods and meals according to the study protocol.

Foodservice Assistant/Food Production Assistant
Assists in preparing and portioning meals and other aspects of food service for study participants.

---

[1]Job titles and assigned responsibilities will vary among research centers. The role of the principal investigator is discussed under The Personnel Organization of Controlled Diet Studies. General Clinical Research Centers follow personnel guidelines provided by the funding agency.

ferent positions are listed in Exhibit 20-1 (exact job titles may vary among institutions). There also may be need for a study coordinator, a recruiter, and a quality assurance specialist.

Nutrition Research Manager

The principal function of the nutrition research manager is to manage the administrative, research, and clinical responsibilities of a nutrition research unit. (A typical position de-

scription is shown in Exhibit 20-2.) Responsibilities include protocol design and implementation; management of the research kitchen; and participant nutritional care (Table 20-4). Many GCRC units have only one research dietitian, who also functions as the nutrition research manager. The diversity of the unit's activities, the number of protocols, and the required nutrition services will all have the potential to influence professional staffing needs. Functional time analyses are often required to justify additional professional staff

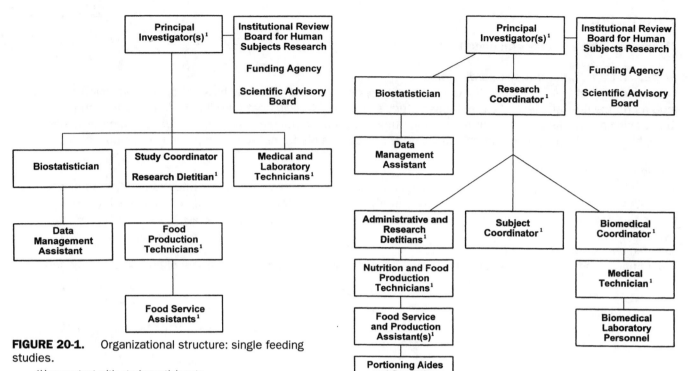

FIGURE 20-1. Organizational structure: single feeding studies.

[1]Has contact with study participants.

FIGURE 20-2. Organizational structure: multiple concurrent feeding studies

[1]Has contact with study participants.

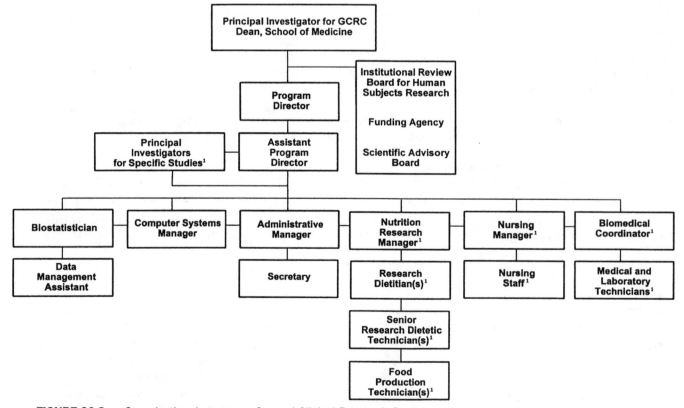

FIGURE 20-3. Organizational structure: General Clinical Research Center.

[1]Has contact with study participants.

EXHIBIT 20-2

Position Description: Nutrition Research Manager

PRINCIPAL FUNCTION

Manages the administrative, research, and clinical nutrition responsibilities of a nutrition research unit. Responsible for designing and implementing dietary protocols, managing the research kitchen, and providing nutritional care to study participants.

DUTIES AND RESPONSIBILITIES

Administrative

- Manages the operation of the research kitchen to ensure accurate delivery of diets as defined by research protocols.
- Develops all policies and procedures for the nutrition research unit.
- Recruits, hires, trains, supervises, and evaluates nutrition research personnel.
- Prepares annual budget for personnel, equipment, and supplies.
- Maintains standards for sanitation, safety, and quality assurance.
- Prepares reports of activities of the nutrition research unit for annual reports, site visits, and grant applications and renewals.
- Serves on the clinical research center advisory committee and evaluates the nutrition aspects of research protocols.
- Evaluates, uses, and maintains computer systems to manage food purchasing and preparation and to analyze food consumption data.
- Consults with architects and kitchen design consultants to plan for remodeling and/or expansion of the nutrition research facility as needed.

Research and Clinical

- Collaborates with clinical investigators to plan, organize, conduct, and evaluate the nutrition component of research protocols.
- Designs and implements research diets consistent with the scientific purpose of each project, general nutrition principles, and the needs of individual research participants.
- Performs nutritional assessments, makes recommendations regarding nutritional care, and records data in the medical record.
- Collects and interprets nutrition-related data; participates in the publication and presentation of research findings to the scientific community and the lay public.
- May develop and conduct independent nutrition research projects.
- Informs research participants of the dietary aspects of research protocols, and evaluates compliance.
- Develops individualized nutrition education materials for research projects and provides nutrition counseling.
- Attends conferences and educational symposiums to maintain current knowledge in clinical nutrition, food science, and research methodology.
- Trains clinical investigators, graduate students, dietetic interns, and support personnel in nutrition research design and methodology.
- Establishes and maintains positive interdisciplinary professional relationships to facilitate planning and implementation of research projects and effective participant nutrition care.

QUALIFICATIONS

Education

- Masters or doctoral degree in nutrition or related field.
- Undergraduate concentration in clinical dietetics preferred.

Job Knowledge and Skills

- Must possess thorough knowledge of theory and practices of dietetics and nutritional sciences.

Experience and Training

- Completion of an approved dietetics education program and registration by The American Dietetic Association.
- Three years of clinical experience.
- Exposure to clinical research preferred.
- Managerial or supervisory experience highly desirable.

TABLE 20-4

Task Descriptions: Nutrition Research Manager

Task	Activities
Protocol design	Review scientific literature. Hold conferences/teleconferences with investigators and other research dietitians. Develop data collection instruments and/or nutrition education materials.
Research diet design	Calculate nutrient composition by computer analysis. Verify nutrient content by chemical analysis. Develop and standardize recipes.
Subject interviews	Screen subjects. Collect data to calculate energy needs. Review research diet, protocol, and compliance issues. Schedule meal pickup times for outpatient studies.
Data collection	Obtain diet history and 24-hour recall. Provide instructions for food records and other questionnaires. Clarify data recorded.
Individualized diet calculations	Adapt designed research diets for individual subjects as needed (primarily for energy level).
Nutritional care	Assess nutritional status of subjects. Plan, implement, and monitor care for subjects. Conduct nutritional counseling, document medical records, and refer for discharge.
Communications	Hold conferences with investigators, other research dietitians, nurses, and subjects. Annotate charts in the medical record.
Employee training	Hire, recruit, and train employees to: prepare food in accordance with research methodology; prepare diet composites for chemical analysis; interview subjects and instruct them in compliance procedures; and enter food intake data using nutrition software.
Employee supervision	Provide ongoing training and supervision specific to varied protocols. Counsel and implement disciplinary action.
Quality assurance	Establish and maintain an integrated quality assurance program.
Computer resources	Manage periodic improvements of nutrient databases and software.
Data preparation	Prepare dietary intake data for analysis.
Publications and presentations	Participate in data analysis and writing groups with other investigators. Prepare scientific manuscripts for publication. Present data and other study information at professional meetings.

(Table 20-5). Because the production and delivery of research diets are so costly and labor-intensive, it is critical that estimates of time requirements and staff needs be available when the overall research budget is being developed and when funding applications are being written.

Nutrition Research Staff

The principal function of the senior research dietetic technician is the management of the nutrition research kitchen. This includes supervision of staff, production and service of research diets, inventory and purchase of food and supplies, and quality assurance. Some units may employ an administrative dietitian with the management responsibilities of both the senior research dietetic technician and the nutrition

research manager. Position tasks and functional time analysis estimates for nutrition research staff are found in Tables 20-6 and 20-7. (Position descriptions are shown in Exhibits 20-3 and 20-4.)

Other Staff

The exact job titles and position descriptions can vary considerably for the staff who prepare and portion foods, deliver food to study participants, and handle many of the logistical aspects of the research kitchen and dining room. Some responsibilities for data collection also may be included. These staff members may have the job titles of cooks, chefs, food-service assistants, food production technicians, nutrition technicians, portioning aides, and sanitation workers.

TABLE 20-5

Functional Time Analysis Estimates for Different Types of Research Diets: Nutrition Research Manager[1]

Task	Formula Diet	Weighed Diet	Constant Diet	All Diets
Protocol design	1–3 hr/protocol	5 hr/protocol	10 hr/protocol	—
Research diet design	10 hr/diet	20 hr/diet	40 hr/diet	—
Subject interviews				
Inpatient (IP)	0.50–0.75 hr/subject	0.50–0.75 hr/subject	0.50–0.75 hr/subject	
Outpatient (OP)	—	—	—	Add 25% to IP diet estimates
Data collection				
Anthropometric measurements	—	—	—	0.25–0.5 hr/subject
Dietary assessment and history	—	—	—	0.5 hr/subject
Food record instruction	—	—	—	0.5 hr/subject
Clarification	—	—	—	0.17 hr/day of recorded intake
Food frequency questionnaires	—	—	—	0.5–1 hr/subject
Individualized diet calculations				
IP protocols	0.17 hr/menu[2]	0.17 hr/menu[2]	0.17 hr/menu[2]	—
OP protocols	—	—	—	Add 25% to IP diet estimates
Nutritional care	—	—	—	2 hr/subject
Communications	0.25 hr/subject/wk	0.50 hr/subject/wk	0.25 hr/subject/wk	—
Employee training				
Research methods	—	—	—	20 hr/staff member; 1 hr/protocol
Entry of dietary intake data	—	—	—	40 hr/staff member; 1 hr/protocol
Compliance	—	—	—	1 hr/staff member; 0.25 hr/protocol
Quality assurance	—	—	—	1 hr/protocol
Employee supervision				
Orientation	0.25 hr/protocol	0.5 hr/protocol	0.5 hr/protocol	—
Menu design	0.5 hr/protocol	0.5 hr/protocol	1 hr/protocol	—
Recipe standardization	0.5 hr/protocol	2 hr/protocol	2 hr/protocol	—
Subject instruction	0.25 hr/protocol	0.5 hr/protocol	0.5 hr/protocol	—
Quality assurance	1 hr/protocol	10 hr/protocol	20 hr/protocol	—
Computer resources	1 hr/protocol	2 hr/protocol	2 hr/protocol	—
Diet preparation	0.5 hr/subject	1 hr/subject	1 hr/subject	Add 2 hr/month for all diets
Publications and presentations	—	—	—	[3]

[1]The various types of research diets are described in Chapter 10, "Planning Diet Studies."

[2]0.17 hr = 10 min.

[3]See the Conclusion and Exhibit 20-9 of this chapter for further discussion of publications and presentations.

TABLE 20-6

Task Descriptions: Nutrition Research Staff

Task	Activities
Protocol development	Assess personnel needs. Determine freezer and refrigeration capacity for storage. Prepare written procedures for nutrition protocols.
Recipe testing and standardization	Assist in menu development. Develop, test, and standardize recipes. Determine product shelf-life. Prepare standardized forms for quality assurance using computer software.
Nutritional care	Instruct research subjects in procedures necessary for compliance with research studies. Monitor and record food intake. Write menus. Obtain food preferences. Perform anthropometric measurements.
Dietary assessment	Enter food intake data using nutrition software. Assist in analyzing nutrient content of research diets and recipes. Assist in other calculations as necessary.
Quality assurance	Assist in the development of data collection forms. Tabulate and prepare data for analysis. Record and monitor food intake and compliance. Record and monitor weight to ensure weight stabilization. Prepare diet composites for chemical analysis.
Communications	Maintain telephone, interpersonal, and written communication among participants, research dietitians, nutrition research staff, nurses, and investigators.
Employee training	Train employees in procedures required for nutrition protocols, including food preparation techniques, sanitation and food safety, use of computer software, food record and menu analysis.
Employee supervision	Schedule and direct the activities of the nutrition research staff. Maintain continuous quality assurance checks on procedures for weighing food items, methods for preparing foods, and records for data collection.
Ordering and inventory	Order food items and maintain inventory of food and supplies.
Preparing and portioning food	Weigh, measure, and prepare food portions and ingredients using standardized methods. Wrap, label, and store food items using standardized procedures.
Sanitation	Clean work areas and equipment using established procedures.
Food safety	Portion food for cooling and storing into appropriate containers. Label and date food items. Monitor refrigerator and freezer temperatures.
Outpatient study activities	Coordinate meal pickup times with subjects' schedules. Pack and label meals using established procedures.

TABLE 20-7

Functional Time Analysis Estimates for Different Types of Research Diets: Nutrition Research Staff[1]

Task	Formula Diet	Weighed Diet	Constant Diet	All Diets
Protocol development	1 hr/protocol	2 hr/protocol	5 hr/protocol	—
Recipe testing and standardization	2–3 hr/protocol	5–10 hr/protocol	60 hr/protocol	—
Nutritional care	0.25 hr/subject	0.5 hr/subject	1 hr/subject/wk	—
Dietary assessment	—	—	—	0.33–0.50 hr/recorded day
Quality assurance				
Develop protocols	0.25 hr/protocol	0.50–1 hr/protocol	20 hr/protocol	—
Monitor compliance	0.25 hr/protocol	0.50–1 hr/subject	1 hr/subject/wk	—
Prepare diet composites	1 hr/composite	4–8 hr/composite	4–8 hr/composite	—
Communications	0.25 hr/subject/day	0.25 hr/subject/day	0.25 hr/subject/day	—
Employee training	0.50 hr/protocol	1 hr/protocol	8 hr/protocol	—
Employee supervision	0.50 hr/protocol	0.50 hr/protocol	2 hr/day	—
Ordering and inventory	—	—	—	6–8 hr/week
Preparing and portioning food	0.5 hr/formula	0.25 hr/meal	0.75 hr/meal	—
Sanitation	—	—	—	0.50–1 hr/day
Food safety	—	—	—	0.25–0.50 hr/day
Outpatient study activities	—	—	—	Add 0.33 hr/subject/day

[1]The various types of research diets are described in Chapter 10, "Planning Diet Studies."

A typical position of this type is that of the food production technician (sometimes termed research dietetic technician). The principal function of the food production technician is the preparation and service of meals to research subjects on controlled nutrient diets in accordance with established methods and procedures. This staff member also assists with the collection and entry of dietary intake data using computer software. (For a position description see Exhibit 20-5.)

Planning Considerations

To determine staffing needs, it is important to identify the tasks to be performed ("task descriptions") and to estimate the time required for each ("functional time analysis estimates"). Task descriptions for the nutrition research manager and the nutrition research staff are shown in Tables 20-4 and 20-6. Functional time analysis estimates for various aspects of nutrition protocols, particularly for three commonly used types of research diets, are shown in Tables 20-5 and 20-7. These are provided as examples of time requirements and can be altered to fit specific situations. Because each research center will develop its own unique experience of the time and effort required to carry out various activities, planning activities for new protocols can benefit greatly from information gained during recently completed projects.

There are several ways to estimate total research kitchen staff effort for a controlled diet protocol. Small studies and inpatient studies often must allot 1 to 2 full-time employees (FTE) for each 3 to 4 participants who are receiving weighed, constant, controlled nutrient, or metabolic balance diets. It may be necessary to distribute the effort among several individuals to ensure that all work shifts are covered and there are no gaps when a staff member is on leave. Some large-scale studies (n > 25), which serve half of the meals on site with the other half packed for off-site consumption, allocate 1 FTE per 5 to 6 participants.

Staffing needs also are affected by the number and complexity of concurrent studies and the total number of participants engaged in all studies. Large studies may require staffing patterns that vary greatly through the course of the week. Some nutrition research units have found that using an evening shift can yield an increase in production without requiring a concomitant increase in kitchen space and equipment.

Another approach is to conduct a task analysis to determine the estimated production time per meal. This exercise is shown for a sample protocol ("Protocol 809: Adipose Tissue Distribution and Adrenergic Mechanisms in Aging"). The first step is to describe the key features of the protocol (see Exhibit 20-6). Next, the study's design elements and methods are summarized (see Table 20-8). Information from this summary, in conjunction with worksheets that link specific professional tasks to required effort, can be used to

EXHIBIT 20-3

Position Description: Senior Research Dietetic Technician

PRINCIPAL FUNCTION

Responsible for management of the nutrition research kitchen. This includes supervision of staff, production and service of research diets, inventory and purchase of food and supplies, and quality assurance.

DUTIES AND RESPONSIBILITIES

Administrative

- Ensures accuracy and precision in the preparation of controlled diets for research protocols.
- Plans, directs, and supervises the activities of nutrition research staff.
- Trains employees in appropriate methods and techniques of food preparation for the implementation of nutrition protocols.
- Participates in the performance evaluation of nutrition research staff.
- Inventories and orders food and supplies.
- Supervises and assists in the production and delivery of research meals.
- Assists in the development of recipes and menus to meet research protocol specifications.
- Maintains food safety and sanitation standards; monitors quality assurance.
- Updates policy and procedure manuals.
- Supervises the cleaning and maintenance of equipment in work area.
- Maintains communication among subjects, research dietitian, and nutrition research staff.
- Uses computer software for food purchasing and inventory control.

Research and Clinical

- Instructs research subjects in the dietary procedures necessary for compliance with research studies.
- Monitors and records food intake; reinforces compliance with research protocols.
- May write diets, obtain participant food preferences, take anthropometric measurements, and participate in the nutrition education of participants.
- May clarify dietary intake records; gather and prepare data for analysis.

QUALIFICATIONS

Education

- Graduate of an approved dietetic technician program (or equivalent education and experience).

Job Knowledge and Skills

- Must be able to manage the foodservice operation of a nutrition research kitchen.
- Must have knowledge of basic food preparation, nutrition, and food composition.
- Must have good interpersonal skills.

Experience and Training

- One year related work experience.
- Computer literacy desirable.

EXHIBIT 20-4

Position Description: Administrative Dietitian (or Nutrition Research Manager)

PRINCIPAL FUNCTION

Responsible for management of the nutrition research facility. This includes supervision of staff, production and service of research diets, inventory and purchase of food and supplies, and quality assurance.

DUTIES AND RESPONSIBILITIES

Administrative

- Manages the operation of the research kitchen to ensure accurate delivery of diets as defined by research protocols.
- Develops and updates all policies and procedures for the nutrition research service.
- Maintains policy and procedure manuals.
- Recruits, hires, trains, supervises, and evaluates nutrition research personnel.
- Prepares annual budget for personnel, equipment, and supplies.
- Maintains food safety and sanitation standards; monitors quality assurance.
- Ensures accuracy and precision in the preparation of controlled diets for research protocols.
- Inventories and orders food and supplies.
- Assists in the development of recipes and menus to meet research protocol specifications.
- Supervises the cleaning and maintenance of equipment in work areas.
- Maintains communication among subjects, research dietitian, and nutrition research staff.
- Maintains computer systems to manage food purchasing and inventory control.
- Consults with architects and kitchen design consultants to plan for remodeling and/or expansion of the nutrition research facility as needed.

Research and Clinical

- Collaborates in the design and implementation of research diets.
- Collects and interprets nutrition-related data; participates in the publication and presentation of research findings to the scientific community and the lay public.
- May develop and conduct independent nutrition research projects.
- Informs research participants of the dietary aspects of research protocols and evaluates compliance.
- Attends conferences and educational symposiums to maintain current knowledge in management, finance, food-service, clinical nutrition, food science, and research methodology.
- Establishes and maintains positive interdisciplinary professional relationships to facilitate planning and implementation of research projects and effective participant nutrition care.
- Monitors and records food intake, and reinforces compliance with research protocols.
- May clarify dietary intake records and gather and prepare data for analysis.

QUALIFICATIONS

Education

- Bachelor's degree in foods and nutrition or related field.
- Master's degree in nutrition or related field highly desirable if position has research responsibilities.

Job Knowledge and Skills

- Must possess thorough knowledge of theory and practices of management, dietetics, and nutritional sciences.
- Must have good interpersonal skills.

Experience and Training

- Completion of an approved dietetic education program and registration by The American Dietetic Association.
- Three years of administrative experience.
- Exposure to clinical research preferred.
- Managerial or supervisory experience required.

EXHIBIT 20-5

Position Description: Food Production Technician (or Research Dietetic Technician)

PRINCIPAL FUNCTION

Responsible for the preparation and service of meals to research participants on controlled nutrient diets in accordance with established methods and procedures.

DUTIES AND RESPONSIBILITIES

Administrative

- Precisely weighs, measures, and prepares food portions and ingredients for research meals using standardized methods and procedures.
- Prepares duplicate subject diets and/or aliquots for laboratory analysis.
- Assists in the development of recipes and menus to meet research protocol specifications.
- Inventories food and supplies; delivers requisitions; obtains assembled items.
- Maintains food safety and sanitation standards.
- Cleans all work areas in accordance with established procedures.
- Operates and maintains equipment according to prescribed safety and sanitation standards.
- May assist in training new employees or students.
- Maintains communication among subjects, nutrition research staff, nurses, and investigators.

Research and Clinical

- Instructs research subjects in the dietary procedures necessary for compliance with research studies.
- Monitors and records food intake; reinforces compliance with nutrition protocols.
- Uses nutrition software for the analysis of dietary records, research menus, and recipes.
- May write diets, obtain participant food preferences, take anthropometric measurements, and participate in the nutrition education of participants.
- May assist with data collection and data entry.

QUALIFICATIONS

Education

- Graduate of an approved dietetic technician program (or equivalent education and experience).

Job Knowledge and Skills

- Must have knowledge of basic food preparation, nutrition, food safety, and food composition.
- Must have good interpersonal skills.

Experience and Training

- One year related work experience preferred; computer experience desirable.

EXHIBIT 20-6

Example of a Protocol Description for Protocol 809:
"Adipose Tissue Distribution and Adrenergic Mechanisms in Aging"

AIMS

The aims of this study are to compare values at baseline and after a weight-loss diet in young and elderly subjects with respect to measures of sympathetic nervous system activity; adrenergic receptor, lipolytic, and adenylate cyclase activity; glucose tolerance and insulin sensitivity; lipoprotein lipase (LPL) activity; and body fat distribution as measured by circumference and tomography.

OUTLINE OF PROPOSED RESEARCH

Thirty-three elderly (60-yr-old to 80-yr-old) male subjects will be recruited for the 3-month weight loss study (4 months including weight stabilization periods). Subjects must be healthy and taking no regular medications (other than multiple vitamins). They must be between 130% and 170% of ideal body weight, with adult-onset obesity. Subjects entering the study will follow an isocaloric diet similar to Step 1 NCEP of the American Heart Association diet (50% carbohydrate, 30% fat, 20% protein; 300 mg/day cholesterol; and 4 g/day sodium). Following the weight stabilization period, subjects will be instructed in a 1,000 kcal to 1,200 kcal weight-loss diet.

SUBJECT-DAYS

Each subject will participate in the study for 4 months. Twice as many people will be screened as are required for the study. Thirty-three subjects will be enrolled and 66 subjects (33 × 2) will be screened. Each screened subject will require 1 day for medical history and physical examination (66 × 1 day = 66 days). Each enrolled subject will require : 1 day food record review, before and after weight loss (33 × 2 days = 66 days); 1 day for fat biopsy, before and after weight loss (33 × 2 days = 66 days); 1 day for plasma LPL before and after weight loss (33 × 2 days = 66 days); and 3 visits per week for weigh-in and diet counseling (33 × 16 weeks × 3 days/week = 1,584 days).

NUTRITION SERVICES

Type of Diet: During the 2-week pre- and post-assessment phases, subjects will be weight-stabilized on a constant diet as described under the outline. All meals will be cooked, packaged, stored, and distributed to the subjects as out-patients. Adjustments in caloric intake will be made as necessary using a liquid formula of the same composition as the constant diet. Following the weight stabilization period, subjects will be instructed in a 1,000 kcal to 1,200 kcal weight-loss diet. All diets will include a daily multivitamin and mineral supplement.

Nutritional Data and Analysis: Subjects will complete two 3-day food records, once during the preassessment phase and once during the weight-loss phase. These food records will be analyzed for kilocalorie and macronutrient content using a nutrient analysis software program (University of Minnesota Nutrient Data System, NDS).

TABLE 20-8

Example of a Protocol Features Worksheet for Protocol 809:
"Adipose Tissue Distribution and Adrenergic Mechanisms in Aging"

Protocol Features	Specifics
Research diet design	Constant diet provided as a 2-day rotating menu.
Resident or nonresident study	Nonresident (outpatient).
Number and length of study periods	Total time on protocol: 4 mo.
	Two 14-day controlled diet, weight-stabilization periods per subject (one at baseline and one following a 3-mo weight-loss period).
Number of subjects	n = 33 (11 subjects/year for 3 years).
Nutrients to be controlled	Isocaloric diet for weight-stabilization periods. Energy (kcal) distribution: carbohydrate 50%, protein 20%, fat 30%. Cholesterol 300 mg/day, sodium 4 g/day, dietary fiber 15 g/day.
Outpatient nutritional care	1,000–1,200 kcal weight loss diet, individualized for each subject.
	Follow-up counseling and weight monitoring 3 times/wk throughout the 3-mo (12 wk) weight-loss period.
Data collection instruments	Two 3-day food records (one at baseline and one during weight loss period). Data analyzed using NDS software for designated study nutrients.
Quality assurance procedures	Verify composition of diets by chemical assay of composites. Standardize procedures for collecting anthropometric and dietary data. Verify food preparation and storage temperatures. Verify weights of food items on research menus. Calibrate kitchen scales on regular basis and maintain log of results. Check accuracy of packing procedures for outpatient diets. Assess subject compliance with protocol using standardized procedures.
Protocol intensity ranking	High intensity.

estimate professional and other dietary staff needs (see Tables 20-9 and 20-10).

Planning also must account for the designated hours of operation and coverage for staff vacations, holidays, weekends, and sick leave. It is important to be familiar with any employee union contracts because they may stipulate work hours, the tasks allowable for specific job categories, payment for temporary assignment to higher-level duties, employee rights in relation to disciplinary action and grievance procedures, reimbursement for uniforms, and vacation and holiday schedules. Other restrictions may apply if the research kitchen is located within a hospital.

Additional support may be available from nonnutrition personnel, with the caveat that all plans for sharing of responsibilities must be coordinated in advance with the appropriate supervisors or department heads. This may include nursing staff, who might help to facilitate a single shift of nutrition personnel by passing trays and reheating delayed meals, recording heights and weights, and serving one meal on weekends. Assistance with some cleaning tasks may also be available from the environmental services department.

Some institutions are able to use undergraduate or graduate students for certain kitchen and participant management activities, provided this occurs in the context of practicum courses and other educational programs. This valuable option is more likely to be feasible at universities that have undergraduate dietetics programs.

Multiple Concurrent Studies

Most clinical research centers and research kitchens are used simultaneously by many investigators, resulting in heavy demands on the dietary staff. Good communication among the investigators, recruiters, nurses, and laboratory and research kitchen personnel is essential for effective coordination of multiple projects. When carrying out multiple concurrent studies, the number of admissions allowed on each individual study will of necessity be limited. This number must be agreed upon with each investigator and recruiter before the study begins or the capacity of the facility may become overloaded.

A convenient way to facilitate planning and coordinate the activities of various personnel for concurrent projects is to develop individualized flow sheets for each study participant's schedule (Exhibit 20-7). This is particularly helpful if the participant is simultaneously involved in several protocols.

A good quality control system should be in place before investigators launch any study. For multiple concurrent studies, this quality control system must be designed specifically to prevent confusion and errors among studies, as well as among the diets for any one study. In some research centers, each participant is assigned a color and every food item can be marked with colored stickers or tape; for concurrent studies, the colors used for each study must be unique to that study. Similarly, letter and number codes also must be study-specific. Menu items for each study can be packaged and stored on separate shelves in the refrigerator or freezer. If certain items look the same but are made with different ingredients (such as cookies made with different fats), two employees can check each other and initial the quality control sheet before the food is served.

Study participants also can play a crucial role in quality control when multiple studies are being conducted. They can be given a copy of the menu, and when their tray is delivered, the staff member can double-check the tray as participants read their copy of the menu.

The foodservice supervisor or kitchen manager should make an overview of the expected workload for all of the studies and then set priorities for the coordinated production schedule. The work schedule must include the time needed to produce each recipe in each protocol; it is more efficient to prepare quantities that can be used for the whole study or at least several weeks. Recipe-based foods can be prepared ahead, frozen in appropriate portions, and weighed again on the day they are served.

It is essential that kitchen staff working on multiple concurrent studies be given particularly clear instructions regarding their responsibilities. A large erasable work calendar kept in the kitchen is a convenient way to organize this information in a central location; special instructions can be written on it and checked by the staff on a daily basis. It also is helpful to have individualized work schedules for each employee so all are aware of specific duties to be performed during their shift. This will streamline the logistics of food production and distribution and minimize errors.

Job descriptions for the foodservice workers engaged in multiple studies should be written so that staff can be universally trained, meaning that every kitchen staff member should know how to perform all tasks. This arrangement will permit the greatest flexibility because most research facilities are too small to assign one or two foodservice workers exclusively to each protocol. Job descriptions also must be written in explicit detail to avoid contract disputes if the employees are covered under a labor contract. There should be adequate staffing to cover vacation leave, sick leave, holiday leave, and 7-day-per-week kitchen coverage, and to accommodate the specific requirements of each protocol (Exhibit 20-8). Flexibility in staffing is an important aspect of planning for the workload. Quick alterations in work assignments may be needed to accommodate unexpected problems such as sickness, budget shortfalls, or recruitment delays.

The research kitchen staff need to work one of several shifts, depending on the complexity of the multiple protocols. Typical shifts are: 6:00 AM to 2:30 PM, 8:00 AM to 4:30 PM, and 10:30 AM to 7:00 PM. On occasion, when equipment needs to be shared, staff can be scheduled up until 11:00 PM to spread out the work and optimize the use of equipment.

QUALITY ASSURANCE AND TRAINING

Quality assurance programs are critical to the performance of nutrition research units. Such programs protect the

TABLE 20-9

Example of an Effort Estimation Worksheet for the Nutrition Research Manager for Protocol 809: "Adipose Tissue Distribution and Adrenergic Mechanisms in Aging"[1]

Tasks	Time Required per Yr[2]
Protocol design	10 hr
Research diet design @ 40 hr/diet × 2 diets	80 hr
Subject interviews @ 1 hr/subject × 11 subjects	11 hr
Data collection	
Instruction @ 0.5 hr/subject × 11 subjects	5.5 hr
Clarification @ 0.5 hr/food record × two 3-day food records/subject	11 hr
Individualized diet calculations	
First study period: @ 0.17 hr (10 min)/menu × 2 menus/subject	3.75 hr
Second study period: @ 0.17 hr (10 min)/menu × 2 menus/subject	3.75 hr
Add 25% for outpatient diets	2 hr
Nutritional care	
Calculation of weight loss diet @ 1 hr/subject × 11 subjects	11 hr
Instruction on weight loss diet @ 1 hr/subject × 11 subjects	11 hr
Other instruction @ 1 hr/subject × 11 subjects	11 hr
Follow up visits @ 0.25 hr/visit × 3 visits/wk for 12 wk	99 hr
Communications @ 0.5 hr/subject/wk × two 2-wk periods of weight stabilization	22 hr
Employee training	
Research methods	1 hr
Computers	1 hr
Compliance	0.25 hr
Quality assurance	1 hr
Employee supervision	
Orientation	0.5 hr
Menu design	1 hr
Recipe standardization	2 hr
Subject instruction	0.5 hr
Quality assurance	20 hr
Computer resources	2 hr
Data preparation @ 1 hr/subject × 11 subjects	11 hr
Total effort[3]	321.25 hr/yr
% Full-time equivalent (FTE)	15% (321.25 hr/yr/2080 hr/FTE = 0.15)

[1]Protocol 809 will enroll 11 subjects/yr for 3 years. For each subject, there are two 2-wk controlled diet periods/subject/yr.
[2]Effort is rounded to the nearest 0.25 hr.
[3]These figures do not include the additional time that is required for manuscript preparation. The effort expended on this activity will depend on the level of responsibility; primary authorship or co-authorship of multiple manuscripts may require 0.10 FTE or more. (Also see Conclusion: Presentation and Publication of Data; and Exhibit 20-9.)

TABLE 20-10

Example of an Effort Estimation Worksheet for the Nutrition Research Staff[1] for Protocol 809:
"Adipose Tissue Distribution and Adrenergic Mechanisms in Aging"[2]

Tasks	Time Required per Yr
Protocol development	5 hr
Recipe testing and standardization	60 hr
Nutritional care 1 hr/subject/wk × 11 subjects × two 2-wk controlled diet periods	44 hr
Dietary assessment Two 3-day food records/subject @ 0.33 hr (20 min)/recorded day of intake	22 hr
Quality assurance Develop protocols Monitor compliance @ 1 hr/subject/wk × two 2-wk controlled diet periods	20 hr 44 hr
Communications 0.25 hr/subject/visit × 3 visits/wk × two 2-wk controlled diet periods	33 hr
Employee training	8 hr
Employee supervision 1 hr/protocol/day × 154 days	154 hr
Ordering and inventory 2 hr/wk × 44 wk	88 hr
Preparing and portioning food 0.75 hr/meal × 4 meals/day × 14 days/subject × two 2-wk controlled diet periods	924 hr
Sanitation 0.5 hr/day × 154 days	77 hr
Food safety 0.17 hr (10 min)/day × 154 days	26 hr
Outpatient study activities 0.33 hr (20 min)/day × 14 days/subject × two 2-wk controlled diet periods	102 hr
Total effort	1,607 hr per year
% Full-time equivalent (FTE)	77% (1,607 hr/2,080 hr/FTE = 0.77)

[1]Nutrition research staff positions usually are given the job title of senior research dietetic technician, administrative dietitian, or food production technician.

[2]Each year, Protocol 809 will enroll 11 subjects for two 2-wk controlled diet periods. For practical reasons, subjects are enrolled two at a time (ie, 5-6 pairs/yr, average 5.5 pairs/yr). The research kitchen thus will produce and deliver study diets for 154 days/yr (5.5 subject pairs/yr × 4 wk/yr × 7 days/wk).

EXHIBIT 20-7

Example of a Scheduling Flow Sheet for Participants Enrolled in Multiple Concurrent Studies

Name: Doe, J.

Date: 23-Jan-98

Date of Birth:

Height (cm):

Age (yr):

Weight (kg):

PROTOCOL COMPONENTS

High-phosphorus research diet
Vitamin D infusion study (urinary vitamin D metabolite assays)
24-hr diurnal variation (blood calcium and phosphorus assays)
EDTA infusion
Calcium Infusion

Date	Hospital Day		Protocol Day	Scheduled Activities
14-Jan-98	1	Thur	0	Begin high-phosphorus diet at dinner
15-Jan-98	2	Fri	1	Start vitamin D infusion in AM
16-Jan-98	3	Sat	2	
17-Jan-98	4	Sun	3	
18-Jan-98	5	Mon	4	Start 24-hr urine collections
19-Jan-98	6	Tues	5	Assay urine for vitamin D metabolites
20-Jan-98	7	Wed	6	Obtain assay results; adjust vitamin D infusion rate
21-Jan-98	8	Thur	7	
22-Jan-98	9	Fri	8	
23-Jan-98	10	Sat	9	
24-Jan-98	11	Sun	10	
25-Jan-98	12	Mon	11	0800 start 24-hr diurnal variation study (hourly phlebotomy for Ca and P levels)
26-Jan-98	13	Tues	12	0800 end 24-hr diurnal variation study; calcium infusion 0800-1130 (hold breakfast)
27-Jan-98	14	Wed	13	
28-Jan-98	15	Thur	14	EDTA infusion study (hold breakfast)
29-Jan-98	16	Fri	15	
30-Jan-98	17	Sat	16	
31-Jan-98	18	Sun	17	
01-Feb-98	19	Mon	18	
02-Feb-98	20	Tues	19	
03-Feb-98	21	Wed	20	0800 start 24-hr diurnal variation study (hourly phlebotomy for Ca and P levels)
04-Feb-98	22	Thur	21	0800 end 24-hr diurnal variation study; calcium infusion 0800-1130 (hold breakfast)
05-Feb-98	23	Fri	22	
06-Feb-98	24	Sat	23	
07-Feb-98	25	Sun	24	
08-Feb-98	26	Mon	25	EDTA infusion study (hold breakfast)
09-Feb-98		Tues		Discharge

EXHIBIT 20-8

Workday and Leave Coverage for Foodservice Staff Engaged in Multiple Concurrent Studies[1]

I. FTE required to maintain a basic staffing pattern of 3 foodservice personnel on duty 7 days/week.

Basic Coverage

One full-time equivalent (FTE) represents 8 hr/day × 260 working days/yr.
3.0 FTE/day × 7 days/week coverage/5 day standard work week = 4.2 FTE

II. FTE required to provide sick, holiday, and vacation leave for 4.2 FTE (see above):

Sick Leave (SL) Coverage

Based on an average absenteeism rate of 4.6% per year allowed by policy

260 working days/yr/FTE × 4.6%   =   12 SL days/yr
12 SL days/yr × 4.2 FTE   =   50.4 SL days/yr

$$\frac{50.4 \text{ SL days/yr}}{260 \text{ working day/yr/FTE}} = 0.19 \text{ FTE needed for absentee coverage}$$

Holiday Leave (HL) Coverage

Based on 12 holidays/yr/FTE

12 holidays/yr × 4.2 FTE   =   50.4 HL days/yr

$$\frac{50.4 \text{ HL days/yr}}{260 \text{ working days/yr/FTE}} = 0.19 \text{ FTE needed for holiday coverage}$$

Vacation Leave (VL) Coverage

Employees earn VL days based on length of service.
The 4.2 foodservice personnel in the research kitchen would earn a total of 78 VL days/yr.

$$\frac{78 \text{ VL days/yr}}{260 \text{ working days/yr/FTE}} = 0.30 \text{ FTE needed for VL coverage/yr}$$

III. Summary

Total FTE level necessary to provide 3.0 FTE coverage 7 days/wk, including all paid leave:

Basic 7 days/week coverage	4.20 FTE
Sick leave coverage	0.19 FTE
Holiday leave coverage	0.19 FTE
Vacation leave coverage	0.30 FTE
Total	4.88 FTE

[1]Example courtesy of Karen Todd, MS, RD, General Clinical Research Center, University of California, San Francisco.

physical and psychological well-being of the participants and ensure the scientific validity and integrity of the collected data. An integrated plan for continuous evaluation and improvement should be established for the preparation and delivery of research diets, for laboratory assays, and for the collection of dietary intake data. Stringent quality assurance begins with written policies and procedures, establishment of monitoring systems, and ongoing continuing education programs for employees.

A model for the development of a quality assurance program is provided in Figure 20-4; a sample procedure for implementation is shown in Table 20-11. Other aspects of quality assurance programs are discussed throughout this book (particularly in Chapter 18, "Documentation, Record Keeping, and Recipes," Chapter 21, "Performance Improvement for the Research Kitchen," and Chapter 22, "Validating Diet Composition by Chemical Analysis").

Well-chosen training programs for both new and experienced staff can be quite helpful. Considerable time and money can be saved and mistakes can be prevented by shortening the "trial-and-error" phase of the learning process. Some programs, such as those required by departments of health for hospital hygiene certification, are straightforward and readily available in many locations. It also may be desirable to arrange for additional training directed toward the specifics of research diet production in order to provide broader scientific perspectives for the daily work of the food-service workers. Such specialized classes are seldom available as part of regular degree programs in dietetics or nutrition, but they can be conducted effectively using a short-course format. Managers can develop their own on-site programs or can take advantage of courses open to the general community. (The Table of Contents for this book provides a list of topics that might compose such a training program. For examples of short course curricula, contact Director of Metabolic Kitchen, Pennington Biomedical Research Center, 6400 Perkins Road, Baton Rouge, LA 70808; and Director of Nutrition, Clinical Research Center, University of Indiana, 550 North University Boulevard, Indianapolis, IN 46202. See also MM Windhauser, A Ershow, Meeting the need for training on the design, preparation, and delivery of research diets, *J Am Diet Assoc,* in press.)

CONCLUSION: PRESENTATION AND PUBLICATION OF DATA

Research studies are not truly completed until their results are published. The nature of controlled diet studies means that members of the nutrition research staff, particularly those who are registered dietitians or have otherwise completed undergraduate and graduate degrees, usually are familiar with the scientific goals of the study, the protocol methodology, and the data collection activities. Many of the individuals in these positions can make valuable contributions to writing groups engaged in data analysis and manuscript preparation. They also may be interested in presenting the results of the study at scientific and professional meetings. For those wishing to undertake such efforts, activities at this level should be important components of their job descriptions, with appropriate allotments of time (see Exhibit 20-9).

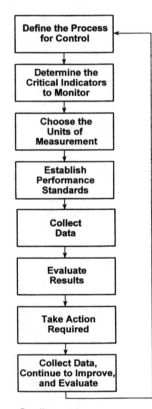

FIGURE 20-4. Quality assurance program: process flowchart.

The authors gratefully acknowledge the contributions of Donna Nickel to the development of tables in this chapter.

TABLE 20-11

Quality Assurance Program: Implementation Procedures

Quality Assurance Step	Procedures
Define the process for control	Develop standardized methods for the collection and analysis of dietary intake data. Use a specific procedure for each protocol.
Determine the critical indicators to monitor	Establish timelines for data entry. Establish guidelines for documentation of data obtained from participants. Establish tracking system to log receipt of data and completion of data analysis. Monitor results.
Choose the units of measurement	Monitor documentation errors (eg, accurate portion sizes, complete food descriptions, recipe yield etc), data entry logs, time lines, and results.
Establish performance standards	90% or better accuracy for documentation. 90% or better adherence to timelines. 10% or lower error rate for data entry and analysis.
Collect data	Conduct pilot study (eg, complete sample set of data or exercises using data collection instruments selected). Peer review and/or double entry of a subset of data. Collect random subset of data to monitor and designate timeline to be used.
Evaluate results	Assess the difference between the data collected and the performance standards.
Take action required	Provide additional training. Modify instruments as necessary. Complete quarterly documentation exercises.
Collect data, continue to improve, and evaluate	Monitor and verify controls.

EXHIBIT 20-9

Preparing Manuscripts and Scientific Presentations

Preparing manuscripts and scientific presentations can be a highly rewarding aspect of conducting research. The required allotment of effort varies greatly from project to project, but there is no question that writing is a skill that improves with practice.[1] The following are some of the issues to consider in planning publication activities:

Clearly define the purpose of the paper and one's role in writing it.

Roles often are given titles that clarify responsibilities (eg, lead author, coauthor, section writer, data verifier).

Review the design and scientific scope of the nutrition project to be described.

Initially it is helpful to review the protocol and consider how the elements of the study design (eg, parallel-arm vs crossover design; number and time course of treatments; enrollment criteria; number and characteristics of participants; pilot studies and methods development) should be reflected in the various sections of the research report (rationale, methods, results, discussion).

In collaboration with a statistician, review the nutrition data that will be reported.

Standardized forms are invaluable for data entry and analysis, although they require time to be developed and tested before the study is implemented.

Review the literature.

The degree of familiarity with the subject matter of the report will influence the time and effort required for this portion of the paper.

Determine which data displays will be developed.

Appropriate visual communication of the quantitative data collected during the study is crucial to the message of the publication. The information displays (ie, tables, charts, graphs, and other figures) are more likely to reinforce the goals of the presentation or manuscript if the following points are considered:[2]

- The data should be presented in a way that is based on the cognitive task at hand. Most authors ask their audiences to make comparisons or assess changes.
- The display should help lead the reader toward the mechanisms and other types of causality that the authors plan to address in the discussion section. Time sequences can provide useful explanations of process but are not always the best way to clarify causal relationships.
- The displays should enforce visual and quantitative comparisons. These comparisons are made more effectively when the data or images are physically adjacent (ie, placed next to each other), rather than separated (ie, within different figures, pages, or slides). It is particularly difficult to compare data presented in multiple pie charts.
- The visual presentation and the original data should have the same degree of complexity. This helps to keep the cognitive message clear, honest, and free of clutter. For example, three-dimensional bar graphs should not be used to convey two-dimensional data (such as frequency counts).

Make realistic forecasts of time estimates.

Many experienced investigators allot one half-day per week (or 10% of effort) or more for working on manuscripts. Drafting and then polishing papers usually takes much longer than originally expected. It often is wise to estimate the time required, and then either double the figure, or round up to the next unit of time (eg, for four hours, round up to one day; for three days, round up to one week).

---

[1]An excellent general guide to scientific writing is: Day RA. *How to Write and Publish a Scientific Paper.* 5th ed. 1998. Oryx Press, 4041 North Central Avenue, Phoenix, AZ 85012.

[2]These principles of information design are explained in a particularly insightful series of books by Tufte ER: *The Visual Display of Quantitative Information* (1983); *Envisioning Information* (1990); and *Visual Explanations* (1997); Graphics Press, Inc, Box 430, Cheshire, CT 06410.

CHAPTER 21

PERFORMANCE IMPROVEMENT FOR THE RESEARCH KITCHEN

ELAINE J. AYRES, MS, RD; MARJORIE BUSBY, MPH, RD; PATTI RIGGS, RD;
MICHELLE SANDOW-PAJEWSKI, MS, RD; AND CYNTHIA SEIDMAN, MS, RD

Performance improvement (PI) is a straightforward approach to ensuring the quality of dietetics and nutrition services for controlled feeding studies. PI programs start with externally imposed standards, such as those of the Joint Commission on the Accreditation of Healthcare Organizations (JCAHO, 1 Renaissance Boulevard, Oakbrook Terrace, IL 60181; [630]792-5000) (1). They are supplemented with the research dietitian's professional knowledge of nutrition, foodservice process control, and research methodology. The goal is to provide the best possible participant-centered service in support of the research protocol.

Performance improvement has two distinct components. The first is quality control. (See Figure 21–1.) The second is customer service and relations. (See Figure 21–2.) Whereas traditional quality control focuses on inspection, the cycle of continuous PI is not complete without the interaction of the customer (in this case, the research participant).

Quality goals for controlled feeding studies are based on state-of-the-art service or product standards. Determinants of quality goals are derived from three sources. First, the dietitian and metabolic kitchen staff have professional standards or specifications for clinical service and foodservice aspects of controlled feeding studies. Second, the principal investigator has standards or expectations for the nutritional aspects of the protocol and how these parameters will affect the outcomes of the study. Lastly, the subject has standards or expectations for both the food and the service received during participation in the study. This interdependence of professionals and participants provides the opportunity for better participant compliance, clearer expectations regarding diets and protocols, and the ability to continuously improve the methodology and the execution of the nutrition component of research studies.

QUALITY CONTROL

Quality control (QC) is the process of measuring the outcome of a procedure, comparing the outcome to a quality goal, and acting on the difference (2). (See Figure 21–1.) Quality control is not a one-time process of inspection; rather, it is a continuous loop where the product or service is measured against a quality standard or specification. Differences between expectations and actual outcome are evaluated, and the product is improved based on the data gathered. Data are then gathered again and evaluated in an ongoing cycle. This cycle leads to better performance through improved outcomes.

From the research dietitian's and research kitchen's perspective, every function that produces a tangible output can be defined in terms of a process. For example, tray assembly is a process made up of defined tasks with a clear beginning and end. The outcome of this process is a completed tray ready for service. The assessment of a participant prior to the start of a study is another process with defined professional tasks, a defined beginning, and a defined end.

The dietitian's role is to understand and control each of the processes of service. The customers of that process, the

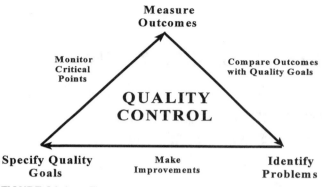

FIGURE 21-1.   The continuous quality improvement cycle for controlled feeding studies—elements of the process.

participant and investigator, see only the outcomes of the process. Therefore, the dietitian guarantees the consistent output of each process so that the customers of that process are satisfied. To achieve true improvement, constant attention to quality control of processes is necessary as well as continuous customer input. (See Figure 21–2.)

From the participant's perspective, the research team operates as a whole, and all of the research processes are integrated. Therefore, quality control is not an isolated procedure for just the nutritional aspects of the study. The research team needs to synchronize all of the critical processes of a particular protocol or work unit with the goal of positive participant outcomes.

In patient care, the patient receives services from the medical team. In the research setting, the relationships among the investigator, the participant, and staff are of a very different nature. The research study participant takes on the role of ensuring positive outcomes for the investigator and therefore becomes a "coproducer" with the research team (3). A triangular relationship is thus established between the investigator, the staff, and the participant, rather than the linear relationship seen in classic patient care situations. The dietitian and kitchen staff play an integral role in helping the participant understand this

relationship. Educational activities for participants should focus on the importance of adherence to meal consumption procedures and how the diet fits into the overall research protocol.

CONSTRUCTING A QUALITY CONTROL PROGRAM: THE SEVEN-STEP APPROACH

The concepts underlying process quality control are applicable to any aspect of controlled feeding studies. The Seven-Step Approach can be used to continuously monitor and improve the processes involved in diet development, food production, tray accuracy, tray delivery, and laboratory verification of diet composition. This approach can also be used to monitor and improve coordinated activities of the research team.

The number of critical points to monitor (ie, the number of indicators) should be determined by the operation. Professional judgment, the nature of the protocol, and the reactions of the customer will provide the best guide to which critical outcomes should be monitored. The JCAHO does not stipulate the number of indicators but advocates performance improvement programs that ultimately promote positive outcomes (1).

Quality control can and should be practiced by everyone who participates in research. Employees should be able to record and tabulate data if the data collection sheets are clear and easy to use. Data on factors such as food temperature, recipe yields, and refusals can be recorded by the staff. The dietitian, however, is responsible for reviewing the data, determining when a process is out of control or needs adjustment, setting the specifications for each critical element, and educating the staff as to these standards. The dietitian is also the liaison to other members of the research team. Indicators that measure protocol outcomes or ongoing processes of the

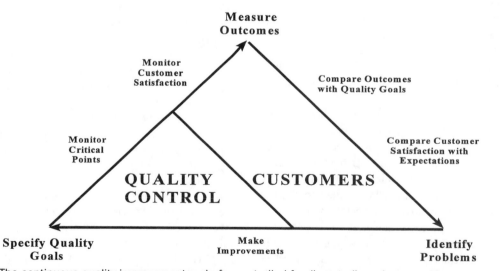

 FIGURE 21-2.   The continuous quality improvement cycle for controlled feeding studies—incorporating customer feedback.

whole research team are useful in improving the entire research process.

Step 1: Define the Process

Choose processes that are high-volume, high-risk, or problem-prone. Typical examples may be production of formula diets, the cook/chill process, or preparation of diet composites.

Step 2: Determine Which Critical Point(s) to Monitor

Any process may have one or more critical points. Choose the critical point or activity that most influences the outcome by constructing a flowchart. All critical points in a process need to be examined if improvements are to be achieved. Exhibit 21–1 describes how to flowchart a process and determine these points (4).

Step 3: Establish a Quality Goal or Specification for Each Critical Point

The critical point serves as the basis for what the JCAHO calls an "indicator" (1). An indicator is a measurement tool for gauging the success of a process. For foodservice procedures, the specification for critical points might be based on an industry standard, such as rethermalizing an entree to 165°F. The study protocol also can serve as a means of identifying goals or specifications. For example, a diet controlled for sodium might be specified to deliver 50 ± 1 mEq.

In the rethermalization example (Exhibit 21–1), a decision must be made when a prepared frozen item is removed from the freezer. Is the item used within the specified time frame? Does the item show signs of thawing or freezer burn? If so, the result would be an unsatisfactory product, with an "off" taste and poor texture. To ensure the desired outcome, the specifications for the critical point must be determined. In this case, specifications can be set for rotations of food in and out of the freezer; items can be dated and rotated accordingly.

Once specifications are determined, a quality control indicator can be identified, and compliance can be monitored. Such a quality control indicator might be stated as follows: Frozen prepared items are to be used within 2 months of production. If the data that have been collected on usage of frozen items indicate that wastage is occurring, then food production and storage practices should be examined and modified. The temperature critical point does not require extensive written documentation, but again, specifications for internal temperature of rethermalized foods need to be established and followed. See Exhibit 21–2 for guidelines (5–7).

Step 4: Collect Data About the Critical Point or Indicator

This step requires that measurable, observable facts be gathered about a particular point in a process. Examples would be the number of accurately assembled trays or the number of samples that meet the specifications for a liquid formula diet as determined by chemical analysis. Each critical point indicator should have a specially designed data collection sheet that reflects the conditions and sequence of activities for the particular operation or study.

Step 5: Determine the Difference Between the Data Collected and the Quality Goal

Some specifications are absolute, allowing no margin for error and no deviance from the standard. This concept of zero defects is necessary in certain situations; for example, a formula diet may not be served if the temperature exceeds 45°F. In other instances, variation is acceptable. For example, temperatures may fall within a certain range of acceptability. As specifications for foodservice and clinical activities are set, acceptable variation needs to be addressed and noted in the protocol. The concept of *threshold* is often used when defining acceptable variation. When variation of a process or outcome exceeds an acceptable level, an opportunity for improvement presents itself. It is at this time that a process is examined in detail for problems, and solutions are developed.

Customers may also signal that there is a problem by indicating dissatisfaction with the outcome; for example, there may be complaints that the food is always cold. Their expectations or standards may be different from the specifications established for the process. If this is the case, the process needs to be improved, and the specifications or quality goals must be set to meet or exceed the expectations of the customer.

Step 6: Improve the Process (Take Action on the Difference)

Improvement activities may include fine-tuning a process or eliminating unnecessary steps. If the process is complicated or the outcomes are poor, it may be necessary to establish a quality improvement team. In many cases, to guarantee the consistent output of a process, the monitoring phase continues even when thresholds are not crossed.

Step 7: Continue Data Collection for Continuous Improvement

Data collection about a critical point should continue until specifications are met or exceeded for at least 3 months. If

EXHIBIT 21-1

Using Process Flowcharts to Determine Critical Points

COMMENTARY

Flowcharts are used to help visualize a process. This enables the manager to specify how the system or process works (4). By definition, a process has a beginning and an end with a tangible output. The goal of the process is uniformity of product and consistent adherence to specifications. Once the critical points in the process have been identified, they can be used to develop performance specifications and can also serve as quality control indicators.

HOW TO CONSTRUCT A FLOWCHART

1. List each step in the process from beginning to end.
2. Identify the decision points (key junctions or critical points) in the process.
3. Enclose each step in a symbol:
   Decision points are enclosed by diamonds, ◇ .
   Other process steps are enclosed by rectangles, ▢.
4. At each decision point, show all possible options.

EXAMPLE OF A PROCESS FLOWCHART: RETHERMALIZATION OF A FROZEN ENTREE

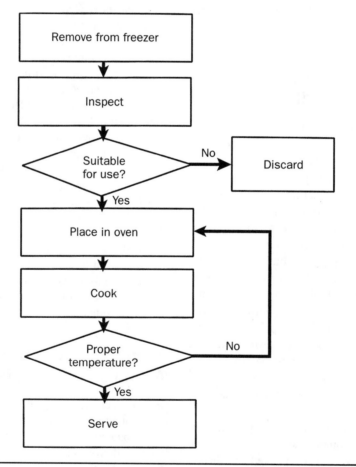

the process is under control, the frequency of data collection can be decreased. For high-volume processes, the sample size can be decreased. Less frequent monitoring will spare the time and staffing required to collect and tabulate data.

If an indicator no longer provides useful information about a process, or if the specifications are met consistently and customers are satisfied, the indicator can be eliminated. It is advisable to archive old data as a reference point for similar protocols or procedures.

EXHIBIT 21-2

Principles of Time/Temperature Control of Potentially Hazardous Foods

Cook food for at least 15 seconds to a required internal temperature:

165°F for poultry, stuffed meats, stuffed pasta.

155°F for ground beef, pork, ham, sausage, bacon.

145°F for beef roasts, fish.

Reheat foods for at least 15 seconds to a minimum of 165°F.

Cool solid foods or liquid formulas rapidly within 4 hours to 45°F using:

Shallow pans (2-in to 3-in depth).

Ice bath.

Agitation.

Loose-fitting covers.

No stacking.

Placement of food in coldest part of cooling unit.

Maintain equipment at proper temperatures:

Refrigeration units at 35°F to 45°F.

Freezer units at 0°F or below.

Provide calibrated thermometers for checking foods for proper and safe temperatures.

THE APPLICATION OF QUALITY CONTROL IN CONTROLLED FEEDING STUDIES

There are many ways in which the principles of quality process control can be applied to feeding studies. The following examples do not constitute a complete quality control program but reflect approaches that can transcend a variety of research settings and protocols. Critical decision points (determined from flowcharts) and potential indicators are identified for each process.

Diet Development

The process of diet development begins with establishing specifications and ends with the successful calculation of diets that meet the requirements of the study. One critical point that must be monitored is the calculation of the diet and/or a specific food item. This is typically done with the help of iterative computer programs that compare the output with the specifications of the protocol. The quality goal of this process is to develop a diet with a nutrient composition that is within the range specified in the protocol. Therefore, diets exceeding this acceptable variation require modification and recalculation. To ensure optimum quality control, appropriate limits for nutrients should be established with the investigator during the development of the protocol.

Another critical point that may be used for diet development is a comparison of the computerized analysis and the laboratory analysis of prepared samples of the study diet. Again, the quality goal would be that the actual composition of the food falls within the levels specified by the research protocol.

The diet development phase of a study does not require an indicator per se. Because each diet will be reworked until it meets the specifications of the protocol, ongoing analysis of the calculation process itself is not necessary. In some cases, however, it may not be possible to meet original protocol specifications for specific foods or menus because of problems with availability, compositional variability, palatability, participant acceptance, difficulty of preparation, or storage. These obstacles should be addressed with the investigator during the protocol development stage.

Food Production

The purpose of food production for research diets is to provide a specialized diet or food product that meets protocol specifications. Because the actual production of the research diet involves multiple steps, a great deal of effort is required to ensure levels of accuracy and efficiency. Even the best planned diet, however, will not produce the desired outcome (ie, high compliance by participants) if it is not prepared safely, or on time, or if the food is so unpalatable that it is not consumed. The critical points to monitor in food production include:

- Procurement of food items that can be prepared to meet specifications.
- Preparation of individual food items according to recipes or research standards.
- Weighing of food items.
- Labeling of food items.

- Packaging of food items.
- Rethermalization of food items.
- Length of time the foods are stored (frozen, refrigerated, or on the shelf).

All of these areas are crucial internal controls for the food production process and applicable to any protocol.

Food Safety

Food safety is a serious concern in the production of research diets. Fortunately, the food industry has provided an excellent model for preventing foodborne illness. The Hazard Analysis Critical Control Point (HACCP) concept was devised by the Pillsbury Company, the US Army Natick Research and Development Laboratories, and the National Aeronautics and Space Administration in the 1960s for providing safe food in outer space (5). HACCP is a widely used systems approach to quality control that focuses particularly on microbial control.

HACCP is a preventive system in which safety checks are designed into the food formulation and production processes. The hazard analysis portion of HACCP as defined by Bauman (6) is "the identification of sensitive ingredients, sensitive areas in the processing of the food or ingredients, people control, etc, from which we can identify the critical points that must be monitored to assure safety of the product. Critical control points are those areas in the chain of food production from raw materials to finished product where the loss of control can result in an unacceptable food safety risk."

When analyzing hazards, Bobeng (7) considers the following factors: (1) potentially hazardous ingredients, (2) biologic and physical hazards in processing, and (3) potential for consumer abuse. Therefore, critical control points commonly fall into the following categories: microbiology, sanitation, time/temperature ranges, and employee cleanliness.

Potentially hazardous foods are usually of animal origin and have high moisture content and neutral pH. Cooked vegetables and legumes and raw bean sprouts also have these characteristics. Other foods fall into this category because they involve multiple preparation steps or major temperature changes (ie, cook/cool/reheat), or are prepared several hours or days before serving.

Compared to other hospital foodservice systems, the production of controlled research diets is distinguished by additional steps. These may include:

1. Precise, time-consuming weighing of food on electronic balances.
2. Freezer, refrigerator, or shelf storage of weighed foods for a period of time before the diet study begins.
3. Overnight thawing of precision-weighed foods.
4. Tray assembly of foods that are inspected for accuracy prior to service.
5. Overnight refrigeration of completed trays.
6. Microwave heating at the time of service.

7. Packing of research diets for consumption away from the research center.

To establish critical control points, determine the production stages at which bacteria can be destroyed, growth minimized, and contamination prevented. Specifications to minimize bacterial growth should be based on time/temperature ranges and sanitation guidelines for equipment and dietary staff.

Monitoring involves checking and verifying proper processing and handling procedures at the identified critical control points. One of the most important monitoring techniques is measuring food temperatures during preparation and storage. Time/temperature analysis should be performed by taking several readings at varied intervals to ensure that potentially hazardous foods reach a safe temperature within the required time period.

Foods used for weighed research diets are usually small portions that readily attain the safe temperature range when refrigerated. However, the time it takes to weigh and prepare these foods must be as short as possible to prevent excessive bacterial growth. The dietary staff needs to be well informed about the relationship of time and temperature ranges to risk of foodborne illness (Exhibit 21–2).

Tray Accuracy

The process of ensuring accuracy of tray contents includes not only accurate delivery of food items to the study participant but also accurate substitutions for foods not consumed at the previous meal. Critical points in this process include:

- **Using the correct utensils to portion foods.** For each food item or group, establish specifications for appropriate utensils that correspond to the desired portion. Consistency and accuracy are crucial in the production of research diets. Quality control for portioning is governed by clear specifications and training of kitchen staff; data collection is not usually necessary.
- **Correctly weighing each food item on the menu.** Again, consistency and accuracy are crucial for research diets.
- **Placing foods on the tray.** The specification or the indicator for this would be that all trays contain all of the items, and only the items, listed on the menu. This can be monitored as the tray leaves the kitchen or at the point of service. The expected standard is 100% accuracy. Monitoring returned trays is useful in delineating compliance to a protocol. For offsite meals, accuracy is extremely important because substitutions are not readily available.
- **Establishing substitutions for each research kitchen's and each protocol's procedures and specifications.** Making inappropriate substitutions may prompt further data collection, or the staff or participants must be educated as to suitable alternatives. When substitutions are needed routinely for a particular research diet, the appropriateness of the diet or the restrictions or the production process should be investigated. Requests for replacement foods

also may signal participant dissatisfaction. Procedures should be established for documenting substitutions.

Tray Delivery

Tray delivery is the process of serving the meal trays in the appropriate location and in a timely fashion. The critical points in tray delivery are:

- The trays must be served to participants either over a particular time period established by the feeding facility or at more precise times specified by a protocol. A common specification is that trays be served within 15 minutes of the established meal times. If a protocol specifies timed meal service, staff must establish a realistic variance on the specified time with the investigator. Once the allowed variance is established, service can be evaluated against this goal.
- The time elapsed between tray assembly and delivery must be in compliance with foodservice standards. Tray assembly and delivery time should not exceed 20 minutes to maintain appropriate food temperatures, appearance, and palatability. This can be easily measured by monitoring the time from the beginning of tray assembly to the time the tray is served to the participant. If this process takes longer than normal variance will allow, the process of assembly and delivery should be examined.

Intake

The goal of the intake process is the full consumption of the research meal. The critical points include: educating the participant about the importance of full consumption; recording intake, substitutions, or discrepancies; and communicating any issues related to intake or discrepancies to the research team. The process begins by determining preferences via questionnaire or interview so that the planned diet reflects participants' wants and needs.

It also is vital to educate participants regarding the importance of intake. The participants' understanding can be increased by providing printed materials about the research diet, written expectations about consumption, and one or more sample research meals. As a general rule, the more information provided to participants, the better the compliance with the research meal. The dietitian must inform the investigator about dietary noncompliers and document each instance of noncompliance.

During the feeding period, the research participant may also be provided with incentives to comply with the diet. By using the behavior modification techniques of reward and withdrawal of privileges, compliance can be increased. For example, adults who consume a research diet can be treated to a gourmet dinner after the protocol is finished. Incentive programs are especially important for the pediatric population; children can be given small trinkets.

Questionnaires about the acceptability of meals can provide documented feedback from the participants. This information then can be used to make adjustments to the research meals as described in the next section.

Refusals

Food refusals may indicate that the research diet is in some way unacceptable to the participant. Collecting data about refusals thus will help investigators decide whether they need to educate the participants, train the staff, or modify the food. Critical points in the process of monitoring food refusals include weighing or estimating food after it is returned to the research kitchen and documenting the episode. Sometimes the refused food is labeled and stored. Each one of these critical points requires standardized procedures with which staff are familiar. Data on the process can then be tracked by participant or by protocol. If specified by the protocol, substitutions may be needed.

Research kitchen personnel are responsible for recording the refusals of all foods. This should be done using the same balance on which the food was originally weighed during production. The dietitian is responsible for collecting the data on refusals and calculating the research participants' actual intake. Once this calculation has been done, a prompt report to the investigator and/or a note on the medical record is required. The dietitian must maintain an accessible record of all intake data to use for development of future research diets.

Diet Composition

Research diets must be prepared to meet the specifications of the protocol. This means that the diet must contain relevant nutrients at the levels required to test the hypothesis. Once the diets are designed and produced, their composition must be verified through an independent method of chemical assay. Food analysis protocols should reflect study design features such as the number of research diets, the length of the menu cycles, and the required degree of precision for nutrients of highest interest (such as the range of dietary sodium values for a study of blood pressure). A detailed discussion of food composition methodology is provided in Chapter 22, "Validating Diet Composition by Chemical Analysis."

Demonstrating that nutrient composition is constant over time is concrete evidence that good quality control has been used in producing the research diet. *Calorimetry,* the science of measuring quantities of heat, can be used as a tool to ensure consistent quality by determining the gross energy of the food (8). This is a particularly convenient way to monitor compositional consistency of formula diets, which are constructed from a small number of constituent components. The oxygen bomb calorimeter is considered the standard method for measuring the caloric value (heat of combustion) of liquid or solid foods. The bomb calorimeter consists of a closed container surrounded by an enclosure with a constant volume of water. The weighed food sample is ignited by an electric spark and burned in an oxygen atmosphere inside the closed chamber. The rise in the temperature of the water after complete burning of the food is used to calculate the heat energy liberated. (Bomb calorimetry is rarely used for assessing the caloric content of whole-food diets.)

The heat energy measured in a bomb calorimeter may be expressed either as calories (cal), British thermal units (Btu), or Joules (J). One calorie is equivalent to the heat energy needed to raise the temperature of one gram of water 1°C (from 15°C to 16°C); 1,000 calories are equivalent to the familiar kilocalorie (kcal). The gross energy is determined by the heat of combustion and is calculated from the initial weight. Conversion factors are used to convert from gross energy to metabolizable energy per gram of test sample (Table 21–1) (9, 10).

There are several critical points in this process which can be monitored to ensure quality data. (See Figure 21–3 for the flow chart of the bomb calorimetry process.) The first critical point is the consistency of the sample. Samples must be homogenized to a uniform consistency. This is best determined by taking aliquots from successive layers of the homogenate and assaying them separately. (This topic is also addressed in Chapter 22, "Validating Diet Composition by Chemical Analysis.") If complete homogenization is not achieved, another sample is prepared.

A minimum of six replicates is run for each food (or diet) and the average taken. There are two other samples that must be used to ensure accuracy. The first is a known standard such as benzoic acid. At this point, if a variance is noted, corrections must be applied to adjust the test sample for any heat transfer occurring during the runs. In addition, a previously analyzed "known" sample is also assayed and compared to the test sample. Results must fall within the specifications or range set by the investigator and the dietitian; usually a 5% variance is allowed. If the analysis indicates that the composition falls outside the limits set by the investigator, it may be necessary to discard the batch and evaluate the process of formula preparation from start to finish.

THE ART OF SERVICE: GUARANTEEING PARTICIPANT SATISFACTION

The transition from traditional quality control to PI is contingent on feedback from individuals who receive a product or service. In PI terminology, those who receive a product or service are called "customers" (2). Therefore, PI for controlled feeding studies should include monitoring the processes of the research kitchen, but it should also reflect the needs and wants of participants and investigators.

Quality of service is measured through "the eye of the beholder," and, in the case of a research study, a dissatisfied participant is a noncompliant participant. The first step in ensuring that participants remain satisfied is to understand that quality service is not the same as quality control. A service is created at the instant of delivery, and it is at that point that the participant decides whether it is good or bad. Albrecht (11) describes this critical point as a "moment of truth." The job of the research kitchen staff is to engineer positive moments of truth for the participant.

The concepts of quality service vs quality products are compared in Table 21–2 (12). The key to quality service revolves around the personnel involved in the research setting. Each time any member of the research team interacts with a participant at any point in the research process, the concept of positive moments of truth should be used. Why? Without the participant, there is no clinical research.

A typical moment of truth for a controlled feeding study occurs when the tray is delivered and the cover removed. It is at this point that the participant experiences the reality of a research diet. A positive moment of truth in this situation would be an attractively arranged tray with foods served at their proper temperatures. Another moment of truth may be the interaction with the staff. Friendly encouragement and a sense of how the diet relates to the study as a whole are crucial elements in participant compliance, especially if the diet is difficult to consume.

The best way to find out whether service is measuring up to expectations of the participant is to ask. It is more difficult to design and complete service measurements than

TABLE 21-1

Energy Value of a Liquid Formula as Determined by Bomb Calorimetry[1]

Source	Nutrient	Gross Energy (Heat of Combustion) (kcal/g)[2]	Metabolizable Energy (Physiological Fuel Value) (kcal/g)[2]
Milk whey (Promix®)	Protein	5.65	4.0
Corn oil	Fat	9.30	9.0
Dextrin (Polycose®)	Carbohydrate	4.10	4.0
Prepared formula (calculated)[3]	—	1.37	1.25

[1]Courtesy of Cindy Seidman, MS, RD, and Jalanta D. Tremaroli, MS, RD, General Clinical Research Center, Rockefeller University, New York.
[2]Energy values are based on the Atwater system as reported in references 9 and 10.
[3]Observed gross energy value of prepared formula = $1.41 \neq 0.02$ kcal/g (n = 102 batches). Distribution of energy: 15% protein, 40% fat, 55% carbohydrate. Recipe: 25 g Promix, 21.2 g corn oil, 58.4 g Polycose, 295.4 g water.

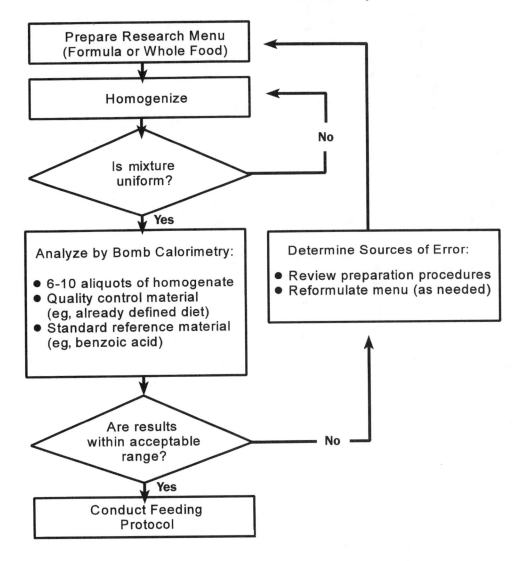

FIGURE 21-3.   Flowchart of the bomb calorimetry process.

TABLE 21-2

Comparison of Quality Control Features for Processes or Products vs Services (12)

Process or Product	Service
The goal is uniformity.	The goal is uniqueness; each participant is "special."
A product can be put into inventory.	A service happens "at the moment"; it cannot be stockpiled.
The participant is an end user who is not involved in the production process.	The participant is a coproducer who is a partner in creating the service.
Managers conduct quality control by comparing output to specifications.	Participants conduct quality control by comparing expectations to experience.
If improperly produced, the product can be discarded.	If improperly performed, apologies are the only means of recourse.
The morale of production employees is important.	The morale of service employees is critical.

to check whether a product meets a specification. The best assessments of quality service measure both customer perceptions and employee behaviors. Participant surveys (verbal or written) are the most direct way of obtaining this information. Participants need not be asked for information that can be measured directly by the staff (eg, the correct serving temperature). Survey tools are best used to ask questions that only the "customer" can answer. Exhibit 21–3 provides a sample participant satisfaction survey.

CONCLUSION: RECOMMENDATIONS OF THE JCAHO

The Joint Commission on the Accreditation of Healthcare Organizations (JCAHO) periodically revises its standards on quality assessment (1). This process has traditionally focused on monitoring mistakes or errors. Performance improvement recognizes that mistakes or errors may occur. However, when management recognizes that the staff are motivated and competent to perform their duties, it becomes the norm to view problems as opportunities to improve processes and therefore improve participant outcomes.

Quality control activities typically have been conducted along departmental or discipline lines. With performance improvement, teams or groups that span different disciplines are encouraged to integrate assessment and improvement activities. The research team provides a natural organizational unit for these activities, and each protocol provides a mechanism for clearly defining desired participant and research outcomes. When these outcomes are well defined, the critical processes can be monitored and improved using the seven-step process described earlier. The protocol states the expected outcome. The indicator simply enables the team to assess whether the study methodology is producing the desired outcomes. If not, corrections in the study can be made.

The JCAHO recommends that processes that are high-risk, high-volume, or problem-prone in terms of participant outcome become the primary indicators for data collection. For a research kitchen or metabolic diet ward these indicators may be designed for a specific protocol or they may transcend multiple protocols. An indicator that might apply to all protocols, for example, addresses adequate prestudy blood work to ensure sound nutritional status. Another might be whether participants actually attained the desired blood level of a nutrient after consuming a depletion diet.

EXHIBIT 21-3

General Clinical Research Center Patient Satisfaction Questionnaire[1]

Date:_____   Type of Diet:_____

How many meals did you eat at the GCRC?

Did you receive enough food?

How would you rate the metabolic research staff?

How would you rate the appearance of your food?

How would you rate the taste of your food?

What did you like best about the meals?

What did you like least about the service?

Other comments:

[1]Provided courtesy of General Clinical Research Center, University of Virginia, Richmond, Va.

The research team should examine the frequency of the event or activity in question, the significance of the event in the context of the research question, and the extent to which an indicator has been demonstrated to be free of problems. Ongoing monitoring and data collection efforts should be focused on critical activities in processes that affect participant or research outcomes. The JCAHO does not specify numbers of indicators, and an indicator need not be continued if it does not reveal the potential for improvement. The goal is to generate meaningful information that can be used to improve the process. If a process is under control, it should be stopped and another critical area examined. If a process is out of control and exceeds a tolerable threshold, the team must plan and implement a solution and continue to monitor the indicator until the outcome reaches the expected level.

REFERENCES

1. Joint Commission on the Accreditation of Healthcare Organizations. *1998 Hospital Accreditation Standards.* Oakbrook Terrace, Ill: JCAHO; 1998.
2. Juran JM, ed. *Juran's Quality Control Handbook.* 4th ed. New York, NY: McGraw Hill; 1988.
3. Barzelay M. *Breaking Through Bureaucracy—A New Vision for Managing in Government.* Berkeley, Calif: University of California Press; 1992.
4. Senge PM. *The Fifth Discipline.* New York, NY: Doubleday Currency; 1990.
5. Sperber W. The modern HACCP system. *Food Technol.* 1991;45:115–120.
6. Bauman H. HACCP: concept, development, and application. *Food Technol.* 1990;44:146.
7. Bobeng GJ, David BD. HACCP models for quality control of entree production in hospital food service systems. *J Am Diet Assoc.* 1978;73:524–529.
8. Greenfield H, Southgate DAT. Analytical methods for the production of food composition data. In: *Food Composition Data: Production, Management, and Use.* New York, NY: Elsevier Applied Science; 1992.
9. US Dept of Agriculture. *Energy Value of Foods: Basis and Derivation.* Agricultural Handbook No 74. Washington, DC: Agricultural Research Service; 1975. (Electronic version can be downloaded from the USDA Web site http:/www.nal.usda.gov/fnic/foodcomp.)
10. US Dept of Agriculture. *Composition of Foods: Raw, Processed, Prepared.* Agricultural Handbook No 8. Washington, DC: Agricultural Research Service; 1963: 159–165.
11. Albrecht K. *At America's Service.* Homewood, Ill: Dow JonesIrwin; 1988.
12. Zemke R. The emerging art of service management. *Training.* January 1992:37–42.

PART 5

Enhancing the Outcome of Dietary Studies

CHAPTER 22

VALIDATING DIET COMPOSITION BY CHEMICAL ANALYSIS

KATHERINE M. PHILLIPS, PHD; AND KENT K. STEWART, PHD

This chapter describes conceptual issues, selected methods, and a general approach to the field of chemical analysis of diets. Readers desiring more specific information on methods and procedures may contact our laboratory (Food Analysis Laboratory Control Center, KM Phillips, Director, Department of Biochemistry, 304 Engel Hall, Virginia Polytechnic Institute and State University, Blacksburg, VA 24060-0308; [540]231-9960 or kmpvpi@vt.edu).

WHY SHOULD DIETS BE CHEMICALLY ANALYZED?

Preliminary estimates of nutrient levels in research diets are made by calculation from food composition databases, but the diets themselves still must be chemically assayed. Why should this be, if composition data are available for the foods and nutrients of interest? This is a reasonable question that deserves a thoughtful response, especially because chemical analysis of diets can be expensive.

There are really three reasons for assaying the diets used in controlled diet studies. The first is to develop diets with the desired nutrient concentrations; the second is to verify, prior to feeding, that the prepared diets have the desired

nutrient levels, and the third is to document the constancy of dietary composition over the course of the study. If experimental diets do not have the designed nutrient levels, and especially if the diets are not chemically distinguishable from each other, the study hypothesis will not have been subjected to a valid test.

DIFFERENCES BETWEEN CALCULATED AND CHEMICALLY ASSAYED NUTRIENT VALUES

Food Composition Databases and Individual Foods

The primary source of food composition data in the United States is the USDA *Nutrient Database for Standard Reference* ("USDA Database") (1), which is the origin of the values in most other widely used food composition tables, computer databases, and menu planning software. The USDA database was developed to provide average (or weighted average) food composition values applicable to the nation as a whole. The data are subject to many sources of variance in sample collection (such as varieties, brands, seasons, and locations) and to many other factors affecting nutrient content values, including plant cultivar and maturity, soil and water composition, feedstock for animals, and postharvest storage and processing/cooking. As a result, it is very likely that the nutrient content of a specific sample of food (as would be purchased for a feeding study) will differ from the average values published in the USDA (or other) database. The greater the naturally occurring nutrient variance in a food item, the greater the potential that the database average will not reflect the composition of a selected sample of that food. For example, in a report by the International Food Biotechnology Council (2), the ratio of the highest level to the lowest level of some common nutrients in commercial vegetables ranged from about 1.5 for potassium to 12.6 for sucrose in green beans to 15 for carotene in tomatoes. For most of the foods, for most of the nutrients, this ratio ranged from 2 to 5. Piironen, Varo, and Coivistoinen (3) found relative standard deviations (RSDs) of up to 50% in the vitamin E content of baked rye breads. Slover, Lanza, and Thompson (4) found RSDs as high as 28% for the total fat content of beef and up to 16% for the cholesterol content of fast foods. In this same study the range of cholesterol content in fast food hamburgers was 26.5 to 48.3 mg/100 g; for french fries the range was 7.2 to 16.4 mg/100 g.

This issue has been examined carefully for vitamin C. Vanderslice and Higgs (5) found the vitamin C content of several major food sources to vary by a factor of two. Consequently, for a later study of the bioavailability of vitamin C from fresh broccoli and oranges, crates of the products, each from a single cultivar and supplier, were assayed. The relative standard deviation of the vitamin C content of broccoli and oranges was, respectively, 16% and 14% among crates and 7% and 13% within crates (6), and these values differed considerably from those reported in the USDA database (Table 22–1).

As a result, the foods for this study were analyzed on a continuing basis and amounts in the diet were adjusted to ensure targeted levels of vitamin C. Had this not been done,

errors and variance in vitamin C intake likely could have impaired the detection of biological effects.

The concentrations of some nutrients in some foods vary with the season of the year or from year to year, for example, fat and protein in soybeans (7), sodium, calcium, and zinc in tomatoes (8), and fatty acids in milk (9). Such variance may lead to changes in levels of experimental nutrients in diets during the course of a feeding intervention. This drift is of particular concern in long-term crossover studies, in which each subject serves as his or her own control.

The composition of the food supply also shifts with time because of changing agricultural production and food-processing practices. For example, the fat content of pork has been declining, presumably because of changes in the production operations of that industry (10). Likewise, there has been a general decrease in the amount of sodium added to processed foods in response to dietary recommendations to limit sodium intake. Some processed foods, such as certain brands of potato chips, may not be consistently made with the same oil, which causes variance in the fatty acid composition of different lots. Updates to food composition tables usually lag well behind these changes.

Assay methodology can also affect the validity of database values. Standard methods for particular nutrients are often applied to foods that are different from those for which the analytical procedure was designed and validated. If an assay method is faulty or inappropriate, data obtained by that method will be inaccurate. Analytical methods are continually being improved, and standard methods are being updated. Such improvements and revisions alter estimates of the composition of foods.

For instance, the studies of Marshall et al (11, 12) demonstrated that cholesterol values measured by gas-liquid chromatography (the current method of choice) were only about 68% of cholesterol values measured colorimetrically. Presumably these differences resulted from inclusion of plant sterols in the (now outdated) colorimetric assay results. Until recently this was the method by which most food da-

TABLE 22-1

Assayed Vitamin C Content of Broccoli and Orange Products Taken from Multiple Crates Within a Single Shipping Lot[1]

| | Vitamin C Content | | | |
| | Assayed Value | | | USDA Database Value[3] |
Sample	Mean (mg/100g)	Range (mg/100g)	RSD[2] (%)	Mean (mg/100g)
Broccoli, raw	121.2	88–163	15.5	93.2
Brocooli, cooked	80.2	55–121	19.0	62.8
Oranges, navel	75.9	65–86	14.0	57.3
Orange juice (frozen, reconstituted)	43.8	42–46	5.0	38.9

[1]Vanderslice JT, Higgs DJ (5):117–119.
[2]RSD = Relative standard deviation (= SD ÷ mean).
[3]US Department of Agriculture database as cited in (5).

tabase values were generated. This issue is also raised by the work of Wills, Balmer, and Greenfield (13), who reported the fat content of a variety of foods determined by five commonly used methods; the fat content of peanut butter ranged from 38.7% to 51.8% and the fat content of soybean flour ranged from 15.8% to 19.5%.

Users of a food composition database often are not able to evaluate its credibility because many databases do not adequately document the quality or source of data. For example, Lurie et al (14) demonstrated that the published copper concentration values for more than half of the foods that are primary contributors of this element in the American diet are based on poor or limited analytical data.

In addition, some of the values in food composition databases are not obtained from direct assays but rather are imputed from "similar" foods or from the raw materials that go into a recipe for a food. The accuracy of values obtained by imputation may well be unacceptable for feeding studies. For commercial products, the 1990 Nutrition Labeling and Education Act (15) allowed and encouraged manufacturers to use an algorithm to adjust analytical values and thereby to derive nutrient label values for a food item. Each and every individual package of the product is also required to *meet or exceed* the labeled nutrient values for some nutrients, but for others, the law requires concentrations to *meet or be less than* the labeled nutrient values. Consequently, nutrition label data may substantially yet legally understate or overstate the actual nutrient content of an individual package of a food (16).

Food identification and preparation practices also result in inconsistencies between calculated and actual dietary nutrient levels. Nomenclature can be a significant problem because the same names may refer to different foods, menus, or products in various regions within a country or in different cultures (17). Even if a particular item is accurately portrayed in the database, if that food is misidentified by those preparing the diets, the calculated composition of the diet may be in error. Misidentifications are not uncommon in the kitchen, and the supervisory dietitian needs to be alert to this possibility. Furthermore, food preparation habits vary widely by cook, by kitchen, by culture, and by region. Recipes for prepared foods (eg, "meat loaf" and "lasagna") also can differ markedly and can considerably affect the composition of prepared foods. Cooking methods, times, and temperatures, trimming of meats, and peeling of fruits and vegetables can influence concentrations and oxidation states of food constituents such as vitamins, fatty acids, dietary fiber, starch, sugars, and cholesterol.

Examples of Calculated and Assayed Nutrient Content of Research Diets

The obvious question raised when planning whole food diets is, how large are differences between the calculated and actual nutrient contents likely to be? Table 22–2 summarizes some of the potential sources of variance and error in the nutrient content of experimental diets. Certainly, deviations will be affected by many factors other than those that influence the actual composition of individual foods, including the quality (ie, accuracy and completeness) of the particular food composition database used, the accuracy with which diets are coded for calculations, control of food procurement, the accuracy and precision of food measurement and preparation, the specific foods used, the duration of the feeding trial, and the particular nutrients studied. Overall nutrient deviations will likely vary, and probably decrease, as one moves from analysis of *individual foods* to analysis of *daily menus* and then *diet cycles*. Few data are available, however, to clarify this issue. Table 22–3 shows tentative qualitative estimates of expected deviations for selected nutrients, based on our own experience in analyzing experimental diets.

Our laboratory has validated diets for both the DELTA (Dietary Effects on Lipoproteins and Thrombogenic Activity) (18) and DASH (Dietary Approaches to Stop Hypertension) (19, 20) studies, two multicenter programs with rigorous diet design and diet composition quality control protocols. Figure 22–1 shows the assayed sodium content as a percent of the calculated level in 12 daily menus developed for the DASH study. In this case, the target sodium concentration was 3,000 mg/day, and the mean assayed content was 92% of target. If the menus had not been assayed, sodium in the diet would have been assumed to be 240 mg/day higher on average than it actually was. Furthermore, sodium in individual menus ranged from 55% to 112% of target, suggesting variable bias in calculated concentrations depending on the particular foods and menu.

Figure 22–2 shows analytical data from the prefeeding phase of the DELTA study. The mean assayed cholesterol content of 12 prepared menus was 87% of the calculated target of 300 mg/day. The menu-to-menu variability in cholesterol content illustrated by Figure 22–2 also suggests that the quality of data for this nutrient may vary by food. Similar results were obtained for total fat (21). In this study, validating menus prior to the feeding phase of the study allowed the investigators to eliminate menus that substantially deviated from target nutrient composition.

The State of Food Analysis Methodology

The state of the art in food analysis is less well developed than the more familiar clinical chemistry. For example, blood and body fluids are reasonably well-defined matrices in which analytes, such as cholesterol, are evenly distributed. Hence, dispensing uniform subsamples is straightforward. In addition, standard methods, commercial kits, and often automated systems are available for rapid determination of many blood or urine components. Concentrations of many analytes are defined by physiological limits, and standard samples for precise quality control are frequently available. Intra- and inter-laboratory reference or calibration samples and systems are

TABLE 22-2

Sources of Error and Variance in Nutrient Content of Experimental Diets

Source	Examples
Features of study design	Number of different diets
	Number of feeding periods
	Number of study sites
	Length of study/feeding periods
	Magnitude of difference in nutrient concentrations of treatment diets
	Number of menus and energy levels in diet cycle
	Nutrient levels that are intended *not* to differ
	Units of target nutrient concentrations (eg, % kcal; g/day)
Menu calculation and nutrient database	Variance across calculated menus vs calculated diets
	Number of different foods used
	Precision of weight specification for food items
	Experience of person calculating the diets
	Quality of data in the food composition database
	Completeness of database (number of missing and imputed values)
	Natural variance in food composition (database values are average values)
Food chemistry	Within-assay coefficient of variation, between-assay coefficient of variation
	Stability of nutrient during storage
	Lability of nutrient during cooking/food preparation
	Accuracy of lab (eg, ability to achieve accurate results for relevant standard reference material)
	Validity of analytical methodology (ie, reliable and accurate vs weak or problematic[1])
	Homogeneity of composites
	Comparability of diet samples assayed to diets as consumed
	Assay quality control (eg, ability of quality control sample to monitor precision and accuracy of analysis system)
Food preparation	Experience of staff preparing foods.
	Food procurement protocol (eg, single lots vs multiple purchases)
	Standardization of preparation and cooking methods
	Accuracy and precision in weighing foods (including calibration of balances)

[1] See Table 22–4.

also available for laboratory calibration and certification. (Reference samples are chosen to have a background matrix similar to that of study samples, like food or plasma, and are well characterized for the analyte of interest.)

Food matrices are usually more complex than the biological fluids and tissues seen in a clinical laboratory. Not only are there hundreds to thousands of different compounds per cell type (as found in clinical samples), but a typical diet has components from numerous plant and animal sources combined with other pure and semipure ingredients. Many foods have active enzyme systems that, when released during food processing, may cause significant chemical transformations. Thermal degradation of some food components also occurs during processing and cooking. Food and diet samples are frequently heterogeneous in texture and composition, and nutrients are not usually distributed uniformly within the sample.

Another difference between food and clinical samples is that metabolite concentrations in clinical samples typically range from about 1 nMolar to 100 mMolar (a 100 million-fold range), whereas nutrient concentrations in foods usually range from 1 nMolar to 1 Molar (a billion-fold range). Thus, compared with clinical methods, the assays used for foods must be able to detect nutrient analytes over a much wider range of concentrations. This makes assays of foods yet more difficult, because analytical methods and quality control materials typically are developed and validated for specific and limited nutrient concentration ranges. If a particular sample has a higher or lower concentration of the analyte, then a different aliquot weight and/or dilutions will be required. Multiple quality control materials and considerable preliminary testing may also be necessary.

Nutrient assay methods are particularly matrix dependent. That is, the same method might yield different results depending on the overall composition of the food or diet. For instance, if acid hydrolysis is used to determine total fat in a sample that is high in carbohydrate, coextraction of the carbohydrate will give falsely elevated fat values (22, p. 95).

TABLE 22-3

Sources of Error and Variance in Nutrient Content of Experimental Diets: Qualitative Estimates of Magnitude for Selected Nutrients[1]

Source	Fat/Fatty Acids	Sugars	Cholesterol	Vitamin E	Selenium
Number of feeding periods/duration of study[2]	M	M	M	M	M
Completeness of database	S	L	S	L	L
Natural variance in food composition[2]	M	M-L	M-L	L	L
Lability of nutrient during storage and cooking/food preparation (also see Table 22–7)	M[3]	L[4]	M[5]	L[5]	S-M[3]
Homogeneity of composites	L	M	M	M	M
Food procurement and preparation standards[2]	L	L	L	L	L
Accuracy and precision of weighing foods[6]	M	M	S-M	S	S
Experience of person calculating the diets	L	L	L	L	L

[1]S = small; M = moderate; L = large. Estimates are based on authors' experience.

[2]Likely interactive influence (number of feeding periods, natural variance in food composition, and food procurement and preparation standards).

[3]Potential loss during cooking (eg, to cooking container or cooking water).

[4]Degradation caused by fermentation or enzyme activity is a potential problem in some menus.

[5]Oxidation.

[6]Depends on how concentrated the nutrient is in its food source(s).

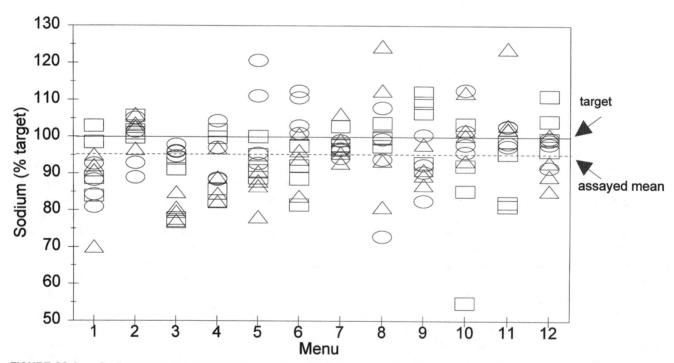

FIGURE 22-1.   Sodium content of 12 daily menus developed for a controlled feeding trial with 3 experimental diets.[1, 2, 3]

[1]The target sodium content for all three diets was 3,000 mg/2,100 kcal.

[2]For each diet, each menu was prepared in duplicate and composited. Two aliquots from each composite were assayed. Datapoints show determinations on these individual aliquots (ie, two sodium values per composite). (Data from authors' laboratory.)

[3]Legend: Diet 1, △; Diet 2, □; Diet 3, ○.

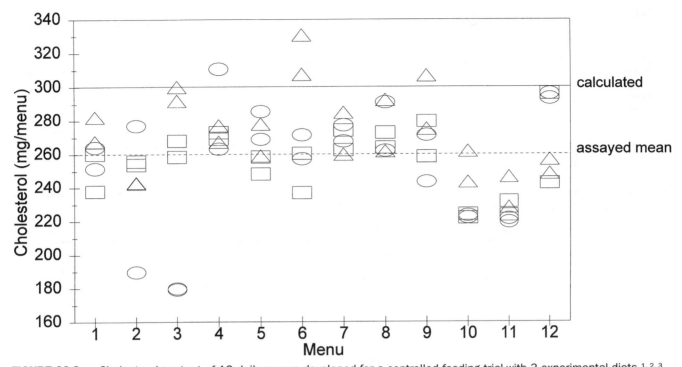

FIGURE 22-2. Cholesterol content of 12 daily menus developed for a controlled feeding trial with 3 experimental diets.[1, 2, 3]

[1]The calculated (target) cholesterol content for all three diets was 300mg/menu.

[2]For each diet, each menu was prepared in duplicate and composited. Datapoints show the cholesterol content of each composite (based on averaged data from analysis of duplicate aliquots). (Data from authors' laboratory.)

[3]Legend: Diet 1, △; Diet 2, □; Diet 3, ○.

In addition, methodology appropriate for analyzing a compound in a clinical sample usually is not applicable for use in food samples. Cholesterol in serum, for example, can be accurately determined using the enzyme cholesterol oxidase; however, if this same assay system is used to determine cholesterol in foods, the values obtained are falsely elevated because plant sterols are quantified in addition to cholesterol. These sterols are not commonly found in blood serum, but they are common components of plant foods. The use of cholesterol oxidase to determine cholesterol in diets would lead to approximately 20% overestimation of the actual levels.

It is therefore important to validate food assays in a matrix identical (or at least very similar) to that of the samples to be analyzed. This validation is complicated by a lack of standard reference materials for verifying the accuracy of nutrient measurements in different matrices, and mixed diets can vary widely in composition and physical properties. Although the National Institute of Standards and Technology (NIST) and the Association of Official Analytical Chemists (AOAC) are currently trying to rectify this deficiency (23), the production of reliable food analysis data require careful in-house validation of the accuracy and precision of methods in the matrices being analyzed.

The quality of current quantitative analytical methodology for various nutrients in foods is described in Tables 22–4 and 22–5. In general, *adequate* methods are those in which a good food analysis laboratory can obtain accurate and pre-cise data on the nutrient content of all significant food sources of that nutrient. *Substantial* methods are those in which a good food analysis laboratory can obtain accurate and precise data on the nutrient content of many (but not all) significant food sources of that nutrient. *Conflicting* methods are those for which different methods yield different results, and there is no agreement among the experts as to which methods (if any) give accurate data. Where methodology is *lacking*, there is agreement among experts that none of the available methods gives accurate results for that nutrient in foods.

The field of food and diet analysis has not enjoyed the type of extensive methodology and instrumentation development that has occurred in clinical chemistry during the past two decades. Thus, there is virtually no automated methodology and almost a complete lack of commercial kits for assays of individual food components. Hence, most existing food analysis methods are still labor intensive. Output is low in terms of the number of assays per analyst and per instrument (frequently less than 10 per day), and unit labor costs are correspondingly high. Additional costs may be incurred because many assay methods have not been validated for use with the wide variety of matrices seen in diet and food analysis; such validations should be done prior to the use of the methodology.

All of these factors lead to the high costs that typically range from $10 to $100 per nutrient assay per sample for routine analyses. Startup costs can also be significant, depending on the nutrients being assayed and the diet matrices.

TABLE 22-4

Criteria for Evaluating the State of Nutrient Analysis Methodology

State	Accuracy	Speed of Analysis	Cost per Analysis
Adequate	Excellent	Fast	Modest (<$100)
Substantial	Good	Moderate	Modest to high
Conflicting	Fair	Slow	High
Lacking	Poor	Slow	Unknown

TABLE 22-5

State of Methodology for Analysis of Specific Nutrients in Foods[1]

Nutrient Category	Adequate	Substantial	Conflicting	Lacking
Carbohydrates	—	Individual sugars Total dietary fiber Starch	Other fiber components	Resistant starch
Available energy	—	Bomb calorimetry	—	Calculated[2]
Lipids	—	Cholesterol Fatty acids: common (C12–C20)	Fat (total) Sterols Fatty acids: short chain (C4–C10), trans, omega-3	—
Mineral nutrients	Calcium Copper Magnesium Phosphorous Potassium Sodium Zinc	Iron Selenium Manganese	Arsenic Chromium Fluorine Iodine	Boron Cobalt Molbydenum Silicon Tin Vanadium Organic Species
Protein and amino acids	Nitrogen (total)	Amino acids (most)	Amino acids (some)	—
Vitamins	—	Niacin Riboflavin Thiamin Vitamin B-6 Vitamin E	Vitamin A Folate Vitamin B-12 Vitamin C Vitamin D Pantothenic acid Vitamin K	Biotin Choline
Other	—	—	Phytate Carotenoids Phytosterols Tocotrienols	Flavonoids Lignins Saponins

[1]Criteria for evaluating the state of nutrient analysis methodology are described in Table 22-4.
[2]Calculated from assayed proximate composition (water, fat, protein, ash, and carbohydrate by difference) and general Atwater factors (4 kcal/g for protein, 4 kcal/g for carbohydrate, 9 kcal/g for fat).

DIET ASSAY AS PART OF THE CONTROLLED FEEDING PROTOCOL

The diet assay component of a controlled diet study can be viewed as having two phases: *prefeeding validation* of the daily menus and *monitoring* of the diets as fed. In our experience the prefeeding validation is clearly the more important because it ensures that the desired nutrient levels are delivered to participants. Diet monitoring documents the nu-

trient levels fed and the degree of drift in the composition of the diets throughout the course of the study. If diet composition is validated prior to intervention *and* appropriate food procurement and preparation protocols are instituted to minimize subsequent nutrient variance (see Chapter 12, "Producing Research Diets," and Chapter 13, "Delivering Research Diets"), then drift is unlikely and the diets probably will meet design criteria throughout the study.

There are other advantages of having a well-designed diet assay component as an integral part of the feeding study protocol. First, the chemical data can provide valuable information for refining the design of subsequent studies, facilitating comparison of results from different investigations, and allowing the precise study of dietary components for which food composition data are lacking (eg, individual sugars, carotenoids, soluble dietary fiber). Second, a frozen archive of diet samples is a natural by-product of the sample preparation process. This archive can be a resource for retrospective studies, including assay of supplementary components that become of interest. Archived samples also might become extremely valuable for further characterization of the experimental diets if unexpected clinical endpoint results are obtained.

The Role of Food Analysts in Feeding Studies

The individuals responsible for chemical analysis of the diets or those with experience in quantitative chemical analysis of food composition should be involved in the overall planning of the diet intervention, as well as in designing various diets. As noted earlier, chemical assay of foods and diets is a specialized field; those with competence in clinical assays may, but do not necessarily, have sufficient expertise in the quantitative assay of diet and food components. Those experienced with food composition analysis will have the background required to suggest where differences between database values and chemically determined values might be a problem. They will appreciate the complexity of diet assays and can evaluate critical factors such as cost, turnaround time, precision of methods, normal nutrient levels in different foods, natural variations in food composition, and potential problems in diet assays. These analysts will frequently be able to suggest alternate approaches to diet design to maximize the accuracy and consistency of the diets delivered to participants.

Which Dietary Components Should Be Assayed?

At a minimum, assays should be planned for those nutrients fundamental to the experimental hypothesis and those nutrients known or suspected to influence the outcome variables. Additional assays may be required to obtain reference points necessary for the nutrient parameters. For example, if total fat will be calculated as a percent of total energy, total energy must be assayed in addition to total fat. The traditional measure of total energy requires ancillary determination of total weight, moisture, and ash. Alternatively, bomb calorimetry can be used to measure total energy, particularly for liquid formula diets. (See Diet Monitoring; also see Chapter 21, "Performance Improvement for the Research Kitchen.") Table 22–6 lists some typical calculated parameters for macronutrients and micronutrients and the corresponding assays needed.

It is also important to precisely define the analytes to avoid misunderstandings within the research team. For example, most chemists define analytes by their specific chemical structure, or sometimes by the assay methodology. In contrast, biomedical scientists may define analytes by their biological activity, which might effectively collapse a large number of individual components into a smaller number of categories. For example, "total saturated fatty acids" is actually the sum of multiple individually measured fatty acids. Similar disparities exist in the definitions of total carbohydrates, fiber, and energy.

As noted earlier, assay costs can be significant and can vary a great deal. Care must be taken not to raise the cost of the study by performing extraneous assays that are not central to the clinical investigation. The "turnaround time" from reception of the sample to the presentation of the results can also vary widely from assay to assay. Turnaround time can affect study timelines, and some assays may be inappropriate because the results may be obtained too late to be useful.

A Paradigm for Diet Analysis

A general paradigm for diet analysis is shown in Figure 22–3. It must be emphasized that this is a general approach, which must be adapted for the special concerns of a particular study. The phases of the diet analysis portion of a dietary intervention study are: (1) planning, (2) prefeeding diet validation, (3) diet monitoring, and (4) follow-up assays of the archived samples.

Planning

The plans for menu validation and diet documentation schemes will depend on the specific requirements of a given study and should be developed after the feeding protocol has been designed. The investigators should first assume that calculated and actual nutrient levels may differ and then think critically about the impact of any variance or inaccuracy in diet composition on the experimental hypotheses and biological measurements. Answering the following key questions during the planning phase will help the researchers determine the most appropriate analytical scheme for a particular study. Failure to address these issues early in the planning phase can lead to expensive mistakes later in the clinical study.

- What are the key nutrients in the study (ie, those fundamental to the experimental hypothesis and those expected to affect biological measurements)?
- Are exact nutrient levels important, or is it more important to maintain the difference between nutrient levels among diets?
- If differences among diets are vital, how far apart are the nutrient levels that are being studied? What are the expected analytical variances for the assay of the key nutrients? Given these differences in nutrient levels, the normal variances in the foods in the diets, and the expected ana-

TABLE 22-6

Assay Profiles for Selected Nutrient Parameters[1]

Nutrient Parameter	Usual Profile	Alternative Profile
Total intake of any nutrient (per menu)	Total food weight (g/menu) Nutrient concentration (g/100 g)	
Energy, total (per menu)	Total food weight (g/menu) Total fat (g/100 g) Moisture (g/100 g) Ash (g/100 g)	Total food weight (g) Bomb calorimetry (kcal or Kj)
Protein (% energy)	Protein (or nitrogen) (g/100 g) Total fat (g/100 g) Moisture (g/100 g) Ash (g/100 g)	Protein (or nitrogen) (g/100 g) Bomb calorimetry (kcal or kJ)
Carbohydrates, total (g/100 g)	Calculated by difference: Protein (or nitrogen) (g/100 g) Total fat (g/100 g) Moisture (g/100 g) Ash (g/100 g)	Assayed: Starch (g/100 g) Sugars (g/100 g) Fiber (g/100 g)
Fat, total (% energy)	Total fat (g/100 g) Moisture (g/100g) Ash (g/100 g)	Total fat (g/100 g) Bomb calorimetry (kcal or kJ)
Fatty acid (individual) (% total fat)	Total fat (g/100 g) Fatty acid (g/100 g)	

[1]These assay profiles are groups of distinct laboratory analyses that must be performed on aliquots from a single composited menu (which could represent one meal, one day, or several days). Additional data manipulations may be needed to generate final results. Examples include: difference calculations (for total carbohydrate), nitrogen-to-protein conversion factors; Atwater factors (for converting protein, fat, and carbohydrate content to energy); and adjustments between gross energy of combustion (by calorimetry) and physiological fuel value (Atwater factors). Energy may be expressed as kilocalories (kcal) or kiloJoules (kJ).

lytical variances, is it feasible that the proposed nutrient differences among the diets will actually be observed?

- Is a temporal relationship between nutrient intake and clinical measurements expected? If so, what unit of the diet (eg, meal, day, week) is significant?
- How much variability is expected in the levels of key nutrients in foods that make up the diet? For example: Are these nutrients susceptible to degradation? Does their concentration in food products have a high natural variance that cannot be controlled? Will foods be prepared at multiple sites?
- What is the scope and quality of available food composition data for the key nutrients? How much information is available about the variance of the nutrient content of the foods to be used in the diets?
- What is the value of definitive chemical data relative to the cost of chemical analyses?

Pilot Studies

Pilot studies should be considered at an early stage, because they can provide critical information for diet design. For instance, if the levels of different fatty acids are of interest and the main source of dietary fat is commercial oils, it would be useful to procure the oils to be used, assay for fatty acid concentrations, and use these data for diet design. In

any case, once menus have been assayed and acceptable menus have been selected, ingredient specifications and preparation procedures should not be changed indiscriminately but only after careful discussion with input from all those involved in diet design, including those responsible for the chemical analysis of the diets.

Diet Validation

The purpose of diet validation is to evaluate by chemical analysis *prior to feeding* whether the prepared diets contain the key nutrients at the levels targeted for the intervention. In this way, unforeseen and correctable deviations from experimental design (and possible overlap of diet treatments during the intervention) are prevented. Our experience suggests that this validation usually is best done at the level of the daily menus. In some cases, it may be necessary to assay individual foods or meals. If assayed nutrient concentrations differ from design specifications, errant menus can be eliminated or reformulated and reassayed before being delivered to participants. Often, examination of the chemical data will reveal a possible source of deviation. Before any chemical assays are done, those responsible for diet preparation should have developed, specified, and standardized the ingredients and food preparation methods. Special attention should be given to the

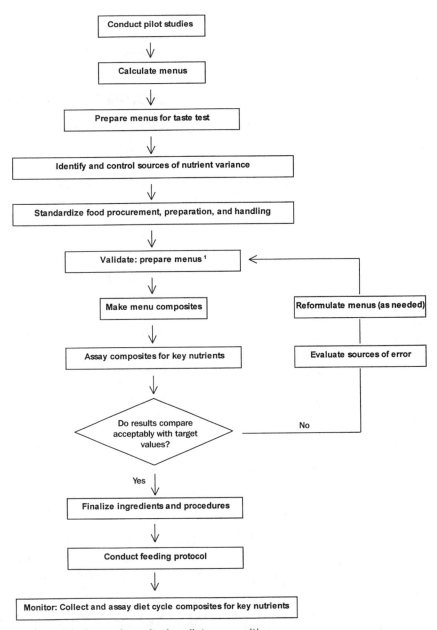

FIGURE 22-3. A scheme for validating and monitoring diet composition.

[1]For validation of diets for multicenter studies, menus should be prepared at 2 or more sites. In a four-site study, menus for 3 experimental diets were prepared as follows: diet 1, sites A and B; diet 2, sites B and C; diet 3, sites C and D (18).

primary sources of key nutrients, and the potential sources of variance should be identified and controlled.

Although prefeeding validation of individual menus is preferable, at least one menu cycle composite (ie, a composite containing all the food in one full rotation of menus) for each experimental diet should also be assayed for composition validation prior to feeding. (For multicenter studies we recommend collecting one of these cycles from each feeding site.) Assaying individual menus is the best way to prevent day-to-day overlap that can blur the distinctions between different dietary treatments. However, some investigators may choose to first check whether the entire menu cycle meets the design target. If not, having a set of frozen individual menus available for assay will allow the outliers

to be identified. This is especially important if there is a large natural variance of the experimental nutrient levels in foods or differences in nutrient levels among diets are small.

Diet Monitoring

The bottom line for any feeding study is ensuring that actual levels of key nutrients fed to participants match the experimental design. Theoretically, diets that have been validated should meet the target composition specifications over the entire study and across all centers, if ingredients and preparation methods match those used in the prefeeding menu validation. In reality, errors or variance in preparation, substitution of ingredients, and seasonal or lot-to-lot variability in food composition are apt to occur, with the potential to cause drift in nutrient levels. The purpose of the diet monitoring is to document that the diets actually met the target specifications, and to document any changes in the diets consumed by participants over the course of the intervention.

The composition of diets as fed can be monitored by collecting and assaying exact replicates of foods eaten by the participants during the intervention. Although one might think it would be ideal to continually monitor each menu during the feeding trial, such intensive sampling can be expensive and not necessarily the best use of money and time. The study investigators should carefully evaluate the sampling plan for the diet monitoring, in the context of potential variance and the clinical measurements.

In the multicenter DELTA study (18, 24) daily menus for a given diet at a given site were collected and composited into individual diet cycle composites—one for each center and sampling period. Each field center sampled one diet energy combination during each menu cycle. In this fashion, we were able to document the composition of the diets across centers, calorie levels, and the duration of the study.

A less intensive sampling plan was used for a second DELTA feeding trial (25). We had found that once ingredient specifications and diet preparation protocols were fixed and menu compositions validated, we had little variance in the key nutrients (fatty acids, cholesterol and total fat) across centers, calorie levels, or time (18). Such information reassured reviewers and was a compelling argument that the study had been done in the intended manner. The goal is to undertake sufficient, but not excessive, sampling and assays in the diet monitoring phase. In general, we recommend that at least one menu cycle from each diet and feeding period be collected, composited, and assayed for monitoring purposes.

For certain limited applications, such as process control in the preparation of liquid formula diets composed of pure ingredients, bomb calorimetry might be used to monitor consistency of diet composition. (Also see Chapter 21, "Performance Improvement for the Research Kitchen.") However, because this technique measures total energy only, changes in the proportion of different nutrients may not be revealed. Also, although bomb calorimetry is not suitable for monitoring the specific nutrient composition of whole-food diets, it can provide useful information on the total energy content of formula diets or of other composited menu samples. In our experience, the total energy content of the diet (kcal/day or kcal/cycle) can vary even when the design targets for relative distribution of macronutrient calories are achieved consistently.

Follow-up Assays of Archived Samples

After the endpoint measurements are completed for a study, investigators often wish that they had information on the composition of diets for some nutrient not originally believed to be important to the study. Proper archiving of composited menu and diet samples can be an invaluable resource

at such times. It is a relatively simple chore to archive composited samples if properly planned for at the beginning of the study. (See Storing Samples.)

PROCEDURES FOR CHEMICAL ANALYSIS OF DIET SAMPLES

Obtaining dependable chemical measurements requires more than simply sending samples to a "black box" food analysis laboratory. Chemical measurements will be assumed to reflect the composition of diets as consumed, and the quality of the entire assay process directly impacts the reliability of the analytical data. Therefore, each phase of diet assay must be controlled and conducted with proficiency and documented if reliable results are to be obtained. This is especially important because any analytical value is generally regarded as the true value, regardless of the quality of the procedure by which it was generated. An overview of the diet assay process is shown in Figure 22–4. *An error at any stage will probably invalidate the results.* The probability of two errors canceling each other is quite small. If assays are performed indiscriminately or without proper quality control, the data will be noisy (imprecise) and misleading (inaccurate). When documentation is inadequate, the diet composition data may be questioned even if they are accurate.

This section will explain how reliable diet composition data can be obtained, from sample collection through evaluation of assay results. Particular emphasis will be placed on quality control of the analytical process. (Also see Chapter 23, "Laboratory Quality Control in Dietary Trials.") Key terms relating to diet assay are defined in Exhibit 22–1. Exhibit 22–2 provides a checklist for investigators preparing to chemically analyze diets.

Importance of Quality Control

Quality control (QC) has been defined as the "overall system of activities whose purpose is to control the quality of a product or service so that it meets the needs of users" (26). Within the controlled diet study, chemical assay of nutrients is part of overall quality control of the clinical results (the product of the study). Similarly, for the assay results to meaningfully reflect actual diet composition, quality control of the analytical process itself is crucial.

There are three basic goals of analytical QC: to minimize the variance of the measurements, to verify the accuracy of the measurements (lack of assay bias), and to document the precision and accuracy of the measurements. Repeated analyses of the same sample (ie, food composite) give an indication of overall assay variance. The total variance in a measured value for a sample is really the sum of actual variance in composition plus analytical variance. Because the goal of diet assay is to determine variance in diet

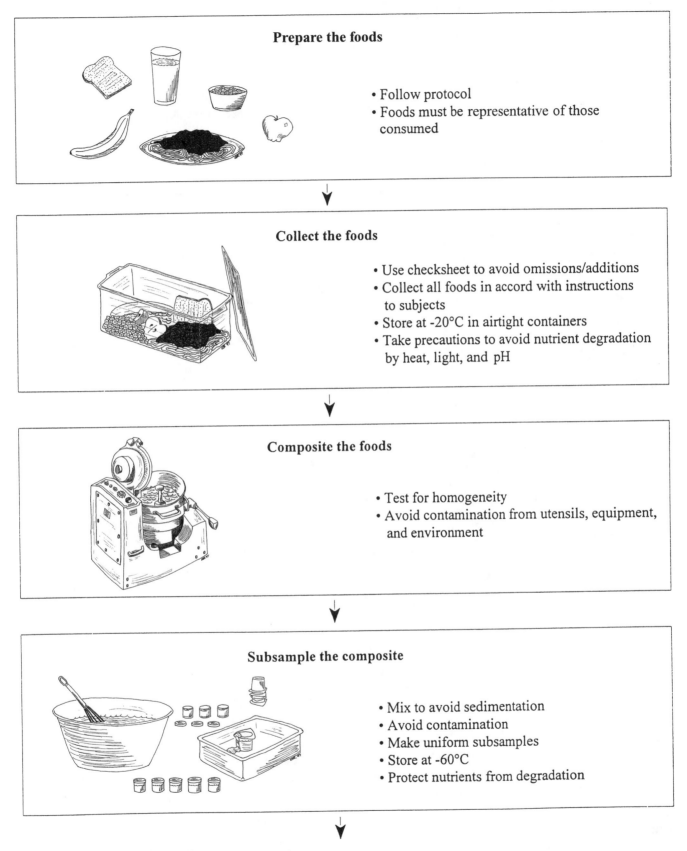

Prepare the foods

- Follow protocol
- Foods must be representative of those consumed

Collect the foods

- Use checksheet to avoid omissions/additions
- Collect all foods in accord with instructions to subjects
- Store at -20°C in airtight containers
- Take precautions to avoid nutrient degradation by heat, light, and pH

Composite the foods

- Test for homogeneity
- Avoid contamination from utensils, equipment, and environment

Subsample the composite

- Mix to avoid sedimentation
- Avoid contamination
- Make uniform subsamples
- Store at -60°C
- Protect nutrients from degradation

FIGURE 22-4.   Overview of the diet assay process.[1]

[1]Illustrations by Karen Richardson, Virginia Polytechnic Institute and State University, Blacksburg, Va.

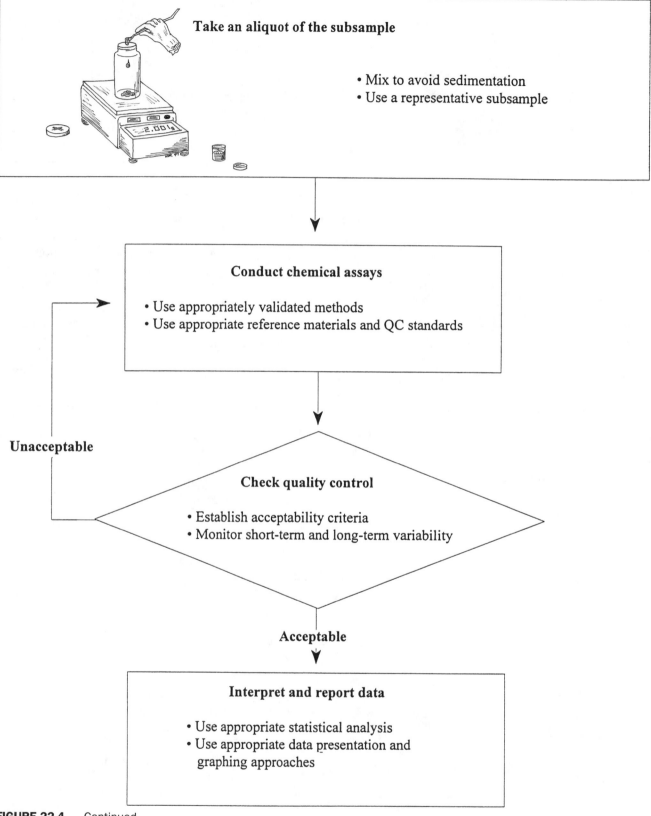

FIGURE 22-4. Continued

EXHIBIT 22-1

Glossary of Analytical Chemistry Terms

Accuracy: The degree of agreement of a measured value with the true or expected value of the quantity of concern.[1]

Aliquot: A measured amount of composite taken for a specific assay.

Archive sample: A subsample placed in long-term storage for study documentation.

Bias: A systematic error in a method or a deviation in the system caused by some artifact or idiosyncrasy of the assay process.[1]

Composite: A homogenized mixture of foods.

Homogeneity: The degree of uniformity of the distribution of analyte(s) throughout the food composite.

Matrix: The food or food composite, with characteristic physical and chemical properties, in which a nutrient analyte occurs.

Method validation: The process of verifying that a given (standardized) method yields results of acceptable precision and accuracy for a given analyte in specified concentration range in the matrices of interest.

Precision: The degree of mutual agreement characteristic of independent measurements as the result of repeated application of the process under specified conditions.[1]

Quality control (QC): The entire system by which accuracy and precision of data are achieved to meet the end use of the data.

Quality control chart: A graph that is used to evaluate precision, accuracy, and drift of the measurement system, for example, a plot of the assayed value of the control sample vs time.

Quality control material (QCM): A material with nutrient levels and matrix similar to food composite samples to be analyzed, and of adequate homogeneity and stability to monitor the precision of the measurement process.

Standard reference material (SRM): A substance for which one or more properties are established sufficiently well to calibrate instrumentation or to validate a measurement process.[2]

Subsample: A portion of the total composite.

[1]Taylor JK (26):7.
[2]Taylor JK (26):159.

EXHIBIT 22-2

Checklist for Planning the Diet Assay Component of a Feeding Study

_____ Decide which nutrients to assay.
_____ Develop a sampling plan for validation and monitoring.
_____ Establish the time lines and budget for all diet assay activities.
_____ Evaluate storage space.
_____ Determine susceptibility of analytes to degradation or contamination and measures for prevention.
_____ Select and document assay methods.
_____ Develop appropriate forms for documenting samples, procedures, and data and for maintaining a complete audit trail.
_____ Gather materials and develop standard procedures for collection, shipping, compositing, and assay.
_____ Perform pilot tests for composite homogeneity.
_____ Procure the appropriate food-based control material(s).
_____ Establish appropriate criteria for precision of assay data for each nutrient.
_____ Select food analysis laboratory.
_____ Validate in-house assays.
_____ Set quality control standards for assay values.
_____ Establish quality control charts for each assay.

composition (the measured value is the estimate), analytical variance must be known and ideally it should be minimized.

Determining the accuracy of an assay is more difficult. Most quantitative analysts believe that although accuracy can be disproved, it cannot be proven. Estimates of assay bias are frequently made by analyzing reference samples of known composition and comparing the results with known values. If the results differ consistently, the assay has bias. However, even if the results for a reference material agree, the result for a particular unknown sample still might be wrong because the unknown sample is not identical to the reference sample.

Analytical errors can arise at any point in the entire diet assay process. *Sampling errors* occur when the aliquots that are assayed are not representative of the original sample. For food composites, sampling errors include nonrepresentative collection of food samples; loss or degradation of nutrients during food collection, storage, or assay; contamination of samples; and composite heterogeneity. *Method bias* contributes to analytical error when different methods designed to measure the same component differ in accuracy and precision and are used interchangeably. Examples of this are the difference in cholesterol determined by gas chromatography and by colorimetry (11); in total fat measured by acid hydrolysis, chloroform/methanol extraction or as the sum of triacylglycerols (22); or in *trans* fatty acids measured by infrared spectrophotometry vs gas chromatography (27). *Measurement error* comprises all factors involved in the chemical determination, such as imprecision in weighing, dilution, extraction, detection, and calculation (28). *Reporting errors* include omissions, transposition of data values, or sample misidentification.

Given the myriad sources of analytical error, proper quality control measures are *essential* to the generation of believable analytical values. The following summarize key aspects of quality (discussed below in more detail).

- Carefully collecting foods, preparing composites, and subsampling composites for analysis.
- Using suitable and validated assay methods.
- Implementing assay quality control and using reference materials.
- Maintaining adequate documentation of samples, methodology, quality control procedures, and results.
- Appropriately evaluating (ie, reviewing and interpreting) analytical data and calculations.

Collecting, Compositing, and Subsampling Diets

Collecting Diet Samples

There are two overriding concerns in food collection: the foods sampled for assay must strictly replicate those consumed by participants, and no nutrient loss or degradation should occur after collection. No special treatment should be afforded "lab" samples during preparation. The foods must be procured from the same sources and prepared, handled, and heated in exactly the same manner as for participants. Inedible portions (eg, apple cores, banana peels, chicken bones, wrappers) must be removed. Generally, water and nonnutritive beverages (coffee, tea, diet sodas) are not included in food samples for assay but may be analyzed separately at the discretion of the investigator (12). For example, tap water could be a significant source of minerals in a trace element study. Usually foods can be collected and stored frozen (at $-20°C$) in clean, airtight containers prior to homogenization (however, see Table 22–7 for considerations for particular nutrients). A well-tested food collection

protocol that has been used in our laboratory for some time is provided in Exhibit 22–3.

If the assayed samples do not accurately represent the food in the menu or diet, if nutrient loss or gain occurs after collection, or if composite aliquots are heterogeneous, then the analytical data will not represent the actual diet composition no matter how accurate and precise the chemical measurements. The following general precautions will minimize errors throughout sample collection, composite preparation, and storage:

- Use carefully cleaned and dried containers and utensils.
- Wear powder-free gloves when manipulating samples.
- Minimize sample handling and transfer.
- Minimize temperature fluctuations (eg, repeated freeze-thaw or exposure to freezer automatic defrost cycles).
- Limit time exposure to temperatures in excess of 4°C or extended storage at greater than $-20°C$.
- Protect samples from contact with extraneous materials.
- Maintain a clean, climate-controlled laboratory environment.

Additional nutrient-specific safeguards may be necessary. (See Table 22–7 for typical causes of sample alteration along with measures for prevention.) An experienced food chemist or the food chemistry literature can be consulted to determine appropriate criteria for other nutrients.

For prefeeding menu validation, all traces of foods should be included in the composite, because the goal at this stage is to verify calculated nutrient levels. Each item is weighed into the collection container or directly into the food processor bowl if the composite is to be prepared immediately. The weight of each item in the composite is recorded on a checksheet. During the feeding intervention, when the goal is to document the nutrient levels as consumed, diet samples should be collected with the same technique used by participants. For example, if subjects are instructed to wipe down and consume all residues of food with bread or muffin, this same procedure should be employed for the assay sample. In the ideal scenario, the extra foods (for the assay composite) are plated and served to one or more additional "participants," with food handlers unaware that the meals are not to be eaten. These "participants" collect rather than consume the foods. In this way, selection biases such as choosing poorer cuts of meat or damaged/mishandled foods for the laboratory sample can be avoided.

The foods should be collected at the same time the corresponding items are consumed by the participants; longer storage, even under refrigeration, can lead to microbiological spoilage or chemical deterioration of nutrients. In addition, the foods collected for the assay sample should be documented in the same manner as participants' menus, for example with a tray assembly checklist. (See Chapter 18, "Documentation, Record Keeping, and Recipes.") Any known deviations from the food preparation protocol must be logged on this or a separate standard form. Deviations include ingredient substitutions, weight differences, and

EXHIBIT 22-3

Procedure for Assembling Foods for Composites

The following is a general procedure for collecting and storing daily menu samples. Modification may be needed for specific foods and/or nutrients (see text and Table 22-7).

A. MATERIALS

Prepared foods from menus (prepared exactly as for consumption by participants)
Airtight food collection containers[1]
Stainless steel spatula(s)
Cryogenic marker[2]
Disposable fat-free powder-free gloves[3]
Refrigerator (0°C to 4°C)
Freezer (-20°C or lower)

B. GUIDELINES FOR FOOD PREPARATION

- Procure the foods from the same sources and prepare, handle, and heat the foods exactly as specified by the menu and recipes. For example, reconstitute dehydrated foods (eg, mashed potatoes) and prepare and cook composite foods (eg, casseroles) and other cooked items (eg, meats) according to the recipe/menu.
- Reconstitute beverage mixes (nondiscretionary) according to menu instructions (ie, as if the drink were to be consumed) before adding to the food collection.
- Remove inedible portions (eg, apple cores, chicken bones, wrappers) when food is collected for analysis.
- Do not include discretionary/*ad libitum* beverages (eg, water, coffee, tea, diet sodas) in the menu samples for assay. (It may be necessary to analyze ad lib beverages for some studies; in most cases they should be assembled as separate samples.)
- For any portion-controlled items: for diet validation, weigh out the exact amount specified by the menu; for monitoring, collect the portion-controlled serving as specified by the menu.
- Protect samples from contact with extraneous materials and maintain a clean environment.
- Use carefully cleaned and dried containers and utensils and wear powder-free gloves to handle and collect foods.
- Include all traces of prepared/weighed foods specified by the menu in the menu collection (because the goal at the diet validation is to verify calculated nutrient levels).
- Record and report any known deviations from the menu preparation protocol. Deviations include ingredient substitutions, weight differences, preparation differences, brand name differences, etc. (This information will be used to evaluate any discrepancies between assayed and calculated nutrient levels.)
- Make sure that each diet sample container is clearly labeled with sample identification information, using a cryogenic marker.

C. TOTAL MENU COLLECTION

1. Assemble all foods from the breakfast menu. *Include* milk and juices but *not* ad lib beverages (eg, coffee, tea, water, diet soft drinks).
2. Retrieve a food collection container and label it, using the cryogenic permanent marker, with the menu number and diet description, date, and your initials (and any other key information).
3. Wear clean, fat-free, powder-free gloves and using a clean stainless steel spatula, scrape *all* of the food into the container. If bread or a muffin is a part of the meal being collected, set it aside and use it to scrape the plate, then add it to the collection container.
4. Completely seal the container and place it in the refrigerator (0°C to 4°C) until collection of total menu is complete (24 hrs or less).
5. Repeat steps 1 through 4 for lunch, dinner, and snacks, adding foods into the same container.
6. After all foods have been collected in the container, completely seal the container and place it in the freezer (-20°C or lower).

---

[1]For example, Rubbermaid™, available from Consolidated Plastics Co (Twinsburg, Ohio): 12-cup rectangular size (#0040) for 2,000-kcal menu; 19-cup square size (#0016) for 3,000-kcal menu.
[2]For example, Nalgene Cryoware™ markers, available from Fisher Scientific (Atlanta, Ga), catalog #13–382–52.
[3]For example, Sup-pli Line antistatic powder-free vinyl gloves, from Fisher Scientific (Atlanta, Ga), catalog #11–393–85B.

TABLE 22-7

Precautions to Minimize Deleterious Effects of Sample Preparation and Storage on the Chemical Composition of Diet Samples[1]

Constituent	Partial Changes	Significance of Change	Precautions
Water	Loss (dehydration)	Affects composition of composite as analyzed. Affects calculated total energy.	Report nutrients on dry weight basis. Determine moisture immediately after measuring total (wet) composite weight.
	Changes in distribution in food	Affects homogeneity of composite especially when freezing/thawing	Mix composites thoroughly before/while taking aliquots. Thaw frozen subsamples completely and thoroughly mix before/while taking aliquots.
	Uptake (hydration)	Important if composite is lyophilized	Keep samples in sealed containers. Devise sampling operations to minimize water uptake. Report nutrients on dry weight basis, measuring water in the assayed aliquot at the same time samples are weighed for nutrient assay.
All organic constituents (including protein)	Microbial degradation	Changes in overall composition	Store at low temperature ($<0°C$).
	Enzymatic degradation (autolysis)	Losses and gains of nutrients	Endogenous enzymes may have to be inactivated.
Fat	Separation	Heterogeneity of composite	Thaw to room temperature. Thoroughly mix before taking aliquots.
	Oxidation	Destruction of polyunsaturated fatty acids	Store at $≤-30°C$ in sealed, air-free containers, preferably flushed with nitrogen or argon gas. Antioxidants may prevent oxidation in some samples.
	Contamination from handling containers	Falsely elevated values	Use thoroughly cleaned containers. Wear clean gloves when handling containers.
Sugars	Caramelization at elevated temperatures	Losses from decomposition	Avoid elevated temperatures ($>60°C$). Analyze fresh or freeze-dried samples.
	Conversion of sucrose to mannitol	Loss of sucrose	Keep sample frozen.
Starch	Retrogradation	Increases resistance to enzymatic attack and decreases starch measured by enzymatic methods	Work on freshly prepared sample with minimal storage. Do not dry samples.
Inorganic constituents	Contamination of original sample by soil, water, storage container	Falsely elevated values	Wash containers and utensils carefully and rinse with distilled deionized water.

(continued)

TABLE 22-7

Continued

Constituent	Partial Changes	Significance of Change	Precautions
Inorganic constituents	Contamination of sample by dust, processing equipment and other metallic sources in laboratory	Falsely elevated values	Use containers cleaned according to strict protocol for trace element analysis (including acid washing). Protect samples from dust contamination in laboratory. Acid wash all containers and utensils. Store subsamples in glass acid-washed containers.
Fat-soluble vitamins	Oxidation	Loss	Store at low temperature ($< -20°C$). Protect from light and O_2. Store samples in dark containers, flushed with nitrogen or argon gas.
Water-soluble vitamins			
Thiamin	SO_2 degradation	Destruction	Exclude SO_2.
Riboflavin	Oxidation Photodegradation	Extensive loss	Protect from light and oxygen. Store at low temperature, in the dark, under nitrogen or argon gas.
Niacin	Microbial activity	Loss and/or synthesis	Store at low temperature ($<0°C$).
Vitamin B-6	Microbial activity	Loss and/or synthesis	Store at low temperature ($<0°C$).
Folates	Enzymatic deconjugation Oxidation	Loss	Inactivate deconjugase enzymes immediately. Protect with ascorbate.
Vitamin B-12	Microbial activity	Loss and/or synthesis	Store at low temperature ($<0°C$).
Vitamin C	Enzymatic oxidation	Loss	Analyze fresh if possible. Extract immediately into metaphosphoric acid.
	Catalysis by trace metals	Loss	Avoid metallic contamination.

[1]Adapted with permission from H Greenfield and DAT Southgate, *Food Composition Data* (New York: Elsevier; 1992), pp 57–59.

preparation differences. This information will be used to evaluate any discrepancies between assayed and calculated nutrient levels. (See Evaluating the Analytical Data.)

Containers used to collect diet samples must be clearly labeled with sample identification information, using a cryogenic marker and labels that are water resistant and adhesive at $-20°C$ (eg, Nalgene Cryoware™ markers and Poly Paper computer labels from Fisher Scientific, Atlanta, Ga). To preserve the composition of collected foods, samples should be stored immediately at $-20°C$ or lower in airtight containers. These conditions will hinder microbial and enzymatic degradation and moisture loss. Additional precautions should be taken for preservation of specific nutrients (Table 22–7). Some components require assay of fresh material and/or addition of stabilizers during composite prep-

aration and storage to prevent nutrient degradation; others may be susceptible to degradation during freeze-thaw, such as sucrose (29). In these instances, appropriate adjustments to the protocol must be made.

If samples are shipped off-site (eg, to the food analysis laboratory) for homogenization, care must be taken to maintain the integrity of the foods and prevent loss during shipment. Foods should be frozen solid at $-20°C$ or lower and shipped on dry ice in a sealed, insulated cooler to prevent thawing during transit. Each shipment should include a transfer form to document which specific samples were shipped, the sample weights, and the condition of samples.

At the receiving end, samples should be inspected immediately upon receipt for signs of thawing or damage, and the condition of samples should be recorded. Weighing containers before and after shipment will ensure the absence of leakage during transit. Any procedural deviations (eg, open or damaged containers, thawed foods, absence of labels, missing samples) should be documented on the sample transfer form, which is then returned to the shipping facility. Clearly adulterated samples should be documented and discarded.

Preparing Composites

The purpose of homogenization is to prepare a uniform slurry from a collection of whole foods with no nutrient gain or loss in the process. Whole diets are heterogeneous and variable mixtures of individual foods in which nutrients are unevenly distributed across widely varying concentration ranges and matrices. Homogenizing the menu or diet samples into a food composite thus is possibly the most critical step in the assay of diets.

A *composite* is a uniform mixture of the foods constituting the unit of the diet to be assayed and is basically a slurry of small particles of these foods. A *menu composite* comprises all foods served in a given day, and a *diet cycle composite* includes all foods from one full rotation of menus. If food is lost or if nutrients are altered during composite preparation or are not uniformly distributed, assay values will not represent nutrient levels in the original foods. Composite preparation can be done in-house or at the food analysis laboratory, but in either case it must be performed carefully by trained personnel.

A typical menu composite has a volume of 2 to 3 liters, and a week's menus will add up to 20 liters or more. Chemical assays are usually performed on small aliquots (1 mL to 10 mL) taken from the larger volumes of these mixtures. Therefore, it is critical that the homogenate is uniform, so that assayed aliquots are representative of the entire composite. Otherwise, no matter how accurate and precise the measurements, the values will be meaningless with respect to the original material.

It can be difficult to prepare a uniform homogenate of a menu or diet sample. The homogenization is affected by many factors, including the types, proportion, and texture of different foods; fat levels and types of fat; water content; and the presence or absence of emulsifiers, all of which vary widely from food to food, menu to menu, and diet to diet. No standard method of homogenization can guarantee acceptable results for all foods or mixtures of foods. For multicenter studies, it might seem that preparing composites at each feeding site would reduce the cost of shipping samples for analysis, because in most cases only a small part of the whole homogenate is used for all the assays. It is best, however, to prepare all composites at a single location to prevent site-to-site variability at this critical stage.

For most diets and nontrace element nutrient assays, menu and diet cycle composites can be prepared using a stainless steel batch food processor to yield a composite with acceptable homogeneity for 3-g to 5-g analytical aliquots (50% to 80% moisture). Nutrients susceptible to degradation or contamination (refer to Table 22–7) require modification

of the basic procedure and/or equipment. For example, trace element analysis for chromium and nickel requires titanium blades and nylon-coated utensils to prevent contamination by elements (eg, chromium) from stainless steel; in the analysis of vitamin C (ascorbic and dehydroascorbic acid), citric or metaphosphoric acid must be added during homogenization (30). Temperature control also is critical during homogenization. Prolonged exposure to elevated temperatures (generally >4°C) potentiates microbial growth and/or nutrient degradation. Even brief exposure to high heat from the processor motor can cause breakdown of some nutrients.

Immediately after homogenization, the composite should be dispensed into sample storage jars. (Although most storage jars are made of plastic, the choice of material for these jars and any other storage container should be made in light of the technical requirements of the protocol. Among the factors that should be considered are size, completeness of seal, resistance to freezing, exclusion of light, and whether any undesirable components can leach into the sample.)

Lichon and James (28) reviewed alternate procedures for preparing food composites. In principle, the less processing the foods are subjected to during homogenization, the more likely the samples will represent the foods as consumed. For this reason, it is recommended that samples be assayed in the fresh or frozen-thawed state. However, in the case of certain components (such as sucrose) further treatment (such as lyophilization) is necessary or preferable to stabilize the nutrient (29). In these instances, these extra processing steps would be carried out only for the aliquots destined for assay of that nutrient.

Preparing Subsamples and Analytical Aliquots of Composites

The terms *subsample* and *aliquot* are often used interchangeably. Specifically, however, a subsample is any portion of the total diet composite; an aliquot is a measured amount of composite taken for a specific assay (see Exhibit 22–1). The use of subsamples considerably reduces multiple freeze-thaw cycles and external contamination of the food composites. For most studies, 4 subsamples (15-g to 25-g jars) per analyte for assays and an additional minimum of 5 subsamples for the study archive are adequate. At the point of subsampling the food composite, the composite temperature should be between 20°C and 25°C; lower temperatures result in congealing of fat and concentrating of solutes; higher temperatures contribute to nutrient loss caused by chemical and enzymatic reactions.

Subsampling should be accomplished rapidly and the subsamples immediately frozen to avoid microbial or enzymatic degradation of nutrients. Frozen samples must be thawed and thoroughly mixed prior to taking aliquots for assays. Portioning the total food composite into subsamples with continual stirring prevents sedimentation. Again, specific considerations may be required for labile nutrients (Table 22–7). If samples are lyophilized, they must be reblended (and at the same time protected from excess heat) after freeze-drying because the process of lyophilization can cause stratification of food components.

Taking aliquots of composites for analysis is a crucial step in an assay, the significance of which is often overlooked by untrained personnel. Typical diet composites are prone to sedimentation and fat separation. Thus, if a composite is not adequately mixed prior to dispensing, assayed aliquots will not be representative of the original material.

Composite Homogeneity

Composites must be homogeneous because settling or incomplete blending can be a source of assay bias (ie, from the analysis of unrepresentative samples). The homogeneity of a composite can be evaluated by assaying a range of aliquots, drawn across the entire subsampling procedure. A suggested sampling plan is shown in Figure 22–5. Moisture content is a useful indicator of homogeneity, and the distribution of key nutrients for a given study should be checked as well. Replicate aliquots from each subsample are assayed, and the standard deviations of the replicate values are calculated for within and among subsamples. A composite can be considered homogeneous for purposes of the assay, if (1) the overall variance for replicate values is acceptable based on the end use of the data, and (2) the variance among subsamples does not exceed variance within subsamples (as determined by a statistical analysis of variance).

A pilot study to check composite homogeneity is recommended. If composites appear heterogeneous, additional blending is recommended. If a composite is still not of acceptable homogeneity and cannot be further blended, one way to improve the confidence of assay data is to analyze a greater number of subsamples (ideally drawn from across the subsampling process) and obtain a mean value based on multiple replicates. This will increase the cost of analysis. Alternatively, one can analyze larger aliquots of the composite if allowed by the assay procedure. It is not necessary to validate the homogeneity of each diet composite when different diets to be assayed are composed of similar foods.

Storing Samples

Proper storage of composited diets is important to retain the original composition. The proximate composition (moisture, ash, protein, total fat), fatty acids, and cholesterol of composited diets appear to be stable for at least 3 years at $-60°C$ when samples are packaged and stored as described earlier (Holden JM, USDA, Beltsville, MD; unpublished data). The lability of other nutrients (Table 22–7) should be considered as necessary. Each jar and its lid should be labeled for identity using a cryogenic marker.

Before investigators initiate the study, they should ensure that adequate freezer space is available for sample storage, and alternate freezer space should be identified for emergency use. Freezers fail and power outages do occur with distressing frequency, so it is desirable to have alarm-wired freezers that are visually inspected *and* electronically monitored for temperature fluctuations. Protocols should be put in place to minimize the damage that might occur if these problems arise.

Assay Methods

Methods must be carefully chosen and validated, performed by trained analysts, and undergo continuous quality control

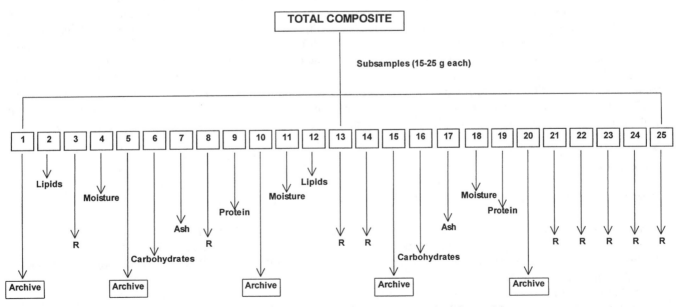

FIGURE 22-5.   Distribution of composite subsamples for nutrient assays: a sample scheme.[1,2]

[1] Subsamples are numbered in chronological order of dispensing from the total composite.

[2] R = Reserve sample (for repeat assays, if needed).

if accurate, precise, and *meaningful* results are to be obtained. These concerns are pertinent whether assays are performed in-house or by an outside laboratory. Most clinical investigators subcontract assays to an experienced food analysis laboratory. By understanding the issues involved in assay methodology, validation, and quality control, investigators will be better prepared to select and interact with the food analysis laboratory and evaluate the resulting data.

Choosing Methods

Most laboratories use "standard" methods or modifications thereof. Standard methods exist for many nutrients and are often the first resource. Such methods are tested and published by several organizations, for example: the Association of Official Analytical Chemists (31), the American Association of Cereal Chemists (32), the American Oil Chemists' Society (33), and the International Union of Pure and Applied Chemistry (34). Excellent discussions of methodology for a wide range of nutrients can be found in Sullivan and Carpenter (35) and Greenfield (36; pp. 81-126). Sullivan and Carpenter (35) also summarize current methods accepted for nutrition labeling in the United States.

Note, however, that standard methods are just that: *standardized* to a set protocol, but not necessarily *accurate* for all possible food matrices or collaboratively studied for precision and accuracy. Currently accepted standard methods vary widely in these qualities (Tables 22–4 and 22–5). Most methods have been verified for only a limited range of matrices. Use of a nonvalidated assay system can result in significant bias, described next.

For novel constituents, the scientific literature is a source of methodology. A selected listing of food analysis journals is given in Exhibit 22–4. Books on methodology for specific nutrients are also available. An appropriate or adaptable method, and possibly an expert laboratory willing to perform the assays on a contractual basis, can usually be located by contacting the authors of articles, abstracts, or books.

Accuracy, precision, cost, quality control, and turnaround time all affect the choice of an ideal method. For each method the investigator should be aware of strengths and limitations and the inherent potential for bias. To minimize variance from analytical bias, it is imperative that for a given nutrient the *same method* is used throughout the study and that all assays are performed at the *same laboratory*.

Method Bias

Often there is more than one standard method for a given nutrient. For example, total fat can be determined by various gravimetric methods: acid hydrolysis (eg, AOAC methods 922.06, 925.12, 925.32, 935.38, 935.39D, 945.44, 948.15, 950.54) (31); Soxhlet (ether) extraction (AOAC methods 920.39B, 920.39C) (31); chloroform/methanol extraction (AOAC methods 983.23) (31); or as the sum of fatty acids measured by gas chromatography (AOAC methods 969.33, 963.22) (31).

The FDA Nutrition Labeling and Education Act (NLEA) (15) defines total fat as the sum of fatty acids C4 to C24 expressed as triglycerides, yet currently there is no corresponding validated methodology for measuring total fat in foods. Because traditional gravimetric total fat methods are known to measure more than fatty acids as "total fat" (22), it can be expected that newer methods standardized to the NLEA definition of total fat will yield different (and in most cases, lower) values for total fat.

There are also several different standard methods utilized to assay *trans* fatty acids, including direct gas chromatography (GC) (AOAC method 985.21) (31), infrared spectrophotometry (AOAC method 965.34) (31), combined GC-infrared spectrophotometry (27), and silver ion thin-layer chromatography or silver ion high-performance liquid chromatography (HPLC) combined with gas chromatography (GC) (37). There are demonstrated biases among different methods. For example, direct GC alone yields values for the total C18:1 *trans* fatty acid content of whole diet composites and food oils that are 5% to 25% lower than values obtained using GC combined with silver ion HPLC (37).

Another source of bias is interlaboratory bias, in which the "same" method yields consistently different results at different laboratories. Interlaboratory variance is well known among chemists (38). Table 22–8 summarizes differences in selected nutrients analyzed in a mixed diet composite at independent laboratories (39). These data illustrate the difference in composition that would be observed simply by sending aliquots to different laboratories. In this study the

EXHIBIT 22-4

Journals Reporting Food Analysis Methods and Results

Journal of Agricultural and Food Chemistry, American Chemical Society (Washington, DC)
Journal of the American Oil Chemists Society, American Oil Chemists Society (Champaign, Ill)
Journal of the Association of Official Analytical Chemists International, Association of Official Analytical Chemists International (Gaithersburg, Md)
Food Chemistry, Elsevier Science Ltd (Oxford, UK)
Journal of Food Composition and Analysis, Academic Press, Inc (San Diego, Calif)
Journal of Food Lipids, Food and Nutrition Press, Inc (Trumbull, Conn)
Journal of Food Science, Institute of Food Technologists (Chicago, Ill)

TABLE 22-8

Nutrient Levels in a Total Diet Composite Assayed at Five Commercial Laboratories[1]

A. Assayed Component per 100 g of Diet Composite[1]

Component		Laboratory				
		A	B	C	D	E
Moisture	(g/100 g)	64.1	64.8	64.8	65.6	65.9
Protein	(g/100 g)	7.8	7.8	7.6	7.4	7.8
Ash	(g/100 g)	1.1	1.2	1.3	1.5	1.3
Total Fat	(g/100 g)	5.2	5.2	5.9	5.6	5.9
Cholesterol	(mg/100 g)	45.8	21.7	25.0	16.9	16.5
Sodium	(mg/100 g)	238.9	219.4	244.4	241.7	258.3
Potassium	(mg/100 g)	188.9	—	197.2	205.6	179.2
Calcium	(mg/100 g)	63.9	58.3	63.9	55.6	60.3

B. Assayed Components per Menu[2]

Component		Laboratory				
		A	B	C	D	E
Moisture	(g)	1,154	1,166	1,166	1,181	1,186
Protein	(g)	140	140	137	133	140
Ash	(g)	20	22	23	27	23
Total Fat	(g)	94	94	106	101	106
Cholesterol	(mg)	824	391	450	304	297
Sodium	(mg)	4,300	3,949	4,399	4,351	4,649
Potassium	(mg)	3,400	—	3,550	3,701	3,226
Calcium	(mg)	1,150	1,049	1,150	1,001	1,085

[1]Holden JM. USDA, Beltsville, MD. Unpublished data, 1994.
[2]Values in Part B are derived from values in Part A.

key nutrients were total fat and cholesterol. Clearly, the values determined for these components varied from laboratory to laboratory. Total fat calculated as grams per daily menu ranged from 93.6 g to 106.2 g.

In the absence of standard reference materials to determine the accuracy of the measurement systems, it is difficult to assess which value is "correct." The previous example underscores the importance of using methods validated for the samples at hand and instituting rigid quality control, including analysis of a food-based control material with each assay. Furthermore, although reputable commercial laboratories routinely employ adequately tested methods, standard methodology does not guarantee accurate results across all food matrices.

The significance of method bias will depend on how the analytical data are used—that is, are the exact nutrient levels of primary concern, or are the differences in the nutrient levels among diets more important? Take, for example, a design in which difference in the nutrient levels among diets is the most important factor, and three diets are studied at levels of 26%, 30%, and 37% of energy as total fat. In this case, the primary parameter is *difference* in fat content; therefore, bias is less critical, and the key concern is consistency throughout the study.

Validating Methods

Validating a method means confirming that the assay measures the concentration of the analyte with acceptable accuracy and precision, in the specific sample type or types to be tested, at a given laboratory (*accuracy* and *precision* are defined in Exhibit 22–1).

Following a standard written method does not guarantee that a given laboratory will obtain acceptable results. The laboratory performing assays must demonstrate that acceptable results can be obtained *in that laboratory* for the relevant nutrient levels *in the appropriate matrices*. Characteristics of a valid method include:

• Produces the same results as a previously accepted method over probable concentrations of the analyte in the matrices to be analyzed.
• Achieves quantitative recovery of pure analyte standards in a total assay.
• Achieves quantitative recovery of analyte standards added to the matrices to be assayed (ie, method of "standard additions").
• Yields a result for appropriate standard reference material(s) within the certified range.
• Has a level of precision for replicate assays (>5 replicates)

of the analyte in the sample matrices to be assayed that is acceptable for the purpose of the study.

- Is free of major sources of interference.
- Has a known limit of detection (LOD) in the matrices to be assayed, and that LOD is acceptable for the study.
- Has a known analytical range in the matrices to be assayed, and that analytical range is acceptable for the study.
- Produces acceptable results with the method when performed by more than one analyst and more than one laboratory.
- Has a built-in quality control protocol.

Detailed discussions can be found in DeVoe (40), Garfield (41), and Dux (42). Even after the laboratory has demonstrated proficiency, the investigator is strongly advised to include blinded control samples along with the diet composite samples submitted for analysis to validate each individual data set.

Assay Quality Control

Assay quality control is the implementation of a system to ensure that the accuracy and precision of chemical measurements meet requirements for the end use of the data. A full discussion of quality control and the statistical treatment of analytical measurements is beyond the scope of this text. Taylor (26), Dux (42), Garfield (41), as well as Chapter 23, "Laboratory Quality Control in Dietary Trials," can help investigators to establish quality control protocols for any in-house assays.

When assays are performed out-of-house, the investigator must still implement quality control measures, and in a sense they are even more important without knowledge of the entire assay system. There are four basic components to quality control of measurements made at an outside laboratory, including use of appropriate control samples with study samples; implementing quality control charts and appropriate standards for precision of measurements; selecting a reputable laboratory that follows Good Laboratory Practice Standards (43); and comprehensively documenting samples, procedures, and data. Other specific components of quality control and quality assurance should be addressed internally by the food analysis laboratory.

Control Materials

A food-based *quality control material* (QCM) is a homogeneous composite consisting of food(s) similar in type and having nutrient concentrations comparable to those in samples to be assayed. Additionally, analyte concentrations in a QCM are well-characterized and known to be stable for the duration of the study. The purpose of the QCM is to ensure the absence of deviations in the routine measurement processes.

Prior to the study, the mean and tolerance limits for the concentration of each key nutrient in the QCM should be established by performing a series of assays using the methods that will be used for the study. (See Quality Control Charts and Standards for Analytical Precision.) Subsequently, an aliquot of the QCM is assayed with each batch of samples, or approximately every 15 samples in a continuous system. A value for the QCM outside the tolerance limits indicates a possible shift in the measurement system; this suggests that results for other samples analyzed in the same batch may be invalid.

Credible laboratories analyze an in-house QCM and/or reference material with each assay run. If the laboratory analyses are done under contract, it also is necessary to include a blinded sample of externally procured, matrix-matched QCM with each batch of diet samples to check consistency of results over time and appropriate handling of samples and data. It is particularly important that at least one of the routinely employed in-house or external QCMs have a matrix and nutrient composition that is similar to the mixed diet composites generated by a particular study. In the worst case, significant errors in the system may not be detected unless a food-based QCM is used.

This point is illustrated in Figure 22–6, which shows data for two QCMs used in the determination of total dietary protein assayed as Kjeldahl nitrogen. Each assay run was conducted using both QCMs. All of the *nitrogen* values for the *nonfood* control material, ammonium oxalate, were well within the acceptable limits (Figure 22–6a). For three of the assay runs (P035, P036, and P037), however, *protein* values for the *food-based* control material were unacceptably low (Figure 22–6b). Review of the data revealed that a mistake had been made in the algorithm that was used to convert assayed nitrogen content to calculated protein content. This calculation step was routine for the food-based control material and for the experimental diet samples but was not necessary for the nonfood control material. Had only the ammonium oxalate control material been used, the mistake would not have been detected, and the reported protein values for the experimental diet would have been erroneously low.

An appropriate food-based QCM is: matrix matched (ie, composed of foods comparable to study samples), with nutrients at concentrations similar to those in samples; homogeneous; stable for the duration of the study; and characterized for key nutrient concentrations. There are a few commercially available mixed-food standard reference materials (SRMs) that have been certified for the concentrations of selected nutrients, and these are sometimes used as QCMs (23). However, because *standard reference materials* are rigorously characterized, they are quite expensive. Most commercial SRMs are freeze-dried and thus present a different matrix than the wet-diet composite. For many nutrients, no mixed-food standard reference material exists. However, an acceptable QCM need not be as rigorously characterized as an SRM because its main purpose is to monitor the precision over time of an assay system that has been validated for accuracy.

One simple way to obtain a QCM for a given diet trial is to prepare a composite of study menus. Sullivan and Carpenter (35) have also discussed the preparation of in-house

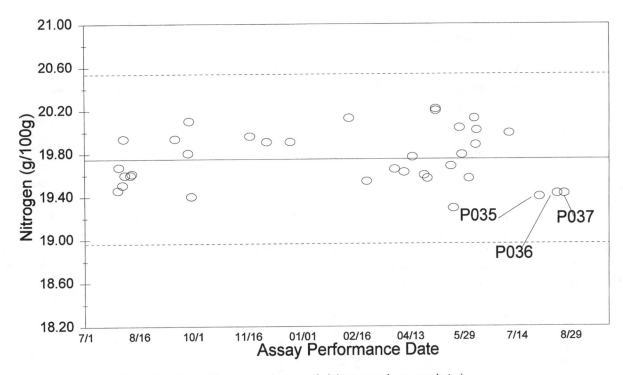

A. Nitrogen content of nonfood quality control material (ammonium oxalate).

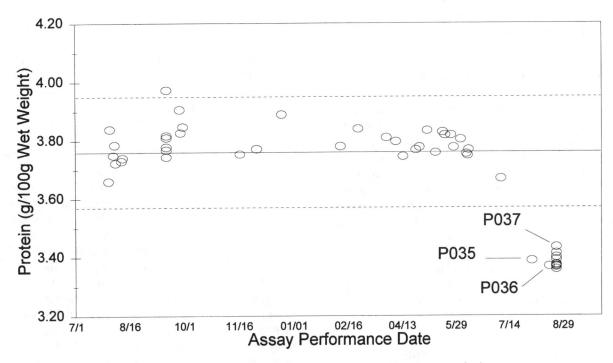

B. Protein content of food-based quality control material (mixed-diet composite).

FIGURE 22-6. Quality control charts for protein assay by the Kjeldahl nitrogen method.[1, 2, 3]

[1] Each oval represents the assay value for one quality control sample (data from authors' laboratory).

[2] _____ Mean, - - - - - Mean ± 3 SD.

[3] P035, P036, and P037 represent three assay runs performed with both quality control materials. Multiple samples of food-based QCM were analyzed in run P037.

control materials. The minimum total amount of QCM that should be prepared can be estimated as

(Total number of composites)
× (Total number of components to be assayed per composite)
× (Number of replicate assays per component)
× (1 QCM subsample per 15 replicate assays)
× (25 grams per QCM subsample)
× 5
= grams QCM required.

The "safety factor" of 5 allows for assays to establish control limits, plus reruns and supplemental assays. However, it is preferable to prepare as much excess QCM as storage and handling allow because unused samples can always be discarded but the exact material cannot be replicated.

For the QCM to be a useful tool for monitoring assay precision, its homogeneity and stability are essential. Because total variance in the QCM measurements comprises both sample heterogeneity and analytical variability, the more homogeneous the QCM, the greater the ability to detect real variance in the assay system. Sample-to-sample variance for the QCM must be lower than the acceptable variance for study samples; otherwise, meaningful deviations in the assay system will be undetectable.

Homogeneity of the QCM can be assessed as described previously (see Composite Homogeneity). If necessary, to optimize uniformity of the QCM, foods that are difficult to composite (eg, fresh vegetables, leafy greens, nuts, and raisins) can be prehomogenized. Alternatively, substitutions can be made with commercially available homogeneous foods of like composition—for example, chicken baby food for whole chicken pieces or breadcrumbs for sliced bread—while maintaining calculated levels of key nutrients. Moisture loss, contamination, and degradation of the key nutrients in QCM samples must also be prevented for the material to be an effective monitoring tool. Again, Table 22–7 lists precautions for preserving labile nutrients. If stability is uncertain, it is best to be extra cautious and store the QCM at −60°C or lower, protect it from freeze-thaw cycles, and limit exposure to light and oxygen by storing in dark containers capped tightly under nitrogen or argon.

Quality Control Charts and Standards for Analytical Precision

A quality control chart (QC chart) is a plot of the assayed values of the QCM vs assay date (see Figure 22–6). A QC chart is specific to a given method and control material. The QC chart depicts assay performance through a period of time and allows the detection of (meaningful) drift or isolated deviations in measurements. QC charts can be used by the investigator to monitor the proficiency of the laboratory and document any assay variance.

Control limits (ie, an acceptable range for the QCM

value) are established and then are used to evaluate data from a given assay. For food analysis, typical control limits are ± 3 times the standard deviation of the mean, approximating the 99% confidence interval (26, pp. 131-132; 43, pp. 19-20). A detailed discussion of establishing and evaluating control limits can be found in Taylor (26).

The mean, standard deviation, and control limits are calculated from a set of preliminary assays (15 or more) of the control material using fixed methodology. It is best for these measurements to span the most possible sources of variance (eg, different analysts, time, new batches of reagents) expected across the duration of the study. To establish a control chart for subcontracted assays, 5 samples of the QCM can be sent on a minimum of three separate occasions as far apart in time as possible.

Details of the statistics and interpretation of QC data are beyond the scope of this discussion, and the reader is referred to one or more textbooks on the subject (26, 41, 42). The concern for the clinical investigator evaluating the QCM control chart is detecting gross shifts in the assay system that might compromise interpretation of the diet composition results. This can be done by assuming that the control limits established from preliminary assays are representative of routine assay precision. If a subsequent value for the QCM is outside the ± 3 SD limits, it is relatively certain that the discrepancy is real, and all samples in that batch should be reassayed. Although the premise is that any factor causing a deviation in the QCM value equally affects other samples in the batch, which may not be true, the risk of falsely rejecting data is small relative to the chance of otherwise accepting errant values. If reassay yields a control value out of range, further analyses should be stopped until the reason for the deviation is investigated and resolved.

Another criterion for the control chart is that all values should be normally distributed about the mean. A rule of thumb is that more than 7 consecutive values on the same side of the mean suggests a statistically significant shift in the system (26, pp. 136-137). Sometimes assay systems will drift slightly up and down over time for no identifiable reason, and this can be considered part of overall analytical variance. Although these shifts may be *statistically* significant, the practical importance of such deviations will be determined by their magnitude and the corresponding impact on the use of the data in a particular study. No general methods have been published for determining acceptable limits for assay drift based on end use of the data and setting corresponding QC criteria, and this is a subject for future study. Although use of quality control samples allows documentation of assay performance, it is incumbent upon the clinical investigator to interpret the significance of any deviations in the context in which the sample data are used.

Replicate assays offer yet another data control measure. It is wise to plan for each composite to be analyzed in replicate (ie, duplicate or preferably triplicate, and occasionally higher). These replicate assays are used to detect and account for isolated, sample-specific, assay errors and/or sample heterogeneity. The investigator should be sure that the food

TABLE 22-9

Key Components of Documentation for Diet Assays

Component	Details Requiring Documentation
Sample identification information	Source Study Description (including details of food preparation procedure) Date Weight
Sample collection information	Date Location Procedures used (including name of person collecting sample) Weight
Sample storage information	Date Location Temperature
Subsampling information	Procedure Date Parent sample
Sample preparation	Detailed description of compositing Description of other procedures performed
Assay procedures performed	Detailed description of each procedure used, including thawing and taking aliquots
Quality control information associated with sample value(s) (eg, QC chart)	Source or description of quality control materials, reference standards, and calibration standards Assay results for these materials
Shipment of samples	Sample identification Sample weights Condition of samples (eg, temperature) at time of shipping and time of receiving
Reported values	Source of data Original sample identification Procedures used

analysis laboratory understands the need for replicates. Commercial laboratories often base the per-sample assay cost on the assumption of a single determination. Single analysis always runs the risk of error because of sample heterogeneity or an isolated error in the assay procedure, despite an acceptable batch QCM value and other data from the laboratory regarding the general precision of the assay. Nonetheless, replicate assays done by a commercial laboratory can be expensive, so the investigator must balance the potential for variance and its impact on the study against cost.

These concerns will be greater in long-term studies or in those requiring high precision. Again, a statistician can be of assistance in this domain. Doing blinded reruns on about 5% of the samples is a good practice that ensures the reproducibility of results for individual composites over the long term.

When a composite is assayed in replicate, we recommend drawing the replicate aliquots from different subsamples (ie, storage jars) that are separated from one another chronologically in the composite subsampling process. Because it is im-

practical to confirm the homogeneity of every composite and settling during composite subsampling is the most likely source of any heterogeneity, assaying replicates in this fashion serves to maximize the chance of detecting any differences. It also renders the mean a better estimate of the true overall composition of the composite. An example of such an assay sampling plan is illustrated in Figure 22–5.

Documentation

Thorough documentation is essential to provide an audit trail linking reported values for a sample to details of the sample description, sample handling, assay methodology used, and associated data (eg, values for quality control samples run in the same assay batch, values for the same sample determined in different assays). It is beyond the scope of this chapter to comprehensively discuss each component of documentation. Interested readers are referred to Good Laboratory Practice Standards for further information (43). A list of key components of documentation for diet assays as part of a well-controlled diet study is given in Table 22–9.

EXHIBIT 22-5

Laboratories That Analyze Nutrients in Foods

Covance Laboratories
3301 Kinsman Boulevard
Madison, WI 53704
Phone: (608) 241-4471
Web site: http://www.covance.com

Eurofins Scientific
2394 Route 130
Dayton, NJ 08810
Phone: (800) 841-1110
Web site: http://www.eurofins.com

Food Analysis Laboratory Control Center (FALCC)
Department of Biochemistry
Virginia Polytechnic Institute and State University
Blacksburg, VA 24061-0308
Phone: (540) 231-9960
Web site: http://www.vt.edu

Lancaster Laboratories
2425 New Holland Pike
Lancaster, PA 17605-2425
Phone: (717) 656-2308
Web site: http://www.lancasterlabs.com

Pennington Food Analysis Laboratory
Pennington Biomedical Research Center
Louisiana State University
6400 Perkins Road
Baton Rouge, LA 70808-4124
Phone: (225) 763-2500
Web site: http://www.pbrc.edu

Ralston Analytical Laboratories
2RS Checkerboard Square
St Louis, MO 63164
Phone: (800) 423-6832
Web site: http://www.ralstonanalytical.com

Southern Testing and Research Labs
3809 Airport Drive
Wilson, NC 27896
Phone: (252) 237-4175
Web site: http://www.strlabs.com

USDA Food Composition Laboratory
Building 161, Room 102
Beltsville Agricultural Research Center
Agricultural Research Service, USDA
Beltsville, MD 20705
Phone: (301) 504-8356
Web site: http://www.usda.gov

Disclaimer: This list is provided for the information of readers and is not intended to be comprehensive. Mention of these laboratories does not constitute endorsement by National Heart, Lung, and Blood Institute, The American Dietetic Association, or the authors.

CHOOSING A FOOD ANALYSIS LABORATORY

The quality of the food analysis laboratory and its product (assayed nutrient levels) will directly affect conclusions about the composition of diets fed to participants. Possibilities for a contract laboratory include government, university, or commercial facilities (see Exhibit 22–5). Certain analyses (for example, *trans* fatty acids, carotenoids) are not standard offerings of most commercial laboratories, and the best approach is to determine (eg, from a literature search) who are the experts in the field and obtain from them recommendations for a subcontractor.

The responsibility for method validation and assay quality control rests with the laboratory itself. Individual laboratories vary widely in quality. Usually, it can be assumed that a reputable commercial laboratory employs well-tested methods. However, the investigator should still request documentation about the exact assay methods used. Although an established method may be in use, this does not necessarily mean the method has been validated for the particular mixed-food composite matrix or for the expected nutrient levels in diet samples from a given study.

The food analysis laboratory should be provided a listing of constituent foods in composite samples to allow the chemist to verify specific methods. The laboratory should also be given the expected concentration range for each nutrient to be assayed so that analytical concentration limits (ie, weight of nutrient per gram of analytical aliquot) can be estimated.

A high-quality laboratory would answer affirmatively to the questions listed in Exhibit 22–6, which test for practices basic to well-conducted chemical analyses. Other pertinent issues are the general reputation of the laboratory, the number of years it has been in business, the usual turnaround time, ability to provide documentation, and potential for flexibility in working with the study and providing continuing support. The relative importance of these factors will be affected by the number of samples, the nature of the analytes, and the duration of the study. Obviously cost is an important consideration, but cost concerns should never compromise data requirements. If accuracy and precision criteria are stringent and standard reference materials are available for analytes, these samples can be sent to the laboratory to test performance. Once a laboratory has been chosen for a given assay, all assays should be performed at that laboratory to eliminate potential bias and interlaboratory variance.

EXHIBIT 22-6

Questions for Assessing the Quality of a Food Analysis Laboratory[1]

_____	Do you use standardized, written methods?
_____	Will you provide descriptions of your methods, any modifications of standard methods, and your internal laboratory quality control procedures?
_____	Do you assay each sample at least in duplicate? Are values for replicate assays reported?
_____	Do you participate in collaborative check sample (ie, reference sample or "round robin") programs when available? Is your performance in these programs within acceptable limits? Can you provide documentation of performance, if requested?
_____	Do you use standard reference materials to validate each method?
_____	Do you use internal standards for chromatographic assays?
_____	Do you develop and implement food-based control materials to monitor the accuracy and precision of all assays in your laboratory?
_____	Are control materials matrices matched to the samples being assayed?
_____	Are summary statistics available for control materials?
_____	Is the control material assayed with each batch of samples?
_____	For each sample value reported, is the control material identity and corresponding assayed value reported?
_____	What is the cost of replicate assays of each nutrient? Do you have any additional costs or service charges? Who pays for shipping?
_____	What is the average time from receipt of the sample to the issuance of an assay report? What is the longest time it will take you to produce an assay report?
_____	How should we prepare the samples for your analysts?

[1] Courtesy of Holden JM, USDA Nutrient Data Laboratory, Beltsville, Md.

EVALUATING THE ANALYTICAL DATA

The first step in evaluating analytical data is to assess the corresponding quality control material data for each assayed value (using a QC chart) and the precision of replicate values, and to reject any data that do not meet the quality control criteria established for the study. Next, assayed nutrient levels are converted to the required units, if necessary. Normally assay values are reported on an as-received basis: for example, grams per 100 g wet weight. The clinical investigator will usually be interested in the nutrient density of the diet, in certain units (eg, g per day, % of kcal). The data can then be compared to the target diet composition and tolerance limits.

For diet validation, if analyzed nutrient concentrations agree with the diet design, no changes should be made to the menus that were assayed. If the analyzed concentration of one or more nutrients deviates meaningfully from the calculated target in a given menu or diet, there are several possible reasons: error(s) in food preparation, analytical error(s), or a true difference in the actual and targeted compositions. Because detection of true differences is the goal of diet analysis, the first step in evaluating any discrepancy is to rule out the other sources of error. Food preparation deviations are suspected when analyses of replicate composites yield different results. Food preparation records should be reviewed to make sure that items were procured and prepared according to specifications and that portions were weighed correctly. In our studies, we have been able to identify the

source of some significant deviations in the composition of prepared menus in this manner (44).

If a preparation error is found, the menu can be prepared again and assayed. Analytical error will be minimized if procedures are properly validated and if composite preparation and assays are performed with strict quality control as outlined in this chapter. The quality control chart can be examined to determine whether assay drift might explain the deviation. Samples of off-target composites can also be reassayed to double-check the data values.

If the actual nutrient concentrations in prepared diets truly deviate from design, there are several possible courses of action. If individual menus were assayed, those erring from target composition can be adjusted and reassayed, or eliminated from the menu cycle. If the diet cycle composite was analyzed, then individual menus (either archived when the cycle composite was prepared or prepared fresh) can be assayed, and those found to differ from target composition can be adjusted (recalculated and cooked) and reassayed, or they can be dropped from the final set of menus.

Finally, there are several other considerations in evaluating the raw analytical nutrient data. First, variance in _moisture content_ will cause variance in nutrient values as percent of wet weight (g/100 g as received), which is the usual unit in which raw data are reported. For example, if the parameter of interest is total fat per day, a 2,000-g daily menu containing 60 g of fat would have an assayed total fat content of 3.0 g/100 g. If an extra 100 g water (with no nutritional value) were inadvertently added, the assayed total fat content would be lower (2.8 g/100 g), even though total fat (60 g) and energy in the menu were unchanged. This difference is corrected when the assayed weight percent of fat is multiplied by total food weight to yield total grams/menu.

Nutrients can also be expressed as percent of dry weight. Errors, bias, and/or variance in the moisture assay will, however, be incorporated into the variance of a nutrient value on a dry-weight basis. The higher the moisture content of the sample, the greater the impact of any error in the moisture measurement. Lyophilized samples are of particular concern. Although they have a low water content, these materials tend to be hygroscopic and the moisture level can fluctuate significantly. Therefore, data for freeze-dried samples should always be reported on a dry-weight basis, and moisture must be assayed in an aliquot of each sample, obtained from the same container, at the same time an aliquot of that material is weighed for the nutrient assay.

Second, all errors or variance in component analytical values will be *additively* incorporated into calculated nutrient parameters (eg, total energy calculated from proximates, nutrients as grams/day or percent of energy). Errors may or may not cancel. Therefore, the precision of calculated parameters will generally be lower than that of assayed values. Furthermore, if analytical nutrient data are converted from weight percent to total weight per day (week, etc), the absolute magnitude of the effect of any analytical deviation will be directly related to the total sample weight. For example, if the total menu weighs 1,500 g or 3,000 g, respectively, differences in assayed cholesterol concentrations of 15 mg/100 g vs 17 mg/100 g in a given composite will translate to differences of 30 mg (225 mg/100 g vs 255 mg/day) or 60 mg (450 mg/100 g vs 510 mg/day).

BUDGET CONSIDERATIONS

Budgets for chemical analysis of research diets are not based solely on assay costs. Aside from expenses typical of any analytical laboratory operation, funds also must be available to purchase basic food supplies and to prepare and collect the individual foods or meal samples. For validation samples, each daily menu for each dietary treatment is prepared in duplicate. For monitoring samples, meals and snacks are prepared for at least one extra participant for each dietary treatment for one or more menu cycles. Such costs must also be anticipated when planning pilot studies.

As a guide for budget preparation, cost components of chemically analyzing diet composition as part of a controlled feeding trial are outlined in Exhibit 22–7. This summary presumes samples will be collected and composited on site, with aliquots shipped to a food analysis laboratory for assays.

CONCLUSION

A key goal of well-controlled feeding studies is to produce and deliver experimental menus that consistently meet the diet design criteria. Diet validation *prior to feeding* ensures that menus contain the targeted nutrient levels. When this prefeeding chemical validation is combined with appropriate and standardized food procurement, handling, and preparation protocols to maintain consistency of diet composition across time (and sites, if the study is multicenter), delivery of the desired diets is likely.

Diet monitoring assays can document what was actually fed to participants. However, by the time the monitoring results are available, the feeding periods usually are finished. Also, it is impractical to sample and analyze enough samples to determine whether a deviation in composition assayed in a single monitoring sample represents an isolated error (in that particular sample), a consistent deviation in the diet composition (which deserves correction), or variance in composition (cycle-to-cycle and/or sample-to-sample). Therefore, the bulk of resources allotted to chemical assays should be used for validating diets prior to feeding and controlling diet preparation during intervention.

This chapter has presented procedures for the implementation of diet assays and has outlined the key components involved in obtaining reliable data from analysis of diet composites. Chemical assay of diets in an intervention study should be considered a control measure, similar in purpose to compliance checks. Although most clinical investigators routinely document their efforts and degree of success in encouraging high compliance, assaying diet composition is a less familiar concept. Both processes, however, serve to ensure desired nutrient intake. Given the limitations of food composition databases and the unpredictability of nutrient variance in prepared diets, prepared experimental diets should be chemically analyzed to definitively link dietary nutrient concentrations with biological measurements. The resulting enhancement of confidence in the validity of the study outcomes suggests that diet analysis should be routinely incorporated into protocols for well-controlled feeding studies.

The authors gratefully acknowledge the artistic skills of Karen Richardson.

REFERENCES

1. US Department of Agriculture. *Nutrient Database for Standard Reference, Release 12*. Nutrient Data Laboratory Home Page http://www.nal.usda.gov/fnic/foodcomp. Riverdale, Md: Agricultural Research Service; 1996.
2. International Food Biotechnology Council. Variability in the composition of traditional foods: nutrients, microorganisms, and toxicants. In: Biotechnologies and food: assuring the safety of foods produced by genetic modification. *Reg Toxicol Pharmacol.* 1990;12(3):S11-S78.

EXHIBIT 22-7

Cost Components for the Chemical Analysis of Diet Composites[1]

LABOR[2]
Designing sampling and analysis plans for diet validation and monitoring
Preparing quality control material
Preparing extra menu/food samples for diet validation and monitoring
Preparing composites
Shipping composite samples for analysis
Receiving, processing, analyzing, and reporting nutrient data
Performing quality control review of analytical data
Maintaining documentation and audit trails
Assaying food samples and quality control samples for nutrients
Establishing and performing data analysis and quality control program

EQUIPMENT
Industrial batch food processors for preparing composites: 25 L or larger for menu cycles (7 to 8 daily menus);
    6 L for individual daily menus
Analytical balance
Other laboratory equipment as needed

SUPPLIES
Containers for food collection
Jars for composite subsamples
Insulated coolers for shipping samples
Dry ice
Supplies for food collection (see Exhibit 22-3)
Supplies for preparing food composites
Chemicals and other laboratory supplies

FOOD[3]
Prefeeding diet validation samples
Diet monitoring samples
Quality control material

STORAGE FACILITIES
Refrigerator
Freezer ($-20°C$) (for storing uncomposited samples)
Ultra-low temperature freezer ($-60°C$) (for short-term storage and archival storage of homogenized samples)

ADMINISTRATIVE EXPENSES
Computer with software and printer
System for logging and tracking samples and associated information, including computer and software
Shipping menus to off-site composite homogenization facility; composited samples to food analysis laboratory

QUALITY CONTROL MATERIAL (QCM) ANALYSES (TO ESTABLISH QUALITY CONTROL CHARTS)
Preparation (food, labor)
Storage
Containers
Assay charges

[1]Cost formulas vary greatly among research units. Some may need to determine per-assay costs that incorporate many categories of expenses. Others will separate labor, equipment, supplies, etc. Overhead rates, fringe benefits, and space and utility charges also vary.
[2]Labor costs are specified as tasks. Job categories and wages or salaries for individuals performing these tasks will vary among laboratories.
[3]Food costs for validation samples will be higher if the daily menu for each diet is prepared and collected in duplicate. Additional costs will be incurred if pilot studies or analyses of individual food items are planned. Food costs for diet monitoring will be determined by the number of extra samples prepared (eg, the food cost for at least one extra participant for each diet cycle and each diet treatment collected).

3. Piironen V, Varo P, Coivistoinen P. Stability of tocopherols and tocotrienols in food preparation procedures. *J Food Comp Anal.* 1988;1:152–158.

4. Slover HT, Lanza E, Thompson RH Jr. Lipids in fast foods. *J Food Sci.* 1980;45:153–159.

5. Vanderslice JT, Higgs DJ Vitamin C content of foods: sample variability. *Am J Clin Nutr.* 1991;54(Suppl):1323S–1327S.

6. Vanderslice JT, Higgs DJ. Vitamin C content variability in samples: implications for dietary studies. In: *Proceedings of the 15th National Nutrient Databank Conference.* Ithaca, NY: The CBORD Group, Inc; 1991:117–119.

7. Hurburgh CR Jr. Long-term soybean composition patterns and their effects on processing. *J Am Oil Chem Soc.* 1994;71:1425–1427.

8. Clarke RP, Merrow SB. Nutrient composition of tomatoes homegrown under different cultural procedures. *Ecol Food Nutr.* 1979;8:37–46.

9. Baer RJ. Alteration of the fatty acid content of milk fat. *J Food Protection.* 1991;54:383–386.

10. Lee SM, Buss DH, Holcombe GD, Hatton D. Nutrient content of retail cuts of beef, pork, and lamb: preliminary results. *J Hum Nutr Diet.* 1995;8:75–80.

11. Marshall MW, Clevidence BA, Thompson RH Jr, Judd JT. Cholesterol and plant sterols in controlled mixed diets: two analytical methods vs food table values. *J Food Comp Anal.* 1989;2:2–12.

12. Marshall MW, Clevidence BA, Thompson RH Jr, Judd JT. Problems in estimating amounts of food cholesterol. Part 2: three methods for self-selected mixed diets. *J Food Comp Anal.* 1989;2:228–237.

13. Wills RBH, Balmer N, Greenfield H. Composition of Australian foods. 2: Methods of analysis. *Food Tech Austr.* 1980;32:198–204.

14. Lurie DG, Holden JM, Schubert A, Wolf W, Miller-Ihli NJ. The copper content of foods based on a critical evaluation of published analytical data. *J Food Comp Anal.* 1989;2:298–316.

15. US Congress. Public Law 101–535 (Nutrition labeling, CFR 21, 1993). Nutrition Labeling and Education Act of 1990. *Code of Federal Regulations.* Vol 21. Washington DC: US Government Printing Office; 1993.

16. Steinke FH. Nutrient composition data uses and needs of food companies. In: Rand WM, Windham CT, Wyse BW, Young VR, eds. *Food Composition Data: A User's Perspective.* Avon, UK: The Bathe Press, United Nations University; 1987:97–100.

17. Foote D. Food composition data and clinical dietetics. In: Uses and Abuses of Food Composition Data. *Food Tech Austr.* 1990;42:S8-S9.

18. Dennis BH, Stewart P, Wang CH, Champagne C, Windhauser M, Ershow A, Karmally W, Phillips K, Stewart K, Van Heel N, Farhat-Wood A, Kris-Etherton PM. Diet design for a multicenter controlled feeding trial: the DELTA program. *J Am Diet Assoc.* 1998;98:766–776.

19. Sacks FM, Obarzanek E, Windhauser MM, Svetky LP, Vollmer WM, McCullough M, Karanja N, Lin P-H, Steele P, Proschan MA, Evans MA, Appel LJ, Bray GA, Vogt TM, Moore TJ, for the DASH Collaborative Research Group. Rationale and design of the Dietary Approaches to Stop Hypertension Trial (DASH): a multicenter controlled-feeding study of dietary patterns to lower blood pressure. *Ann Epidemiol.* 1995;5:108–118.

20. Appel LJ, Moore TJ, Obarzanek E, Vollmer WM, Svetky LP, Sacks FM, Bray GA, Vogt TM, Cutler JA, Simons-Morton D, Lin P-H, Windhauser MM, Lin PH, Karanja N, for the DASH Collaborative Research Group. A clinical trial of the effects of dietary patterns on blood pressure. *N Engl J Med.* 1997;336:1117–1124.

21. Phillips KM, Stewart KK, Champagne CM, Holden JM, for the DELTA Investigators. Assay of menus as part of a multicenter clinical feeding trial: comparison of calculated and assayed fat content. *Proceedings of the 108th Annual Meeting of AOAC International,* Portland, Ore, September 12–15, 1994; Abstract 14–022. Gaithersburg, Md: Association of Official Analytical Chemists International, Inc; 1994.

22. Carpenter DE, Ngeh-Ngwainbi J, Lee S. Lipid analysis. In: Sullivan DM, Carpenter DE, eds. *Methods of Analysis for Nutrition Labeling.* Gaithersburg, Md: Association of Official Analytical Chemists International, Inc; 1993;85–104.

23. Wolf WR. Reference materials. In: Sullivan DM, Carpenter DE, eds. *Methods of Analysis for Nutrition Labeling.* Gaithersburg, Md: Association of Official Analytical Chemists International, Inc; 1993:111–122.

24. Stewart KK for the DELTA Investigators. Diet composition documentation in a multicenter clinical feeding trial. *FASEB J.* 1995;9(3):A289.

25. Phillips KM for the DELTA Investigators. Diet composition validation and monitoring as part of a multicenter clinical feeding trial of Step 1 Diet. *FASEB J.* 1996;10(3):A262.

26. Taylor JK. *Quality Assurance of Chemical Measurements.* Chelsea, Mich: Lewis Publishers, Inc; 1987.

27. Ratnayake WMN. Determination of *trans* unsaturation by infrared spectrophotometry and determination of fatty acid composition of partially hydrogenated vegetable oils and animal fats by gas chromatography/infrared spectrophotometry: collaborative study. *J Assoc Off Anal Chem Int.* 1995;78:783–802.

28. Lichon MJ, James DW. Homogenization methods for analysis of foodstuffs. *J Assoc Off Anal Chem.* 1990;73:820–825.

29. Li BW, Schuhmann PJ, Wolf WR. Chromatographic determinations of sugars and starch in a diet composite reference material. *J Agric Food Chem.* 1985;33:531–536.

30. Vanderslice JT, Higgs DJ, Hayes JM, Block G. Ascorbic acid and dehydroascorbic acid content of foods-as-eaten. *J Food Comp Anal.* 1990;3:105–118.

31. Association of Official Analytical Chemists. *Official Methods of Analysis.* 15th ed. Gaithersburg, Md: Association of Official Analytical Chemists International, Inc; 1990.

32. American Association of Cereal Chemists. *Approved Methods.* 9th ed. St Paul, Minn; American Association of Cereal Chemists; 1995.

33. American Oil Chemists Society. *Official Methods and Recommended Practices.* 4th ed, Vols 1 and 2. Champaign, Ill: American Oil Chemists Society; 1996.

34. Paquot C, Hautfenne A, eds. *Standard Methods for the Analysis of Oils, Fats, and Derivatives.* 7th ed. Boston: International Union of Pure and Applied Chemistry, Blackwell Scientific Publications; 1987. (This is one of a multivolume series comprising analysis methods for a large variety of compounds.)

35. Sullivan DM, Carpenter DE, eds. *Methods of Analysis for Nutrition Labeling.* Gaithersburg, Md: Association of Official Analytical Chemists International, Inc; 1993: 85–104.

36. Greenfield H, Southgate DAT. *Food Composition Data: Production, Management and Use.* New York, NY: Elsevier Science Publishers Ltd; 1992.

37. Phillips KM, Lugogo RD, Harris RF, Tarrago-Trani MT, Bailey JA, Stewart KK. Direct determination of trans-octadecenoic acid in diet composites using a combination of silver ion-high performance liquid chromatography and capillary gas chromatography. *J Food Lipids.* 1997;4:173–188.

38. Wernimont GT. *Use of Statistics to Develop and Evaluate Analytical Methods.* Spendley W, ed. Gaithersburg, Md: Association of Official Analytical Chemists, International, Inc; 1985.

39. Holden JM, Davis CS, Wolf WR, Beecher GR. Variability in nutrient measurements by five commercial laboratories. *Proceedings of the 108th Annual Meeting of AOAC International.* Portland, Ore, September 12–15, 1994. Vol 77; Number 3; abstract number 14–024. Gaithersburg, Md: Association of Official Analytical Chemists International, Inc.

40. DeVoe JR, ed. *Validation of the Measurement Process.* Washington, DC: American Chemical Society; 1977.

41. Garfield FM. *Quality Assurance Principles for Analytical Laboratories.* Gaithersburg, Md: Association of Official Analytical Chemists International, Inc; 1991.

42. Dux JP. *Handbook of Quality Assurance for the Analytical Chemistry Laboratory.* New York, NY: Van Nostrand Reinhold; 1986.

43. Garner WY, Barge MS, Ussary JP, eds. *Good Laboratory Practice Standards.* Washington, DC: American Chemical Society; 1992.

44. Stewart KK, Phillips KM, Champagne CM, Dennis BH for the DELTA Investigators. Menu validation in the DELTA study: the use of total nutrient weights to determine sources of variance and errors. In: Dietary Assessment Methods, Part X (Food Consumption Patterns). *Proceedings of the Second International Conference on Dietary Assessment Methods.* Boston, Mass, January 22–24, 1995, Willett W, ed. *Am J Clin Nutr.* 1995;65(4)(Suppl):1366S.

CHAPTER 23

LABORATORY QUALITY CONTROL IN DIETARY TRIALS

PAUL S. BACHORIK, PHD, AND HENRY J. POWNALL, PHD

Abbreviations

CDC	Centers for Disease Control and Prevention (US Public Health Service, Atlanta, GA)
CV	Coefficient of variation
CV_a	Coefficient of analytical variation
CV_p	Coefficient of physiological variation
$CV_{spec, tot}$	Coefficient of total variation in serial specimens (quantity of biological material obtained on a given occasion; divisible in aliquots or samples that may be analyzed or stored)
EDTA	Ethylenediaminetetraacetic acid
HDL	High-density lipoprotein
LDL	Low-density lipoprotein
NCEP	National Cholesterol Education Program (National Heart, Lung, and Blood Institute, Bethesda, MD)
SD	Standard deviation
TE	Total error
$\bar{x}$	Mean of an individual analytical run
$\bar{\bar{x}}$	Overall mean of the individual run means
$\bar{x}_s$	Mean of serial measurements

The design and implementation of well-controlled diet studies are perhaps among the most demanding scientific endeavors. The logistics and cost of such studies as well as the validity of their conclusions depend in large part on the reliability of the primary measurements. Measurements of diet can include determining the nutrient composition of foods or diet composites and assessing the amount of food consumed by individual participants. Such measurements require a host of analytical methods and can be difficult to make accurately and precisely.

It is also necessary to determine the effects of dietary manipulations on concentrations of components of interest in biological specimens. This process requires measuring these components before and after dietary treatment and determining the magnitude and significance of the changes. Food composition, dietary intake, and measurements of blood and other biological specimens require the collaboration of investigators with different kinds of expertise and are made with a variety of analytical techniques. The one common requirement of the measurements, however, is the assessment of bias and imprecision, and how they affect the study data.

Quality control is fundamental to the conduct of dietary studies. In general, the more reproducible the measurements, the smaller the changes that can be observed in response to treatment, and the more reliably they can be estimated. This, in turn, influences the number of participants that must be enrolled and the number of measurements required per participant. In addition, it is often desirable to compare data collected in different studies. This comparison is facilitated by basing the measurements on accepted reference methods and specifying laboratory bias when the data are reported. For these reasons, it is important that measurement issues be confronted in detail as the study is being planned.

Quality control issues commonly are considered primarily in terms of minimizing laboratory error. This is certainly a major goal of any quality control system, but much broader issues are involved. Laboratory error per se is only one contributor to the error of the measurements; for most measurements, it is not even the major contributor. Issues pertinent to the chemical analysis of diets are discussed in Chapter 22. This chapter uses the example of the major sources of variation associated with lipid and lipoprotein measurements in blood to illustrate how the principles of quality control apply regardless of what is being measured or where the measurements are made.

SOURCES OF VARIATION

The factors that contribute to changes in the measured values of biological parameters such as blood lipids and lipoproteins can be broadly separated into three major categories: (1) laboratory error; (2) normal physiological variation; and (3) response to treatment. Of these categories, the first two determine the reliability with which the third (response to treatment) can be measured.

Laboratory Error

Laboratory error refers to a reported value that is wrong; for example, when the reported cholesterol concentration of a particular specimen does not reflect its true concentration at the time the specimen was drawn. The error can result from measurement error per se but can also result from improper sample preparation, identification, storage, or transport to the laboratory. Such factors can produce inaccurate results but may be beyond the control of the laboratory. The lack of control is not surprising because in many cases the individuals charged with drawing blood specimens, preparing and storing serum or plasma, and transporting or shipping the specimens to the laboratory may not have formal laboratory training and may not be aware of the various factors that can produce an inaccurate result.

This unawareness is of some concern, because the consequences of improper sample handling can be difficult to detect. It is prudent in the initial phase of a study to conduct a training session in which the individuals charged with blood drawing and sample handling are instructed in the proper techniques of patient preparation and specimen collection, and are made aware of how to document and preserve the integrity of the sample until it is received by the laboratory. Instruction should be followed by a small pilot study in which these individuals are asked to obtain, prepare, document, and ship specimens to the laboratory. The performance of these personnel and the condition of the specimens when they arrive in the laboratory are then assessed, and any necessary corrections or alterations of the protocol are made before the main study begins. Such a pilot study also allows the laboratory staff to practice any special handling or documentation procedures that may be specific to the study. Although the pilot study requires some commitment of time and resources, it can prevent unnecessary delays later in the study and help protect the validity of the measurements. The pilot study should be included in the planning phase of the study.

Bias and Imprecision

Errors can also occur after sample collection. Under the best of circumstances there is always some degree of uncertainty associated with a laboratory measurement. *Bias* refers to the proximity of the measured value in a particular specimen to the true concentration in that specimen and depends in large part on proper test calibration. The assessment of bias requires the use of appropriate serum control pools that contain known concentrations of the components of interest and can be analyzed along with the participant specimens.

Imprecision refers to the reproducibility of several measurements in the same specimen. When a component is assayed several times in a specimen, the individual measurements will usually differ somewhat because of variations in the delivery of specimen or reagent volumes, lot-to-lot variations in reagent preparations, instrument function, or other factors. The influence of imprecision can be reduced by making replicate measurements of each specimen and averaging the values. In practice, this is rarely done for either research or routine clinical purposes because of the time and expense involved.

Consider the example of total serum cholesterol. A specimen is generally analyzed once, and the result is assumed to be correct within certain limits that are defined by the bias and imprecision of the analytical procedure. Part of the function of the laboratory quality control system is to define these limits. It is not possible to say with absolute certainty that any particular value is correct. Instead, staff try to minimize the probability that the result is outside the acceptable error limit. The overall reliability of the laboratory results is generally stated in terms of the bias and imprecision of the measurements. Such statements of reliability do not refer to measurements in particular samples but rather to the average proximity of the measurements in specimens during the course of the study to their true values.

For cholesterol, bias and imprecision are monitored through the use of at least two serum control pools with known cholesterol concentrations, one in the 180 mg/dL to 200 mg/dL range and the other in the 240 mg/dL to 280 mg/dL range. Aliquots of each pool are included in each analytical run and each is analyzed at least in duplicate. The mean value for each pool is calculated and the values are used to indicate bias in that run. When considered along with the quality control results from a series of analytical runs, the daily means are also used to estimate run-to-run variation as well as the average bias of the measurements made in specimens in those runs. The difference between the highest and lowest value in a single run, referred to as the *range,* is used as a measure of the reproducibility of the measurements in that run.

Quality control results are displayed visually, as illustrated in Figure 23–1. In the example shown in the figure, the serum control pool is assumed to have a true cholesterol concentration of 200 mg/dL. Each point indicates the mean value of an individual run ($\overline{x}$). The chart also indicates the mean of the individual run means, ($\overline{\overline{x}}$), or the overall mean. In this example this overall mean is 202 mg/dL. The overall mean is usually referred to as the *laboratory mean.* The laboratory bias, in this case +1%, can be calculated from the following equation:

$$\% \text{ bias} = [(\overline{\overline{x}} - \text{true value}) \div \text{true value}] \times 100$$

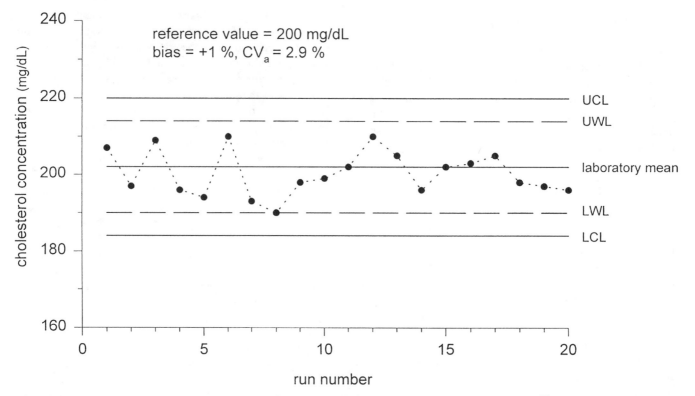

FIGURE 23-1. Sample quality control chart. UCL, LCL, upper and lower control limits, calculated as $\overline{\overline{x}} \pm 2.58$ SD; UWL, LWL, upper and lower warning limits, calculated as $\overline{\overline{x}} \pm 1.96$ SD. In practice, the multipliers are usually rounded to the next whole number. CV_a, coefficient of analytical variation.

The standard deviation (SD) of the run means is 5.9 mg/dL. The imprecision of the measurements is expressed in terms of the coefficient of variation (CV), defined as

$$\%CV = (SD \div \overline{\overline{x}}) \times 100$$

In this case, the CV is 2.9%. The dotted lines on the chart mark the 95% limits, calculated as

$$95\% \text{ limits} = \overline{\overline{x}} \pm 1.96(SD)$$

The heavy solid lines correspond to the 99% limits, which were calculated from the equation

$$99\% \text{ limits} = \overline{\overline{x}} \pm 2.58(SD)$$

In practice, the multipliers are usually rounded to the next whole numbers, 1.96 to 2 and 2.58 to 3.

The laboratory mean and control limits are calculated when sufficient data have been accumulated for the pool, generally after 20 to 50 runs. The true value (also called the reference value) for the pool is assigned using a recognized reference method if available. In the case of total cholesterol, the basis for assigning true values is the reference method for cholesterol (1) used by the Clinical Chemistry Standardization Section, Centers for Disease Control and Prevention (CDC), Atlanta, Ga. Bias estimates determined from the

control pools are used to describe the average accuracy of measurements for the specimens analyzed in those particular analytical runs. When investigators report study data, it is common to summarize the bias estimates for the entire data set from the quality control measurements made during the course of the entire study. The CV expresses the SD of the individual run means as a percent of the laboratory mean. This is a convenient way of expressing the imprecision without having to specify the concentration of the particular serum pool used. For cholesterol, CV values are fairly similar over the concentration range of interest. It should be noted, however, that %CV defines the range in which approximately two-thirds of the measurements can be expected to fall, ie, %CV reflects $\overline{\overline{x}} \pm 1$ SD.

Limits of Acceptability

Limits of acceptable laboratory performance for the measurement of total cholesterol have been defined by the National Cholesterol Education Program (NCEP) Laboratory Standardization Panel (LSP) (2). Subsequently, the NCEP Working Group on Lipoprotein Measurement defined limits of acceptbability for triglyceride and HDL- and LDL-cholesterol measurements (3). These guidelines are summarized in Table 23–1. For cholesterol, acceptable *bias* was defined as $\pm$ 3% with respect to CDC reference values; acceptable *precision* was defined as a CV $\leq$ 3% (2). This means that

TABLE 23-1

National Cholesterol Education Program Recommendations for Lipid and Lipoprotein Measurement

Component[1]	% Bias	% CV_a[2]	Total Error[3]
Total Cholesterol	≤ 3%	≤3%	≤ 9%
Triglyceride	≤ 5%	≤5%	≤15%
HDL-cholesterol	≤10%	≤6%[4]	≤22%
LDL-cholesterol	≤ 4%	≤4%	≤12%

[1]From US Department of Health and Human Services (2) and Working Group on Lipoprotein Measurement (3).
[2]CV_a: coefficient of analytical variation.
[3]NCEP recommendations use total error as the primary criterion to determine the limits of acceptable performance. Total error accounts for bias and imprecision at the same time, and in each case, the bias and CV_a shown are examples of values that would satisfy the limits for total error. A greater bias requires a lower CV_a in order to satisfy the goal for total error. Conversely, a larger CV_a would require a smaller bias to meet the requirements for total error. Laboratories that operate within the bias and imprecision limits shown also meet the goal for total error. The values shown for total error assume maximum allowable bias and CV_a, and a 95% confidence limit for CV_a.
[4]CV_a ≥42 mg/dL; at lower HDL concentrations, it is recommended that SD ≤2.5 mg/dL.

average laboratory bias should be within 3% of true values and that two-thirds of the run means should be no more than 3% from the laboratory mean ($\overline{\overline{x}}$). If measurement error is completely random and the laboratory measurements are stable, the individual run means ($\overline{x}$) are expected to fall above and below the laboratory mean ($\overline{\overline{x}}$) with equal frequency (Figure 23–1).

By definition, 1% of the values would be expected to fall outside the 99% limits when the assay procedures are operating properly. The laboratory control limit is generally set at the 99% limit. Although the results are expected to exceed this limit occasionally, such an occurrence would be uncommon, and it is usual practice to consider any analytical run that falls outside this limit to be "out of control." The results from such a run would not be accepted, and the analyses would be repeated. The 95% limits define the warning zone; a single analytical run falling above the 95% limit and below or on the 99% limit would be accepted; however, two or more sequential runs falling in this area would be cause for concern. The second and subsequent runs would be considered "out of control," and the laboratory would initiate troubleshooting procedures.

Total Error

The overall reliability of a laboratory measurement can also be expressed in terms of *total error* (TE), which is a single parameter that accounts for bias and imprecision at the same time. TE is calculated as follows:

$$TE = \% \text{ bias} + (1.96 \times \%CV)$$

For a laboratory operating at the extremes of the NCEP criteria (Table 23–1), the total error for cholesterol would be 8.9%:

$$TE = 3\% + (1.96 \times 3\%)$$

Again, 1.96 can be rounded to 2, producing a total error estimate of 9%.

In actual practice, most well-controlled laboratories that use modern automated methods to measure total cholesterol are capable of accuracy within 1% to 2% of reference values and CV values in the range of 1% to 2%. (There are many other types of measurements that cannot achieve the level of precision that is possible for cholesterol assays.) Figure 23–2 illustrates the analytical variation for a laboratory with a positive bias of 1% and a CV of 1.1%. The bias and CV used for this example were obtained in one of the authors' (PSB) laboratories. In this case, TE would be:

$$TE = 1\% + (.96 \times 1.1\%) = 3.2\%$$

Normal Physiological Variation

When an individual is in a steady state (ie, consuming a regular diet, not losing or gaining weight, pursuing a normal routine of activity), and a component such as cholesterol is measured in different specimens taken on several occasions, the measured values will differ somewhat but cluster around a mean value that can be considered the "usual value" for that individual. As shown earlier, part of this variation arises from the process of making the measurements. In addition, however, lipid and lipoprotein concentrations fluctuate throughout the course of normal daily activity, contributing to the temporal fluctuations observed in a particular individual (4). This would occur even in the absence of analytical error. Such normal fluctuations occur for various reasons, including recent food intake, postural changes that occur throughout the day, and small seasonal variations (5–13).

For this reason, it is incorrect to speak of the participant's cholesterol concentration as a fixed value. Rather, it is more accurate to consider the participant's usual (ie, average) cholesterol concentration or, better, his or her range of concentrations. The factors that contribute to normal physiological variation are not completely understood, but several, including postural and postprandial changes, have been examined.

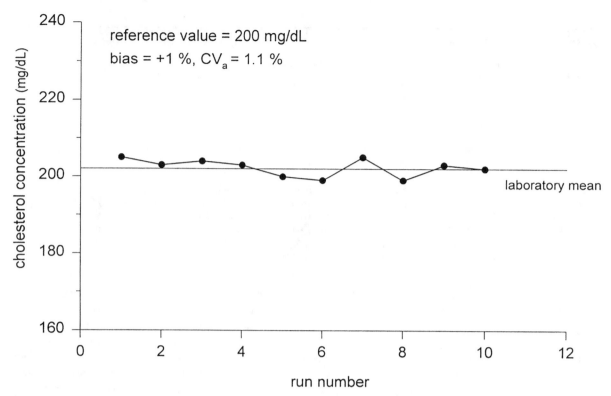

FIGURE 23-2.   Analytical variation. The values represent the cholesterol concentration of a serum control pool with a reference value of 200 mg/dL as measured in a laboratory with a 1% positive bias. The laboratory mean is shown by the horizontal line at 202 mg/dL. CV_a, coefficient of analytical variation.

Postural and Postprandial Effects

The changes that can occur in lipid and lipoprotein concentrations when a standing participant assumes a sitting or recumbent position are shown in Table 23–2. The magnitudes of posture-related changes can vary among individuals, but on average, cholesterol concentration decreases approximately 5% when a standing participant sits and about 10% when a standing participant reclines (13). Similar changes are observed for HDL cholesterol. Triglyceride changes, however, are larger; triglycerides decrease almost 10% when a standing individual sits and almost 20% upon reclining. These changes begin to occur immediately, are about half-maximal after 5 to 10 minutes, and maximal after about 20

to 40 minutes. The changes are reversed over similar periods when the individual resumes the standing position (13).

Recent intake of a fat-containing meal has no measurable effect on total cholesterol (2), but can cause a marked transient increase in triglycerides, as well as smaller but significant transient decreases in LDL and HDL cholesterol (5–7). Triglycerides rise because chylomicrons are released to the circulation. Lipoprotein cholesterol decreases as the consequence of compositional changes that occur in the plasma lipoproteins as the chylomicrons are metabolized (5, 6). The magnitudes of the changes depend on the amount of fat ingested and are greater when the fat is administered in the form of a liquid mixture (5, 6) than when presented

TABLE 23-2

Postural Changes in Plasma Total Cholesterol, Triglycerides, and HDL Cholesterol[1]

Component	Decrease Relative to Standing Subjects (%)[2]	
	Sitting	Reclining
Total cholesterol	5	10
HDL cholesterol	7	8
Triglycerides	10	18

[1]Data from Bookstein L, Gidding SS, Donovan M, et al (11).
[2]Maximal changes are observed 20 min to 40 min after changing position.

in the usual form as a meal (7). Plasma triglyceride and lipoprotein cholesterol levels eventually return to baseline after the chylomicrons are removed from the circulation.

In the case of lipid and lipoprotein measurement, postural and postprandial changes are of sufficient magnitude that they can influence study findings if they are not taken into account. In order to minimize physiological variations from these sources, the participant is asked to fast before blood is drawn. As a matter of convenience for the patient, the NCEP Expert Panel on the Detection, Evaluation, and Treatment of Hypercholesterolemia in Adults (14) has recommended a fasting period of at least 9 hours. This is sufficient for *clinical* purposes but, as discussed by the NCEP Working Group on Lipoprotein Measurement (3), can produce some degree of systematic error in estimating fasting triglyceride and lipoprotein concentrations.

For *research* purposes, we recommend using a 12-hour fasting period. Water can be taken during this period, and required medications are generally not restricted. The posture used for blood sampling should be standardized. The sitting position is usually used, and the participant should be allowed to sit quietly for 5 or 10 minutes before blood sampling. When circumstances require drawing blood from a reclining participant, the same position should be used each time that participant is sampled.

Measurements in Serum vs Plasma

Lipoprotein concentrations can also differ depending on whether the measurements are made in serum or EDTA plasma (15, 16). EDTA (ethylenediaminetetraacetic acid) is the anticoagulant of choice for lipoprotein measurement, because it inhibits oxidative and other changes in the lipoproteins. Measurements in EDTA plasma, however, are 3% to 5% lower than in serum (15, 16). This is because of the osmotic effect of EDTA, which causes a slight shift of water from blood cells to the plasma. Anticoagulants such as citrate or oxalate, or additives such as fluoride, exert much larger osmotic effects and should not be used when lipids or lipoproteins are to be measured.

Lipid and lipoprotein measurements can be made in heparin plasma, however, because heparin exerts no significant osmotic effect when used in concentrations needed to prevent coagulation. Lipid and lipoprotein measurements made in heparin plasma are equivalent to those obtained in serum. For many clinical and research purposes, cholesterol, triglycerides, and HDL and LDL cholesterol can be measured either in serum or plasma. The two should not be used interchangeably, however; either serum or plasma should be used in any particular study.

Venous vs Capillary Samples

For research purposes lipid and lipoprotein measurements are best made in venous samples. Normal physiological variations observed in capillary (or whole blood) specimens appear similar to those in venous specimens (17). The analytical variation associated with capillary or whole blood measure-

ments, however, is greater for venous measurements (17–19). This generates higher total variability for capillary and whole blood measurements, which may be particularly relevant for feeding studies in which the effects of dietary intervention may be modest.

The Comparative Magnitude of Physiological and Analytical Variation

Physiological variations cannot be eliminated, but they can be minimized by controlling preanalytical factors such as posture, fasting, and the time of day the sample is obtained. It is useful to have some idea of the average magnitude of normal physiological variation and the extent to which physiological variation itself can vary among individuals.

Normal physiological variation in an individual can be determined by measuring the component of interest on several occasions when the individual is in a steady state. For total cholesterol, the measurements would be made in serial specimens taken from the individual at least 1 or 2 weeks apart. The mean ($\overline{x}_s$) and standard deviation (SD) of the serial measurements is calculated and a coefficient of variation for that individual is derived:

$$CV_{spec,tot} = SD/\overline{x}_s \times 100$$

where $\overline{x}_s$ is the mean of the measurements in serial samples and $CV_{spec,tot}$ is the coefficient of *total variation* for specimens from that individual, which includes both physiological and analytical sources of variation. Physiological variation can be estimated by adjusting $CV_{spec,tot}$ for the analytical component of variance, as determined by the laboratory from the quality control measurements (2, 3). The adjusted value, CV_p, represents the coefficient of *physiological variation* for the participant and can be approximated fairly closely from the equation:

$$CV_p = [(CV_{spec,tot})^2 - (CV_a)^2]^{1/2}$$

where CV_a is the coefficient of *analytical variation* and is fairly constant with concentration.

The data in Table 23–3 illustrate the 50th (median), 75th, and 95th percentiles for the CV_p values of lipids and lipoproteins as estimated by Kafonek, Derby, and Bachorik (4). The median CV_p for total cholesterol was 5%; those for HDL and LDL cholesterol were 7.1% and 7.8%, respectively, and that for triglycerides was about 18%. As is evident from the table, though, the CV_p values in many individuals were considerably higher.

Figure 23–3 illustrates the contribution of laboratory variation to the total variation observed in cholesterol values analyzed in serial samples from the same individual. The figure assumes a mean measured cholesterol concentration of 202 mg/dL, CV_a of 1.1%, and $CV_{spec,tot}$ of 5.1%. This corresponds to CV_p of 5.0%. The dotted line illustrates the variation that would be observed if normal physiological variation were zero, that is, if the participant's true choles-

TABLE 23-3

Coefficients of Physiological Variation (CV$_p$) for Lipids and Lipoprotein Cholesterol[1,2]

Component	CV$_p$ (%)		
	50th Percentile	75th Percentile	95th Percentile
Total cholesterol	5.0	9.0	14.0
HDL cholesterol	7.1	13.7	24.5
LDL cholesterol[3]	7.8	11.5	20.0
Triglycerides	17.8	26.3	43.6

[1] Data from Kafonek SD, Derby CA, Bachorik PS (4).
[2] 128 participants, 3 specimens/participant taken over an average period of 20 weeks.
[3] Calculated using the Friedewald equation (20).

terol concentration were the same on each occasion. In the absence of physiological variation, fluctuations in the values reported in serial samples would be entirely attributable to measurement error and would be expected to fall within a 95% confidence interval of (202 ± 1.96 × 1.1) mg/dL, or 198 mg/dL to 206 mg/dL. On the other hand, the measured values, marked by the symbols and solid line, illustrate the variation that would be observed when the measurements include the contributions of both analytical and physiological sources of variation. The measured values would fall within a 95% confidence interval of (202 ± 1.96 × 5.1)

mg/dL, or 181 mg/dL to 223 mg/dL. From the figure it can be appreciated that laboratory error, on average, would contribute relatively little to the observed differences in cholesterol values on different occasions. Indeed, it can be calculated for the present example that the analytical variance would contribute about 5% to the total variance of measurements made in serial specimens from the same individual.

Table 23–4 illustrates the expected contributions of laboratory error to the overall variance of the measurements for total cholesterol, triglycerides, and HDL and LDL cholesterol assuming median values for CV$_p$.

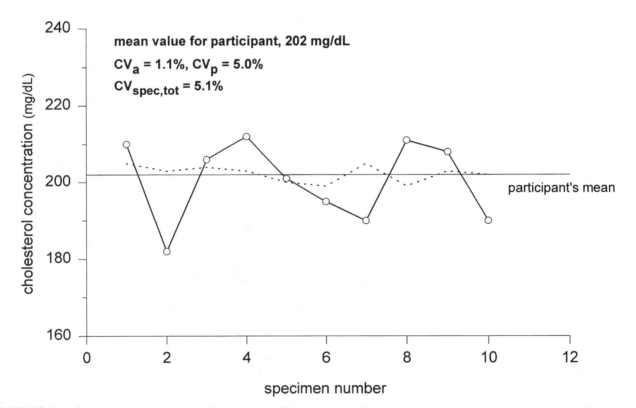

FIGURE 23-3. Serial measurements in 10 specimens from a single individual (o–o). Also shown (.....) is the expected contribution of the analytical component of variation to the overall variation of the serial measurements, ie, the variation that would be observed if physiological variation were zero. The figure assumes the coefficients of variation indicated. CV$_a$, CV$_p$, and CV$_{spec,tot}$, coefficients of analytical, physiological, and total variation, respectively.

TABLE 23-4

Contribution of Analytical Variance to Total Variance of Lipid and Lipoprotein Cholesterol Measurements in Participants with Median CV_p Values

Component	% CV_p[1]	% Variance Contributed by Analytical Variation[2]
Total cholesterol	5.0	4.6
HDL cholesterol	7.1	8.0
LDL cholesterol	7.8	14.6
Triglycerides	17.8	1.2

[1] Data from Kafonek SD, Derby CA, Bachorik PS (4).

[2] Assumes CV_a values as follows: total cholesterol, 1.1%; HDL cholesterol, 2.1%; LDL cholesterol, 3.1%; triglyceride, 2.0%, as observed in one of the authors' (PSB) laboratories.

Response to Treatment

The effects of normal physiological variation discussed earlier assume that the participant is in the steady state. Participation in any study, however, can be expected to alter the steady state to a greater or lesser extent, depending on how much the participant must change his or her usual, day-to-day routine. For this reason, a "run-in" period should be used to allow the participants to reach the new steady state before taking any measurements. Measurements should then be made in two or more serial specimens taken at least 1 or 2 weeks apart and the values averaged to estimate the participant's baseline lipid and lipoprotein concentrations.

After treatment is begun, it should be continued long enough for the participant to reach a posttreatment steady state. For dietary studies, this may require 6 or 8 weeks. It is then advisable to make posttreatment measurements in two or more specimens, again taken 1 or 2 weeks apart. The measurements are averaged to provide an estimate of the posttreatment value. Tables 23–5 through 23-8, respectively, illustrate the $CV_{spec,tot}$ values to be expected for the mean cholesterol, triglyceride, and HDL and LDL cholesterol concentrations determined from measurements in 1 to 10 serial specimens. $CV_{spec,tot}$ values are calculated using the estimates for median and 75th percentile CV_p values shown in Table 23–3. The $CV_{spec,tot}$ values indicated may be of use for estimating the size of the study population needed for dietary intervention studies.

It should be pointed out that for each component, most of the reduction in $CV_{spec,tot}$ is achieved after the first three to four serial specimens. The number of serial specimens to be used for any particular study, however, will be influenced by several factors. These include the purpose of the measurements, the number of participants in the study, the magnitudes of the minimum changes the investigator wishes to detect, and the logistics and cost of the measurements.

THE EVIDENTIARY CHAIN

Laboratory quality control is only one of the issues to be confronted in planning a study. The specimens usually pass through a series of sequential steps that are accomplished by different individuals and in different locations, and procedural mistakes can occur before the specimens reach the laboratory. Specimens can be misidentified, mishandled, or misdirected. As a consequence, a specimen may be lost; the analysis may be delayed to the point that changes have occurred in the analyte of interest; data collection and transmission may be delayed, preventing their timely use by the researcher or physician; or the analytical results for one participant might be identified as originating from another.

Although these problems can be minimized by proper planning, development of detailed study protocols, adequate staff training, and appropriate pilot studies, it is nonetheless important to document that established procedures are actually being followed. This is particularly important in long-term studies during which staff turnover can occur and incoming staff may not have received adequate training by their predecessors. It is therefore necessary to develop a system for tracking specimens through the various steps beginning with sample collection and ending with the laboratory report. This system should provide procedures for documenting the date each step is accomplished and the identity of the staff member performing that task. The steps that should be well documented include: specimen collection and preparation; temperature and length of storage before shipment; when and by whom the specimens were shipped to the laboratory; date specimens are received by the laboratory and by whom; the condition upon arrival; dates of analysis and identities of technicians performing each analytical run; and dates of data transmission.

A reliable way of identifying specimens must also be provided. One fairly straightforward approach is to develop, in advance, a master list of study numbers that can be assigned to the participants as they are enrolled. The study coordinating center or the laboratory can then provide multiple copies of computer-generated labels to be used for the specimen collection tubes, transport vials, and log sheets that accompany the specimens when they are shipped. Specimen identification information should include, as a minimum, the participant identification number and specimen collection date, and this information should be transmitted by electronic means to minimize transcription and data entry errors. Participants should not be identified by name. Information that links the specimen to a particular individual should be

TABLE 23-5

Observed Coefficient of Total Variation for Mean Cholesterol Concentrations in Serial Specimens

Number of Specimens	$CV_{spec,tot}^{1}$ at	
	50th Percentile CV_p^2	75th Percentile CV_p^2
1	5.1	9.1
2	3.7	6.5
3	3.1	5.3
4	2.7	4.6
5	2.5	4.2
6	2.3	3.8
7	2.2	3.6
8	2.1	3.4
9	2.0	3.2
10	1.9	3.1

[1] $CV_{spec,tot}$, or observed total CV, includes both physiological and analytical components of variation. CV_p, coefficient of physiological variation; CV_a, coefficient of analytical variation.
[2] Values shown assume $CV_a = 1.1\%$ and are calculated for median (5.0%) and 75th percentile (9.0%) estimates for CV_p. Based on data from the Working Group on Lipoprotein Measurement (3).

TABLE 23-6

Coefficient of Total Variation for Mean Triglyceride Concentrations in Serial Specimens

Number of Specimens	$CV_{spec,tot}^{1}$ at	
	50th Percentile CV_p^2	75th Percentile CV_p^2
1	17.9	26.4
2	12.7	18.7
3	10.5	15.3
4	9.1	13.3
5	8.2	11.9
6	7.5	10.9
7	7.0	10.1
8	6.6	9.5
9	6.3	9.0
10	6.0	8.6

[1] $CV_{spec,tot}$, or observed total CV, includes both physiological and analytical components of variation. CV_p, coefficient of physiological variation; CV_a, coefficient of analytical variation.
[2] Values shown assume $CV_a = 2.0\%$ and are calculated for median (17.8%) and 75th percentile (26.3%) estimates for CV_p. Based on data from the Working Group on Lipoprotein Measurement (3).

safeguarded and should be made available to staff on a need-to-know basis only, and staff should be instructed on the general principles of confidentiality of patient results.

The study protocols serve to document how the study is conducted. They should include procedures that minimize the effects of physiological variations; specify proper specimen collection, storage, and transportation procedures; describe how laboratory performance will be monitored; and indicate the frequency and format of the laboratory reports, and how study data will be transmitted. To facilitate the development of these protocols, the study team should include investigators with the appropriate laboratory expertise.

Finally, provisions should be made for easy communication between the laboratory and other components of the study. This is particularly important when specimens will be sent from a remote specimen collection site(s). Occasional problems will arise that need to be addressed quickly. For example, a shipment may be delayed in transit, a specimen may be identified incorrectly, or its integrity may be compromised during shipment. Formal procedures should also be put in place to follow up all such verbal communications with written documentation.

Provisions should also be made to monitor compliance with the study protocols, ensure that specimens move through the system on schedule, and collect and transmit study data, including quality control data, in a timely manner. Required turnaround times should be decided upon, although they may vary according to the complexity of the test, stability of the analyte, and the urgency of the report. For example, nonesterified fatty acid levels change during

TABLE 23-7

Coefficient of Total Variation for Mean HDL Cholesterol Concentrations in Serial Specimens

Number of Specimens	$CV_{spec,tot}$[1] at	
	50th Percentile CV_p[2]	75th Percentile CV_p[2]
1	7.4	13.9
2	5.4	9.9
3	4.6	8.2
4	4.1	7.2
5	3.8	6.5
6	3.6	6.0
7	3.4	5.6
8	3.3	5.3
9	3.2	5.0
10	3.1	4.8

[1]$CV_{spec,tot}$, or observed total CV, includes both physiological and analytical components of variation. CV_p, coefficient of physiological variation; CV_a, coefficient of analytical variation.
[2]Values shown assume $CV_a = 2.1\%$, and are calculated for median (7.1%) and 75th percentile (13.7%) estimates for CV_p. Based on data from the Working Group on Lipoprotein Measurement (3).

TABLE 23-8

Coefficient of Total Variation for Mean LDL Cholesterol Concentrations in Serial Specimens

Number of Specimens	$CV_{spec,tot}$[1] at	
	50th Percentile CV_p[2]	75th Percentile CV_p[2]
1	8.4	11.9
2	6.3	8.7
3	5.5	7.3
4	5.0	6.5
5	4.7	6.0
6	4.4	5.6
7	4.3	5.3
8	4.1	5.1
9	4.0	4.9
10	4.0	4.8

[1]$CV_{spec,tot}$, or observed total CV, includes both physiological and analytical components of variation. CV_p, coefficient of physiological variation; CV_a, coefficient of analytical variation.
[2]Values shown assume $CV_a = 3.1\%$, and are calculated for median (7.8%) and 75th percentile (11.5%) estimates for CV_p. Based on data from the Working Group on Lipoprotein Measurement (3).

storage, and the analysis should be initiated on the day the specimen is collected, if possible. There is less urgency with cholesterol, triglycerides, or HDL or LDL, provided the specimens are properly handled and stored.

Documentation of the methods and procedures used in studies, particularly in large studies, is important for a number of reasons. First, long-term studies may not be completed by the same individuals who initiated them. Written documentation is essential to ensure that procedures are not inadvertently changed in ways that could introduce systematic errors affecting the interpretation of the data. Second, data analysis may begin years after the study started, and accurate documentation of methods and procedures will be required when publishing the findings. Finally, the data analysis for large studies may proceed for many years after the formal termination of the study. These analyses may be conducted by individuals who took no actual part in the planning or conduct of the investigations. The valid interpretation of such add-on analyses will depend on the availability of proper study documentation.

SPECIMEN BANKING

The issue of specimen banking should be addressed at the outset of the study. Can the specimen be discarded after it has been analyzed and the data have been finalized? Should aliquots of the specimens be collected for long-term storage? If so, how many should be prepared from each participant, from how many participants should they be collected, and how long should these samples be retained? Are storage facilities available or can they be acquired? What is the cost of maintaining a specimen bank, and what will be done with the specimens when the study has concluded?

In general, any remnants of the particular aliquots used for the primary measurements should be discarded because they can be expected to suffer some degree of evaporation or other changes during the period of handling and storage required to make the primary measurements. If specimens are to be banked, separate aliquots should be prepared specifically for this purpose. A number of factors must be considered. These include the number of aliquots to be stored, the likely availability of sufficient specimen volumes, the stability of components that may be of interest in the future, and the availability of storage space. Considerable investments of time and resources are made recruiting, characterizing, and randomizing the study population. The availability of stored specimens from the study populations can be useful if certain measurements are to be delayed because of logistical, technical, or economic constraints. They also can afford particularly cost-effective opportunities to make additional measurements as new components of interest may emerge, because the study population will have already been characterized. It is therefore common practice, particularly in large studies, to provide for the permanent storage of one or more aliquots of each specimen. This practice is worthwhile for dietary studies, and should be considered in the planning phase of the study.

REFERENCES

1. Myers GEL, Cooper GR, Winn CL, et al. The Centers for Disease Control-National Heart, Lung and Blood Institute Lipid Standardization Program. An approach to accurate and precise lipid measurements. *Clin Lab Med.* 1989;9:105–135.

2. Laboratory Standardization Panel, National Cholesterol Education Program. *Recommendations for Improving Cholesterol Measurement.* US Department of Health and Human Services, NIH publication 90–2964; February 1990.

3. Working Group on Lipoprotein Measurement. *National Cholesterol Education Program Recommendations on Lipoprotein Measurement.* Bethesda, Md: NHLBI; NIH publication 95–3044; September 1995.

4. Kafonek SD, Derby CA, Bachorik PS. Biological variability of lipoproteins and apolipoproteins in patients referred to a lipid clinic. *Clin Chem.* 1992;38:864–872.

5. Cohn JS, McNamara JR, Cohn SD, et al. Postprandial plasma lipoprotein changes in human subjects of different ages. *J Lipid Res.* 1988;29:469–479.

6. Cohn JS, McNamara JR, Schaefer EJ. Lipoprotein cholesterol concentrations in the plasma of human subjects measured in the fed and fasted states. *Clin Chem.* 1988;34:2456–2459.

7. Wilder LB, Bachorik PS, Finney CA, Moy TF, Becker DM. The effect of fasting status on the determination of low density and high density lipoprotein cholesterol. *Am J Med.* 1995;99: 374–377.

8. Buxtorf JC, Baudet MF, Martin C, et al. Seasonal variations of serum lipids and apoproteins. *Ann Nutr Metab.* 1988;32:68–74.

9. Gordon DJ, Trost DC, Hyde J, et al. Seasonal cholesterol cycles: the Lipid Research Clinics Coronary Primary Prevention Trial placebo group. *Circulation.* 1987;76:1224–1231.

10. Mjos OD, Rao SN, Bjoru L, et al. A longitudinal study of the biological variability of plasma lipoproteins in healthy young adults. *Atherosclerosis.* 1979;34:75–81.

11. Bookstein L, Gidding SS, Donovan M, et al. Day-to-day variability of serum cholesterol, triglyceride, and high-density lipoprotein cholesterol levels. *Arch Intern Med.* 1990;150:1653–1657.

12. Warnick GR, Albers JJ. Physiological and analytical variation in cholesterol and triglycerides. *Lipids.* 1976;11:203–208.

13. Miller M, Bachorik PS, Cloey TA. Normal variation of plasma lipoproteins: postural effects on plasma concentrations of lipids, lipoproteins and apolipoproteins. *Clin Chem.* 1992;38:569–574.

14. National Cholesterol Education Program. Second report of the National Cholesterol Education Program Expert Panel on Detection, Evaluation, and Treatment of High Blood Cholesterol in Adults (Adult Treatment Panel II). *Circulation.* 1994;89:1329–1445.

15. Laboratory Methods Committee, Lipid Research Clinics Program of the National Heart, Lung, and Blood Institute. Cholesterol and triglyceride concentrations in serum/plasma pairs. *Clin Chem.* 1977;23:60–63.

16. Cloey T, Bachorik PS, Becker D, et al. Reevaluation of serum-plasma differences in total cholesterol concentration. *JAMA.* 1990;263:2788–2789.

17. Kafonek SD, Donovan L, Lovejoy KL, Bachorik PS. Biological Variation of Lipids and Lipoproteins in Fingerstick Blood. *Clin Chem.* 1996;42:2002–2007.

18. Bachorik PS, Cloey TA, Finney CA, et al. Lipoprotein-cholesterol analysis during screening: accuracy and reliability. *Ann Intern Med.* 1991;114:741–747.

19. Bachorik PS, Rock R, Cloey T, et al. Cholesterol screening: comparative evaluation of on-site and laboratory-based measurements. *Clin Chem.* 1990;36:255–260.

20. Friedewald WT, Levy RI, Fredrickson DS. Estimation of the concentration of low-density lipoprotein cholesterol in plasma without use of the preparative ultracentrifuge. *Clin Chem.* 1972;18:499–502.

CHAPTER 24

BIOLOGICAL SAMPLE COLLECTION AND BIOLOGICAL MARKERS OF DIETARY COMPLIANCE

JANIS F. SWAIN, MS, RD

Biological samples are collected in virtually every controlled feeding protocol; their analysis provides the *primary outcome data* for evaluating the effects of the defined dietary manipulation. Many feeding study hypotheses are tested by evaluating changes in physiologic pools of nutrients or metabolites in response to the research diet. The concentrations or half-lives of various compounds in the pools are determined by laboratory assay, and estimation of pool volume is achieved for internal compartments (such as blood) using algorithms, whereas for excretory compartments (such as urine and feces) pool volumes can be measured directly. (Also see Chapter 16, "Compartmental Modeling, Stable Isotopes, and Balance Studies.")

Biological samples are also collected in search for an objective measure of *compliance* with diet. Every controlled feeding study raises the question "Did the participant eat all of the study food, and no other foods?" Investigators can make observations of the behavior of the participants, and they can ask questions of the participants, but this information is subject to bias. Thus, it is valuable to have an independent laboratory-based indicator of compliance as well.

Valid interpretation of data for any of these measurements, whether as study outcomes or as measures of compliance, requires assurance that the collection of the biological sample was complete. When members of the research staff collect the sample (such as during phlebotomy) and otherwise have control of the collection process, it is relatively easy to provide the assurance that no sample was lost. Collection of urine and feces presents a different set of challenges, however; the study participant "collects" the samples at intervals that may extend for hours or days, and sometimes in a variety of locations. Verification that collection is complete likely will require use of markers of the completeness of collection.

A variety of markers and measurements can be used to provide qualitative and quantitative estimates of dietary compliance and sample collection. A biological marker has been defined by Bingham as "any biochemical index in an easily accessible biological sample that in health gives a predictive response to a given dietary component" (1). Markers used for measuring dietary compliance and collecting biological specimens can be either naturally occurring nutrients ingested within the diet or physical or chemical markers taken orally or added to the food. A good biomarker is nontoxic, accurately and easily measurable, excreted rapidly without being metabolized, minimally invasive, and inexpensive. When the marker is added to food, it should be colorless, odorless, and tasteless, and it should not change the appearance of the food.

When planning the study protocol and its associated laboratory analyses, investigators must consider which analytes in which samples will serve as primary endpoints, as markers of compliance, and, if urine and fecal samples are to be collected, as markers of completeness of collection. To avoid confounded interpretations of data, it is crucial that each purpose be achieved through analysis of a different component; that is, the various measures must be independent of each other. The components can be analyzed in the same biological sample, but they cannot serve two purposes at once. For example, a study evaluating fecal calcium levels as a primary outcome variable should not also use fecal calcium levels to determine compliance with research diets containing various levels of calcium; yet another marker would be needed to assess whether all of the fecal samples had been collected.

This chapter will review several currently used measures of compliance with diet and will discuss, for several of the most frequently analyzed tissues and body pools, the logistics of sample collection in the context of feeding protocols and the assurance of completeness of this sampling. These additional procedures not only add time and cost to the study, but also may affect adherence to the overall protocol. All methods have their limitations for application and effectiveness, and their usefulness must always be evaluated within the context of individual research projects.

BIOLOGICAL MARKERS OF DIETARY COMPLIANCE

At present there is no ideal biomarker of compliance with a research diet regimen. Such a marker would be easily measured in an easily obtained specimen, and the resulting data could be readily compared with expected values based on available information about the diet. This ideal marker would indicate, with perfect sensitivity and specificity, whether any study foods were not consumed ("omissions"), whether any unauthorized foods were consumed ("additions"), and whether any study foods had been replaced with unauthorized foods ("substitutions"). The available methods for evaluating compliance generally permit a judgment to be made about whether omissions have occurred, but it is difficult to detect additions or substitutions with any certainty.

It would be convenient to have compliance markers that could be measured in blood samples, but the metabolic transformations associated with nutrient metabolism, and the homeostatic regulation of metabolite pools among the blood and other compartments, mean that there are few dietary components whose intakes are reflected in blood levels with sufficient precision to meet the purposes of feeding studies. Thus, as a method of monitoring compliance, blood samples at present are of little value in "catching" those who have not complied with the dietary protocol. Similarly, many of the classic nutritional status indicators are seldom useful as markers of dietary compliance. These indicators may be more useful in epidemiological studies that require the assessment of nutrient status over long periods of time to classify subjects into broad categories of intake (2–4). For feeding studies whose duration is relatively long (for example, several months), however, some nutritional status in-

dicators might be useful for indicating compliance with a specific treatment; the sensitivity of the measure will be increased if the dietary treatments are markedly different.

Even though the composition of plasma or blood generally does not reflect dietary intake with sufficient specificity to serve as a *quantitative* measure of dietary compliance, blood samples occasionally can be used as *qualitative* markers of dietary compliance for certain nutrients. For example, participants taking fish oil are expected to have a plasma fatty acid profile that reflects this intake. The presence of the marker fatty acids indicates dietary compliance; unexpectedly low levels or the absence of a given marker is more difficult to interpret, however, because it is impossible to distinguish noncompliers from nonresponders under the circumstances of most dietary interventions.

Role of Compliance Markers in Feeding Studies

One of the greatest challenges in conducting well-controlled feeding studies is ensuring and then documenting dietary compliance. This is particularly true for metabolic studies in which food is consumed outside the research facility. Subjective methods such as oral reporting, written records, and visual observation can enhance compliance, but objective methods are necessary to verify dietary adherence. Biological collections can provide the medium for such quantitative determinations and documentation.

The most commonly used methods for evaluating compliance entail the collection and analysis of 24-hour urine samples (see below). Fecal samples are seldom used in monitoring compliance with diet, although this can be considered if feces are being collected for other required analyses. (In the case of either urine or feces, additional markers indicating the completeness of sample collection would be needed, as described later.)

When evaluating the results of a compliance assessment and before concluding the study participant is "guilty" of noncompliance, investigators must rule out other reasons for the findings. These include the potential for interference from other physiologic processes, as well as various types of protocol errors, such as errors in laboratory processing and analysis, omission of the marker from the food, errors in sample collection, and wrong dosage given to the participant. Nevertheless, quantitative markers add another level of confidence to controlled feeding studies, which otherwise have to rely upon subject compliance and subjective measures only.

Urinary Measures of Dietary Compliance

Most qualitative and quantitative measures of dietary compliance require measurements made from 24-hour urine collections. Commonly used methods involve measuring the urinary excretion of para-aminobenzoic acid, urinary osmolality, or individual nutrients such as sodium.

Para-aminobenzoic Acid

The potassium salt of para-aminobenzoic acid (PABA) is a physiologically inert indicator that is readily excreted in the urine.

Advantages of using PABA as a biological indicator of dietary compliance are (1) it is excreted in the urine within 24 hours; (2) it may be taken orally in tablet or liquid form; (3) it can be added to individual foods; and (4) it has no detectable taste. In addition, PABA is inexpensive and can be analyzed by colorimetric assay with a minimum of technical expertise. It is also used as a means of assessing the completeness of 24-hour urine collections.

Limitations include the time-consuming procedures needed to incorporate PABA into the different foodstuffs and the fact that the method only assesses the intake of foods that have been marked with the PABA. The consumption and omission of unmarked foods will go undetected.

The PABA solution is incorporated into foods in exact amounts delivered by pipette. It can be added to many different foods such as beverages, bread products and other baked goods, meats, and salads. The appearance of the food does not change. It is difficult, however, to add PABA to high-fat foods such as peanut butter, cream cheese, margarine, and oils, because the water-based PABA solution tends to separate. There does not appear to be any difference in recovery if the PABA is incorporated into the food item such as a cookie before baking or afterward.

Because PABA and its metabolites are subject to degradation by ultraviolet light, the PABA solution should be kept in dark containers, and all foods containing the added PABA need to be covered immediately with foil or placed in a dark area. Collected urine should be kept in brown jugs or opaque containers and away from light. Certain drugs (such as acetaminophen, furosemide, paracetamol, phenacetin, and sulphonamides) and vitamins (such as folic acid) can interfere with the assay for determining PABA recovery; study participants should be instructed to avoid these compounds.

The usefulness of PABA to verify food intake in controlled dietary studies was first described by Bingham and Cummings (5) and further developed by Roberts et al (6). Roberts et al (6) concluded that PABA was a sensitive index of dietary compliance when multiple-day collections are pooled. In a 3-day validation study the recovery of the PABA, administered daily in 4 test foods, was 98.7%. The between-participant variability was much greater in individual collections (coefficient of variation [CV] 9%) than in combined 3-day collections (CV 3.7%). Therefore, multiple-day collections are recommended to monitor actual compliance.

Osmolality

The measurement of urine osmolality to monitor dietary compliance in metabolic studies has been described by Roberts et al (7). This method is based on the hypothesis that the urine osmol excretion rate (OER), which reflects the urinary solute load (made up primarily by nitrogen-containing compounds, sodium, and potassium), can be compared to the OER predicted from a known nitrogen, sodium, and potassium intake. A complex series of polynomial-regression equations is used for the calculations. The OER predicted from dietary intake is reported (7) to be most precise for dietary periods of more than 6 days (CV 6.9%).

Using OER as a compliance measure of dietary intake requires that all known sources of sodium, potassium, and nitrogen be controlled and measured. Advantages of using urinary osmolality to monitor dietary compliance are (1) both over- and underconsumption of food intake can be determined with high accuracy; (2) chemical analysis is simple and relatively inexpensive; and (3) there is no need to add an extrinsic marker to the food. Disadvantages include the need for multiple 24-hour urine collections and the inability to detect food substitutions that either have a similar nitrogen, sodium, and potassium content or unauthorized foods that are void of these nutrients. Also, the calculations for determining the predicted dietary OER can be time consuming.

Sodium

Twenty-four hour urinary sodium levels can be used as an indicator of dietary compliance when the dietary sodium intake is known and kept constant. This measure is based on the body's homeostatic tendency to maintain "sodium balance" in which urinary sodium output is equivalent to that of intake after several days on a constant sodium intake. For example, a participant living under controlled conditions, consuming 10 mEq of sodium per day, and in a state of sodium balance will excrete in the urine approximately 10 mEq or less of sodium per day. Typical urinary sodium recovery is approximately 95%; 2% is accounted for by fecal loss, and the remainder by sweat. Depending on environmental temperature and level of physical activity, however, the amount of sodium lost in sweat can vary from 2% to 5%, making it difficult to determine sodium balance in free-living participants. This loss should be considered and controlled when investigators use urinary sodium as a compliance marker.

Advantages of urinary sodium monitoring are its simplicity, speed of laboratory measurement, and its minimal cost. For certain types of investigations, such as endocrinology studies requiring controlled sodium intake, this simple measure is all that is needed for checking dietary compliance.

The primary limitation of urinary sodium as an indicator of dietary compliance is that it reflects only total sodium intake. Because sodium is a natural component of almost all foods and water, both in the natural state and as an additive, intake of actual food items consumed may not be discernable unless weighed salt is incorporated into selected foods. Likewise, overconsumption or failure to eat foods not containing sodium goes undetected.

Sodium concentrations in drinking water, whether from a municipal water supply or a well, can vary considerably because of various environmental factors. Therefore, the sodium content of the water supply should be known and accounted for in evaluating sodium balance. Providing distilled or deionized water for drinking can eliminate this variable; however, bottled water can be cumbersome to supply for extended periods of time.

Other Measures: Riboflavin, Potassium, Nitrogen

Riboflavin (vitamin B-2) excretion in urine can serve as a marker of dietary compliance. Riboflavin is a yellow to orange-yellow crystalline powder having a slight odor. When a high dose is added to foods, the excess vitamin appears in the urine and can be detected by fluorometric methods. Wolraich et al (8) reported the addition of 16.7 mg riboflavin to 100 g sugar that was then incorporated into a variety of foods. This was estimated to provide about 10 times the RDA for riboflavin when sweetened foods are consumed in typical quantities. Although this technique is not quantitative, it does verify that specific test foods are consumed.

Riboflavin has the advantages of being water-soluble and being easy to incorporate into foods. Because of its color, riboflavin is difficult to incorporate into a blinded study; its deep yellow color can easily be observed in lightly colored foods and in the urine. Participants do not usually know, however, what causes the yellow color. In the study by Wolraich et al (8), most thought a dye was added to the diet.

Riboflavin should be stored in airtight containers and protected from light to prevent degradation. The recovery of the load dose of riboflavin must be evaluated against the expected recovery from the 1 mg to 2 mg riboflavin present in an ordinary, riboflavin-adequate diet. The use of multivitamins, especially therapeutic doses of riboflavin, should be avoided. Also, certain drugs or substances found in food such as quinine or tonic water should be avoided because they can result in the excretion of fluorescent compounds, which may give false positive assay results.

Urinary *potassium* excretion can be compared with intake to qualitatively or semiquantitatively assess dietary compliance. Approximately 30% of potassium intake is excreted in the stool, however, reducing its accuracy as a urinary compliance measure.

Measurement of urinary nitrogen often is performed for studies of protein metabolism. Protein is not the sole source of urinary nitrogen; nonprotein nitrogen sources must also be considered. However, if total dietary nitrogen can be measured, urinary nitrogen can provide a means of assessing compliance.

URINE SAMPLES

Urine is analyzed in feeding studies to obtain primary outcome data and evaluate compliance with a specific dietary protocol.

An advantage of using urine for measuring biological parameters is that the collection procedure is noninvasive and can be done in free-living participants. Interpreting the resulting data, however, also requires documenting the completeness of the urine collection.

Collection Procedures

In some research studies, random daytime or morning urine samples are used. More often, however, urine samples collected in feeding studies are obtained over 24-hour periods. Usual urine output ranges between 1,200 ml and 2,500 ml per day and depends on individual fluid intake, temperature, exercise, and kidney function. Some investigators using 24-hour urine measures encourage a fluid intake of 2,000 ml to 2,500 ml per day to ensure adequate hydration, renal perfusion, and a good urine output.

Over- or undercollection of urine samples results in data that are difficult to interpret. Overcollection can occur when a participant collects urine beyond the time frame specified in the protocol, whereas undercollection can result from missed collections or spillage. The protocol should incorporate methods to estimate the completeness of the collection, such as urinary creatinine or para-aminobenzoic acid. The accuracy of a complete 24-hour urine collection requires that the participant understand thoroughly the collection technique and the timing of the sample. The collection procedure should be explained orally to the participant, who should then have an opportunity to ask questions. Written instructions must also be provided (Exhibit 24–1).

The process of collecting 24-hour urine samples can be tedious and awkward. Participant cooperation may be easier to obtain if there is some flexibility as to the day(s) the urine is to be collected. For example, a weekend day may not be better than a week day because schedules may be less predictable. Participants' motivation can also can be enhanced if they are told they will be informed of the results of the analyses and what those results mean to them or in the context of the study. Some potential participants may find urine collections difficult because of problems with motor coordination or remembering and following procedures accurately.

A research participant involved in 24-hour urine collections usually is encumbered with a gallon jug, and, for females, some type of collection device. If this equipment presents a particular problem, it may be helpful to provide several smaller collection containers from which urine can be pooled. A brown paper shopping bag, gym bag, or opaque plastic bag with handles can be used to carry containers.

As with all biological sample collections, storage and processing techniques for urine must be appropriate to the analytes of interest. Samples collected for analysis of ascorbic acid, for example, require cold storage and stabilization with acid to prevent oxidation. Some organic analytes require protection from ultraviolet light; some are destroyed by bacterial growth, a process that can be prevented or decreased by refrigerating urine samples. Interfering sub-

EXHIBIT 24-1

Procedure for 24-hour Urine Collection

Materials: Collection container—1 gallon brown jug or several smaller collection containers (labeled and preservatives added, if necessary); funnel, urinal, or collection "hat"; large safety pin to attach to undergarment as a reminder; brown paper or opaque plastic bag with handles; written instructions to give to participant; cooler; and ice.

Instructions

1. The collection time begins immediately after the first void of the morning. Do *not* save that first specimen as part of the beginning day's collection. For multiple-day collections, this void should complete the collection from the previous day, otherwise, it should be discarded. Write the time of the first void (that you threw away or that you saved as the end of the previous day's collection) on the collection container as your START TIME. Remember also to put the date that you began the collection.
2. Collect each sample in the urinal or "hat," then pour it into the brown jug. Females can also use a funnel to urinate directly into a container when it is inconvenient to carry around a gallon jug. Males can void directly into the collection container.
3. Keep the brown jug on ice in the cooler provided and replenish ice as needed.
4. The final specimen collected will be the first void upon awakening on the second morning (24 hours after you began). Be *sure* to write this date and the time on the jug.
5. Be especially careful not to spill any of your collection. Keep the jug upright to prevent leaking. All urine, except the first void, is to be collected.
6. If a collection is missed or spilled, estimate the amount, if possible, and be sure to report *any* uncollected urine to the investigator.
7. Upon completion of your 24-hour collection, bring the container to the _____. Be sure that the label is filled out completely indicating your name, the date and time of starting the collection (the time you threw the specimen away), and the date and time of finishing the collection.
8. If you have any questions, please call us at _____.

Remember: the accuracy of your collection determines the accuracy of your results.

SAMPLE LABEL FOR 24-HOUR URINE COLLECTION

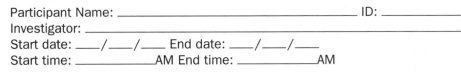

Participant Name: _____ ID: _____
Investigator: _____
Start date: ___/___/___ End date: ___/___/___
Start time: _____AM End time: _____AM

stances can leach from urine collection containers. Glass containers are required when certain analytical techniques are used because many plastics contribute fluorescent compounds or minerals to samples. Specific instructions for collection, storage, and processing of urine and other biological specimens are available from reference texts (eg, *Clinical Guide to Laboratory Tests* by Toetz [9]).

Urine Collection Markers

The two most commonly used markers for assessing the completeness of urine collection are creatinine (an intrinsic physiologic marker) and para-aminobenzoic acid (an extrinsic dietary marker).

Creatinine

Creatinine is the most frequently used quantitative measure of complete 24-hour urine collections in participants con-

suming a controlled diet. Urinary creatinine is a by-product of muscle metabolism and reflects lean body mass. Its excretion by a given healthy individual is expected to be consistent from day to day when dietary intake of protein is held constant. Age, sex, body mass, and kidney function affect creatinine excretion, making it invalid for interparticipant comparisons. Creatinine excretion may be less suitable for long-term studies with participants who are in positive nitrogen balance, such as children or pregnant women.

Multiple consecutive 24-hour urine collections are necessary to use urinary creatinine as a measure of sample completeness. The coefficient of variation for creatinine excretion in consecutive daily urine collections was reported as 4% and 3.2% in studies by Bingham and Cummings (10) and McCullough et al (11). Other investigators, however, have found a much greater variability, ranging from 21% to 24% (12).

Advantages of using urinary creatinine to assess completeness of 24-hour urine collections are:

- Creatinine is excreted in the urine as a naturally occurring, measurable metabolite.
- No inert substances need to be taken by the research participant.
- No additional work or measures are necessary on the part of the research team.
- The measurement of urinary creatinine is inexpensive and can be done easily on standard laboratory autoanalyzers.

The usefulness of urinary creatinine as a collection marker is limited in studies that allow a varying dietary intake because of the sizable effect of protein intake on creatinine excretion.

Para-aminobenzoic Acid

In addition to its use as a marker of dietary intake compliance, PABA has also been used to validate the completeness of 24-hour urine collections. The use of PABA for this purpose was first described by Bingham and Cummings (5) based on the hypothesis that the amount of PABA excreted in the urine is directly related to the dose. An advantage of using PABA to determine completeness of 24-hour urine collections is that it is physiologically inert, unaffected by food intake or physiological characteristics of the participant, easily analyzed, and relatively inexpensive. Because PABA is light sensitive, urine collections must be stored in brown jugs or opaque containers and in a dark area.

Bingham and Cummings (5) showed that in a group of four individuals, 93% of a single 80-mg tablet of PABA given with a single meal was recovered after 5 hours. In order for a marker to represent a complete 24-hour collection, the marker must be present in significant quantities in each individual specimen. These same researchers determined that 240 mg PABA given by mouth with the day's three meals was an effective dose to monitor 24-hour urine collections. A recovery of less than 205 mg PABA (85%) was considered to represent an incomplete collection.

Because of the large measurement variance for PABA, a single 24-hour urine collection may not be as useful as a sample pooled from 3 to 4 days of collection. As mentioned earlier, Roberts et al (6) reported a CV of 9% for 1-day collections but only 3.7% for pooled 3-day measurements. Therefore, PABA may be more useful in evaluating the completeness of multiple-day, pooled collections.

STOOL SAMPLES

Controlled diet studies frequently collect and analyze stool samples (13, 14). Such analyses provide information about the digestion, absorption, bioavailability, and balance of nutrients, as well as about the actions of colonic flora and other aspects of gastrointestinal physiology. Fecal markers are an important component of stool collection protocols because, as Davignon, Simmonds, and Ahrens explained, "In metabolic balance studies stools collected during a given period of time do not necessarily reflect the biological events that

take place in the intestine during the collection period; even 4-day collections rarely represent exactly 96 hr in the transit of any particular portion of the intestinal contents. Hence there is a need for an inert marker which can be incorporated into the food intake, the excretion of which can indicate the completeness of stool collections and permit corrections for variations in fecal flow" (15).

Collection Procedures

Fecal collections are physically and psychologically demanding for research study participants. For many prospective participants, stool collection goes against cultural norms and years of social conditioning. Carrying collection containers and samples can be embarrassing, awkward, and tedious; and cooperation of participants can be difficult to achieve. For these reasons, extra financial incentives may be necessary for participants in studies requiring fecal collection.

It is particularly important to realize that stool collections are difficult if a participant is prone to diarrhea or constipation or if either is a complication of the study. As with urine collections, some individuals may have difficulty in understanding the protocol and physically collecting the specimen.

Participant cooperation is imperative in obtaining a complete stool collection. Careful and detailed instructions, both verbal and written, as well as all the collection materials and storage containers should be provided. As with urine collections, compliance is enhanced when there is some flexibility about the timing of the collections.

Stool collections usually need to be frozen. The temperature ($0°C$, $-20°C$, $-70°C$) will vary depending on which analytes will be assayed. Some study investigators provide a small home freezer to their free-living participants, particularly if daily collections are made over a significant time period. Other investigators provide participants with an insulated food storage style or Styrofoam container (48 qt to 54 qt) containing dry ice (frozen CO_2). Fifty pounds of dry ice (pellets or block) will last approximately 5 to 7 days in a tightly sealed insulated container; however, in warm weather, dry ice will need to be replenished more frequently. Care should be taken not to handle dry ice without gloves because direct skin contact can cause frostbite. Dry ice should be held in a tightly sealed box in a well-ventilated room; the CO_2 vapors can reduce oxygen concentrations to dangerous levels.

When specific freezing temperatures are required, participants must understand the distinction between the freezing temperatures of dry ice ($-78.5°C$) and water ice ($-0°C$). Otherwise a participant might mistakenly "thaw" the sample in his or her home freezer when the dry ice runs out.

Finally, containers for storing stool collections need to be designated for that use only and should never be used for storing or transporting food. Containers must also be tested in advance to make sure that there is no leaching of interfering compounds into the sample. Stool collection procedures are outlined in Exhibit 24–2.

Fecal Collection Markers

Criteria for a good fecal marker were described by Whitby and Lang (16). The substance should be inert, nontoxic, and easily measured. It should have very little bulk, mix well with the intestinal contents, be completely unabsorbed, and not undergo any metabolism in the body or the intestinal lumen. Many years later, these criteria still hold.

Two types of markers have proved themselves useful in controlled feeding studies. *Intermittent markers* such as inert colored dyes and radio-opaque pellets are given in single bolus doses to define the *timespan* (ie, the beginning and end) of the fecal collection period. Occasionally dyes of differing colors or pellets of differing shapes are used to distinguish between time points or collection periods. Some

dyes may contain minerals and thus may not be suitable for trace element studies (13); laboratory analysis in advance is recommended to avoid generation of confounded data.

Continuous markers such as polyethelene glycol, chromic oxide, and barium sulphate are given in multiple doses at regular intervals throughout the feeding period to determine the *completeness* of fecal collection. By defining the quantity of feces in relation to a given quantity of food, they allow the investigator to account for intra- and inter-individual differentials in fecal flow due to variability in transit time and intestinal pooling (intraluminal sequestration of intestinal contents).

The type of fecal marker should be selected judiciously for a given study so that the desired time course, collection, and endpoint can be measured according to the study design. For example, not all fecal markers traverse the gastrointestinal tract at the same rate, and some are more lipid- or water-soluble than others. Likewise, different luminal contents,

EXHIBIT 24–2

Procedure for Fecal Collections

Materials: Underseat collection frame (''hat''), clear plastic collection bags with twist ties (numbered and labeled) or ''deli-style'' pint containers with lids, resealable bags (eg, Ziploc®), disposable gloves, brown paper or opaque plastic bag with handles, insulated or Styrofoam container containing dry ice (if necessary).

Procedure

1. Obtain a numbered, large plastic collection bag or container, being careful that it is in numerical order. Complete label with date and time.
2. Urinate (if necessary) and collect as usual prior to bowel movement.
3. Put on disposable gloves.
4. Open the large plastic bag/container (in numerical order) and place inside collection ''hat.'' If a collection container is not available, attach the bag to the outside of the toilet bowl or hold the bag, whichever is easier.
5. During the bowel movement, make sure that the entire stool falls into the bag/container *without any urine.*
6. *After the bowel movement, remove the plastic bag/container, remove air from collection bag (air insulates sample and slows the freezing process), gently twist the top and place the bag inside the self-sealing freezer bag.*
7. *Seal the freezer bag and immediately place the bag inside the dry ice chest or the freezer provided by the study.*
8. Remove and discard gloves.
9. Replace ice chest lid tightly.
10. Use a new large plastic bag in numeric sequence for each stool sample.

Important:

• Immediately freeze stool sample.
• No urine in stool sample.

Caution: Do not let dry ice come in contact with your skin. It can cause burns! Keep dry ice tightly sealed and in a well-ventilated room.

SAMPLE LABEL FOR FECAL COLLECTION

Stool Sample Number _____
Participant Name: _____ ID: _____
Investigator: _____
Date: ___/___/___
Time: _____ AM/PM (Please circle AM or PM)

such as fats, move through the intestinal tract at different rates than those transported in an aqueous medium.

There may be occasions when an investigator does not want the subject to take biochemical marker capsules or wants the subject to be unaware of a specific collection period. Real foods, such as corn kernels, which are usually only partially digested and readily visible in the stools; beets, which usually color the stool red; or seeds can be used to mark a diet intake period without the subject's being aware of the intent.

Extrinsic markers given in capsule or added to food must have food- and pharmaceutical-grade sanitary clearances and handling procedures so that they cannot be a source of illness (as described later).

Intermittent Markers

Coloring Agents (Inert Dyes)

The inert dyes *carmine red (CI Natural Red 4)* and *brilliant blue (FD&C Blue 1)* are two of the most commonly used fecal markers for defining dietary periods. They are usually administered in powdered form (available from Spectrum Chemical, New Brunswick, NJ). They are not absorbed in transit and do not undergo secondary metabolism by gastrointestinal bacteria, and thus are recovered fully in the stool. Another dye, *methylene blue*, is also used as an intermittent fecal marker, although it is partially absorbed in the gut, with some urinary excretion and less than complete recovery in the stool sample. Methylene blue can be administered in two forms, a dark green crystalline powder and a deep blue liquid (available from Fisher Scientific, Pittsburgh, Pa).

Capsules containing dye markers can be purchased commercially. They can also be prepared to study specifications by the investigators. The dyes are obtained from laboratory suppliers, mixed with methylcellulose microcrystals (Avicel), and encapsulated in size 00 or 000 capsules. The methylcellulose helps to keep the dye stationary and prevents the blending of colors. Carmine red is frequently autoclaved before being encapsulated, as contamination with *Salmonella* has been reported. (Formulations for carmine red and methylene blue capsules are shown in Exhibit 24–3.)

Radio-opaque Pellets

The use of radio-opaque pellets (ROP) for measuring stool transit was first described by Hinton, Leonard-Jones, and Young (18) and further described by Cummings and Wiggins (19). Radio-opaque pellets have since been used successfully by a variety of investigators (20, 21). The method provides a valid quantitative measure of a complete fecal collection because 100% recovery of the pellets is expected. As with all human feeding studies, however, the unexpected can happen. For example, in a study where all participants were to receive 40 pellets, one participant excreted only 20 while another excreted 60 pellets, suggesting a dosage error.

Barium-impregnated radio-opaque polyethylene pellets may be obtained from Konsyl Pharmaceutical Co, Fort Worth, Texas (Sitzmark brand pellets). Using pellets of differing geometric shapes allows more specific demarcation of time periods (13). The tiny ROP are incorporated into gelatin capsules and swallowed at the beginning and end of each collection period or with certain meals. All stools for a designated time period are then collected and examined under fluoroscopy for retrieval of the pellets. An advantage of using ROP is that this method of measurement, which uses X-rays, does not alter the stool, and fecal handling is kept to a minimum. Disadvantages of using ROP include the additional cost of fluoroscopy and participant reluctance to swallow the pellets.

Continuous Markers

Polyethylene Glycol

Polyethylene glycol (PEG) (Spectrum Chemical, New Brunswick, NJ) is a white, crystalline, water-soluble, high molecular weight polymer. It is neither absorbed nor decomposed by the intestinal tract during transit. PEG has been used as a fecal marker to follow time and completeness of collections, to determine when experimental diets have been eliminated, and to correct for differences in the day-to-day variation of fecal transit time (22, 23).

PEG is easily dissolved in water, juice, or other fluids and has little taste. PEG is not the marker of choice when study participants are taking vitamin and mineral supplements because it is used as an inert filler in some prepara-

EXHIBIT 24-3

Formulations for Fecal Dye Markers

Courtesy of General Clinical Research Center, Massachusetts Institute of Technology, Cambridge, Mass

Carmine Red Markers	Methylene Blue Markers
10 g sterilized carmine red dye	5 g methylene blue
10 g Avicel (methylcellulose)	20 g Avicel (methylcellulose)
Size 00 gelatin capsules	Size 00 gelatin capsules
(approximately 500 mg dye each)	(approximately 250 mg dye each)
Yield: 20 capsules	Yield: 20 capsules
Dose: 1–2 capsules	Dose: 1 capsule

tions. A typical dosage schedule for PEG is 3.0 g per day provided as 1.0 g dissolved in 120 cc water and given at breakfast, lunch, and dinner.

Barium Sulphate

Barium sulphate ($BaSO_4$) is a nonabsorbable, nontoxic, insoluble compound (Spectrum Chemical, New Brunswick, NJ; Fisher Scientific, Pittsburgh, Pa) that can easily be measured and given in capsule form. Its usefulness for correcting the variability of fecal flow in metabolic balance studies was described by Figueroa, Jordan, and Bassett (24). A 0.5-g dose of flocculating $BaSO_4$ was divided equally among 3 capsules and administered at 3 daily meals. Recovery of the barium sulphate from 5 participants throughout the 5-day balance was 97.7% to 103%, indicating its usefulness in validating complete collections. Barium sulphate should not be used in the presence of antacids containing aluminum hydroxide and magnesium hydroxide as they are partially recoverable in the stool and may interfere with subsequent chemical assays.

Chromium Oxide

Chromium oxide (Cr_2O_3, chromium sesquioxide, Fisher Scientific Company, Pittsburgh, PA) is a bright green continuous fecal marker delivered in capsular form. Its usefulness in metabolic balance studies for calculating fecal pool size, turnover rates of unexcreted intestinal contents, and attainment of a steady state was well documented by Davignon, Simmonds, and Ahrens (15). Although varying doses in the range of 250-mg to 500-mg capsules or tablets have also been used, these authors determined that 300 mg per day given as one 60-mg tablet 5 times per day was an adequate dose for recovery determinations.

Radioisotopic chromium (as $^{51}CrCl_3$) has also been used as a fecal marker in balance studies, although it may undergo partial absorption in the gut (13).

BLOOD SAMPLES

Blood samples in feeding studies often provide the main vehicle for assessing the effects of the controlled diet intervention. They can also provide information about nutrient utilization, nutritional status, and dietary patterns. An advantage of using blood samples is that they are less demanding of the research participant's time than are urine and stool collections. The sample can be collected quickly and in almost any off-site location. Another advantage of blood samples is that they can sometimes be obtained with no additional discomfort to the participant by increasing the volume drawn during an already scheduled venipuncture.

Blood drawing should only be done by a well-trained technician, nurse, or physician. Although there are no regulations governing who can draw blood, a good training program covering technique, infection control, and processing is critical, not only for the safety of the participants and staff

but also for accurate data collection. Most medical facilities can provide training for researchers who will be drawing blood specimens. Technicians responsible for blood sampling should have this task written into their job descriptions. Such documentation will ensure that liability for any accident or resultant injury, although rare, would be covered by the insurance of the affiliated institution and/or researcher.

The informed consent document should clearly state that blood sampling will be a part of the study and should detail the associated risk. A simple venipuncture under sanitary conditions carries minimal risk; this risk is typically limited to minor discomfort during the blood draw and to the possibility of a slight hematoma. The frequency of the blood sampling and the amount to be drawn should also be clearly stated in the informed consent document, and blood sampling to be conducted outside the research facility (eg, at home, school, work) should be identified.

It is important to keep blood drawings to the necessary minimum. Overly frequent blood draws may become an aversive experience and make it hard for the participant to complete the protocol. In addition, study costs may be increased by the need for extra financial incentives for the participants. Finally, total volume of blood must be limited to prevent anemia, especially in children and reproductive-age women.

No person enjoys undergoing a venipuncture; therefore, rapport with the subject is important for compliance and participation. Some participants become light-headed or faint during or shortly after blood collections. A reclining chair, bed, or couch should be available so that a dizzy or faint individual may lie down. In addition, smelling salts and a supply of food and juice should be kept close to the blood drawing area. A source of rapidly absorbed carbohydrate, typically fruit juice, can quickly counter the light headedness that some people experience. Similarly, participants should be provided with a meal or snack if blood has been drawn under fasting conditions so that they are not in danger of fainting after they leave the facility. If a controlled food intake is part of the study, part of the participant's daily food should be reserved for this purpose.

Meticulous collection and processing of blood samples is critical for generating accurate data. The laboratory responsible for analyzing the sample should be consulted prior to the study for detailed collection, processing, and storage guidelines. These guidelines may entail the addition of various chemicals to stabilize the specimens; the temperature at which centrifugation should take place; and sample storage details such as temperature, light, and stability.

Both the day of the week and the timing of blood samples should be considered in the context of the study protocol. If fasting is required, participants should understand the exact time after which they can consume no food in the evening. They must also understand that they can eat no food the following morning until after the sample has been drawn. Some investigators elect not to collect blood samples on Monday mornings because participants who have take-out meals for weekends may eat their Sunday evening meals late and therefore not comply with the typically required 12-hour fast. Others avoid collecting blood on Fridays or the day before holidays because this may delay the laboratory analysis of time-sensitive samples.

Blood specimen labels should be as detailed as possible with the participant's identification number, date, time of sample collection, and any other pertinent information. Other variables to consider are whether the participant should be supine or sitting, fasting, the time of day, and any medications the participant may be taking.

OTHER BIOLOGICAL SAMPLES

Other types of samples, such as saliva, sweat, breast milk, and expired CO_2, are sometimes used for endpoint measurements, as indicators of nutrient intake, or for assessing nutrient status. Their range of applications is relatively narrow, but may include studies of mineral balance, energy balance, and endocrine physiology.

Subcutaneous adipose tissue samples obtained by either a needle or skin biopsy punch have been used to provide information on long-term fatty acid storage. A noninvasive technique using cheek cell membranes was developed by McMurchie, Potter, and Hetzel (25) to investigate tissue fatty acid composition reflective of a shorter duration. Cheek cell turnover is approximately 5 days; cells can be collected by having a participant lightly scrape the cheeks with the side of a plastic spoon, rinse the mouth with distilled water, and collect the sample in a container.

Hair and nail samples have the advantage of being easily collected. However, their use in nutrition research is limited primarily to assessing the status of long-term dietary intake or toxic exposure of trace elements and heavy metals. Contamination of hair and nails with cleaning agents, shampoos, and environmental pollutants can provide misleading data unless identified and controlled in advance.

CONCLUSION

Biologic samples, particularly of blood, urine, and feces, are commonly analyzed in feeding studies to assess primary endpoints of interest and to monitor dietary compliance. Valid interpretation of the analytical results depends on proper collection and storage of these biological samples. The data must also be interpreted with the knowledge that human motivation and compliance with collection procedures can be difficult to achieve. When selecting measures to use for assessing dietary compliance, one must carefully assess the application of the techniques as well as their advantages and logistics.

Most studies documenting the use of markers for dietary compliance and biological collections have been conducted using small, limited population groups with results about

their usefulness extrapolated to the general population. More extensive studies are needed that include men and women, children, the elderly, and minorities, as well as clinical subpopulations. For example, individuals with impaired renal function and renal abnormalities could have altered excretion of urinary markers. Given the importance of verifying dietary adherence in human feeding studies, further research is greatly needed to expand the roster of specific and sensitive biochemical/biological indicators.

REFERENCES

1. Bingham S. The dietary assessment of individuals; methods, accuracy, new techniques, and recommendations. *Nutr Abstr Rev (Series A).* 1987;57:705–742.
2. Hunter D. Biochemical indicators of dietary intake. In Willett W, ed. *Nutritional Epidemiology, Monographs in Epidemiology and Biostatistics.* Vol 15. New York, NY: Oxford University Press; 1990:143–216.
3. Bates CJ, Thurnham DI, Bingham SA, Margetts BM, Nelson M. Biochemical markers of nutrient intake. In M. Margetts and M. Nelson (ed.) *Design Concepts in Nutritional Epidemiology.* New York, NY: Oxford University Press; 1991:192–265.
4. Riboli E, Ronnholm H, Saracci R. Biological markers of diet. *Cancer Surveys.* 1987;6, 685–715.
5. Bingham S, Cummings JH. The use of 4-aminobenzoic acid as a marker to validate the completeness of 24-hr urine collections in man. *Clin Sci.* 1983;64:629–635.
6. Roberts SB, Morrow FD, Evans WJ, Shepard DC, Dallal GE, Meredith CN, Young VR. Use of p-aminobenzoic acid to monitor compliance with prescribed dietary regimens during metabolic balance studies in man. *Am J Clin Nutr.* 1990;51:485–488.
7. Roberts SB, Ferland G, Young VR, Morrow F, Heyman MB, Melanson KJ, Gullans SR, Dallal GE. Objective verification of dietary intake by measurement of urine osmolality. *Am J Clin Nutr.* 1991;54:774–782.
8. Wolraich ML, Lindgren SD, Stumbo PJ, Applebaum MI, Kristsy MC. Effects of diets high in sucrose or aspartame on the behavior and cognitive performance of children. *N Engl J Med.* 1994;330:301–307.
9. Toetz NW. *Clinical Guide to Laboratory Tests.* 2nd ed. Philadelphia, Pa: WB Saunders Company; 1990.
10. Bingham SA, Cummings JH. The use of creatinine output as a check on the completeness of 24-hour urine collections. *Hum Nutr Clin Nutr.* 1985;39C:343–353.
11. McCullough ML, Swain JF, Malarick C, Moore TJ. Feasibility of outpatient electrolyte balance studies. *J Am Coll Nutr.* 1991;10:140–148.
12. Knuiman JT, Hautvast JG, van der Heijden L, Geboers J, Joossens JV, Tornqvist H, Isaksson B, Pietinen P, Tuomilehto J, Flynn A, Shortt C, Boing H, Yomtov B, Angelico F, Ricci G. A multi-centre study on within-person variability in the urinary excretion of sodium,

potassium, calcium, magnesium, and creatinine in 8 European centres. *Hum Nutr Clin Nutr.* 1986;40C:343–348.

13. van Dokkum W, Fairweather-Tait SJ, Hurrell R, Sandström B. Study techniques. In: Mellon FA, Sandström B, eds. *Stable Isotopes in Human Nutrition.* San Diego, Calif: Academic Press; 1996.

14. Haack VS, Chesters JA, Vollendorf NW, Story JA, Marlett JA. Increasing amounts of dietary fiber provided by foods normalizes physiologic response of the large bowel without altering calcium balance or fecal steroid excretion. *Am J Clin Nutr.* 1998;68:615–622.

15. Davignon J, Simmonds, W, Ahrens EH, Jr. Usefulness of chromic oxide as an internal standard for balance studies in formula-fed patients and for assessment of colonic function. *J Clin Invest.* 1968;47:127–138.

16. Whitby LG, Lang D. Experience with the Cr_2O_3 method of faecal marking in metabolic balance investigations in humans. *J Clin Invest.* 1960;39:854–863.

17. Morgan J. Use of non-absorbable markers in studies of human nutrient absorption. *Human Nutrition: Applied Nutr.* 1986;40A:399–411.

18. Hinton JM, Lennard-Jones JE, Young AC. A new method for studying gut transit times using radio-opaque markers. *Gut.* 1969;10:842–847.

19. Cummings JH, Wiggins HS. Transit through the gut measured by analysis of a single stool. *Gut.* 1976;17:219–223.

20. Branch WJ, Cummings JH. Comparison of radio-opaque pellets and chromium sesquioxide as inert markers in studies requiring accurate faecal collections. *Gut.* 1978;19:371–376.

21. Carmichael RH, Crabtree RE, Ridolfo AS, Fasola AF, Wolen RL. Tracer microspheres as a fecal marker in balance studies. *Clin Pharmacol Ther.* 1973;14:987–991.

22. Wilkerson R. Polyethylene glycol 4000 as a continuously administered non-absorbable faecal marker for metabolic balance studies in human subjects. *Gut.* 1971;12:654–660.

23. Allen LH, Raynolds WL, Margen S. Polyethylene glycol as a qualitative fecal marker in human nutrition experiments. *Am J Clin Nutr.* 1979;32:427–440.

24. Figueroa WG, Jordan T, Bassett SH. Use of barium sulphate as an unabsorbable fecal marker. *Am J Clin Nutr.* 1968;21:1239–1245.

25. McMurchie EJ, Potter TE, Hetzel BS. Human cheek cells: a non-invasive method for determining tissue lipid profiles in dietary and nutritional studies. *Nutr Rep Int.* 1984b;29:519–526.

CHAPTER 25

THE MULTICENTER APPROACH TO HUMAN FEEDING STUDIES

MARLENE M. WINDHAUSER, PHD, RD, FADA; ABBY G. ERSHOW, SCD, RD;
EVA OBARZANEK, PHD, MPH, RD; BARBARA H. DENNIS, PHD, RD;
JANIS F. SWAIN, MS, RD; PENNY M. KRIS-ETHERTON, PHD, RD;
WAHIDA KARMALLY, MS, RD; AND SUSAN E. BLACKWELL

Feeding studies form an essential link in the lines of evidence that establish causal relationships between diet and disease risk factors because the degree of dietary control is unparalleled by any other type of nutrition intervention. Along with other nutrition studies, feeding studies provide data that subsequently are used by health professionals to develop dietary recommendations for the public. At times, however, study findings are inconsistent because human feeding studies usually have small sample sizes and often use different experimental designs. The result is that the public may perceive a mixed message that can lead to confusion about optimal nutrition.

One strategy to minimize conflicting scientific reports is to conduct large, well-controlled feeding studies, using the model of the multicenter clinical trial in which several field centers follow a common dietary protocol. This approach allows for human feeding studies with adequate sample size and broad representation of the population.

This chapter describes several recently completed multicenter studies; provides information on the rationale, organization, and function of such studies; considers issues of quality control and cost; and discusses implementation of the dietary component of multicenter feeding studies.

EXAMPLES OF MULTICENTER FEEDING STUDIES

To date, few multicenter feeding studies have been conducted and they vary considerably in size and scope. Two large-scale studies were Dietary Effects on Lipoproteins and Thrombogenic Activity (DELTA) and Dietary Approaches to Stop Hypertension (DASH), both sponsored by the National Heart, Lung, and Blood Institute (NHLBI), National Institutes of Health. Throughout the chapter, examples from DELTA and DASH are used to illustrate the multicenter feeding study approach.

The DELTA program (1992-1996), a multicenter, collaborative human feeding study with rigorous standardization and monitoring of diet composition (1), was initiated to study the effects of dietary fat modifications on plasma lipids and lipoproteins and markers of thrombogenesis. The need for this study derived from uncertainties about the efficacy of reduced-saturated-fat diets for all segments of the population. There were numerous clinical investigations of the effectiveness of a reduced-saturated-fat diet in lowering blood cholesterol levels in men. However, far fewer studies had been conducted in women. In addition, little information was available for different age and ethnic groups, and for individuals with clinical disease or other elevated risk factors. This paucity of information highlighted the need for larger studies, which could be achieved by using a multicenter collaborative effort.

In DELTA, two protocols were developed to answer separate research questions for two distinctly defined populations. The first DELTA protocol examined the effects on blood lipids and hemostatic factors of three levels of total and saturated fat in 103 normolipidemic participants from several demographic subgroups, including pre- and post-menopausal women, men, Caucasians, and African-Americans (2). The second protocol evaluated the response to diet of lipids and hemostatic factors in 86 adults with biomarkers of dyslipidemia/insulin resistance (low high-density lipoprotein cholesterol and elevated triglyceride and serum insulin levels). Three experimental diets were fed: an average American diet, a diet low in saturated fat and high in total fat and monounsaturated fatty acids, and another low-saturated fat diet that was also low in total fat and high in carbohydrate and fiber (3).

The DASH study (1993-1997) tested the effect of three dietary patterns on blood pressure in 459 adults using a randomized controlled human feeding trial design (4). The DASH study fed its participants an average American diet, a high-fruit-and-vegetable diet, and a low-fat, "combination" diet high in fruits, vegetables, and dairy products.

Based on many previous studies, the efficacy in lowering blood pressure of caloric restriction for weight reduction and of reduced consumption of alcohol and sodium is generally well accepted and forms the basis for nutritional recommendations for preventing and treating high blood pressure (5, 6). Epidemiologic studies on other diet-related factors and blood pressure have reported significant associations. These factors included micronutrients such as potassium, calcium, and magnesium (inversely related to blood pressure); macronutrients such as amount of dietary fat (directly related) and protein (inversely related); and dietary fiber (inversely related). However, the results from randomized controlled clinical trials testing these dietary factors singly have been inconsistent and equivocal. In contrast, the blood pressure-lowering effect of a vegetarian dietary pattern has been consistent. This evidence provided the basis for the DASH study to test the efficacy of dietary patterns in reducing blood pressure. To achieve a sample size sufficient to allow adequate representation of women and minorities, particularly African-Americans for whom high blood pressure is a major public health problem, a collaborative multicenter effort was required.

The multicenter approach was also used recently for a large industry-sponsored study examining the efficacy of commercially prepared complete diets for nutritional management of cardiovascular risk factors (7). Food prepared at a central location (Campbell Center for Nutrition and Wellness, Campbell Soup Company, Camden, NJ) was shipped to 10 clinical centers, where it was distributed to 283 adults with hypertension, dyslipidemia or diabetes. The participants in the active intervention group were instructed to supplement the centrally prepared breakfast, lunch, dinner, and snack menus with specific quantities of self-obtained fruit, vegetables, and dairy products. Values for risk factors (such as blood pressure, weight, plasma lipids, and plasma glucose) during baseline and treatment periods in these subjects were compared with values for 277 control subjects whose treatment was a completely self-selected version of a similar therapeutic diet.

Other multicenter human feeding studies that have been reported were smaller in scope. A NASA-sponsored study of zinc and copper balance during long-term bedrest enrolled a total of 7 participants at two centers because of limited bed

availability and the high amount of care required for study participants. To ensure similar food preparation between the centers, both dietary staffs were trained to use the same techniques for weighing and preparing the foods (8). Food aliquots were analyzed before and throughout the 29-week study, confirming the good correlation in the mineral content of the experimental diets prepared between the metabolic kitchens.

Another example is a four-center randomized crossover feeding study that examined the effects of carbohydrate content on glycemia and plasma lipoproteins in 42 patients with non-insulin-dependent (type 2) diabetes mellitus (9). Standardized diets were prepared in four metabolic kitchens and plasma samples from each site were shipped to various laboratories for analyses of lipids, lipoproteins, and insulin levels.

SCIENTIFIC RATIONALE FOR MULTICENTER STUDIES

The typical single-center human feeding study has a small sample size from a narrowly defined population. Because these studies are expensive and require a large investment of time, labor, and space, it generally is difficult for a single investigator funded by a research grant to enroll, feed, and study more than 20 to 25 participants at one time. This maximum imposes constraints on study duration and design. Consequently, many human feeding studies lack sufficient statistical power to detect small, but biologically meaningful, differences among groups or treatments. The relationship between sample size and the ability to detect small effects has been described in Chapter 2, "Statistical Aspects of Controlled Diet Studies."

One way of accruing sufficient sample size to estimate the quantitative effect of diet on physiological parameters is through meta-analysis techniques that combine data from different studies that sought to answer the same scientific question. However, often the various studies are not comparable. They employ different experimental designs and vary with respect to dietary modification, length of intervention, participant inclusion and exclusion criteria, and inclusion of control groups. These factors, among others, affect the findings and conclusions made in each study. A multicenter feeding study, by using a common protocol, is able to pool data collected at different centers and thus has a large sample size and high statistical power to detect a small effect size.

The DASH investigators wanted high statistical power (power = 85%) to detect a reduction of 2.0 mm Hg in diastolic blood pressure in response to the dietary treatments (4). To detect this difference a minimum of 405 participants, or 135 in each of three treatment groups, was required. During a 2-year period each field center was required to randomize a total of approximately 120 participants, allowing for dropouts. Five cohorts of 20 to 30 participants were studied at each of the 4 field centers. This allowed feasible management of the participants by the staff.

Because they can accommodate a large sample size, multicenter studies can complete a protocol in a shorter time period overall than would be possible for a single study site. For example, a crossover design requiring 80 to 100 participants for adequate statistical power would take 4 years to complete if only 20 persons could be studied at a time, but only 1 year if 4 centers worked simultaneously. With a multicenter study design participants are enrolled concurrently among the centers, and the entire study can be completed in a shorter time period than in single-center studies.

The small sample size in single-center studies also places constraints on the population groups that can be included. To minimize sources of variability and factors that might affect the dietary response and reduce statistical power, investigators usually study a homogeneous population. For example, many previous diet studies were conducted with young Caucasian males. Much less is known, therefore, about how other population groups respond to dietary changes. Studies of dietary response as affected by sex, age, race, comorbid conditions (such as obesity), genetic profiles, and other factors ultimately provide evidence for dietary recommendations that are applicable to a broader population. The DELTA protocols found that plasma lipid responses to the experimental diets were similar for men and women of different ages and for Caucasians and African-Americans (2). Similarly, the results of DASH showed that the experimental diets lowered blood pressure in men and women, in minorities and nonminorities, and in individuals who had and did not have hypertension (10).

THE MULTICENTER MODEL: ORGANIZATION AND OPERATION

The organization and operation of randomized controlled trials stems from their overall purpose, testing the effectiveness of an experimental drug, procedure, or other treatment (11), and when several clinical centers are needed to meet large sample size requirements, a multicenter study is instituted (12). These trials vary in size and extent, have a complex organizational structure, and are costly. However, they have the potential to yield data of high validity and detect small but important effects. Rigorous adherence to the protocol and manual of operations is central to performing the tasks in a standardized manner.

Multicenter feeding studies have a structure similar to that of multicenter clinical trials in that they include field centers in different geographical locations, centralized laboratories, a data coordinating center, and central coordination of activities (12). Figure 25–1 illustrates the organizational structures of the DELTA and DASH studies.

The operation of multicenter feeding studies also parallels that of multicenter clinical trials. In general, study investigators design one or more collaborative research protocols. *Field center* personnel prepare standardized experimental diets, feed participants, and use identical methods for data collection. *Central laboratories* may be used to ensure standardized analyses of food and biological samples and minimize interlaboratory variations. A *coordinating center* standardizes management and data collection procedures, oversees a centralized quality control program for all aspects of the study, and provides expertise in biostatistics to ensure sound approaches to study design and data analysis. For smaller multicenter studies, one field center also may act as the coordinating center. Table 25–1 summarizes the functions of the multicenter feeding study organizational units.

The primary governing body is the *steering committee,* which is composed of the principal investigator of each field center and the coordinating center and a sponsoring agency representative also known as the project officer or scientist. The steering committee members are responsible for developing the study protocol, making scientific and policy decisions, facilitating the conduct of the study, and interpreting and reporting the study results. Members of the steering committee define rules regarding access and analysis of data from collaborative studies. Subcommittees of the steering committee are formed to address such issues as protocol development or design and analysis, recruitment, measurement, quality control, diet design and management, and publications. Work is managed through numerous conference calls and periodic meetings. Additionally, an independent *data and safety monitoring board* usually is appointed by the sponsor to review progress, monitor safety, and assess the significance of preliminary results. Administrative and scientific oversight of the entire study are provided by the *sponsoring agency.*

The coordinating center staff make a major contribution to the statistical design of the study, the organization of study activities, and the preparation of the study protocol and the manual of operations. They have responsibility for developing and implementing standardized procedures to collect data from the field centers so that the data can be pooled for analysis. The coordinating center often arranges for centralized laboratory analyses of the biological specimens and experimental diet nutrient composition, and may play a role in developing plans for specimen and food composite transfer. The coordinating center oversees a study-wide quality control program, which ensures comparability and reliability of data and includes site visits, staff training and certification, and data monitoring. These quality assurances add to the higher costs for a multicenter project. Finally, the coordinating center personnel have the responsibility for analyzing data generated by the field centers and the centralized laboratories.

Field center interdisciplinary teams comprise senior investigators and coinvestigators; research dietitians; a study coordinator; recruiters; and kitchen, technical, and clerical staff. The main functions are to recruit and feed study participants and collect data. To do these tasks, they must have experience in recruiting and managing participants, preparing the diets, handling the food, evaluating compliance,

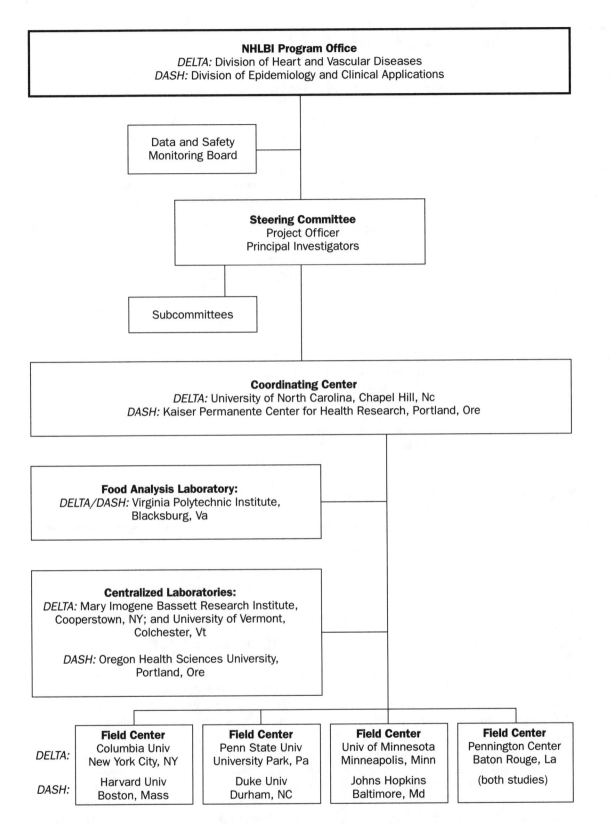

FIGURE 25-1.   Organizational chart of multicenter feeding studies, DELTA and DASH, sponsored by the National Heart, Lung, and Blood Institute, Bethesda, Md.

TABLE 25-1

Functions of the Multicenter Feeding Study Organizational Units

Unit	Functions
Program office	Oversee administration and provide scientific oversight of project
Steering committee	Make policy decisions for the study
	Design study protocol, including dietary treatments and endpoint measurements
	Interpret data and report study results
Subcommittees	Develop procedures for implementing protocol
	Provide input to steering committee for design of study protocol, including dietary treatments, measurements, and data analyses
Coordinating center	Standardize data collection procedures
	Arrange for centralized laboratory analyses
	Prepare protocol and manual of operations
	Prepare and distribute forms
	Oversee quality control and staff training and certification
	Control data transfer and management
	Monitor and analyze data
	Arrange meetings and conference calls
Centralized laboratories	Analyze biological samples
	Conduct nutrient analyses of diets
Field centers	Adhere to all aspects of the protocol
	Recruit and enroll participants
	Prepare experimental diets
	Feed study participants
	Assess and ensure participant compliance
	Collect data
	Ship samples to centralized laboratories
	Transfer data to coordinating center
Data and safety monitoring board	Review study progress, monitor safety, and assess significance of preliminary results

collecting and handling biological specimens, and maintaining masked (blinded) designs.

Maintaining these designs is a critical element of all clinical trials. At the field centers, masking is preserved by keeping measurement staff unaware of the diet assignment and by keeping kitchen staff who know the diet assignment unaware of measurement results. Standardized laboratory analyses often are conducted at the field centers but may also be performed at a central laboratory. The field center personnel also are responsible for the shipment of food composites and biological samples to analytical laboratories outside the field center and for the expedient transfer of data to the coordinating center.

The Diet Subcommittee is composed of dietitians and nutritionists from the various study centers, as well as the individuals responsible for the food composition analyses. This subcommittee is instrumental in developing the dietary component of the protocol, including menus, standardized food preparation procedures, participant feeding procedures, and techniques for monitoring dietary compliance (Exhibit 25–1).

COSTS AND QUALITY CONTROL IN MULTICENTER STUDIES

The cost of conducting multicenter feeding studies is substantial. In addition to the high cost of laboratory analyses, there are expenses, similar to any feeding study, associated with labor, supplies, and time. Although there are some cost savings, expenditures are usually multiplied when several sites work together. Principal investigators, dietitians, study coordinators, and other professionals must meet to plan the study, develop a common protocol, and produce a manual of operations that specifies in detail how the study is to be implemented. Decisions must be made regarding which activities to centralize, how to standardize procedures, and how to monitor quality control. Unlike single-center studies, these decisions require considerable coordination, including frequent travel and conference calls. Study information and data must be mailed, faxed, or sent electronically to a coordinating center. The addition of a coordinating center, not

EXHIBIT 25-1

Issues Addressed by the Diet Subcommittee During the Planning Stage of the DASH Study

DIETARY TREATMENTS

Calculate costs of feeding
    3 vs 4 diet treatments
    8-week vs 12-week trial
Define "usual" or control nutrient levels
Recommend use of absolute nutrient levels or nutrient intakes indexed to energy needs
Establish nutrient targets
    fatty acids, cholesterol
    protein
    micronutrients
    fiber
    sodium

MENU DEVELOPMENT

Identify commonly used food sources for micronutrients
Consider soft drink micronutrient content
Determine how to control sodium intake
Discuss restrictions on water supply, if needed
Identify types of fruits/vegetables that will be acceptable to the study participants
Determine use of specific foods
    types of dairy products
    complex vs simple carbohydrates
    fortified foods
    margarine/*trans* fatty acids
    dietetic jelly and syrup
Set calorie levels
Develop unit foods as calorie adjustors
    define nutrient and calorie content
Select nutrient database
Develop recipes/menus according to guidelines
Taste-test recipes

MENU AND FOOD GUIDELINES

Define menu cycle
Specify portion control items
Select fresh, canned, or frozen fruits and vegetables
Establish consumption allowances
    alcohol
    caffeinated and other beverages
    spices and seasonings
Determine whether to adjust beverage consumption according to caloric needs

MENU VALIDATION STUDY

Determine nutrients to assay
Identify menus and calorie levels to prepare
Draft schedule
    cooking
    shipping
    chemical analysis
Specify diet preparation assignments
Obtain procedures, containers, and supplies from food analysis laboratory

(continued)

EXHIBIT 25-1
Continued

FEEDING LOGISTICS

Determine on-site and off-site meals
Discuss special meal situations
    weekend meals
    emergency meals
    holidays
Discuss procedures for packaging and serving foods
Discuss food safety precautions for staff and participants

FOOD PROCUREMENT AND PREPARATION

List foods with brand names/specifications
Specify centrally procured foods
Determine food industry participation
    identify and contact companies
    match company food items with menu items
    estimate amounts
Estimate food storage requirements
Decide on batch preparation techniques
Define cooking procedures
Calculate cooked weight portions
Establish guidelines for weighing foods

DIET ASSESSMENT PRIOR TO ENROLLMENT

Determine what type of information to gather
Select best method to gather information
Consider cost of administration, labor, materials, data evaluation
Decide when to collect information

SCREENING VISIT ACTIVITIES

Determine what information is required
    food allergies
    lactose intolerance
Determine how to assess whether the person will comply
    discuss menus
    assess food preferences, general dietary information
    assess usual eating habits (food frequency questionnaire; 3-day food record; other)
Decide when to administer forms and review data

CALORIC REQUIREMENTS OF PARTICIPANTS

Determine how to assess and calculate requirements
    equation to use
    physical activity assessment

WEIGHT MANAGEMENT DURING FEEDING

Define ''baseline weight''
Define ''stable weight''
Determine frequency of weight measurements
Decide when and how to adjust calories

(continued)

EXHIBIT 25-1

Continued

DIETARY COMPLIANCE

Describe compliance assessment
>foods not consumed
>nonstudy foods consumed
>missed meals
>sodium intake
>alcohol consumption
>attendance for on-site meals

Determine monitoring methods
>biochemical measures
>self-report

Define "adequate compliance" during run-in
Define noncompliance with intervention diet
Specify actions to take with noncompliance
Decide how to handle refusals to eat foods or meals
Prepare retrospective compliance questionnaire

MISCELLANEOUS ISSUES

Prepare study orientation meeting for participants
>when to conduct
>activities and issues to discuss
>prepare video about study and procedures

Establish exit interview and diet counseling at end of trial
Discuss incentives for participants
Discuss whether toothpaste with baking soda should be controlled
Determine interval needed between diet assignment and commencement of feeding
Design forms needed
Propose manuscripts

---

necessary in a single-center study, also adds considerable costs to the overall study. Nevertheless, in return, data collected from multicenter feeding studies are of the highest quality because of the great deal of attention paid to quality control.

For any feeding study, chemical analyses of experimental diets strengthen the validity of the findings because the actual composition of the study diets may differ from the nutrient targets. Such discrepancies in nutrient composition (due to variations in food sources or errors in databases) may be sufficient to bias the results toward the null, ie, finding no effect, especially if the experimental diets have small contrasts (eg, 30% vs 26% kcal from total fat). For a multicenter study, however, validation and monitoring of the experimental diets are indispensable components of quality control, ensuring not only that the actual nutrient composition reflects the target goals but, perhaps even more importantly, that the study results can be pooled because the diets are the same at all centers.

OVERVIEW OF MULTICENTER TRIAL ACTIVITIES

The decision to launch a multicenter study is based on the significance of the problem, the need for a trial, and the feasibility of conducting the research (13). Once the study is initiated, it comprises a planning phase, an implementation phase, and a closeout phase.

During the planning phase the study protocol is designed through collaborative effort among scientists, clinicians, dietitians, and statisticians. If the study was initiated in response to a sponsor's solicitation, the protocol usually is derived from the research designs proposed in the successful grant applications or proposals but modified as necessary to develop a single common protocol. The investigators in multicenter feeding studies must agree to a common protocol in order to answer the research question(s).

Protocol development includes defining or refining the main hypotheses or research questions of the study. This will guide decisions related to experimental design, sample size calculations, randomization procedures, dietary treatments, eligibility criteria, duration of intervention, endpoint measurements, and statistical analyses. Subsequently, recruitment strategies, data forms, manual of operations, and quality control procedures are developed. Exhibit 25–1 lists the diet-related issues and tasks discussed during the planning phase of DASH. The entire planning process is lengthy, detailed, and often tedious in that it requires careful consideration of many proposed approaches, but it ultimately yields a study design that is based on the strengths and experiences of all the people involved.

In finalizing the study design and protocol, a pilot study might be necessary. For example, in DELTA the question arose about whether diet composition could be standardized to a sufficiently precise degree among the four field centers. Consequently, a pilot study was carried out to evaluate two approaches to food procurement and preparation (14). The first approach employed central procurement of primary food sources of fat and cholesterol, with preparation of cooked entrees and baked goods at a single location. All other foods were procured and prepared locally according to standard specifications. The second approach had central procurement of the fat- and cholesterol-containing foods, local procurement of all other foods, and local preparation of all foods. Each field center prepared several menus using both approaches. The chemical analysis results showed that the second approach achieved nutrient targets and yielded sufficiently standardized diet composition among the field centers. The steering committee subsequently decided that the study kitchens should *locally prepare* all foods but *centrally procure* the key foods that might be major sources of variability in fat and cholesterol content.

Following the planning stage, the field center staff implements the protocol. Activities include recruitment, random assignment of study participants to the treatments, compliance monitoring, measuring implementation and outcomes, and monitoring quality control and results. Food preparation procedures and methods of determining participant compliance to the diets are observed closely by the kitchen and dietary staffs. Standardized data collection procedures, including the methods and frequency of acquisition and transfer of data, are followed. To ensure compliance with the protocol all procedures and data collection forms are monitored during regular site visits by the coordinating center.

After all participants complete the study, a number of activities occur during the final phase or "close-out" period. Field center investigators review and interpret their data in collaboration with the coordinating center staff who continue data management activities, verify the accuracy of the data, and conduct the statistical analysis. The coordinating center personnel also support manuscript preparation efforts through data analysis, statistical consultation, editorial activities, and coordination of meetings. At the conclusion of the trial, field centers usually inform the participants of the study results.

IMPLEMENTING THE MULTICENTER DIETARY INTERVENTION

The steps described here for planning and implementing the dietary components of multicenter feeding trials are similar to those for all well-controlled feeding studies. However, several unique issues must be considered with respect to staffing, facilities, equipment, menu development, food procurement and storage, food preparation, and participant management. Field center dissimilarities offer challenges both in implementing a common protocol and in standardizing methods of food preparation and delivery.

Facilities and Staff

Most likely, field center kitchens will differ in staffing patterns, size, production capacity, and equipment. Facilities can range from a metabolic kitchen at a clinical research center to a university food preparation teaching laboratory. At some research institutions the kitchens are designed specifically for conducting large-scale feeding studies. Field centers without an on-site kitchen may contract with a nearby hospital or another facility for use of the institutional kitchen. For DASH, Johns Hopkins University in Baltimore, Md, contracted with the Human Studies Facility at the US Department of Agriculture Human Nutrition Research Center, Beltsville, Md, to prepare the foods. Those foods then were transported to the feeding facility in Baltimore.

Every research kitchen has its own unique system of staffing. Facilities with a small number of foodservice employees may hire temporary or student help as needed for each project, but at some locations labor union rules may prohibit this practice. Sites with multiple funding sources may use their foodservice staff for consecutive projects. As for all grant-supported projects, it is imperative that the staff realize that their positions and length of employment are dependent on the funding period. Careful planning determines the number of staff required and their period of employment.

For example, if a site is required to feed 60 participants per year for 12-week periods, either two cohorts of 30 people or three cohorts of 20 people may be completed. The total number of weeks for study activity will be minimized by feeding two cohorts per year. Between cohorts the kitchen staff will become unemployed or available for another study. Alternatively, three smaller cohorts will use fewer staff more consistently, and the weeks between cohorts can be used for vacations, holidays, or other short assignments. Although some multicenter feeding studies will allow flexibility when the cohorts are completed, others may dictate the start and end dates for every cohort.

Food preparation procedures must be evaluated with respect to available facilities and staff at each field center. Menus that include many baked items might be problematic for field centers with limited access to ovens. For research kitchens with limited staff, it might be difficult to prepare complicated recipes. Similarly, precision weighing of many food items translates into higher labor costs and may place another burden on some field centers. The use of items that are packaged in discrete portion sizes for noncritical foods alleviates the burden. Batch preparation of homogeneous foods or the use of pre-prepared foods such as muffins also may minimize labor efforts.

Menu Development

Perhaps the most challenging aspect of multicenter feeding studies is menu development. The menus and methods of food preparation must permit implementation of a common protocol in different settings. Field center dietitians must select the optimal approach for preparing and delivering research diets to the participants in terms of nutrient control, acceptability, and feasibility. For example, the meals must be easy to prepare within the constraints of the budget and of the research kitchen staff and facilities. The approach that meets these criteria, and also provides acceptable foods and minimal nutrient variability, is the best choice for multicenter feeding trials.

As with all feeding studies, the foods presented to the research volunteers must be acceptable or dietary compliance will suffer. In multicenter studies, regional and cultural food preferences may have considerable impact on menu development. To address this issue in DELTA and DASH, each field center dietitian developed several menus for possible use in the weekly cycle. The menus were then entered into one nutrient database program and were adjusted to meet target nutrients. After all diet subcommittee members reviewed the menus, modifications were made as needed. Selected food items were taste-tested at all field centers, and those foods found unacceptable were modified or replaced.

For example, in DELTA, the Louisiana participants preferred spicier foods than participants in the other field centers. Therefore, individuals were allowed to add seasonings (eg, hot pepper sauce). The Louisiana dietitians also originally developed a menu in which cornbread was served with chili, but taste testers at one northern center found that combination odd. As a result, cornbread was removed from the menu because it was not acceptable to all prospective participants.

The availability of foods at each field center also affects menu planning for a multicenter feeding trial. To provide diets that are as consistent as possible in nutrient composition, brand names are specified. However, not all brand name foods are available in each region of the country. Alternate brands that are similar in nutrient composition must be identified. The use of fresh, frozen, or canned foods also must be compared for possible nutrient variability, cost, preparation, and acceptability. For example, some kitchen managers prefer to use fresh mushrooms; others prefer the cost and time savings of canned mushrooms. For a study such as DELTA in which fats were the nutrients of interest, the type of mushroom used did not matter. However, if sodium were to be controlled, the food product specifications would have to indicate the form of mushrooms (canned, dried, fresh).

Finally, the inherent variability of food components provides challenges for maintaining identical experimental diets. Various combinations of central or local procurement and preparation provide several options for controlling the diet. Centralized procurement and preparation of foods offer the greatest control of nutrient variability but could result in higher cost, increased efforts in distribution coordination, and foods of lower acceptability. Foods highly variable in a critical nutrient are the most likely to require central procurement with distribution to the feeding sites.

The experimental treatments for DELTA required manipulations in the fatty acid composition of the diets. To minimize the considerable variability of this nutrient, all major sources of fat in the experimental diets were procured centrally (1, 15, 16). Those foods included meat, fish, poultry, margarine, butter, oils, dairy products except fluid milk, bread, and other grain products. Each field center was required to identify a local dairy that provided both skim and whole milk within the study specifications. All other foods were procured locally or were obtained through donations. (Also see Overview of Multicenter Study Activities.)

Chemical Verification of Diets

The food composition laboratory in a multicenter feeding trial establishes the effective premise of the study, that the nutrient content of the experimental diets will be sufficiently comparable across the feeding centers to be considered identical (1). This assurance is developed in two stages. First, during menu development the nutrient content of the diets is estimated with food composition databases and chemically analyzed to verify that the actual chemical composition meets the target values established by the study design.

Second, throughout the study the food analysis laboratory conducts ongoing quality assurance monitoring of each field center by assessing critical nutrients in randomly assigned composites of the experimental diets. Sources of variance in diet composition include daily differences among menus, market turnover, seasonal food supplies, commercial food product packaging, preparation techniques, assay procedures, and variation among calorie levels. The potential for variation among the field centers is unique to multicenter feeding studies. Each center may experience each source of variation but not necessarily to the same extent. This complicates the process of preparing identical diets but does not necessarily hinder the provision of experimental diets that meet nutrient specifications (1, 14).

Food Procurement

Procurement of food for multicenter studies requires careful planning and implementation because all sites must use the same food items. Food specifications must be reviewed by all to ensure that there are no regional differences in interpretation that might affect nutrient composition. For example, two of the four DELTA centers purchased parboiled rice when "rice, white, uncooked" was specified because in their geographical regions, parboiled rice is most commonly used. The other two centers purchased white uncooked (not parboiled) rice. As noted previously, during menu development all sites should be familiar with their possible food procurement options to avoid using food items that cannot be procured by all field centers. Food source options include national institutional or retail distributors, individual retail grocers, or food companies.

Although food donations might appear to be a way of saving funds, the time necessary to make contacts and to orchestrate deliveries to each field center location is extensive. Based on our experience with DELTA and DASH, coordination can take easily 6 to 9 months of planning and follow-up and may require a half-time person depending on the number of contacts and companies being solicited and the number of field centers involved. The principal investigators must commit this time in advance. There may be additional costs to the field centers associated with shipping the foods and with renting storage space. These expenses must be considered in deciding whether to solicit food donations. It may be less expensive to purchase some foods directly than to incure the hidden costs of donated items.

Unique problems with food procurement arise during a multicenter feeding study. For example, food usage may vary across centers. Several donated foods for the DELTA study were shipped to one field center, and the staff at that site packaged and sent the foods to the other field centers. One field center used more of the centrally procured foods than anticipated. Therefore, the other sites had to ship specified quantities of their supplies to that field center to make up the shortfall. When feeding studies span several years, food product composition must be monitored for consistency. Frequently, manufacturers redesign their food products and the nutrient composition may be modified. The feeding periods for DASH spanned two years, and during that time, a commercial zucchini lasagna used in a menu was discontinued by the company. An alternate product that closely matched the nutrient composition of the lasagna had to be identified for the remaining cohorts.

Food Storage

Every field center has differing sizes of storage areas available. For a multicenter feeding study, ample storage space must be available on site, but off-site storage can be used creatively. Adequate storage space is required when a particular food item, such as meat, is purchased for an entire feeding period before the study begins. In addition, storage space becomes a significant issue when foods are donated in large quantities because food companies prefer to minimize shipments to save money on transportation costs.

Dry goods storage space may be available at the research facility or obtained through negotiations elsewhere at the institution. Off-site storage is an option but must be suitable for food in terms of temperature and rodent control. The amount of refrigerated space also may be satisfactory in the research kitchen or readily available within the institution. Frequent deliveries of food, when possible, will decrease the amount of storage space required.

Sufficient freezer space was a major problem for all field centers participating in both DELTA and DASH. All meats for each DELTA feeding protocol were distributed once to each field center. At each DASH field center, twice yearly food donations of frozen fruits and vegetables required significant frozen storage space. Options for acquiring freezer space included negotiating the use of freezer space from within the institution, renting freezer space from a frozen food warehouse, leasing a generator refrigerator/freezer unit and maintaining it on site, or soliciting donated freezer space. With an off-site location, an employee with a vehicle must transfer the food items. In the DELTA study, off-site food storage locations posed a significant problem for the field center located in New York City and for the other northern field centers during heavy snow storms. Some frozen food warehouses will charge a fee for retrieving the food in addition to the monthly rental fee.

Food Preparation

In a multicenter feeding study, not only must menus and foods be similar at each field center, but also all foods must be prepared identically and cooking procedures must be standardized across the field centers.

Detailed food preparation procedures are essential. For example, draining times for canned fruits and cooling times for cooked vegetables must be defined. Conversely, it may be specified to weigh fruit with the liquid using a nonslotted spoon and to weigh vegetables in the frozen state. In the DASH trial, which controlled dietary potassium levels, it was important to specify whether potatoes were to be boiled with the skin on and then peeled, or boiled without the skin. The potassium content of the potatoes differed according to the technique used.

Food preparation techniques will vary with the type of equipment available in the research kitchens. Rice, for example, may be prepared on a cooktop or in a plug-in steamer. The yield of cooked rice from raw rice must be similar regardless of cooking method to ensure equality in the portions served among the field centers. Similarly, cooking procedures for other foods such as vegetables must be equivalent. The finished cooked product at each field center must be similar regardless of the method used.

Meal Delivery and Compliance Assessment

All study participants at the field centers must follow similar guidelines for allowed "free foods," beverages, and seasonings. Limits for alcohol and caffeine consumption must be identical among field centers. Guidelines also are needed for discretionary or mandatory use of unit foods, which are specially prepared foods that have the same nutrient composition as that of the diet and provide needed calories. Dietitians in multicenter feeding studies may follow established methods to adjust participants' calorie levels for weight maintenance. The number of on-site meals may be specified, as well as which meal(s) must be consumed on-site.

Departures from the feeding protocol should be handled similarly among the field centers. For example, dietary compliance before randomization was assessed in DASH during a 3-week run-in period. The number of missed meals and foods allowed before removing a participant from the trial prior to randomization was defined (17). During intervention, specific guidelines for foods not consumed and non-study foods consumed were used to assess compliance to the diet.

To assist with compliance assessment, methods for recording dietary intake and adherence information are established by the diet subcommittee, and the forms needed are provided by the coordinating center. Daily food diaries that are completed by the study participants may be designed to identify deviations from the experimental diet, and other information such as number of unit foods eaten, the amount of alcohol consumed, or the number of salt packets used. Forms to monitor weight and calories consumed also are helpful in providing clues about dietary adherence.

Planning Time Line

A time line facilitates the coordination of planning activities. Much of the impending work depends on the completion of other activities. For example, menus cannot be designed until the nutrients of interest are defined. In turn, the nutrient composition of the experimental diets is guided by the study hypothesis. Figure 25–2 illustrates the time line used for planning the dietary component of the DASH study.

It is essential that the study hypothesis and the dietary treatments be defined as early as possible. Menu develop-

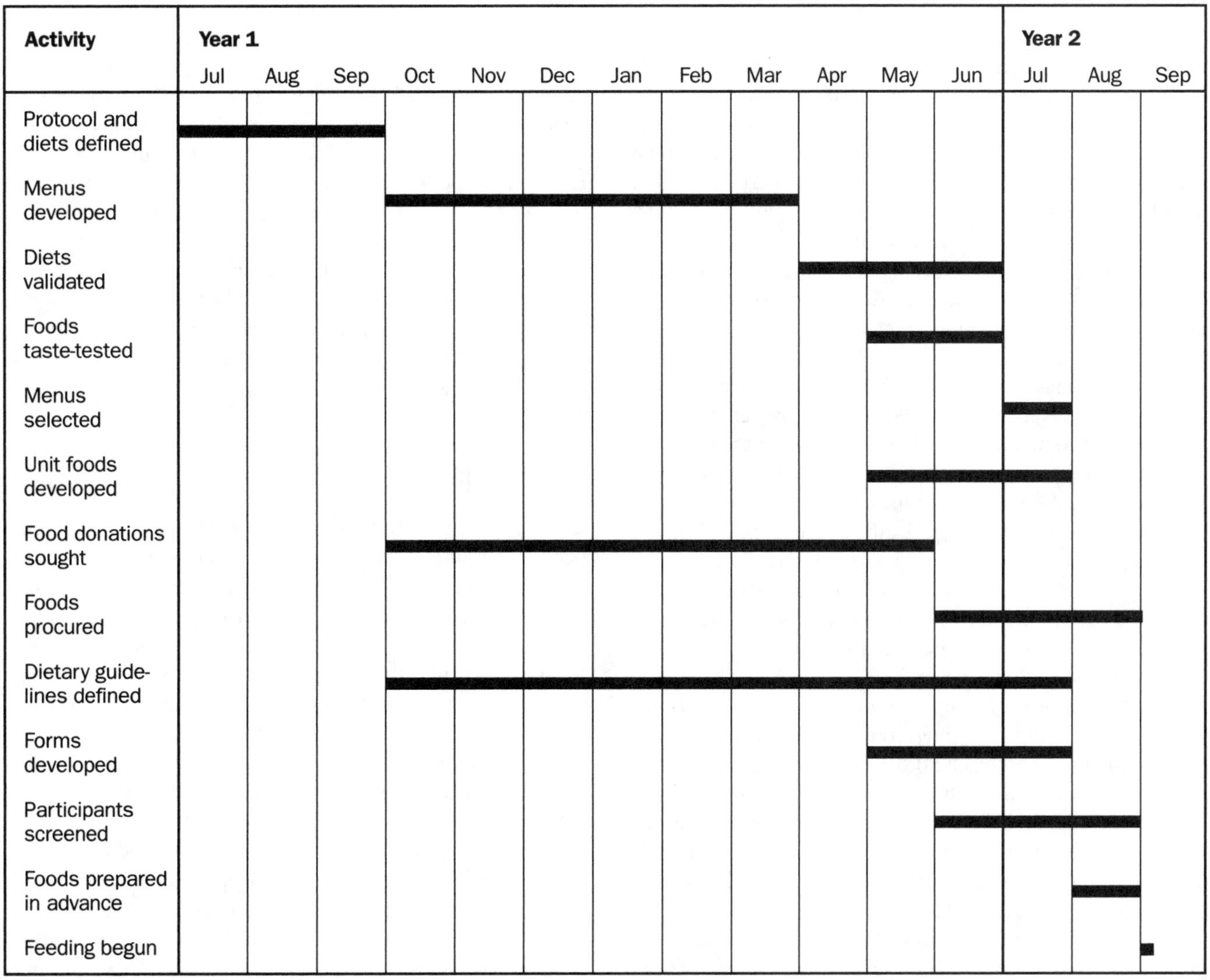

FIGURE 25-2. Planning time line for the dietary component of the DASH study.

TABLE 25-2

Diet-Related Forms Used for the DASH Study[1]

Form	Purpose
Study Food Checklist	Screening
General Dietary Information Questionnaire	Screening
Food Frequency Questionnaire	Screening/data collection
Study Menus	Screening/participant study information
Food Donation Tracking Form	Foodservice/procedural
Food Donation Contact Form	Foodservice/information
Food Inventory Control Form	Foodservice/procedural
Foodservice Sanitation Self-Inspection Checklist	Foodservice/quality assurance
Food Production Form	Foodservice/procedural/quality assurance
Tray Assembly Form	Foodservice/procedural/quality assurance
Orientation Form	Participant study information
Guidelines for Beverages and Seasonings	Participant study information
Safe Foods to Go	Participant study information
Daily Diary	Data collection
Compliance Assessment Form	Data collection
Body Weight and Energy Adjustment Form	Data collection
Post-study Anonymous Survey	Data collection

[1]Dietary Approaches to Stop Hypertension. *Forms Study Manual for DASH.* Portland, Ore: Dash Coordinating Center, Kaiser Permanente, Center for Health Research; 1995.

ment can take 6 months or more, depending on the complexity of the nutrient modifications. Time is needed to standardize food preparation techniques and recipes. Menus then are prepared for chemical validation, which may take 3 to 4 months to complete. Taste-testing may be conducted while the diets are analyzed, but menu modifications must not alter the nutrient composition. Otherwise, the chemical validation of the menu must be repeated. Based on the taste-testing and nutrient composition results, menus may be selected, deleted, or modified.

If food donations are pursued, possible contributors can be identified during menu development. Initial contacts can be made, but companies usually will not commit to donating foods until they know exact amounts that will be needed. Depending on the structure of the company, food donations may be approved and shipped quickly (within 2 months), but this process can take as long as 6 months.

Regardless of the procurement method, adequate time is needed to obtain foods before feeding begins. Arrangements must be made for purchasing foods from distributors or grocers. Depending on the facility, it could take several months to approve a billing system. For some institutions, such as the Pennington Center, foods must be placed on bid through the state purchasing office. The entire process takes approximately 3 months. It may be necessary to place food items on the bid, then remove them before the bid is awarded if the foods were on a deleted menu. Other foods needed because of menu changes but not on the original bid must be purchased separately or placed on a subsequent bid.

While menus are developed and validated, standardized guidelines may be established for allowed intakes of free and restricted foods and beverages, and procedures are de-

veloped for diet delivery and compliance assessment. Forms needed for the study are also designed and completed at this time. A list of diet-related forms used for the DASH study is given in Table 25–2. Field center dietitians most likely will be involved in participant recruitment and screening procedures. Then, a month before feeding, kitchen staff members are trained and may begin to prepare some foods that can be stored until needed. Finally, the day arrives when participant feeding begins. The unexpected may occur, but a multicenter feeding study that is carefully planned can be executed efficiently and effectively.

CONCLUSION

Similar to well-controlled single-center feeding studies, multicenter feeding studies seek to answer research questions about how diet affects metabolic parameters and disease risk factors. Their unique feature is that they are modeled after standard multicenter clinical trials. They have multiple feeding sites, usually located in different geographic areas, and thus can have a large sample size drawn from a diverse population, resulting in increased statistical power and enhanced generalizability. With this advantage, small, but biologically meaningful, differences among treatments have a higher likelihood of being detected.

Following the model of multicenter clinical trials, multicenter feeding studies have centralized laboratories and a coordinating center. Steering committees, composed of principal investigators and other professionals, design a common protocol and define the treatments and outcomes. The protocol is followed closely and the dietary treatments and procedures are the same for all centers. At the field centers, study participants are recruited and fed, and biological samples are collected and shipped to the centralized laboratories for analysis. The coordinating center provides administrative support, maintains quality control throughout the trial, and is responsible for the statistical analysis of the data. Quality control is a major component of study implementation and includes pre-feeding verification of the nutrient composition of study diets, during-feeding monitoring of the diets as fed at all field centers, and standardization of all data collection procedures. Although complex in design, costly, and time-demanding, multicenter feeding studies are good models for examining important and timely nutritional issues and controversies. The information gained from these studies can provide critical evidence necessary for developing dietary recommendations.

REFERENCES

1. Dennis BH, Stewart P, Wang CH, Champagne C, Windhauser M, Ershow A, Karmally W, Phillips K, Stewart K, VanHeel N, Farhat-Wood A, Kris-Etherton PM, for the DELTA Research Group. Diet design for a multicenter controlled feeding trial: the DELTA Program. *J Am Diet Assoc.* 1998;98:766–776.

2. Ginsberg HN, Kris-Etherton P, Dennis B, Elmer PJ, Ershow A, Lefevre M, Pearson T, Roheim P, Ramakrishnan R, Reed R, Stewart K, Stewart P, Phillips K, Anderson N, for the DELTA Research Group. Effects of reducing dietary saturated fatty acids on plasma lipids and lipoproteins in healthy subjects: the DELTA Study, Protocol 1. *Arterioscler Thromb Vasc Biol.* 1998;18: 441–449.

3. Ershow A, for the DELTA investigators. Dietary effects on lipoproteins and thrombogenic activity in subjects with markers for insulin resistance (DELTA-2): study design and recruitment. *FASEB J.* 1996;10:A262.

4. Sacks FM, Obarzanek E, Windhauser MM, Svetkey LP, Vollmer WM, McCullough M, Karanja N, Lin P-H, Steele P, Proschan MA, Evans MA, Appel LJ, Bray GA, Vogt TM, Moore TJ. Rationale and design of the Dietary Approaches to Stop Hypertension Trial (DASH): a multicenter controlled-feeding study of dietary patterns to lower blood pressure. *Ann Epidemiol.* 1995;5:108–118.

5. National High Blood Pressure Education Program, Joint National Committee on Detection, Evaluation, and Treatment of High Blood Pressure. *The Sixth Report of the Joint National Committee on Detection, Evaluation, and Treatment of High Blood Pressure.* NHLBI, NIH, PHS, USDHHS. NIH publication 98–4080. 1997.

6. National High Blood Pressure Education Program. *Working Group Report on Primary Prevention of Hypertension.* NHLBI, NIH, PHS, USDHHS. NIH publication 93–2669; 1993.

7. McCarron DA, Oparil S, Chait A, Haynes RB, Kris-Etherton P, Stern JS, Resnick LM, Clark S, Morris CD, Hatton DC, Metz JA, McMahon M, Holcomb S, Snyder GW, Pi-Sunyer FX. Nutritional management of cardiovascular risk factors: a randomized clinical trial. *Arch Intern Med.* 1997;157:169–177.

8. Krebs JM, Schneider VS, LeBlanc AD, Kuo MC, Spector E, Lane HW. Zinc and copper balances in healthy adult males during and after 17 wk of bed rest. *Am J Clin Nutr.* 1993;58:897–901.

9. Garg A, Bantle JP, Henry RR, Coulston AM, Griver KA, Raatz SK, Brinkley L, Chen I, Grundy SM, Huet BA, Reaven GM. Effects of varying carbohydrate content of diet in patients with non-insulin-dependent diabetes mellitus. *JAMA.* 1994;271:1421–1428.

10. Appel LJ, Moore TJ, Obarzanek E, Vollmer WM, Svetkey LP, Sacks FM, Bray GA, Vogt TM, Cutler MA, Windhauser MM, Lin P-H, Karanja N. A clinical trial on the effect of dietary patterns on blood pressure. *N Engl J Med.* 1997;336:1117–1124.

11. Feinstein AR. The scientific and clinical tribulations of randomized clinical trials. *Clin Res.* 1978;26:241–244.

12. Friedman LM, Furberg CD, DeMets DL. *Fundamentals of Clinical Trials.* Boston, Mass: John Wright/PSG Inc; 1981.

13. Higgins MW. Conducting clinical trials. *Am J Res Dis.* 1980;122:3–9.

14. Stewart K, for the DELTA investigators. Diet composition documentation in a multicenter clinical feeding trial. *FASEB J.* 1995; 9:A289.

15. Dietary Effects on Lipoproteins and Thrombogenic Activity. *Manual of Operations, Protocol 1.* Chapel Hill, NC: DELTA Coordinating Center, Department of Biostatistics, The University of North Carolina; 1994.

16. Dietary Effects on Lipoproteins and Thrombogenic Activity. *Manual of Operations, Protocol 2.* Chapel Hill, NC: DELTA Coordinating Center, Department of Biostatistics, the University of North Carolina; 1994.

17. Dietary Approaches to Stop Hypertension. *Manual of Operations.* Portland, Ore: DASH Coordinating Center, Center for Health Research; 1995.

Index